Respiratory Medicine

Respiratory Medicine

Edited by Elijah Jones

hayle medical

New York

Hayle Medical,
750 Third Avenue, 9th Floor,
New York, NY 10017, USA

Visit us on the World Wide Web at:
www.haylemedical.com

ISBN: 978-1-63241-753-4

The publisher's policy is to use permanent paper from mills that operate a sustainable forestry policy. Furthermore, the publisher ensures that the text paper and cover boards used have met acceptable environmental accreditation standards.

Printed in China.

Cataloging-in-Publication Data

Respiratory medicine / edited by Elijah Jones.
p. cm.
Includes bibliographical references and index.
ISBN 978-1-63241-753-4
1. Respiratory organs--Diseases. 2. Respiratory organs--Diseases--Diagnosis.
3. Respiratory organs--Diseases--Treatment. 4. Respiratory infections. I. Jones, Elijah.
RC731 .R47 2019
616.2--dc23

Table of Contents

Preface

It is often said that books are a boon to mankind. They document every progress and pass on the knowledge from one generation to the other. They play a crucial role in our lives. Thus I was both excited and nervous while editing this book. I was pleased by the thought of being able to make a mark but I was also nervous to do it right because the future of students depends upon it. Hence, I took a few months to research further into the discipline, revise my knowledge and also explore some more aspects. Post this process, I begun with the editing of this book.

The human respiratory system is a biological system that facilitates the exchange of gases between the organism and the environment. In humans, the respiratory tract is involved in respiration and is divided into the upper and lower respiratory tract. The upper tract comprises of the nose, nasal cavities, pharynx, sinuses and the part of the larynx that is above the vocal folds. The lower tract includes the trachea, larynx, bronchi, bronchioles and alveoli. The disorders of the respiratory system affect these parts and can be classified into several groups, namely airway obstructive conditions, vascular diseases, pulmonary restrictive conditions, infectious and environmental diseases, cancers and surfactant deficiency disorders. Emphysema, asthma and bronchitis are airway obstructive conditions. Pulmonary restrictive conditions are fibrosis, pleural effusion, sarcoidosis, etc. while some vascular diseases are pulmonary embolism, pulmonary edema and pulmonary hypertension. Respiratory distress syndrome is a condition that occurs in premature babies due to a structural immaturity in the lungs and due to the developmental insufficiency of pulmonary surfactant production. All disorders of the respiratory system are treated with respiratory medicine. Various surgical and therapeutic strategies are employed for the treatment of these conditions. This book contains some path-breaking studies in the domain of respiratory medicine. It will also provide interesting topics for research, which interested readers can take up. It is appropriate for students seeking detailed information in this area as well as for experts.

I thank my publisher with all my heart for considering me worthy of this unparalleled opportunity and for showing unwavering faith in my skills. I would also like to thank the editorial team who worked closely with me at every step and contributed immensely towards the successful completion of this book. Last but not the least, I wish to thank my friends and colleagues for their support.

Editor

Comparison of Mask Oxygen Therapy and High-Flow Oxygen Therapy after Cardiopulmonary Bypass in Obese Patients

Mazlum Sahin,[1] Helin El,[2] and Ibrahim Akkoç[3]

[1]*Department of Cardiovascular Surgery, Haseki Teaching and Research Hospital, Istanbul, Turkey*
[2]*Department of Cardiovascular Surgery, Sisli Teaching and Research Hospital, Istanbul, Turkey*
[3]*Department of Anesthesia and Reanimation, Haseki Teaching and Research Hospital, Istanbul, Turkey*

Correspondence should be addressed to Mazlum Sahin; mzlmshn@gmail.com

Academic Editor: Panfeng Fu

Background. To clarify the efficiency of mask O_2 and high-flow O_2 (HFO) treatments following cardiopulmonary bypass (CPB) in obese patients. *Methods.* During follow-up, oxygenization parameters including arterial pressure of oxygen (PaO_2), peripheral oxygen saturation (SpO_2), and arterial partial pressure of carbon dioxide ($PaCO_2$) and physical examination parameters including respiratory rate, heart rate, and arterial pressure were recorded respectively. Presence of atelectasia and dyspnea was noted. Also, comfort scores of patients were evaluated. *Results.* Mean duration of hospital stay was 6.9 ± 1.1 days in the mask O_2 group, whereas the duration was significantly shorter (6.5 ± 0.7 days) in the HFO group ($p = 0.034$). The PaO_2 values and SpO_2 values were significantly higher, and $PaCO_2$ values were significantly lower in patients who received HFO after 4th, 12th, 24th, 36th, and 48th hours. In postoperative course, HFO leads patients to achieve better postoperative FVC ($p < 0.001$). Also, dyspnea scores and comfort scores were significantly better in patients who received HFO in both postoperative day 1 and day 2 ($p < 0.001$, $p < 0.001$ and $p = 0.002$, $p = 0.001$, resp.). *Conclusion.* Our study demonstrated that HFO following CPB in obese patients improved postoperative PaO_2, SpO_2, and $PaCO_2$ values and decreased the atelectasis score, reintubation, and mortality rates when compared with mask O_2.

1. Introduction

According to World Health Organization, obesity is defined as excessive and abnormal fat accumulation that creates risk for health, and a person with a body mass index (BMI) greater than or equal to 30 kg/m^2 is considered obese [1]. Incidence of sedentary lifestyle with high-fat diet intake and comorbidities including metabolic syndrome, diabetes mellitus, and hypertension are common among obese patients. Also, it is well known that obesity and obesity-related disorders are risk factors for severe coronary artery diseases which may require cardiopulmonary bypass (CPB) [2]. Additionally, obese patients are more vulnerable to pulmonary complications following CPB due to decreased total lung capacity, functional residual capacity, forced vital capacity, and expiratory reserve volume. Moreover, anesthetic agents and sedatives aggravate the respiratory instability in obese patients [3].

Previous studies had demonstrated that severe hypoxemia, hypercapnia, and prolonged apnea periods deteriorate healing after CPB. To avoid these undesirable conditions, some authors recommended oxygen therapy which had a key role in improving respiratory functions and patient comfort by decreasing desaturation episodes and reintubation rates after cardiac surgery [4, 5]. In a prospective randomized study, Zhu et al. showed significant reduction of the reintubation rate after cardiac surgery with mask O_2 [5]. In contrast, Stéphan et al. reported insufficiency of mask O_2 therapy for oxygen treatment following cardiac surgery-supported high-flow O_2 (HFO) treatment [6]. Therefore, the most appropriate method of oxygen therapy is still under investigation, especially in obese patients who are at high risk for respiratory problems following CPB.

Although previous studies investigated the role of mask O_2 and HFO treatments following CPB, none of these studies have compared these two different treatment modalities in patients with BMI more than 30 kg/m^2. In this study, we, for the first time, aimed to clarify the importance of mask O_2 and HFO treatments following CPB in obese patients.

2. Materials and Methods

In this prospective randomized study, charts of patients who underwent CABG in a tertiary academic center between January 2015 and January 2017 were analyzed. Ethical approval for the study was obtained from the Haseki Teaching and Research Hospital's Regional Ethical Committee, with study ID number 499. Patients with BMI > 30 kg/m^2 were enrolled in the study. Randomization was done by a computer-based random number-sequencing program. Exclusion criteria were hemodynamic instability, patients younger than 18 years of age, and patients with tracheostomy, obstructive sleep apnea, and active pulmonary disease. Also, patients with low cardiac output and operations who were held under emergency conditions were excluded from the study. Written consent was obtained from patients and/or relatives.

2.1. Study protocol. In Cardiovascular Surgery Intensive Care Unit (ICU), every patient, who underwent CABG, was followed up by a well-trained ICU nurse and a cardiovascular surgeon in the postoperative period. Hemodynamically stable patients, who had a sufficient oxygenation (SpO_2 (peripheral oxygen saturation) > 92, FiO_2 (fraction of inspired oxygen) ≤ 0.4, PEEP (positive end-expiratory pressure) ≤ 8 mmHg, and PaO_2 (arterial pressure of oxygen)/FiO_2 ≥ 150), were weaned by the spontaneous breathing trial (SBT) with low-level pressure support or oxygen T-piece for 90–120 minutes. Endotracheal extubation was performed in patients who have tolerated the SBT.

After endotracheal extubation, patients were randomly divided into two groups. In patients ($n = 50$) who received HFO treatment, high-flow humidified oxygen (44 mm/H_2O/L and 37°C) was released through a nasal cannula continuously with Optiflow (Vapotherm, New Hampshire, USA). The preliminary flow rate was 25–40 L/min, and the initial FiO_2 was 50% to maintain $SaO_2 > 93$. In the other group ($n = 50$ patients) who underwent oxygen therapy, oxygen was delivered from a simple face mask (Orya Medikal, Istanbul, Turkey) with a flow of 2–4 liters in a minute to maintain $SpO_2 > 93\%$. Active respiratory physiotherapy was performed for all patients during the postoperative period. The patients were encouraged for early mobilization.

2.2. Atelectasis Scoring. Presence of atelectasis was evaluated by a postoperative chest X-ray and classified according to the radiological atelectasis score system (RAS) [7]. The RAS is divided into five categories (0: clear lung fields, 1: plate-like atelectasis or slight infiltration, 2: partial atelectasis, 3: lobar atelectasis, and 4: bilateral atelectasis), and chest X-rays were evaluated by a single radiologist who was blinded to mask O_2 and HFO outcomes.

After the surgery, respiratory parameters and physical examination findings were recorded in 4th, 12th, 24th, 36th, and 48th hours, respectively. Patients' comfort and relief was evaluated once per day (1, very poor; 2, poor; 3, sufficient; 4, good; and 5, very good). Also, patients were assessed about the effectiveness of treatment once per day (2, marked improvement; 1, slight improvement; 0, no change; −1, slight deterioration; and −2, marked deterioration) [6].

Discontinuation of mask O_2 or HFO therapy due to the side effects, requirement of additional treatment, or necessity of reintubation for mechanical ventilation was accepted as failure of the current treatment. Reintubation criteria were cardiovascular instability, respiratory arrest or respiratory acidosis (pH < 7.30 and $PaCO_2 \geq 50$ mmHg), encephalopathy, and clinical findings of exhaustion and refractory hypoxemia (arterial oxygen saturation < 88% with $FiO_2 = 100\%$). Reintubation was performed according to the physician's decision, if required. The length of ICU and hospital stay was recorded. Lastly, respiratory complications, extrapulmonary complications, and presence of mortality were documented.

During statistical analyses, values were evaluated as numbers, means, percentages, and intervals. Numbers and percentages were compared using the chi-square test. Before the comparison of means of values, the values were evaluated for homogeneity. Homogeneously distributed values were compared using Student's t-test, and heterogeneously distributed values were compared using the Mann–Whitney U test.

3. Results

During the study period, 137 patients underwent the CABG procedure, and 100 patients were enrolled in the study. Other 37 patients were excluded from the study according to study exclusion criteria (Figure 1). These patients were divided into two groups; 50 patients were treated with mask O_2, and 50 patients were treated with HFO. The mean age was 61.3 ± 8.5 in patients who received mask O_2 and 62.0 ± 6.7 in patients who received HFO ($p = 0.660$). Sex, BMI, and history of smoking were similar between groups ($p = 1.000$, $p = 0.259$, and $p = 0.842$, resp.). The operative parameters in terms of duration of surgery, myocardial ischemia period, and extubation time were comparable between patients who received mask O_2 and HFO ($p = 0.709$, $p = 0.740$, and $p = 0.529$, resp.). Preoperative and operative parameters are summarized in Table 1.

Among the patients who have received mask O_2, 11 patients required continuous positive airway pressure (CPAP) and four patients required reintubation due to the increased arterial carbon dioxide value and mental deterioration despite extensive pulmonary rehabilitation maneuvers. In patients who have received HFO, CPAP was required in six patients; however, none of these patients required reintubation ($p = 0.187$ and $p < 0.001$). The duration of ICU stay was 2.8 ± 1.7 days in patients with mask O_2 and 2.4 ± 0.5 days in patients with HFO ($p = 0.130$). The duration of hospital stay was 6.9 ± 1.1 days in the mask O_2 group, whereas it was significantly shorter (6.5 ± 0.7 days) in the HFO group

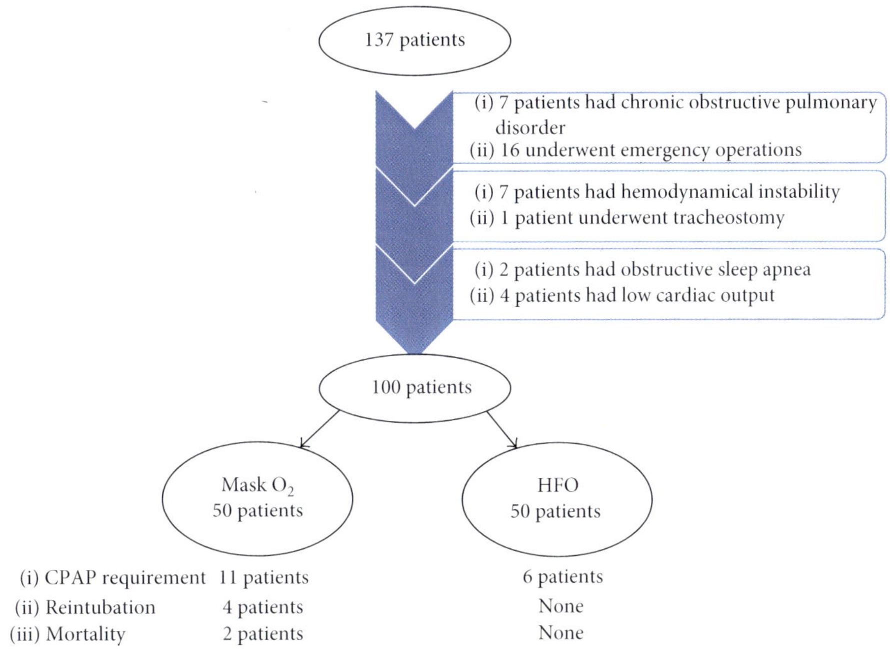

FIGURE 1: Flow chart scheme of the study.

TABLE 1: Preoperative and operative characteristics of patients.

	Group		p value
	Mask O_2 ($n = 50$)	High-flow O_2 ($n = 50$)	
Sex (female/male)	32/18	32/18	1.000
Age (years)*	61.3 ± 8.5	62.0 ± 6.7	0.660
Body mass index (kg/m^2)*	32.3 ± 1.1	32.5 ± 1.2	0.259
Comorbidities			
Diabetes mellitus	20	19	0.840
Hypertension	29	30	0.841
Chronic kidney disease	3	3	1.000
Smoking history	21	22	0.842
Ejection fraction (%)*	51.3 ± 6.8	50.3 ± 6.2	0.445
Number of CPB*	3.2 ± 0.7	3.2 ± 0.7	0.786
CPB duration (min)*	90.5 ± 12.1	91.4 ± 13.0	0.709
Clamping duration (min)*	41.0 ± 11.8	41.8 ± 12.8	0.740
Duration of extubation (hour)*	8.2 ± 4.3	7.8 ± 1.4	0.529

*Mean ± standard deviation; CPB: cardiopulmonary bypass; min: minutes.

($p = 0.034$). Moreover, the atrial fibrillation rate and mortality rate were significantly lower in patients who were treated with HFO ($p < 0.001$ and $p < 0.001$, resp.). Death was observed in only two patients who have received mask O_2 (Table 2).

The respiratory parameters PaO_2 value and SpO_2 value were significantly higher and $PaCO_2$ value was significantly lower in patients who have received HFO. The PaO_2 value was 104.3 ± 5.6, 96.2 ± 7.4, 96.6 ± 6.7, 97.1 ± 6.3, and 99.4 ± 7.1 after 4th, 12th, 24th, 36th, and 48th hours in patients with mask O_2 and 112.3 ± 8.8, 106.9 ± 7.5, 100.0 ± 4.5, 104.9 ± 5.9, and 106.0 ± 6.9 after 4th, 12th, 24th, 36th, and 48th hours in patients with HFO ($p < 0.001$, $p < 0.001$, $p = 0.004$, $p < 0.001$, and $p < 0.001$, resp.). Similarly, SpO_2 values were 98.0 ± 0.7, 97.5 ± 1.1, 97.4 ± 4.3, 97.5 ± 1.2, and 97.5 ± 1.2 after 4th, 12th, 24th, 36th, and 48th hours in patients with HFO. SpO_2 values were statistically better in patients who have received HFO when compared with the mask O_2 group ($p < 0.001$, $p < 0.001$, $p = 0.001$, $p < 0.001$, and $p < 0.001$, resp.). In contrast, patients with mask O_2 faced with worse $PaCO_2$ values (43.1 ± 2.8 versus 41.2 ± 2.1, 43.7 ± 1.9 versus 41.2 ± 2.1, 43.5 ± 1.8 versus 40.7 ± 2.2, 43.3 ± 1.6 versus 39.3 ± 2.8, and 42.3 ± 2.2 versus 37.9 ± 2.6 after 4th, 12th, 24th, 36th, and 48th hours, resp.). The mean heart rate was significantly lower in the HFO group in 4th, 12th, 24th, and 36th hours after CPB ($p < 0.001$, $p = 0.009$, $p = 0.001$,

TABLE 2: Postoperative complications, treatment failure, and mortality rates of patients.

	Group		
	Mask O_2 ($n = 50$)	High-flow O_2 ($n = 50$)	p value
CPAP requirement	11	6	0.187
Reintubation	4	0	**<0.001**
Pneumonia	2	0	**<0.001**
ICU stay (day)*	2.8 ± 1.7	2.4 ± 0.5	0.130
Hospitalization duration (day)*	6.9 ± 1.1	6.5 ± 0.7	**0.034**
Atrial fibrillation	12	7	**<0.001**
Transfusion rate*	1.8 ± 0.7	2.0 ± 0.7	0.080
Mortality	2	0	**<0.001**

*Mean ± standard deviation; CPAP: continuous positive airway pressure; ICU: intensive care unit.

and$p < 0.001$, resp.). In addition, patients who have received HFO had higher blood pressure values in 4th and 12th hours (98.0 ± 2.2 versus 94.5 ± 3.3 after 4th hour and 98.0 ± 2.2 versus 96.1 ± 3.2 after 12th hour). The respiratory rate following endotracheal extubation was significantly lower at the 4th hour in patients who have received HFO ($p < 0.001$); however, it did not differ significantly at the other follow-up intervals. Postoperative atelectasis score in the 4th hour was similar between groups ($p = 1.000$); however, patients who have received HFO had significantly better atelectasis scores in 12th, 24th, 36th, and 48th hours ($p = 0.004$, $p < 0.001$, $p < 0.001$, and$p < 0.001$, resp.). Preoperative FEV_1 (forced expiratory volume) and FVC (forced vital capacity) were comparable between groups ($p = 0.650$and$p = 0.228$). However, during postoperative follow-up, HFO leads patients to achieve better FVC ($p < 0.001$) values. The dyspnea scores were significantly better in patients with HFO in both postoperative day 1 and day 2 ($p < 0.001$ and $p < 0.001$). The comfort scores of patients who have received HFO were better in postoperative day 1 and day 2 ($p = 0.002$and$p = 0.001$, resp.). Postoperative parameters are summarized in Tables 3 and 4.

4. Discussion

Acute respiratory failure is still a challenging and life-threatening complication in patients who underwent open heart surgery with CPB. During respiratory insufficiency, respiratory support is a critical step to maintain patient comfort, prevent invasive mechanical ventilation, and decrease mortality [8]. Therefore, choosing the most appropriate device for oxygen therapy is a crucial decision to maintain adequate oxygenation especially in patients who are at high risk for acute respiratory failure such as patients with sleep apnea syndrome, advanced stage heart failure, and high BMI.

Obese patients are prone to hypoxia development due to several risk factors. Obese patients have extensive adipose tissue with high metabolic activity that is associated with increased oxygen consumption and carbon dioxide production. Due to breathing difficulties in obese cases, supportive muscles spend more oxygen and produce more carbon dioxide to overcome the workload. Additionally, compliance of respiratory organs and lung volumes are decreased in obese patients [9]. Due to the lower resting functional residual capacity, obese patients have an increased respiratory rate to compensate the ventilation-perfusion mismatch especially at the base of the lungs. Furthermore, postoperative atelectasis is common and more prominent in obese patients when compared with nonobese patients [10]. Thus, the best treatment modality to overcome postoperative oxygenation problems in obese patients is a critical problem and still under investigation.

The simple face mask and HFO nasal cannula are used for oxygen delivery in patients with hypoxia and/or hypercarbia. However, there is a trend in use of HFO especially in high-risk patients. Costello et al. stated that delivering oxygen through a face mask leads to dryness of the mouth and respiratory tract, and this situation leads to displacement of the face mask. Also, displacement of the mask is associated with the decrease in oxygen concentration [11]. On the other hand, HFO generates a dead space and creates a reservoir for oxygen in the respiratory system. In patients with tachypnea, delivered O_2 may decrease due to the increased respiratory frequency, and HFO overcomes this by adequate and stable oxygenation. Moreover, HFO with positive pressure prevents the formation of atelectasis [12].

Previous reports on the efficiency of mask O_2 and HFO in the management of acute respiratory failure had controversial results. Lemiale et al. investigated the effect of HFO in immunocompromised patients and found that HFO neither decreased the need for mechanical ventilation nor improved patients' quality of life [13]. In contrast, Schwabbauer et al. found significantly better dyspnea and patient comfort scores with HFO [12]. In another study, Maggiore et al. compared HFO and mask O_2 in patients who were mechanically ventilated for more than 24 hours. They stated that high-flow O_2 provided better oxygenation, fewer desaturation episodes, and lower reintubation rates [14]. Rittayamai et al. suggested HFO to overcome dyspnea and improve physiologic parameters [15]. In the present study, we achieved better PaO_2, SpO_2, and PCO_2 levels in the first 48 hours with HFO in our obese patient cohort.

Pulmonary atelectasis is a common and undesired condition which is associated with oxygen impairment, decrease in lung compliance, increase in vascular resistance, and infectious complications [16]. To achieve more accurate classification of atelectasis and to evaluate treatment response, the Radiological Atelectasis Score was developed and validated. Parke et al. evaluated the effect of mask O_2 and HFO by using Radiological Atelectasis Score, in 340 patients who underwent heart surgery. They claimed that prophylactic HFO improved the atelectasis scores [7]. Zarbock et al. analyzed 500 patients who underwent elective cardiac surgery and were supported by HFO to prevent atelectasis in the postoperative period [17]. In accordance with the literature, we have obtained better atelectasis scores in patients

Table 3: Postoperative respiratory characteristics, physical examination findings, and atelectasis scores of groups.

	Group		p value
	Mask O_2 ($n = 50$)	High-flow O_2 ($n = 50$)	
*Postoperative 4th hour**			
PaO_2	104.3 ± 5.6	112.3 ± 8.8	**<0.001**
SpO_2	96.8 ± 1.3	98.0 ± 0.7	**<0.001**
$PaCO_2$	43.1 ± 2.8	41.2 ± 2.1	**<0.001**
Heart rate (beats/min)	105.7 ± 8.0	98.4 ± 3.3	**<0.001**
Mean arterial pressure (mmHg)	94.5 ± 3.3	98.0 ± 2.2	**<0.001**
Respiratory rate (breaths/min)	21.6 ± 1.6	20.2 ± 0.8	**<0.001**
Atelectasis score	1 ± 0	1 ± 0	1.000
*Postoperative 12th hour**			
PaO_2	96.2 ± 7.4	106.9 ± 7.5	**<0.001**
SpO_2	95.7 ± 1.4	97.5 ± 1.1	**<0.001**
$PaCO_2$	43.7 ± 1.9	41.2 ± 2.1	**<0.001**
Heart rate (beats/min)	99.3 ± 6.1	96.4 ± 3.3	**0.009**
Mean arterial pressure (mmHg)	96.1 ± 3.2	98.0 ± 2.2	**0.001**
Respiratory rate (breaths/min)	20.1 ± 1.9	20.0 ± 0.9	0.845
Atelectasis score	1.7 ± 0.5	1.4 ± 0.5	**0.004**
*Postoperative 24th hour**			
PaO_2	96.6 ± 6.7	100.0 ± 4.5	**0.004**
SpO_2	95.7 ± 1.3	97.4 ± 4.3	**0.001**
$PaCO_2$	43.5 ± 1.8	40.7 ± 2.2	**<0.001**
Heart rate (beats/min)	100.7 ± 4.4	97.5 ± 4.9	**0.001**
Mean arterial pressure (mmHg)	96.6 ± 2.5	97.7 ± 6.5	0.277
Respiratory rate (breaths/min)	19.9 ± 1.7	19.9 ± 0.8	0.697
Atelectasis score	2.2 ± 0.5	1.7 ± 0.7	**<0.001**
*Postoperative 36th hour**			
PaO_2	97.1 ± 6.3	104.9 ± 5.9	**<0.001**
SpO_2	95.8 ± 1.2	97.5 ± 1.2	**<0.001**
$PaCO_2$	43.3 ± 1.6	39.3 ± 2.8	**<0.001**
Heart rate (beats/min)	100.6 ± 4.5	96.2 ± 4.3	**<0.001**
Mean arterial pressure (mmHg)	96.7 ± 2.5	95.4 ± 4.9	0.119
Respiratory rate (breaths/min)	19.6 ± 1.2	19.4 ± 0.9	0.322
Atelectasis score	2.2 ± 0.5	1.4 ± 0.5	**<0.001**
*Postoperative 48th hour**			
PaO_2	99.4 ± 7.1	106.0 ± 6.9	**<0.001**
SpO_2	95.7 ± 1.3	97.5 ± 1.2	**<0.001**
$PaCO_2$	42.3 ± 2.2	37.9 ± 2.6	**<0.001**
Heart rate (beats/min)	94.7 ± 4.6	95.1 ± 3.5	0.612
Mean arterial pressure (mmHg)	96.8 ± 2.4	97.0 ± 2.2	0.219
Respiratory rate (breaths/min)	19.5 ± 1.1	19.3 ± 0.9	0.451
Atelectasis score	1.7 ± 0.4	1.3 ± 0.5	**<0.001**

*Mean ± standard deviation; PaO_2: arterial pressure of oxygen; SpO_2: peripheral oxygen saturation; $PaCO_2$: arterial partial pressure of carbon dioxide; min: minutes.

who received HFO. Thereby, we recommend HFO to prevent atelectasis in obese patients.

During oxygen therapy, patients' subjective response and patients' satisfaction have important roles in continuing oxygen treatment and mostly evaluated by scoring systems. Delclaux et al. analyzed patients who have received mask O_2 treatment for acute hypoxemic respiratory insufficiency according to dyspnea scores. They found that applying O_2 through a face mask had an impact on healing of dyspnea scores [18]. In another study by Stéphan et al., both mask O_2 and HFO were found as beneficial tools to improve dyspnea scores to overcome hypoxia problem after cardiothoracic surgery. Also, Stéphan et al. emphasized that the two treatment modalities were not superior to each other according to dyspnea scores [6]. Kramer et al. demonstrated that 18% of mask O_2 treatment failure was associated with mask discomfort [19]. Similarly, Calderini found mask discomfort as a reason for the cessation of treatment [20]. In our study, patients who received HFO had significantly better dyspnea and comfort scores. We analyzed only a specific group with BMI > 30 kg/m^2, and this is emphasized to be the explanation of better dyspnea and comfort scores with HFO. Obese patients spend more effort on breathing and are more vulnerable to hypoxia. Thus, adequate oxygenation is mandatory to improve symptoms. Moreover, the treatment failure rate was higher with mask O_2 and may have contributed to lower dyspnea and comfort scores in our patients.

Although the current study is a prospective randomized study in which we investigated the efficiency of HFO and compared HFO with conventional mask O_2 in the postoperative period of obese patients who underwent open heart surgery, the research has certain limitations. The sample size in both groups in the study is modest. The cost of mask O_2 and HFO treatments in obese patients was not investigated. Lastly, we have only evaluated the short-term results of both treatment modalities in statistically similar groups, and further researches with long-term follow-up outcomes may be helpful to strongly support the superiority of the technique to another.

In conclusion, we demonstrated that HFO therapy following CPB in obese patients improved postoperative PaO_2, SpO_2, and $PaCO_2$ values and decreased atelectasis scores, reintubation, and mortality rates when compared

Readability and Suitability of COPD Consumer Information

Kathryn Fullmann,[1] David F. Blackburn,[1] Mark E. Fenton,[2] and Holly Mansell[1]

[1] *College of Pharmacy and Nutrition, University of Saskatchewan, Saskatoon, SK, Canada*
[2] *Division of Critical Care and Sleep Medicine, Department of Medicine, University of Saskatchewan, Saskatoon, SK, Canada*

Correspondence should be addressed to Holly Mansell; holly.mansell@usask.ca

Academic Editor: Isabella Annesi-Maesano

Background. Information leaflets have been shown to positively or negatively impact adherence, depending on their content. The objective of this study was to perform an appraisal of the consumer information provided in COPD inhaler monographs. *Methods.* COPD inhalers were identified from the Health Canada Drug Product Database. Medication information and instructions for inhaler use were analyzed for readability by seven formulas, with an acceptability threshold of grades 6–8. Three researchers rated suitability using a modified Suitability Assessment of Materials (SAM) tool and assessed leaflets for explicit warnings. *Results.* Twenty-six inhalers with a COPD indication were evaluated. Medication information sections were rated as "difficult to read" or "hard," and 85% (22/26) had a reading level above grade 8. The instructions for inhaler use were rated as "easy" or "fairly easy" to read and 63% (16/26) met the threshold by all formulas. While all leaflets achieved superior suitability ratings, extreme warnings included risk of premature death ($n = 12$), risks of serious injury ($n = 26$), serious interactions ($n = 26$), and statements that convey a serious consequence to therapy ($n = 26$). *Conclusion.* While COPD information leaflets in Canada performed well in terms of readability and suitability, overemphasis on side effects, warnings, and precautions may contribute to patient fear and nonadherence.

1. Background

Information leaflets are considered an important facet of patient education for all types of prescription medications [1]. In the case of inhaled agents for COPD, printed information not only serves to provide basic education about the drug but also contains detailed instructions about proper technique for administration. Indeed, administration of inhalers requires a certain degree of technical competence and suboptimal technique has been associated with an increased risk of hospitalizations, along with increased use of antibiotics and corticosteroids [2, 3].

In Canada alone, at least $1.5 billion dollars are spent on COPD hospitalizations annually [4], and COPD is the 4th leading cause of death in Canada and the only major chronic health condition where mortality rates are actually increasing [4, 5]. Although many medications were shown to reduce the risk of hospitalization [6], their use is clearly suboptimal. An average of 60% of patients with COPD do not adhere to prescribed therapy and up to 85% of patients use their inhalers ineffectively [7].

Patient information leaflets have the ability to positively enhance medication knowledge, patient satisfaction, and medication adherence [8]. On the other hand, poorly presented information in monographs can lead to misinterpretations of adverse effects and nonadherence to the prescribed therapy [9, 10]. Guidelines have been suggested on how to write patient friendly information appropriate for the general public [11]. Nevertheless, the readability of these materials often exceeds the recommended grade level [12]. Moreover, information leaflets have frequently been criticized for their potential to increase patient fears over drug safety [10].

The purpose of this study was to conduct an appraisal of the quality of information provided in the product monographs of COPD inhalers available in Canada.

2. Methods

2.1. COPD Inhalation Devices Identification. A search was conducted to identify all inhaled medications marketed in Canada for COPD using the national Drug Product Database [13]. Search terms were selected within each field of the online

Table 1: Readability interpretation.

(i) Flesch Reading Ease	(i) Gunning Fog	(i) Flesch-Kincaid Grade Level (ii) Coleman-Liau Index (iii) SMOG Index (iv) Automated Readability Index (v) Linsear Write Formula
90–100: very easy 80–89: easy 70–79: fairly easy 60–69: standard 50–59: fairly difficult 30–49: difficult 0–29: very confusing	5: readable 10: hard 15: difficult 20: very difficult	Number is considered equivalent to grade level. Anything above 12 is considered college level.

SMOG: simple measure of Gobbledygook.

database as follows: Status: "marketed and approved"; (i) Class(es): "human"; (ii) Route(s) of administration: "inhalation"; (iii) Dosage form(s): "all"; and (iv) Schedules: "prescription". Monographs were reviewed to identify devices specifically indicated for the treatment of COPD. Nebulized products were excluded.

For each product monograph identified, the consumer information section written in English (i.e., Part 3) was assessed for readability and suitability. In addition, a subjective assessment was undertaken to identify potential messages that might exaggerate the perception of risk associated with regular use.

2.2. Readability. While there are a variety of methods used to assess the readability of written materials, there is no consensus as to which formula is best suited for assessing patient education materials. To improve the validity of the results, it is favourable to use a variety of methods [14]. As such the readability of each leaflet was assessed with seven formulas: the Flesch Reading Ease formula [15], the Flesch-Kincaid Grade Level readability formula [16], the Gunning Fog Index [17], the SMOG Index [18], the Automated Readability Index [19], the Coleman-Liau Index [20], and the Linsear Write Formula [21]. These formulas use average sentence length, number of syllables, or average word length to calculate a reading ease or a reading grade level (Table 1). It is suggested that health information should be written no higher than grades 6–8 reading level to accommodate patients with poor health literacy [11].

Consumer information in each monograph was separated into "medication information" and "instructions on inhaler use." Each of these sections was entered separately into an online readability calculator [22]. Sections pertaining to reporting side effects to Health Canada and supplemental information were excluded.

2.3. Suitability. A suitability assessment was conducted on the leaflets to evaluate additional factors that may impact health literacy [11]. Two different researchers independently assessed each document using a modified version of the Suitability Assessment of Materials (SAM) tool [23, 24]. A third researcher was used to make a final decision in the event of a discrepancy. The modified SAM tool consisted of 16 items after removal of irrelevant elements ("cultural appropriateness", "summary reviews", "cover graphics", "lists/tables", and "interaction used") (Table 2). The Flesch-Kincaid Grade Level formula [16] was used to assess item (2)(a): Reading Grade Level.

Each factor was given a rating of "superior," "adequate," or "not suitable," which has a value of 2, 1, or 0, respectively [11, 23]. The values for each inhaler were summed and divided by the maximum score of 32 to produce a percentage. The percentages were categorized as 70–100% ("superior" material), 40–69% ("adequate" material), and 0–39% ("not suitable" material) [11, 23].

2.4. Medication Risks. Finally, a subjective review of each monograph was conducted to identify messages that appeared to exaggerate the risk posed to patients. Messages were categorized as highlighting (a) risks of premature death; (b) risks of serious injury; (c) risks of serious interactions; (d) statements that convey a serious consequence to therapy.

3. Results

One hundred and fifty-one medications met the search criteria on the Drug Product Database. After excluding the nebulized medications ($n = 40$), 26 inhalers were found to have a COPD indication and were assessed for readability and suitability (Table 3). Of these, 22 were branded products and four were produced by generic companies.

3.1. Readability. Readability of the medication information sections from each of the 26 leaflets was rated as "fairly difficult," "difficult," or "hard." None of the monographs were assessed within the recommended grade level of 6–8 by all formulas, and only 26% (7/26) met the target by at least one method (Table 4). In contrast, sections relating to inhaler use instructions were rated as "easy" or "fairly easy" to read and the most complex monographs were rated as "average." The majority of the instructions for inhaler use (77%, 20/26) met the target grade level of 6–8 by all formulas. (Table 5).

Table 2: Modified Suitability Assessment.

Category	Element
(1) Content	(a) Purpose (the purpose is evident) (b) Content topics (suggests behaviors that will help solve a problem) (c) Scope (scope is limited to the purpose of objective)
(2) Literacy demand	(a) Reading grade level (reading grade level score) (b) Writing style (text is written in a conversational style and active voice) (c) Vocabulary (vocabulary uses common words) (d) Sentence construction (context is given first) (e) Advanced organizers (advanced organizers are used to tell what is next)
(3) Graphics	(a) Type of illustrations (graphics are appropriate for the communication) (b) Relevance of illustrations (illustrations provide key ideas and messages) (c) Graphic captions (graphics have a corresponding caption)
(4) Layout and type	(a) Layout (layout factors) (b) Typography (font size and style) (c) Subheading (subheadings are used)
(5) Learning stimulation and motivation	(a) Behavior (behaviors are modeled and specific) (b) Motivation (actions are achievable promoting self-efficacy)

Table 3

Inhaler	Type	Manufacturer
Advair Diskus	DPI	GlaxoSmithKline
Airomir*	MDI	Valeant Canada LP
Anoro Ellipta	DPI	GlaxoSmithKline
Apo-Salvent CFC Free*	MDI	Apotex
Atrovent HFA	MDI	Boehringer Ingelheim
Breo Ellipta[a]	DPI	GlaxoSmithKline
Bricanyl Turbuhaler	DPI	AstraZeneca
Combivent Respimat	SMI	Boehringer Ingelheim
Duaklir Genuair	DPI	AstraZeneca
Foradil Aerolizer	DPI	Novartis Pharmaceuticals
Incruse Ellipta	DPI	GlaxoSmithKline
Inspiolto Respimat	SMI	Boehringer Ingelheim
Novo-Salbutamol HFA*	MDI	Teva Canada
Onbrez Breezhaler	DPI	Novartis Pharmaceuticals
Salbutamol HFA*	MDI	Sanis Health
Seebri Breezhaler	DPI	Novartis Pharmaceuticals
Serevent Diskhaler Disk	DPI	GlaxoSmithKline
Serevent Diskus	DPI	GlaxoSmithKline
Spiriva	DPI (handihaler)	Boehringer Ingelheim
Spiriva Respimat	SMI	Boehringer Ingelheim
Striverdi Respimat[b]	SMI	Boehringer Ingelheim
Symbicort Turbuhaler[b]	DPI	AstraZeneca
Tudorza Genuair	DPI	AstraZeneca
Ultibro Breezhaler	DPI	Novartis Pharmaceuticals
Ventolin Diskus	DPI	GlaxoSmithKline
Ventolin HFA	HFA	GlaxoSmithKline

*Generic products; [a]only 100/25 mcg/dose indicated in COPD; [b]approved by Health Canada but not currently marketed; MDI: metered dose inhaler; DPI: dry powdered inhaler; SMI: soft mist inhaler.

Table 4: Readability of patient medication information.

Inhaler	Flesch Reading Ease	Gunning Fog	Flesch-Kincaid Grade Level	Coleman-Liau Index	SMOG Index	Automated Readability Index	Linsear Write Formula
Advair Diskus	58.9	11.2	8.5	11	8.3	8.4	8
Airomir	44.8	14.2	12.5	11	12	12.5	15.4
Anoro Ellipta	54.1	11	9.6	10	9.6	8.7	10.6
Apo-Salvent CFC Free	48.8	14.1	12.2	10	10.7	12.4	15
Atrovent HFA	42.6	15.6	12.8	12	11.8	13.4	15.1
Breo Ellipta	55.9	11.8	10	10	9.5	10.1	11.8
Bricanyl Turbuhaler	44.3	13.5	11.8	13	10.8	12.3	12.9
Combivent Respimat	30.6	17.3	14.9	14	13.5	15.6	17.3
Duaklir Genuair	35.5	15.7	13.9	13	12.9	14.5	16.2
Foradil Aerolizer	46.4	13	10.8	12	10.2	10.5	11.1
Incruse Ellipta	58.2	10.7	8.9	10	8.6	8.4	8.7
Inspiolto Respimat	33.1	15.4	13.9	13	12.5	14.2	15.3
Novo-Salbutamol HFA	45.2	13.7	12.1	11	11	12.2	13.8
Onbrez Breezhaler	51.3	11.7	10.1	13	8.8	11	9.4
Salbutamol HFA	50	13.2	11.4	11	10.5	11.6	13.7
Seebri Breezhaler	49.1	12.5	11	12	9.1	11.9	11.6
Serevent Diskhaler Disk	58.7	10.7	8.5	11	8.4	8.7	8
Serevent Diskus	58.1	10.9	8.6	11	8.5	8.4	8.1
Spiriva	46.5	13.4	11.5	12	10.9	11.8	13.1
Spiriva Respimat	42.3	14.2	12.4	12	11.6	12.5	14.1
Striverdi Respimat	41.1	13.9	12.3	13	11.7	12.9	13.6
Symbicort	58.9	9.8	8.6	10	8.6	8.1	8.3
Tudorza Genuair	47.5	13.5	11	12	10.8	11	12.3
Ultibro Breezhaler	45.6	12.7	11.4	13	10.1	12.1	12.1
Ventolin Diskus	45.1	14.3	12.9	11	11.2	13.7	15.7
Ventolin HFA	51.4	13.2	11.3	10	10.5	11.5	13.7

3.2. Suitability. All patient information documents achieved a "superior" rating in the categories of purpose, content topics, scope, sentence construction, and behaviors but were deemed "not suitable" for their suboptimal reading grade level. The number of graphics in each leaflet ranged from 3 to 14, with a mean number of 8.5. Nevertheless, all documents received "superior" ratings for containing applicable information on what the medication was for and how to use the devices.

3.3. Medication Safety. None of the monographs contained a section dedicated to the benefits of the medication but all contained explicit information on potential risks. Twelve of the 26 inhalers (46%) contained a highlighted warning about the risk of asthma-related deaths associated with the use of the product (i.e., all products containing long-acting beta-2 agonists). All products (26/26) contained risks of serious injury, serious interactions, and statements that convey a serious consequence to therapy. For instance, warnings about dizziness or blurred vision were frequently present and included cautions about driving or operating machinery ($n = 11$). All leaflets had warnings on excessive use, using strong language such as *"extremely dangerous,"* or to *"contact a health care provider immediately if you think you have taken too much."* A statement indicating that *"the safety and effectiveness in children under the age of 4 years is not known"* was found on all salbutamol inhalers ($n = 6$) (and in one leaflet the "safe age" was listed at 6). Some of the warnings are not supported in the literature, such as advising consumers to avoid contact with anyone with measles or the chickenpox, in the case of inhaled corticosteroids ($n = 3$).

In general, warnings, precautions, and drug interactions were a major focus of the information provided for each product, often taking up the majority of the space in the leaflet.

4. Discussion

The provision of patient education is a critical factor for the success of inhaler medications in patients with COPD [25]. Although written information is no substitute for face-to-face education, it has an undeniable influence on the use and perceptions of medications [25]. Health Canada mandates that drug manufacturers develop a detailed consumer information leaflet to educate patients on each medication's purpose, proper administration, and potential side effects [26]. The document should be written using the "simplest,

Table 5: Readability of inhaler use instructions.

Inhaler	Flesch Reading Ease	Gunning Fog	Flesch-Kincaid Grade Level	Coleman-Liau Index	SMOG Index	Automated Readability Index	Linsear Write Formula
Advair Diskus	81.6	6.1	4.2	7	4.6	3.2	4.3
Airomir	80.8	7.5	5.4	7	6.2	5.2	6.9
Anoro Ellipta	74.3	7.3	5.5	7	6.7	3.9	5.6
Apo-Salvent CFC Free	81.2	7.6	5.4	7	5.9	5.2	7
Atrovent HFA	66.8	10.7	7.4	9	8.4	7	8
Breo Ellipta	77.8	7.5	5	7	6.5	3.5	5.5
Bricanyl Turbuhaler	74.8	8.6	6.4	7	7	5.9	7.5
Combivent Respimat	80.3	6.8	4.8	7	5.9	3.8	5.6
Duaklir Genuair	65.8	9.8	8.3	9	8.4	8.7	10.5
Foradil Aerolizer	79	7.1	4.7	8	5.4	4.4	4.8
Incruse Ellipta	74.9	7.5	5.5	7	6.8	3.9	5.6
Inspiolto Respimat	79.4	6.8	5	7	5.8	3.8	5.5
Novo-Salbutamol HFA	71.7	9.8	6.6	8	7.5	6	7.4
Onbrez Breezhaler	69.8	7.2	6.2	10	5.8	6.3	5.4
Salbutamol HFA	72.8	8.8	6.2	9	6.9	5.8	6.6
Seebri Breezhaler	73.6	6.7	5.5	9	5.1	5.4	4.7
Serevent Diskhaler Disk	81.2	6.5	4.8	8	4.9	4.8	5.4
Serevent Diskus	82.6	5.7	4	7	4.4	2.8	4
Spiriva Handihaler	79.9	5.7	4.4	8	5.3	4	4.4
Spiriva Respimat	80.4	6.7	4.8	7	5.8	3.6	5.5
Striverdi Respimat	81.2	6.5	4.6	7	5.7	3.6	5.2
Symbicort	82.5	6.9	4.3	6	5.7	3	5
Tudorza Genuair	64.1	10.3	8.6	10	9	9.1	11
Ultibro Breezhaler	71.1	6.7	5.7	10	5.8	5.5	4.9
Ventolin Diskus	80.4	5.8	4.6	7	5.6	3.5	5
Ventolin HFA	73.8	8.8	6.1	8	6.9	5.7	6.6

shortest words possible," using a language and format that is appropriate for the general public [27].

In general, COPD inhaler monographs contained highly readable instructions for use while more complex language was found in their patient information sections. Achieving an acceptable reading level is important, since approximately 60% of Canadians over age 16 have a low level of health literacy and lack the necessary skills to properly manage their health independently [28]. Poor health literacy in COPD is associated with increased disease severity, frequent hospitalizations, and a decrease in quality of life [29]. Low education levels are also a predictor of poor or incorrect inhaler technique [3, 30]. Improved outcomes in COPD will not be achievable if patients cannot understand how to use the devices. Although we find it encouraging that the instructions for inhaler use were generally rated as acceptable, there is certainly room for improvement with respect to patient information.

The suitability of COPD inhaler monographs was rated as "superior" for the applicability of information and how to use the devices. Nevertheless, all of the leaflets dedicated substantial space to the issue of medication safety, including explicit warnings about the risk of premature death. In many cases, more space was dedicated to warnings than correct administration technique. Not one of the leaflets we analyzed had a section dedicated to benefits. Including such information is arguably as important [31], since patients often do not recall all of the information provided by their health care provider regarding the rationale for use [32].

It has previously been suggested that written sources of drug information *"seem designed more to satisfy [governments and liability lawyers than] to teach patients..."* [33]. In our study, all monographs for inhalers containing long-acting beta-agonists ($n = 12$) warned about a risk of premature death. A recent systematic review of randomized studies in adult asthma patients found 46 deaths in 17,572 patients randomized to salmeterol or formoterol (0.26%) compared to 33 deaths in 16,380 patients randomized to control (0.20%) for a pooled OR of 1.37 (95% CI: 0.88 to 2.13) [34]. Although it must be acknowledged that signals of risk need to be clearly communicated to patients, the tone and severity of the monographs examined in this study far exceeded the objective risks identified in clinical trials [34]. Furthermore, in the treatment of COPD, LABAs used as monotherapy are recognized as safe and effective therapeutic options [6].

Several other examples of excessive warnings were discovered as well. Despite the fact that inhaled short-acting beta-agonists are widely used as first-line therapy for the treatment of bronchospasm in pediatric patients [35, 36], one of the first warnings on salbutamol leaflets was a statement indicating that *"the safety and effectiveness in children under the age of 4 years is not known."* Leaflets for anticholinergics warned patients to exercise caution when operating machinery or avoid driving due to the risk of dizziness or blurred vision. The risk of systemic absorption from inhaled anticholinergics is negligible [37], and these adverse effects have been reported at an incidence of 3% or less (which in most cases was similar to placebo) [37–41]. Furthermore, we are unaware of any studies that have tested the effects of inhaled anticholinergics on the ability to drive.

Even more alarming is the fact that several of the warnings in the monographs are not consistent with current literature. For instance, all inhaled corticosteroids advised consumers to avoid contact with individuals with measles or chicken pox. While the risk of acquiring these illnesses is increased in immunocompromised individuals taking oral corticosteroids, this does not hold true for inhaled formulations [42].

Several studies have indicated that negative information may cause fear and provoke nonadherence to medications. In one study in Australia, a third of consumers (35%, 242/691) indicated they had concerns after reading the consumer medication information [43], while in another study in Copenhagen 32% of patients (35/111) stated that they had stopped taking medication due to information about adverse effects [44]. Recently, a qualitative study ($n = 35$) discovered that the vast amount of side effects and drug interactions reported in package leaflets of commonly prescribed medications provoked fear and anxiety and caused patients to stop their medication or alter their dosage regimen without consulting a health care provider [10].

Studies have shown that confidence in drug therapy could be low among patients with COPD [45], and medication underuse is the most prevalent type of nonadherence with this illness [46]. Rather than emphasizing the (often unfounded) risks, manufacturers should aim to encourage adherence by describing the medication's potential benefits. Studies have demonstrated that patients want information that is encouraging to read and how much a medicine will assist them [10, 47]. We realize that drug manufacturers have a duty to warn patients about foreseeable side effects of medications but argue that the risk/benefit approach should be used. Product warnings should only be included in the leaflet, if it is reasonable and substantial enough to warrant concern. Furthermore, manufacturers should make an effort to consult with the ultimate stakeholder—the consumer—prior to publishing the product monographs.

There are several limitations that should be acknowledged with this study. First, only Canadian monographs written in English were included in this evaluation. The patient medication information sections were retrieved from the Health Canada Drug Product Database, so we were unable to assess the layout of the information that is dispensed with the devices. (Health Canada archives the monographs in pdf. format, whereas the information provided with the devices may be in the format of a booklet.) Readability and suitability tests were used as surrogate markers to evaluate the likelihood of patient comprehension of the materials, and a subjective assessment was used to identify explicit warnings. A study involving actual patients would be needed to directly assess patient comprehension and to truly understand the perceptions and consequences associated with the information presented in the leaflets.

5. Conclusion

Consumer information intended to educate patients on medications for COPD provides adequate instructions for use; however, the main messages contained in the documents were negative, severe, and sometimes inappropriate. In addition, improvements in the readability of the patient information sections are possible since none of them were rated at the appropriate reading level. Previous calls to improve the design of educational materials have not been acted upon.

References

[1] M. Yamamoto, "Patient drug information leaflets for risk/benefit communication," *Journal of Pharmacovigilance*, vol. 3, article e132, 2015.

[2] J. Sanchis, I. Gich, and S. Pedersen, "Systematic Review of Errors in Inhaler Use: Has Patient Technique Improved Over Time?" *Chest*, vol. 150, no. 2, pp. 394–406, 2016.

[3] A. S. Melani, M. Bonavia, V. Cilenti et al., "Inhaler mishandling remains common in real life and is associated with reduced disease control," *Respiratory Medicine*, vol. 105, no. 6, pp. 930–938, 2011.

[4] N. Mittmann, L. Kuramoto, S. J. Seung, J. M. Haddon, C. Bradley-Kennedy, and J. M. FitzGerald, "The cost of moderate and severe COPD exacerbations to the Canadian healthcare system," *Respiratory Medicine*, vol. 102, no. 3, pp. 413–421, 2008.

[5] S. Benady, *THe Human And Economic Burden of COPD: A Leading Cause of Hospital Admission in Canada*, Canadian Thoracic Society, 2010.

[6] *Global Initiative for Chronic Obstructive Lung Disease Global Strategy for the Diagnosis*, Management and Prevention of COPD-2016, http://goldcopd.org/global-strategy-diagnosis-management-prevention-copd-2016/.

[7] R. D. Restrepo, M. T. Alvarez, L. D. Wittnebel et al., "Medication adherence issues in patients treated for COPD," *International Journal of Chronic Obstructive Pulmonary Disease*, vol. 3, no. 3, pp. 371–384, 2008.

[8] M. Sustersic, A. Gauchet, A. Foote, and J.-L. Bosson, "How best to use and evaluate Patient Information Leaflets given during a consultation: A systematic review of literature reviews," *Health Expectations*, 2016.

[9] N. Carrigan, D. K. Raynor, and P. Knapp, "Adequacy of patient information on adverse effects: An assessment of patient information leaflets in the UK," *Drug Safety*, vol. 31, no. 4, pp. 305–312, 2008.

[10] O. R. Herber, V. Gies, D. Schwappach, P. Thürmann, and S. Wilm, "Patient information leaflets: Informing or frightening? A focus group study exploring patients' emotional reactions and subsequent behavior towards package leaflets of commonly prescribed medications in family practices," *BMC Family Practice*, vol. 15, no. 1, article no. 163, 2014.

[11] *National Literacy and Health Program Good Medicine for Seniors: Guidelines for Plain Language and Good Design in Prescription Medication*, Canadian Public Health Association, 2002.

[12] C. Pires, M. Vigário, and A. Cavaco, "Readability of medicinal package leaflets: A systematic review," *Revista de Saude Publica*, vol. 49, no. 1, 2015.

[13] Health Canada Drug and Health Products. Drug Product Database. Available at: http://www.hc-sc.gc.ca/dhp-mps/prodpharma/databasdon/index-eng.php.

[14] S. Badarudeen and S. Sabharwal, "Assessing readability of patient education materials: current role in orthopaedics clin orthop relat res," *Clinical Orthopaedics and Related Research*, vol. 10, pp. 2572–2580, 468.

[15] R. Flesch, "A new readability yardstick," *Journal of Applied Psychology*, vol. 32, no. 3, pp. 221–233, 1948.

[16] J. P. Kincaid, R. P. Fishburn, R. L. Rogers, and B. S. Chissom, "Derivation of new readability formulas (automated readability index, fog count, and flesch reading ease formula) for navy enlisted personnel," *Institute for Simulation and Training*, 1975.

[17] R. Gunning, *The Technique of Clear Writing*, McGraw-Hill, New York, NY, USA, 1952.

[18] H. G. McLaughlin, "SMOG Grading: a new readability formula," *J Read*, vol. 12, no. 8, pp. 639–646, 1969.

[19] E. A. Smith and R. J. Senter, "Automated readability index," *AMRL-TR Journal*, pp. 1–14, 1967.

[20] M. Coleman and T. L. Liau, "A computer readability formula designed for machine scoring," *Journal of Applied Psychology*, vol. 60, no. 2, pp. 283-284, 1975.

[21] A. E. M. Eltorai, S. S. Naqvi, S. Ghanian et al., "Readability of Invasive Procedure Consent Forms," *Clinical and Translational Science*, vol. 8, no. 6, pp. 830–833, 2015.

[22] Readability Formulas. Available at: http://www.readabilityformulas.com. Accessed: 25 January 2017.

[23] C. Doak, L. G. Doak, and J. H. Root, "Assessing suitability of materials," in *Teaching Patients with Low Literacy Skills*, M. Belcher, Ed., J. B. Lippincott Company, Philadelphia, Pa, USA, 2nd edition, 1996.

[24] M. LeBrun, J. DiMuzio, B. Beauchamp, S. Reid, and V. Hogan, "Evaluating the health literacy burden of canada's public advisories: a comparative effectiveness study on clarity and readability drug saf," *Drug Safety*, vol. 36, no. 12, pp. 1179–1187, 2013.

[25] S. C. Lareau and R. Hodder, "Teaching inhaler use in chronic obstructive pulmonary disease patients," *Journal of the American Academy of Nurse Practitioners*, vol. 24, no. 2, pp. 113–120, 2012.

[26] Health Canada Drug and Health Products. Frequently Asked Questions: Product Monographs Posted to the Health Canada Website. 2014. Available at: http://www.hc-sc.gc.ca/dhp-mps/prodpharma/applic-demande/guide-ld/monograph/pm_qa_mp_qr-eng.php. Accessed: 7 February 2017.

[27] Health Canada Drug and Health Products. Guidance document: product monograph. (2013). Available at: http://www.hc-sc.gc.ca/dhp-mps/prodpharma/applic-demande/guide-ld/monograph/pm_mp_2013-eng.php#a110. Accessed: 7 Feb 2017.

[28] *Health Literacy in Canada: A Healthy Understanding*, Canadian Council on Learning, Ottawa, Canada, 2008.

[29] T. A. Omachi, U. Sarkar, E. H. Yelin, P. D. Blanc, and P. P. Katz, "Lower health literacy is associated with poorer health status and outcomes in chronic obstructive pulmonary disease," *Journal of General Internal Medicine*, vol. 28, no. 1, pp. 74–81, 2013.

[30] C. Pothirat, W. Chaiwong, N. Phetsuk, S. Pisalthanapuna, N. Chetsadaphan, and W. Choomuang, "E valuating inhaler use technique in COPD patients," *International Journal of COPD*, vol. 10, pp. 1291–1298, 2015.

[31] R. Dickinson, D. K. Raynor, P. Knapp, and J. MacDonald, "Providing additional information about the benefits of statins in a leaflet for patients with coronary heart disease: A qualitative study of the impact on attitudes and beliefs," *BMJ Open*, vol. 6, no. 12, Article ID e012000, 2016.

[32] R. P. C. Kessels, "Patients' memory for medical information," *Journal of the Royal Society of Medicine*, vol. 96, no. 5, pp. 219–222, 2003.

[33] J. Avorn and W. H. Shrank, "Communicating drug benefits and risks effectively: There must be a better way," *Annals of Internal Medicine*, vol. 150, no. 8, pp. 563-564, 2009.

[34] C. J. Cates, L. S. Wieland, M. Oleszczuk, and K. M. Kew, "Safety of regular formoterol or salmeterol in adults with asthma: an overview of Cochrane reviews," *The Cochrane Database of Systematic Reviews*, vol. 6, no. 2, Article ID CD010314, 2014.

[35] F. M. Ducharme, S. D. Dell, D. Radhakrishnan et al., "Diagnosis and management of asthma in preschoolers: A Canadian Thoracic Society and Canadian Paediatric Society position paper," *Paediatr Child Health*, vol. 20, pp. 353–371, 2015.

[36] Global Initiative for Asthma (GINA) Global Strategy for Asthma Management and Prevention. [Updated 2016]. Available at: http://www.ginasthma.org; Accessed 28 February 2017.

[37] J. E. Scullion, "The development of anticholinergics in the management of COPD," *International Journal of COPD*, vol. 2, no. 1, pp. 33–40, 2007.

[38] *Atrovent HFA (Ipratropium) [Product Monograph]*, Boehringer Ingelheim (Canada) Ltd, Burlington, Ontario, Canada, February 2016.

[39] *Spiriva HandiHaler (Tiotropium Bromide) [Prescribing Information]*, CT: Boehringer Ingelheim, Ridgefield, Conn, USA, January 2016.

[40] *Incruse Ellipta (Umeclidinium) [Product Monograph]*, GlaxoSmithKline Inc, Mississauga, Ontario, Canada, March 2016.

[41] *Seebri Breezhaler (Glycopyrronium) [Product Monograph]*, Novartis Pharmaceuticals Canada, Dorval, Quebec, Canada, January 2016.

[42] M. J. Welch, "Inhaled steroids and severe viral infections," *Journal of Asthma*, vol. 31, no. 1, pp. 43–50, 1994.

[43] K. K. Hamrosi, D. K. Raynor, and P. Aslani, "Pharmacist, general practitioner and consumer use of written medicine information in Australia: Are they on the same page?" *Research in Social and Administrative Pharmacy*, vol. 10, no. 4, pp. 656–668, 2014.

[44] A. Horwitz, L. Reuther, and S. E. Andersen, "Patient information leaflets seen through the eyes of patients in a general practice," *Ugeskr Laeger*, vol. 171, no. 8, pp. 599–602, 2009.

[45] J. George, D. C. M. Kong, R. Thoman, and K. Stewart, "Factors associated with medication nonadherence in patients with COPD," *Chest*, vol. 128, no. 5, pp. 3198–3204, 2005.

3

Effects of Fasudil on Patients with Pulmonary Hypertension Associated with Left Ventricular Heart Failure with Preserved Ejection Fraction: A Prospective Intervention Study

Xiang Zhang,[1] Xueming Zhang,[2] Saihua Wang,[1] Jun Luo,[1] Zhihong Zhao,[1] Changzhu Zheng,[1] and Jieyan Shen[2]

[1]*Shanghai Zhoupu Hospital, Shanghai, China*
[2]*Renji Hospital, Shanghai Jiaotong University School of Medicine, Shanghai, China*

Correspondence should be addressed to Jieyan Shen; shenjieyan@renji.com

Xiang Zhang and Xueming Zhang contributed equally to this work.

Academic Editor: Alberto Ruano-Ravina

Background. Pulmonary hypertension due to left ventricular heart failure with preserved ejection fraction (PH-HFpEF) is an increasingly medical problem. The aim of the study was to evaluate the clinical efficacy of fasudil on PH-HFpEF elderly patients and to figure out the subtype of PH-HFpEF which may be the therapeutic object of fasudil. *Method.* 58 PH-HFpEF elderly patients were enrolled. Patients were diagnosed with passive pulmonary hypertension (PPH) or reactive pulmonary hypertension (RPH) by right heart catheterization and all receiving Rho kinase inhibitor fasudil for 2 weeks. The endpoint includes changes in SpO2, NT-pro BNP, cardiac functional classification, and echocardiography measurements after 2 weeks treatment. *Results.* The course of disease in the RPH group was longer than the PPH group ($p < 0.05$). Cardiac output was found to be worse in the RPH group than the PPH group ($p < 0.01$). Besides, the RPH group demonstrated a greater transpulmonary pressure gradient (TPG) and pulmonary vascular resistance (PVR) than the PPH group ($p < 0.01$ for both) as well as pulmonary arterial systolic pressure (PASP) and mean pulmonary arterial pressure (mPAP) ($p < 0.01$ for both), which fits the feature of RPH. After treatment of fasudil, in RPH group, PASP significantly decreased ($p < 0.01$) with decreased E/E' and increased E/A ($p < 0.05$ for both), indicating that pulmonary haemodynamics and cardiac diastolic function were ameliorated, but the measurements in the PPH group had no significant changes. NT-pro BNP and 6 MWD of both groups were improved ($p < 0.05$). The total effective rate of the RPH group was 74.29%, which was higher than 47.83% of the PPH group ($p < 0.05$). *Conclusion.* The Rho kinase inhibitor fasudil can improve pulmonary and left ventricular haemodynamics in patients with PH-HFpEF. The total effective rate was higher in the RPH group. Fasudil may be a promising targeted drug for the RPH in PH-HFpEF patients. This trial is registered with ChiCTR-INR-16009511.

1. Introduction

Despite the increasing number of patients with heart failure with preserved ejection fraction (HFpEF), currently there is no proven therapy for HFpEF [1]. The long-term and sustained backward hemodynamic transmission increases the right ventricle afterload and the pulmonary artery pressure [2]. Pulmonary hypertension (PH) is recognized as one of the characteristics of HFpEF and is indeed prevalent in HFpEF patients. Thus, PH is used as a predictor of morbidity and mortality in HFpEF patients [3]. However, the optimal treatment of PH in conjunction with HFpEF is currently unknown [4].

Based on transpulmonary pressure gradient (TPG = mPAP − PAWP), pulmonary hypertension due to left heart disease (PH-LHD) could be classified into two groups: passive PH (PPH; TPG < 12 mmHg) and reactive PH (RPH, also known as the out of proportion PH; TPG ≥ 12 mmHg). The 2015 European Society of Cardiology (ESC) guidelines for the diagnosis and treatment of PH further separated PH-LHD into isolated postcapillary PH and mixed pre- and postcapillary PH. This classification was based on whether the diastolic pressure gradient (DPG = DPAP − PAWP) is lower or higher than 7 [5, 6], which is similar to the RPH and PPH classification of PH-LHD. Earlier studies had reported the roles of TPG and pulmonary vascular resistance (PVR) in predicting outcomes in heart failure. In a study of 463 patients with LV ejection fraction <40%, the mortality rate was significantly higher in patients with pulmonary vascular resistance (PVR) ≥3 WU [7], suggesting that RPH is more severe than PPH and RPH may be involve pulmonary vasculature remodeling.

Fasudil is a Rho-kinase inhibitor that blocks the activity of Rho kinase by competing the ATP binding site of the Rho-kinase catalytic domain with ATP and thus plays an important role in relaxing pulmonary vasculature. A variety of clinical studies suggested that the Rho-kinase pathway is involved in many cellular functions including proliferation, migration, and contraction of the vascular smooth muscle cell [8–10], and fasudil is considered to be a novel drug for the treatment of PH, which has been approved in Japan and China, but currently not in the US.

To date, few clinical trials of Rho kinase inhibitors have been reported in PH associated with left ventricular HFpEF. The goal of this study is to investigate the effects of fasudil on PH-HFpEF and determine the response differences to treatment between RPH and PPH.

2. Methods

2.1. Screening with Echocardiography. The study population was prospectively recruited from patients with heart failure (HF) symptoms from August 2014 to February 2017 in Zhoupu Hospital and Shanghai Renji Hospital. According to the 2016 ESC guidelines for heart failure, all symptomatic HF patients who underwent echocardiography with left ventricular ejection fraction (LVEF) ≥50% [11] were diagnosed with HFpEF. These HFpEF patients with pulmonary artery systolic pressure (PASP) >40 mmHg determined by echocardiography were suspected to be pulmonary hypertension [12].

As proposed by the ASE [13], linear internal measurements of the left ventricle and its walls are performed in the parasternal long-axis view with a two-dimensional (2D) echocardiography-guided M-mode approach, including left atrial systolic diameter (LAD), left ventricular end-diastolic diameter (LVEDD), left ventricular end-systolic diameter (LVESD), interventricular septal thickness (IVST), and left ventricular posterior wall thickness (LVPW). Fractional shortening (FS) was derived from linear measurements obtained from 2D images, and LVEF was calculated by the modified Simpson method.

Mitral valve peak E-wave velocity (E) and peak A-wave velocity (A) were obtained in the apical four-chamber view with color flow imaging for optimal alignment of pulsed-wave (PW) Doppler with blood flow. And mitral annular lateral E velocity (E') was obtained in the apical four-chamber view with proper alignment to acquire septal and lateral mitral annular velocity using tissue Doppler [14]. Left ventricular diastolic dysfunction is reflected by E', E/A, and E/E'.

According to ASE guidelines for the assessment of right heart [15], in the absence of a gradient across the pulmonic valve or right ventricular outflow tract, PASP is equal to right ventricular systolic pressure (RVSP). RVSP was estimated by adding transtricuspid pressure gradient to the right atrial pressure. Transtricuspid pressure gradient can be determined from the peak velocity of the tricuspid valve regurgitant jet, and right atrial (RA) pressure was estimated from IVC diameter and its collapse during inspiration under the long-axis subcostal view.

2.2. Confirmation with RHC and Patient Enrollment. All HFpEF patients suspected with PH by echocardiography had received optimal treatment for HFpEF and other primary diseases for 2–4 weeks, including adequate drug therapies (i.e., diuretics, nitrates, ACEI/ARB, and beta blockers) and/or interventional therapies (i.e., coronary artery stenting or pacemaker implantation). Following the above initial treatment of primary cardiac diseases, right heart catheterization (RHC) was performed, and the patients with mPAP ≥25 mmHg and PAWP >15 mmHg were confirmed as PH-HFpEF [6].

Right atrial pressure, right ventricular pressure, pulmonary artery pressure including PASP, mean pulmonary artery pressure (mPAP), diastolic pulmonary arterial pressure (DPAP), and pulmonary artery wedge pressure (PAWP) were measured by RHC using a 6-lumen Edward catheter. We replaced PAWP by LVEDP when there was PAWP measurement error caused by incomplete balloon incarceration. Cardiac output (CO) was measured in triplicate by the thermodilution technique. TPG was calculated as mPAP minus PAWP, and PVR was calculated using the following formula: (mPAP − PAWP)/CO. Among these PH-HFpEF patients, those TPG ≤12 mmHg were considered as PPH, whereas TPG >12 mmHg were classified as RPH.

The PH-HFpEF patients aged 60–80 years with HFpEF secondary to coronary disease, hypertension, degenerative valvular heart disease (except for patients with severe mitral or aortic valvular organic disease), cardiomyopathy, and New York Heart Association (NYHA) functional class II–IV were enrolled.

The exclusion criteria include the following:

(1) Severe liver or kidney diseases, malignant tumor, and cerebrovascular disease

(2) Restrictive cardiomyopathy, hypertrophic obstructive cardiomyopathy, constrictive pericarditis, moderate-to-severe mitral stenosis, or aortic stenosis

(3) PH caused by congenital heart disease, rheumatic heart disease, autoimmune disease, chronic obstructive pulmonary disease, chronic thromboembolism, pulmonary vascular abnormalities, and idiopathic PAH (IPAH)

(4) Patients who are treated with calcium blockers, prostacyclin, or endothelin receptor antagonists

(5) Patients with incomplete data

A total of 58 PH-HFpEF patients were enrolled, of which 35 were diagnosed with RPH while 23 patients were confirmed as PPH.

2.3. Treatment and Efficacy Evaluation. These enrolled patients were treated with fasudil (fasudil injection solution from the Tianjin Hongri Pharmaceutical Ltd by Share Ltd), 30 mg intravenous drip twice a day for 2 weeks. During the treatment, the heart rate, blood pressure, liver function, renal function, and electrolytes were closely monitored in case adverse events or background therapy remained unchanged.

Data collection was undertaken and compared pre- and posttreatment results in all patients, including Doppler echocardiography, measurement of 6MWD, NYHA heart failure functional classification, and laboratory tests results, such as NT-pro-BNP and SvO_2.

We evaluated the cardiac function of patients based on NYHA classification and 6-minute walking distance (6MWD). The efficacy of fasudil was determined according to the changes of NYHA classification: (1) markedly effective: heart failure is basically controlled or cardiac functional classification increased by 2 and above; (2) effective: cardiac functional classification increases by 1, but less than 2; (3) ineffective: cardiac function is better than before, but its classification did not change; and (4) deterioration: cardiac functional classification decreases by 1 or more.

2.4. Statistical Analyses. Continuous variables are expressed as mean ± SEM unless otherwise stated. The differences of baseline and baseline changes between RPH and PPH were compared using Student's t-test for normally distributed data, and the differences of examination data between pre- and posttreatment were evaluated using the paired t-test. The Wilcoxon test was used for continuous nonnormally distributed variables. Enumeration data were presented in terms of the rate and test by χ^2 or exact probability method, and the rank sum test was used for ranked data.

Two-sided p value < 0.05 was considered to indicate statistically significant. Statistical analyses were performed using SAS and SPSS version 17.0.

3. Results

3.1. Baseline Characteristics and Pulmonary Hemodynamics by RHC. The patients' demographic and etiological data and pulmonary hemodynamic measurements, as well as the medication used for basic diseases and heart failure treatment, are summarized in Table 1. Baseline characteristics of the two groups were comparable except for the course of disease and pulmonary hemodynamics.

The disease course in the RPH group was longer than that in the PPH group (3.69 ± 2.64 years versus 3.09 ± 2.22 years, $p < 0.05$), and the TPG and PVR in the RPH group were higher than those in the PPH group (TPG: 22.11 ± 2.25 mmHg versus 10.08 ± 1.88 mmHg, $p < 0.01$; PVR: 5.24 ± 2.55 WU versus 2.15 ± 0.88 WU, $p < 0.01$), which are the characteristics of patients with RPH. Meanwhile, compared to the PPH group, PASP and mPAP in RPH patients were also higher (PASP: 62.9 ± 17.47 mmHg versus 47.17 ± 8.47 mmHg, $p < 0.01$; mPAP: 45.26 ± 14.96 mmHg versus 33.82 ± 7.26 mmHg, $p < 0.01$) while CO was lower (4.19 ± 1.26 versus 4.84 ± 1.56, $p < 0.01$), suggesting that pulmonary hypertension in RPH patients is more severe than that in PPH and leads to CO decrease.

3.2. Echocardiography. As shown in Table 2, there was no significant difference in echocardiography baselines between RPH and PPH groups except for PASP (64.37 ± 13.82 versus 49.87 ± 8.50 mmHg, $p < 0.05$).

After 2 weeks of therapy with fasudil, the left ventricular diastolic function in RPH group, as indicated by decreased E/E' and increased E/A, was improved (E/E' 16.89 ± 1.11 versus 13.19 ± 1.79, $p < 0.05$; E/A 0.78 ± 0.19 versus 0.98 ± 0.12, $p < 0.05$), and PASP in the RPH group significantly decreased from 64.37 ± 13.82 mmHg to 63.51 ± 13.79 mmHg ($p < 0.05$). However, there was no change in E/E', E/A, and PASP in the PPH group.

3.3. Cardiac Function Evaluation and Laboratory Tests. At baseline, there were no statistical differences between the study groups in SvO_2, NT-pro-BNP, 6MWD, and NYHA classification.

In both groups, NT-pro-BNP and 6MWD were improved after treatment as summarized in Table 3 ($p < 0.05$). In terms of NYHA classification, the RPH group had a better outcome in comparison to the PPH group: 8 cases of the RPH group were markedly effective, effective in 18 cases, and invalid or deteriorated in 9 cases. The total effective rate in RPH group was 74.29%, whereas the total effective rate was 47.83% in the PPH group including markedly effective in 2 cases, effective in 9 case, and invalid or deteriorated in 12 cases (Table 4, Figure 1). Fasudil was more effective for RPH patients, indicated by a significant difference in the total effective rate between the two groups ($p < 0.05$).

3.4. Safety Analysis. During the 2-week treatment, no adverse event was observed in either group; patient's liver function, renal function, electrolyte, blood, urine, and stool routine tests were all normal. Two patients in the PPH group and 3 patients in the RPH group reported some mild side effects including slightly decreased heart rate and blood pressure, dizziness, and fatigue, which were all reported tolerable to the patients and thus fasudil treatment was not discontinued.

Table 1: Baseline characteristics and pulmonary hemodynamics by RHC.

Variable	PPH group ($n = 23$)	RPH group ($n = 35$)	p
Demographics			
Male, n (%)	16 (69.57)	23 (65.71)	0.783
Female, n (%)	7 (30.43)	12 (34.29)	0.684
Age (years)	69.78 ± 10.22	70.60 ± 11.14	0.891
Medical history			
Coronary artery disease (%)	9 (39.13)	13 (37.14)	0.965
Hypertensive heart disease (%)	2 (8.70)	3 (8.57)	0.974
Coronary heart disease with hypertension (%)	7 (30.43)	10 (28.57)	0.862
Dilated cardiomyopathy (%)	2 (8.69)	3 (8.57)	0.975
Degenerative valvular heart disease (%)	3 (13.04)	6 (17.14)	0.763
Course of disease (years)	3.09 ± 2.22	3.69 ± 2.64*	0.012
Medication, n (%)			
Diuretics	22 (95.65)	33 (94.29)	0.912
Hydrochlorothiazide 25 mg qd	15	24	
Torasemide 20 mg qd	7	9	
Antisterone	22	31	
Nitrates	17 (73.91)	26 (74.29)	0.893
ACEI/ARB	19 (82.61)	29 (82.86)	0.981
β-Blockers	20 (86.96)	28 (80.00)	0.261
Pulmonary hemodynamics			
PASP (mmHg)	47.17 ± 8.47	62.9 ± 17.47	0.003
mPAP (mmHg)	33.82 ± 7.26	45.26 ± 14.96	0.007
PAWP (mmHg)	23.26 ± 5.26	23.14 ± 5.26	0.947
TPG (mmHg)	10.08 ± 1.88	22.11 ± 2.25	0.000
PVR (WU)	2.15 ± 0.88	5.24 ± 2.55	0.003
CO (L/min)	4.84 ± 1.56	4.19 ± 1.26	0.000
Cardiac function (n/n)			
NYHA I-II/III-IV	5/18	8/27	0.9426

Data are presented as number and rate or mean ± standard deviation; Student's t-test was used for continuous normally distributed variables; the Wilcoxon test was used for continuous nonnormally distributed variables; ranked data were tested by rank sum test; PASP, pulmonary artery systolic pressure; mPAP, mean pulmonary artery pressure; PAWP, pulmonary artery wedge pressure; TPG, transpulmonary pressure gradient; PVR, pulmonary vascular resistance; CO, cardiac output; NYHA, New York Heart Association; the change from baseline, $^* p < 0.05$.

Table 2: Cardiac effect of fasudil treatment determined by echocardiography.

Variable	PPH ($n = 23$)			RPH ($n = 35$)		
	Pretreatment	Posttreatment	p	Pretreatment	Posttreatment	p
LAD (mm)	46.50 ± 4.75	45.50 ± 4.51	0.987	47.00 ± 6.25	46.63 ± 5.50	0.379
LVEDD (mm)	45.10 ± 6.14	46.07 ± 8.12	0.697	47.14 ± 8.40	47.63 ± 7.73	0.497
LVESD (mm)	27.91 ± 3.16	28.21 ± 2.88	0.378	29.02 ± 3.64	29.91 ± 4.06	0.788
IVST	11.01 ± 1.56	10.98 ± 1.96	0.916	11.85 ± 2.03	11.35 ± 1.96	0.895
LVPW	10.82 ± 1.16	10.01 ± 0.96	0.816	11.01 ± 1.76	10.87 ± 1.86	0.941
E (cm/s)	49.97 ± 6.85	52.59 ± 8.37	0.062	50.35 ± 8.22	53.43 ± 9.22	0.059
A (cm/s)	62.03 ± 10.31	63.36 ± 9.37	0.096	64.5 ± 11.80	54.52 ± 12.65*	0.016
E' (cm/s)	2.89 ± 1.03	3.03 ± 1.11	0.074	2.98 ± 1.16	4.05 ± 1.02	0.071
E/A	0.80 ± 0.11	0.83 ± 0.14	0.069	0.78 ± 0.19	0.98 ± 0.12*	0.011
E/E'	17.29 ± 2.21	17.36 ± 1.89	0.098	16.89 ± 1.11	13.19 ± 1.79*	0.011
EF (%)	61.64 ± 10.31	64.83 ± 12.37	0.069	62.43 ± 11.80	64.24 ± 9.65	0.485
PASP (mmHg)	49.87 ± 8.50	49.48 ± 8.64	0.444	64.37 ± 13.82†	63.51 ± 13.79*	0.017

Data are presented as mean ± standard deviation; differences in change from baseline between groups were evaluated using Student's t-test; LAD, left atrial systolic diameter; LVEDD, left ventricular end-diastolic diameter; LVESD, left ventricular end-systolic diameter; IVST, interventricular septal thickness; LVPW, left ventricular posterior wall thickness; E, early diastolic transmitral flow velocity; A, late diastolic transmitral flow velocity; E', early diastolic mitral annular velocity; †the comparison of PASP between groups before treatment, $p < 0.01$; the change from baseline, $^* p < 0.05$.

4. Discussion

Heart failure with preserved ejection fraction originates from left ventricular diastolic dysfunction secondary to impaired relaxation and stiffened myocardium. The increased load of left ventricle exposes the lung vasculature to pressure-induced challenges. In the long term, the sustained pulmonary hemodynamic change not only leads to pulmonary hypertension but also increases the pulsatile loading on the right ventricle [2], which determines the patient's outcome.

Table 3: Effect of fasudil on SpO_2, NT-pro-BNP, and 6MWD.

Variable	PPH ($n = 23$)			RPH ($n = 35$)		
	Pretreatment	Posttreatment	p	Pretreatment	Posttreatment	p
SpO_2 (%)	92.89 ± 3.97	93.15 ± 5.13	0.071	91.30 ± 4.68	93.07 ± 4.80	0.052
NT-pro-BNP (ng/ml) (min, max)	3664 (789, 21150)	1149 (750, 4651)*	0.031	3980 (1312, 24000)	1287 (155, 8210)**	0.004
6MWD (m)	361.75 ± 50.24	401.34 ± 59.56*	0.042	345.60 ± 44.55	400.7 ± 59.41**	0.001

Normally distributed data are presented as mean ± standard deviation; nonnormally distributed data are presented as minimum and maximum; normally distributed variables were evaluated using Student's t-test; nonnormally distributed data were tested by the Wilcoxon test; ; 6MWD, 6-minute walking distance; the change from baseline,* $p < 0.05$ and ** $p < 0.01$.

Table 4: The number of cases of NYHA classification change.

Efficacy	PPH ($n = 23$)	RPH ($n = 35$)	p
Markedly effective (%)	2 (8.70)	8 (22.86)	
Effective (%)	9 (39.13)	18 (51.43)	
Ineffective or deterioration (%)	12 (52.17)	9 (25.17)	
Total effective (%)	11 (47.83)	26 (74.29)	0.040

Data are presented as patient number and %; enumeration data are tested by χ^2 test or exact probability method.

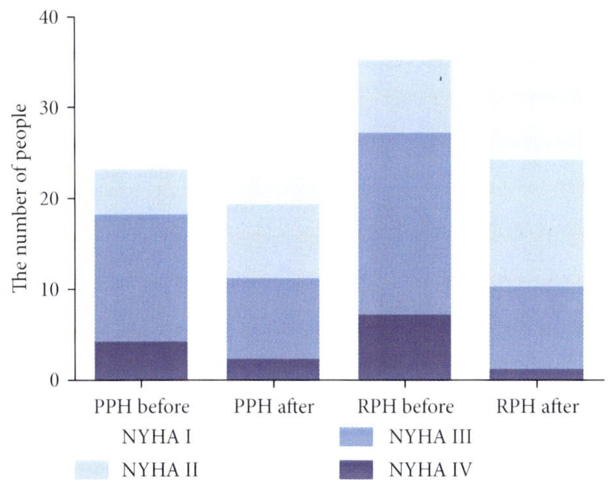

Figure 1: Fasudil treatment-induced changes of patient's NYHA classification in the RPH and PPH groups.

The management of pulmonary hypertension due to left heart disease (PH-LHD) focuses on treating the primary left heart disease and improves left ventricular function, thereby alleviating PH. However, even with optimal treatment, the clinical symptoms and mortality of this disease cannot be improved. Aronson et al. [16] performed a survival analysis of 242 patients with acute decompensated heart failure and observed that the mortality of RPH patients was significantly higher than those of PPH patients or patients without PH. Meanwhile, a population-based report by Lam et al. [3] revealed that, in hypertensive patients with HFpEF, the increased pulmonary artery pressure may not be attributable to the passive venous PH and there may be an additional precapillary pulmonary artery hypertension mediated by functional or organic arteriolar disorders, which may need a novel therapeutic strategy for PH-HFpEF.

Recently, whether PH caused by pulmonary vascular remodeling in late PH-LHD can be treated with targeted drugs has drawn much attention. FIRST [17] and ENABLE [18] studies proved that pulmonary vascular targeting therapy is not suitable for PH due to left heart failure. However, these studies had selected the patients with severe left ventricular systolic dysfunction without evidence of PVR elevating, so these results are not enough powerful to prove that pulmonary vascular targeting therapy is not effective for RPH-HFpEF on the basis of optimal treatment for HFpEF. A previous study of sildenafil [19] effects on PH-HFpEF proved that sildenafil improves pulmonary pressure, vasomotility, and RV function, as well as LV relaxation and distensibility. However, this study did not perform right heart catheterization and subgroup PVR analysis. Recently, there were two randomized placebo-controlled trials of sildenafil's effects in patients with HFpEF and predominantly isolated post-capillary PH reported by Hoendermis et al. [20] and Liu et al. [21], respectively. Both trials showed similar results suggesting that sildenafil is ineffective in improving pulmonary and systemic hemodynamics. Currently, there is little evidence on target therapy for RPH-HFpEF.

The results of our current prospective controlled trial show that fasudil can reduce pulmonary artery pressure and improve cardiac function more significantly in RPH-HFpEF than in PPH-HFpEF patients. We found that RPH patients had a longer course of heart failure, higher levels of PASP, mPAP, TPG, and PVR than those of PPH patients. These findings may be explained by the hypothesis that RPH and PPH have different pathophysiology, and PPH and RPH may be two different stages of PH-HFpEF. PPH is the early stage due to passive transduction of the increased pulmonary venous pressure, whereas RPH is the advanced stage characterized by vascular constriction and proliferation caused by chronic progressive increase of pulmonary artery wedged pressure and pulmonary artery pressure, which leads to the elevation of TPG and PVR, as well as pulmonary vasculopathy. In contrast, there was no significant difference between RPH and PPH in NT-pro-BNP, 6MWD, NYHA, and other cardiac functional indexes suggesting that the cardiac functional impairment of RPH might not be proportional to the increase of pulmonary artery pressure.

Fasudil is a potent selective inhibitor of Rho kinase. Several trials studying the acute- or long-term effects of fasudil on PAH have demonstrated that fasudil improves pulmonary hemodynamics [22–24], which is consistent with our finding that fasudil reduced pulmonary artery systolic pressure in the RPH group. In contrast, pulmonary hemodynamic in the PPH group had no significant change. In terms of cardiac function, there is a significant posttreatment improvement in both groups with higher overall effectiveness in the RPH group.

In animal studies, fasudil was reported to decrease the mean pulmonary arterial pressure, right ventricular hypertrophy, and pulmonary arteriolar medial thickness and augment pulmonary expression of endothelial nitric oxide synthase (eNOS) in rats with PH secondary to left ventricular dysfunction [25]. Furthermore, fasudil was also reported to attenuate pulmonary arteriole endothelial cell injury and the proliferation of smooth muscle cells and collagen fibers [26], as well as lessened the expression of thioredoxin-1 (Trx-1) and hypoxia inducible factor-1α (HIF-1α) [27] in monocrotaline or chronic hypoxia-induced rat PH models. Our findings demonstrated the beneficial effects of fasudil in RPH patients that could be explained by alleviation of pulmonary vasculopathy of RPH-HFpEF and reduction of PVR and PASP.

With regard to the left heart, Guo et al. [28] reported that fasudil improves short-term echocardiographic parameters of left ventricular diastolic function in patients with type-2 diabetes with preserved left ventricular ejection fraction, which is consistent with our results that fasudil therapy leads to improvement in diastolic function as reflected by increase in E/A ratio and decrease in E/E'. Several lines of evidence have revealed that Rho/ROCK inhibitors not only increase eNOS expression both in vivo and in vitro but also regulate the activity of myosin phosphatase activity by inducing the phosphorylation of its myosin-binding subunit [9, 29], which may affect left ventricular (LV) relaxation and LV filling pressure. Moreover, the changes in LV diastolic function may result from the interaction between the LV and RV. Due to the PAH, the distension of patient's RV and atrium may impair LV relaxation and compliance properties. Fasudil may help relieve the compression of the LV by reducing right heart pressure and volumes. Further trials are needed to identify the precise effect of fasudil on LV diastolic function.

In terms of study limitations, the main limitations of the current study include the relatively small number of trial size, the lack of RHC reexamination, and the data of RV function improvement, which limit the precision for estimation of the magnitude of effects. In addition, there is no placebo control group in this study which restricts the accuracy of the efficacy estimation of fasudil. Lastly, the long-term effect of fasudil on RPH or PPH-HFpEF is still unknown.

In summary, Newman et al. had proposed that redefining pulmonary hypertension through pulmonary vascular disease phenomics and resolving the heterogeneity of the PH syndrome will allow for more targeted therapeutics [30]. PH-LHD is also a complex clinical syndrome with complex pathophysiology, and precision medicine indication may have a good therapeutic effect on PH-LHD. Our study provides evidence that fasudil has a better therapeutic effect on RPH-HFpEF than PPH suggesting that fasudil could be an effective precise treatment of RPH-HFpEF. A multicenter, randomized, placebo-controlled trial with optimizing inclusion criteria and dose selection is needed to further investigate the efficacy and safety of fasudil as a potential targeted drug therapy in PH-LHD.

Authors' Contributions

Xiang Zhang and Xueming Zhang contributed equally to this work.

Acknowledgments

This study was supported by grants from National Natural Science Foundation of China (no. 81570040) and Health and Family Planning Commission of Pudong New Area (PW2014A-45).

References

[1] J. J. McMurray, "ESC guidelines for the diagnosis and treatment of acute and chronic heart failure 2012: the Task Force for the Diagnosis and Treatment of Acute and Chronic Heart Failure 2012 of the European Society of Cardiology, developed in collaboration with the Heart Failure Association (HFA) of the ESC," *European Journal of Heart Failure*, vol. 14, no. 8, pp. 803–869, 2012.

[2] R. J. Tedford, P. M. Hassoun, S. C. Mathai et al., "Pulmonary capillary wedge pressure augments right ventricular pulsatile loading," *Circulation*, vol. 125, no. 2, pp. 289–297, 2012.

[3] C. S. Lam, V. L. Roger, R. J. Rodeheffer, B. A. Borlaug, F. T. Enders, and M. M. Redfield, "Pulmonary hypertension in heart failure with preserved ejection fraction: a community-based study," *Journal of the American College of Cardiology*, vol. 53, no. 13, pp. 1119–1126, 2009.

[4] K. Hogg, K. Swedberg, and J. McMurray, "Heart failure with preserved left ventricular systolic function; epidemiology, clinical characteristics, and prognosis," *Journal of the American College of Cardiology*, vol. 43, no. 3, pp. 317–327, 2004.

[5] J. L. Vachiery, "Pulmonary hypertension due to left heart diseases," *Turk Kardiyoloji Dernegi Arsivi*, vol. 42, no. 1, pp. 130–141, 2014.

[6] N. Galie, M. Humbert, J.-L. Vachiery et al., "2015 ESC/ERS guidelines for the diagnosis and treatment of pulmonary hypertension: the Joint Task Force for the Diagnosis and Treatment of Pulmonary Hypertension of the European Society of Cardiology (ESC) and the European Respiratory Society (ERS): endorsed by: Association for European Paediatric and Congenital Cardiology (AEPC), International Society for Heart and Lung Transplantation (ISHLT)," *European Heart Journal*, vol. 37, no. 1, pp. 67–119, 2016.

[7] A. H. Rapp, R. A. Lange, J. E. Cigarroa, E. C. Keeley, and L. David Hillis, "Relation of pulmonary arterial diastolic and mean pulmonary arterial wedge pressures in patients with and without pulmonary hypertension," *American Journal of Cardiology*, vol. 88, no. 7, pp. 823-824, 2001.

[8] A. P. Somlyo and A. V. Somlyo, "Ca^{2+} sensitivity of smooth muscle and nonmuscle myosin II: modulated by G proteins, kinases, and myosin phosphatase," *Physiological Reviews*, vol. 83, no. 4, pp. 1325–1358, 2003.

[9] A. P. Somlyo and A. V. Somlyo, "Signal transduction by G-proteins, rho-kinase and protein phosphatase to smooth muscle and non-muscle myosin II," *Journal of Physiology*, vol. 522, no. 2, pp. 177–185, 2000.

[10] C. P. Mack, A. V. Somlyo, M. Hautmann, A. P. Somlyo, and G. K. Owens, "Smooth muscle differentiation marker gene expression is regulated by RhoA-mediated actin polymerization," *Journal of Biological Chemistry*, vol. 276, no. 1, pp. 341–347, 2001.

[11] P. Ponikowski, "2016 ESC guidelines for the diagnosis and treatment of acute and chronic heart failure: the Task Force for the diagnosis and treatment of acute and chronic heart failure of the European Society of Cardiology (ESC), developed with the special contribution of the Heart Failure Association (HFA) of the ESC," *European Journal of Heart Failure*, vol. 18, no. 8, pp. 891–975, 2016.

[12] N. Galie, M. M. Hoeper, M. Humbert et al., "Guidelines for the diagnosis and treatment of pulmonary hypertension: the Task Force for the Diagnosis and Treatment of Pulmonary Hypertension of the European Society of Cardiology (ESC) and the European Respiratory Society (ERS), endorsed by the International Society of Heart and Lung Transplantation (ISHLT)," *European Heart Journal*, vol. 30, no. 20, pp. 2493–2537, 2009.

[13] R. M. Lang, L. P. Badano, V. Mor-Avi et al., "Recommendations for cardiac chamber quantification by echocardiography in adults: an update from the American Society of Echocardiography and the European Association of Cardiovascular Imaging," *Journal of the American Society of Echocardiography*, vol. 28, no. 1, pp. 1–39 e14, 2015.

[14] S. F. Nagueh, O. A. Smiseth, C. P. Appleton et al., "Recommendations for the evaluation of left ventricular diastolic function by echocardiography: an update from the American Society of Echocardiography and the European Association of Cardiovascular Imaging," *Journal of the American Society of Echocardiography*, vol. 29, no. 4, pp. 277–314, 2016.

[15] L. G. Rudski, W. W. Lai, J. Afilalo et al., "Guidelines for the echocardiographic assessment of the right heart in adults: a report from the American Society of Echocardiography endorsed by the European Association of Echocardiography, a registered branch of the European Society of Cardiology, and the Canadian Society of Echocardiography," *Journal of the American Society of Echocardiography*, vol. 23, no. 7, pp. 685–713, 2010.

[16] D. Aronson, A. Eitan, R. Dragu, and A. J. Burger, "Relationship between reactive pulmonary hypertension and mortality in patients with acute decompensated heart failure," *Circulation: Heart Failure*, vol. 4, no. 5, pp. 644–650, 2011.

[17] R. M. Califf, K. F. Adams, W. J. McKenna et al., "A randomized controlled trial of epoprostenol therapy for severe congestive heart failure: the Flolan International Randomized Survival Trial (FIRST)," *American Heart Journal*, vol. 134, no. 1, pp. 44–54, 1997.

[18] P. R. Kalra, J. C. Moon, and A. J. Coats, "Do results of the ENABLE (Endothelin Antagonist Bosentan for Lowering Cardiac Events in Heart Failure) study spell the end for non-selective endothelin antagonism in heart failure?," *International Journal of Cardiology*, vol. 85, no. 2-3, pp. 195–197, 2002.

[19] M. Guazzi, M. Vicenzi, R. Arena, and M. D. Guazzi, "Pulmonary hypertension in heart failure with preserved ejection fraction: a target of phosphodiesterase-5 inhibition in a 1-year study," *Circulation*, vol. 124, no. 2, pp. 164–174, 2011.

[20] E. S. Hoendermis, L. C. Y. Liu, Y. M. Hummel et al., "Effects of sildenafil on invasive haemodynamics and exercise capacity in heart failure patients with preserved ejection fraction and pulmonary hypertension: a randomized controlled trial," *European Heart Journal*, vol. 36, no. 38, pp. 2565–2573, 2015.

[21] L. C. Liu, Y. M. Hummel, P. van der Meer et al., "Effects of sildenafil on cardiac structure and function, cardiopulmonary exercise testing and health-related quality of life measures in heart failure patients with preserved ejection fraction and pulmonary hypertension," *European Journal of Heart Failure*, vol. 19, no. 1, pp. 116–125, 2017.

[22] H. Fujita, Y. Fukumoto, K. Saji et al., "Acute vasodilator effects of inhaled fasudil, a specific Rho-kinase inhibitor, in patients with pulmonary arterial hypertension," *Heart Vessels*, vol. 25, no. 2, pp. 144–149, 2010.

[23] Y. Fukumoto, N. Yamada, H. Matsubara et al., "Double-blind, placebo-controlled clinical trial with a Rho-kinase inhibitor in pulmonary arterial hypertension," *Circulation Journal*, vol. 77, no. 10, pp. 2619–2625, 2013.

[24] X. Jiang, Y.-F. Wang, Q.-H. Zhao et al., "Acute hemodynamic response of infused fasudil in patients with pulmonary arterial hypertension: a randomized, controlled, crossover study," *International Journal of Cardiology*, vol. 177, no. 1, pp. 61–65, 2014.

[25] Z. K. Dai, B.-N. Wu, I.-C. Chen et al., "Attenuation of pulmonary hypertension secondary to left ventricular dysfunction in the rat by Rho-kinase inhibitor fasudil," *Pediatric Pulmonology*, vol. 46, no. 1, pp. 45–59, 2011.

[26] X. Z. Sun, X. Y. Tian, D. W. Wang, and J. Li, "Effects of fasudil on hypoxic pulmonary hypertension and pulmonary vascular remodeling in rats," *European Review for Medical and Pharmacological Sciences*, vol. 18, no. 7, pp. 959–964, 2014.

[27] M. Liu, Y. Wang, L. Zheng et al., "Fasudil reversed MCT-induced and chronic hypoxia-induced pulmonary hypertension by attenuating oxidative stress and inhibiting the expression of Trx1 and HIF-1α," *Respiratory Physiology & Neurobiology*, vol. 201, pp. 38–46, 2014.

[28] R. Guo, Y. Su, J. Yan et al., "Fasudil improves short-term echocardiographic parameters of diastolic function in patients with type 2 diabetes with preserved left ventricular ejection fraction: a pilot study," *Heart and Vessels*, vol. 30, no. 1, pp. 89–97, 2015.

[29] M. Dong, B. P. Yan, J. K. Liao, Y.-Y. Lam, G. W. K. Yip, and C.-M. Yu, "Rho-kinase inhibition: a novel therapeutic target for the treatment of cardiovascular diseases," *Drug Discovery Today*, vol. 15, no. 15-16, pp. 622–629, 2010.

[30] J. H. Newman, S. Rich, S. H. Abman et al., "Enhancing insights into pulmonary vascular disease through a precision medicine approach, a joint NHLBI-cardiovascular medical research and education fund workshop report," *American Journal of Respiratory and Critical Care Medicine*, vol. 195, no. 12, pp. 1661–1670, 2017.

4

The Relation between Pregnancy-Associated Plasma Protein A and Obstructive Sleep Apnea Syndrome

Ali Cengiz,[1] Suat Konuk ,[2] and Tuncer Tuğ[2]

[1]*Pulmonology Department, Ağrı State Hospital, Ağrı, Turkey*
[2]*Pulmonology Department, Faculty of Medicine, Abant Izzet Baysal University, Bolu, Turkey*

Correspondence should be addressed to Suat Konuk; suatkonukk@windowslive.com

Academic Editor: Dario Olivieri

Aim. We aimed to investigate the relationship between serum pregnancy-associated plasma protein A (PAPP-A) levels and obstructive sleep apnea syndrome (OSAS). *Materials and Method.* 44 patients with OSAS and 44 healthy adults were included in this study. The participants having rheumatic or systemic inflammatory disease, advanced liver or kidney failure, diabetes, heart failure, hypertension, pregnancy, prerenal azotemia, known history of coronary artery disease, any pulmonary disease, rhinitis, or atopy, history of major trauma or surgery within the last six 6 months, and inhaled nasal or systemic corticosteroid use or other anti-inflammatory medications and those with <18 years of age were excluded. Serum PAPP-A levels were determined by the Elisa method with the immune sandwich measuring method. Statistical analysis of the study was performed with SPSS 17.0 statistical analysis package program, and $p < 0.05$ was considered as significant. *Results.* Serum PAPP-A levels of patients with OSAS (2.350 ng/ml (0.641–4.796)) were significantly higher ($p < 0.001$) when compared with healthy controls (0.971 ng/ml (0.109–2.679)). There was a statistically significant difference in serum PAPP-A levels between groups of OSAS patients according to the classification of OSAS severity. Between the groups of patients with OSAS, serum levels of PAPP-A in moderate group was significantly higher when compared with severe OSAS group ($p < 0.001$). There was positive correlations between PAPP-A levels and night minimum ($p = 0.042$, $r = 0.309$), and average oxygen levels ($p = 0.006$, $r = 0.407$). There was a negative correlation between PAPP-A levels and AHI ($p = 0.002$, $r = 0.460$). *Conclusion.* Higher PAPP-A levels in OSAS patients that were found in this study show inflammatory component in OSAS.

1. Introduction

Obstructive sleep apnea syndrome (OSAS) is characterized by permanent recurrent obstruction of the upper airways during sleep. Obstructive apnea is the respiratory effort in response to a totally or partially obstructed airway. Apnea results in loud snoring or arousal when the airway passage is enable again [1, 2]. OSAS is seen in approximately 1–5% of adult men and 1.2–2.5% of women [3–8].

Although the pathogenesis of OSAS could not exactly be clarified, there are studies reporting that chronic inflammation plays a role. It is asserted that recurrent hypoxia attacks in OSAS cause the release of various inflammatory mediators and the initiation of inflammatory process. Chronic inflammation, vasoconstriction as a result of endothelial dysfunction and vascular damage, and hypercoagulability-thrombotic tendency occur. In this case, it leads to cardiovascular and cerebrovascular complications in OSAS patients. In people with OSAS, soluble adhesion molecules like intercellular adhesion molecule 1 (ICAM-1), vascular adhesion molecule 1 (VCAM-1), and acute phase proteins like C-reactive protein (CRP), interleukin-6 (IL-6), retinol binding protein (RBP), and isoprostane are reported to be high [9, 10]. It is known that many factors such as advanced age, male sex, obesity, medications, genetic factors, airway configuration and diameter, sleep position, upper airway muscle and reflexes, and cytokines contribute to the development of OSAS [11, 12].

Pregnancy-associated plasma protein A (PAPP-A) was first defined by Lin et al. in 1974 [13]. PAPP-A is a high molecule weighted zinc binding proatherosclerotic metalloproteinase

[14, 15]. PAPP-A is first synthesized by placenta trophoblasts during pregnancy. It is used for Down Syndrome screening in pregnancy [16]. In addition to trophoblasts, PAPP-A is reported to be synthesized in endometrium, testicle, kidney, bone, colon and other adult and fetal tissues [15]. It is reported that PAPP-A is an inflammatory marker and detected in high levels in patients with asthma, allergic rhinitis, lung cancer, and chronic obstructive pulmonary disease (COPD) [15, 17–19]. In some studies, a relation between insulin-like growth factor 1 (IGF-1) and PAPP-A levels in patients with acute coronary syndrome (ACS) was revealed. It was asserted that PAPP-A may be a new acute coronary syndrome indicator showing the atherosclerotic plaque instability [16, 20].

In this study, we aimed to investigate the relation of PAPP-A levels and OSAS.

2. Materials and Methods

This study was conducted at the Abant İzzet Baysal University, Department of Chest Diseases, Sleep Disorders Center, between December 2015 and July 2016. The ethical committee approval was obtained from the corporate ethical committee (no. 2016/07). Written informed consent was obtained from all participants.

2.1. Patients and Controls. Forty-four patients subjected to a polysomnographic test at the sleep laboratory for OSAS prediagnosis and 44 healthy controls were included to the study. The inclusion criteria for OSAS patients were determined as apnea-hypopnea index (AHI) higher than 5, no previous treatments for OSAS, no other systemic diseases, no major surgical interventions or trauma during last 6 months, no administration of inhaled or systemic medications, and age above 18 years. Healthy controls were chosen among the individuals who were relatives or friends of the hospital staff.

2.2. Polysomnography. Patients were evaluated using Epworth Sleepiness Scale (ESS) and polysomnography (PSG) that was applied all night (Grass Technologies Comet Series EEG/PSG with AS40 Amplifier System). The Epworth Sleepiness Scale (ESS) is a quantitative method to evaluate sleepiness or the propensity to fall asleep in eight everyday life situations, through a Likert scale [21–23]. This instrument has been used in different contexts, populations, and clinical conditions, with particular interest in respiratory sleep disorders [21, 24].

As standard measurement parameters, three-channel electroencephalogram (EEG) (F4-M1, C4-M1, O4-M1), two-channel electrooculogram (EOG), electromyogram (EMG) (jaw, right, and left tibialis anterior), body position, oronasal thermal sensors, nasal pressure sensor, thoracoabdominal respiration movements, electrocardiography (ECG), respiratory sound recording, oxygen saturation measurements from the fingertip, and synchronous video recording were taken. Abnormal respiration events related to sleep were scored manually according to American Association of Sleep Medicine (AASM, 2012) criteria.

Obstructive sleep apnea was defined as decrease in airflow by more than 90% or total interruption for at least 10 seconds while chest and abdominal wall movements continued. Hypopnea was defined as at least 30% decrease in oronasal airflow for 10 seconds or more together with at least 3% oxygen desaturation compared to the level before respiratory event or the development of arousal. AHI was calculated by dividing the sum of obstructive apnea and hypopnea to total sleep duration. Independent from the symptoms, those with AHI >15 were immediately accepted to have OSAS. Besides, subjects who have any one of apnea and/or snoring, excessive daytime sleepiness, fatigue, insomnia, or nonrestorative sleep symptoms together with AHI >5 were also accepted to have OSAS.

Patients with OSAS were evaluated in three groups as mild (5–15), moderate (16–30), and severe (>30) OSAS in terms of AHI and in two groups as low (<10) and high (≥10) according to Epworth score.

2.3. Pulmonary Function Tests. Pulmonary function tests (PFT) was conducted with Vmax Sensormedics 229 spirometry device. After the subjects performed three acceptable maneuvers, the best pulmonary function test result was recorded. The exhaling activity was observed to last at least 6 seconds. At the end of the activity, FEV1, FVC, FEV1/FVC, FEF 25–75, and PEF values of the patients were measured and recorded.

2.4. The Measurements of PAPP-A Levels. Fasting blood samples were collected from the patient and control groups in the morning. Hemogram, CRP, and erythrocyte sedimentation rate (ECR) were studied. Blood samples collected for PAPP-A level were transferred into vacuumed tubes containing coagulation activator (BD Vacutainer®, Franklin Lakes, NJ, USA). After coagulation, blood samples were centrifuged at 1200 G for 15 min and stored at −80°C. PAPP-A levels of the thawed samples were studied according to the directions of the manufacturer on UniCel® DxC 600i (Beckman Coulter, Fullerton, CA) using enzyme-linked immunosorbent assay (ELISA) kits (detection range: 20 ng/ml–0.312 ng/ml, sensitivity: 0.06 ng/ml, intra-assay precision: <8%). All the samples were run in the same assay.

2.5. Statistics. Data obtained in the study were analyzed using SPSS 17.0 (SPSS for Windows, Chicago, USA) statistics program. The Kolmogorov–Smirnov test was used to evaluate whether the distribution of continuous variables was normal or not. Categorical data were given as frequency and percentage. Continuous variables were given as either (mean ± standard deviation) or as (median (minimum–maximum)) according to the results of the normality tests. A chi-square test was used for the comparison of categorical data. An independent sample *t*-test was used for the continuous variables with normal distribution. The Mann–Whitney *U* test was used for the continuous variables with abnormal distribution.

Table 1: Demographic and some clinical characteristics of the groups.

	OSAS (n = 44)	Control (n = 44)	p
Age (years)	44 ± 10	44 ± 12	0.791*
Gender (male/female)	32/12	33/11	0.808*
Body mass index (median (min–max))	29.41 **(23.89–40.44)**	28.58 **(22.42–45.70)**	0.166*
Smoking (n, %)	18, 41%	23, 51%	0.549†

*Mann–Whitney U test; †chi-square test.

Table 2: Hematologic parameters of the groups.

	Control (n = 44), median (min–max) or mean ± SD	OSAS (n = 44), median (min–max) or mean ± SD	p
Leucocyte (K/ul)	6515 (3350–12800)	6885 (3460–10500)	0.981†
Lymphocyte (K/ul)	2145 ± 683	2267 ± 630	0.392*
Neutrophils (K/ul)	3685 (1560–10200)	3895 (1410–7370)	0.893†
Eosinophils (K/ul)	147 (17–436)	178.5 (55–622)	0.124†
NLR	2.11 ± 0.97	1.86 ± 0.64	0.152*
Haemoglobin (g/dl)	14.5 (12.1–17.3)	14.3 (10.3–17.1)	0.733†
Haematocrite (%)	43.1 (37.5–52.6)	44.1 (33.9–52.0)	0.935†
Mean corpuscular volume (fL)	91 (81–103)	91 (67.5–99.1)	0.823†
Red cell distribution width (%)	15.91 ± 0.98	16.11 ± 1.40	0.452*
Mean platelet volume (fL)	7.86 ± 1.28	7.86 ± 1.02	0.994*
Platelet distribution width	18 (16.5–20.8)	17.7 (16–22)	0.449†

†Mann–Whitney U test; *İndependent sample t-test.

Table 3: Respiratory function test results.

	Control (n = 44) (mean ± SD)	OSAS (n = 44) (mean ± SD)	p
Forced vital capacity (FVC) (L)	4.18 ± 0.99	4.21 ± 1.09	0.913
Forced vital capacity (FVC) (%)	101.32 ± 10.47	102.14 ± 13.52	0.757
Forced expiratory volume (FEV1) (L)	3.31 ± 0.79	3.34 ± 0.87	0.843
Forced expiratory volume (FEV1) (%)	96.93 ± 10.53	97.64 ± 13.18	0.78
Forced expiratory volume/forced vital capacity (FEV1/FVC)	79.14 ± 5.51	79.41 ± 5.38	0.819
Forced expiratory flow (FEF 25–75) (L/sn)	3.27 ± 1.09	3.40 ± 1.12	0.594
Forced expiratory flow (FEF 25–75) (%)	81.91 ± 22.43	84.61 ± 22.33	0.570
Peak expiratory flow (L)	6.64 ± 1.88	6.69 ± 1.78	0.902
Peak expiratory flow (%)	79.93 ± 16.18	81.05 ± 15.61	0.748

Independent sample t-test.

The Kruskal–Wallis test was used for the comparison of PAPP-A levels in OSAS patients categorized into 3 groups according to their AHI levels. Bonferroni correction was applied to compare two groups. For this result, p value below $0.05/3 = 0.017$ was considered significant. Spearman correlation analysis was used for the correlations between continuous variables. For all other comparisons, $p < 0.05$ was accepted significant.

3. Results

The study comprised 44 patients with OSAS and 44 healthy control subjects. The age, gender, body mass index, and smoking ratio differences between the groups were statistically insignificant (Table 1). The ratios of snoring, apnea, daytime sleepiness, morning headache, morning fatigue, daytime fatigue, night sweating, and nocturia were 96%, 84%, 75%, 41%, 66%, 64%, 61%, and 55%, respectively. None of the control subjects had any of those complaints on a regular basis.

Patients and control subjects had similar hematologic parameters (Table 2). Both groups had similar respiratory function test results (Table 3).

Both groups had similar ESR and CRP. However, patients with OSAS had significantly higher PAPP-A levels (Table 4).

In OSAS patients, a significant positive correlation was detected between oxygen levels (minimum and mean) at night and PAPP-A levels. A significant negative correlation was detected between the AHI score and PAPP-A levels. No significant correlations were detected between the other parameters (BMI, NREM, Epworth score, ESR, CRP, and PAPP-A levels (Table 5).

A significant difference was detected in PAPP-A levels between the three groups categorized according to the AHI score. It was determined that the significant difference was caused by the higher PAPP-A levels in moderate severity group compared to low and high severity groups (Table 6). In terms of Epworth score, no significant differences were detected in PAPP-A levels between low and high score groups.

TABLE 4: Erythrocyte sedimentation rate, C reactive protein, and PAPP-A levels in the groups.

	Control ($n = 44$) (median (min–max))	OSAS ($n = 44$) (median (min–max))	p
Erythrocyte sedimentation rate (mm/sa)	9 (2–30)	9 (1–26)	0.517
C-reactive protein (mg/l)	1.55 (0–52.8)	2.10 (0–19.1)	0.509
PAPP-A (ng/ml)	0.971 (0.109–2.679)	2.350 (0.641–4.796)	<0.001

Mann–Whitney U test.

TABLE 5: The correlations between PAPP-A levels and clinical parameters.

Parameters	r^*	p
Body mass index	0.126	0.241
Minimum O_2 level in night	**0.309**	**0.042**
Mean O_2 level in night	**0.407**	**0.006**
NREM1 (%)	0.136	0.377
NREM2 (%)	−0.143	0.356
NREM3 (%)	0.149	0.333
REM (%)	0.159	0.302
Epworth score	0.058	0.710
AHI score	**−0.460**	**0.002**
C-reactive protein	−0.002	0.988
Erythrocyte sedimentation rate	−0.088	0.415

*Spearman correlation analysis.

TABLE 6: PAPP-A levels in groups organized according to AHI score and Epworth score.

Parameter	Groups	PAPP-A levels (median (min–max))	p
AHI score	Low (5–15)	1.26 ng/ml (0.64–2.99)	p < **0.001**, p^1 and p^3: **<0.001**, p^2: 0.854
	Average (16–30)	4.26 ng/ml (2.75–4.79)	
	High (>30)	1.74 ng/ml (1.00–2.65)	
Epworth score	Low (<10)	1.89 ng/ml (0.64–4.79)	0.279
	High (≥10)	2.42 ng/ml (1.00–4.73)	

AHI: apnea-hypopnea score; p^1: significance related to low-average groups; p^2: significance related to low-high groups; p^3: significance related to average-high groups.

4. Discussion

In our study, we found that PAPP-A levels were significantly higher in OSAS patients compared to the control group. PAPP-A levels were significantly higher in patients with moderate severity group compared to other groups. While a positive correlation between minimum and mean oxygen levels at night and PAPP-A levels was observed, a negative correlation with AHI was detected.

In the first studies with PAPP-A, Bayes-Genis et al. reported that PAPP-A levels were significantly higher in patients with acute coronary syndrome [25]. Conti et al. reported that hypoxic, oxidative, and inflammatory stresses increased the bioactivity of PAPP-A and that the PAPP-A levels were correlated with myocardial damage [26]. Likewise, Eickhoff et al. and McAllister et al. also reported that risk factors like hypoxia and chronic inflammation are correlated with vascular endothelial dysfunction and atherosclerosis [27, 28].

Studies reported high PAPP-A levels in asthma, COPD, lung cancer, and chronic renal diseases where oxidative stress and inflammation play a role in pathogenesis [15, 17, 29]. Bulut et al. reported that PAPP-A levels were higher in lung cancer compared to the control group [15]. Similarly, Talay et al. showed that PAPP-A levels were significantly higher in patients with COPD compared to the control group [19]. Fialova et al. found a positive correlation between PAPP-A and CRP levels in patients who underwent dialysis [30]. In patients diagnosed with pulmonary embolism, it was reported that there were no correlations between the PAPP-A levels and inflammatory markers [16].

In a study, no correlation between CRP levels and PAPP-A levels was detected in COPD patients [19]. It is known that the increased sympathetic activity caused by hypoxia repeating through the night in OSAS leads to cardiovascular and metabolic changes. OSAS is among the known risk factors for ischemic heart disease, arrhythmia, hypertension, and metabolic syndrome. Many mechanisms like increased sympathetic activity, inflammation, endothelial dysfunction, metabolic disregulation, and oxidative stress play a role in OSAS pathogenesis. In the previous studies with OSAS patients, inflammatory cytokines like CRP, IL-6, and TNFα were reported to be correlated with the disease pathogenesis. A positive correlation was detected between IL-6 and isoprostane levels and the intensity of inhalation [31, 32]. In our study, while the PAPP-A levels were found higher in patients with OSAS compared to the control group, no differences were detected between CRP levels. No correlations were detected between PAPP-A levels and ESR and CRP levels. As far as we know, our study is the first study in the literature conducted about PAPP-A levels in OSAS.

In our study, surprisingly, a negative correlation was detected between PAPP-A levels and AHI. It was observed that PAPP-A levels significantly decreased as AHI moved above 30. In the meantime, a positive correlation was detected between minimum O_2 and mean O_2 levels at night and PAPP-A levels. In severe OSAS patients with significantly lower O_2 levels, PAPP-A levels were also seen to decrease significantly. It made us think that the period when the PAPP-A levels decrease in severe OSAS may correspond to the period when the comorbidities are significant and when the compensatory mechanisms could not overcome oxidative stress and inflammatory activities. The comorbidites may be confounding factors in such a correlation between AHI/O_2 levels and PAPP-A levels. However, a second possibility may be that the low number of participants included in our study may not be sufficient to explore the exact relationship between O_2 levels and PAPP-A levels.

There were no correlations between PAPP-A levels and the duration of sleeping stages and Epworth sleep scale. In the light of these findings, high PAPP-A levels may assist in predicting the comorbidities which may occur in patients with OSAS, they may also be useful biomarkers in the management of patients with OSAS.

There are some limitations in our study. First of all, the number of patients is limited. Studies with larger cohorts may reveal the reasons for higher PAPP-A levels. Secondly, the distribution between patient groups while comparing the severity of disease was not equal. Thirdly, the study did not contain long-term follow-up data and PAPP-A data after treatment of the patients. Besides, there are no data to analyze the biopsy samples to exactly determine the role of PAPP-A levels in indicating especially the endothelial dysfunction in compensatory repair mechanisms.

References

[1] O. Kokturk, "Uykunun izlenmesi (1) Normal uyku," *Tüberküloz ve Toraks*, vol. 47, pp. 372–380, 1999.

[2] C. Guilleminault, A. Tilkian, and W. C. Dement, "The sleep apnea syndromes," *Annual Review of Medicine*, vol. 27, no. 1, pp. 465–484, 1976.

[3] T. Young, M. Palta, J. Dempsey, J. Skatrud, S. Weber, and S. Badr, "The occurrence of sleep-disordered breathing among middle-aged adults," *New England Journal of Medicine*, vol. 328, no. 17, pp. 1230–1235, 1993.

[4] T. Gislason, B. Benediktsdottir, J. K. Bjornsson, G. Kjartansson, M. Kjeld, and H. Kristbjarnarson, "Snoring, hypertension, and the sleep apnea syndrome: an epidemiologic survey of middle-aged women," *Chest*, vol. 103, no. 4, pp. 1147–1151, 1993.

[5] N. M. Punjabi, "The epidemiology of adult obstructive sleep apnea," *Proceedings of the American Thoracic Society*, vol. 5, no. 2, pp. 136–143, 2008.

[6] E. O. Bixler, A. N. Vgontzas, H. M. Lin et al., "Prevalence of sleep-disordered breathing in women: effects of gender," *American Journal of Respiratory and Critical Care Medicine*, vol. 163, no. 3, pp. 608–613, 2001.

[7] H. Bearpark, L. Elliott, R. Grunstein et al., "Snoring and sleep apnea: a population study in Australian men," *American Journal of Respiratory and Critical Care Medicine*, vol. 151, no. 5, pp. 1459–1465, 1995.

[8] J. Duran, S. Esnaola, R. Rubio, and A. Iztueta, "Obstructive sleep apnea-hypopnea and related clinical features in a population-based sample of subjects aged 30 to 70 yr," *American Journal of Respiratory and Critical Care Medicine*, vol. 163, no. 3, pp. 685–689, 2001.

[9] M. S. Ip, H. F. Tse, B. Lam, K. W. Tsang, and W. K. Lam, "Endothelial function in obstructive sleep apnea and response to treatment," *American Journal of Respiratory and Critical Care Medicine*, vol. 169, no. 3, pp. 348–353, 2004.

[10] K. Chin, T. Nakamura, K. Shimizu et al., "Effects of nasal continuous positive airway pressure on soluble cell adhesion molecules in patients with obstructive sleep apnea syndrome," *American Journal of Medicine*, vol. 109, no. 7, pp. 562–567, 2000.

[11] S. Yim, A. S. Jordan, and A. Malhotra, "Obstructive sleep apnea: clinical presentation, diagnosis and treatment," in *Sleep Apnea Current Diagnosis and Treatment*, W. J. Randerath, B. M. Sanner, and V. K. Somers, Eds., pp. 118–136, Karger International, Basel, Switzerland, 2006.

[12] H. İ. Köseoğlu, O. Köktürk, T. U. Çiftçi, and İ. Etikan, "The importance of sleep position in obstructive sleep apnea syndrome," *Turkish Thoracic Journal*, vol. 15, pp. 23–26, 2014.

[13] T. M. Lin, S. P. Galbert, D. Kiefer, W. N. Spellacy, and S. Gall, "Characterization of four human pregnancy-associated plasma proteins," *American Journal of Obstetrics and Gynecology*, vol. 118, no. 2, pp. 223–236, 1974.

[14] C. Oxvig, O. Sand, T. Kristensen, L. Kristensen, and L. Sottrup-Jensen, "Isolation and characterization of circulating complex between human pregnancy-associated plasma protein-A and proform of eosinophil major basic protein," *Biochimica et Biophysica Acta*, vol. 1201, no. 3, pp. 415–423, 1994.

[15] I. Bulut, A. Coskun, A. Ciftci et al., "Relationship between pregnancy-associated plasma protein-A and lung cancer," *American Journal of the Medical Sciences*, vol. 337, no. 4, pp. 241–244, 2009.

[16] S. Berk, O. T. Dogan, E. I. Aydemir, A. Bingol, S. L. Ozsahin, and I. Akkurt, "Diagnostic usefulness of pregnancy-associated plasma protein-A in suspected pulmonary embolism," *Multidisciplinary Respiratory Medicine*, vol. 8, no. 1, p. 49, 2013.

[17] A. Coskun, O. Balbay, S. Duran et al., "Pregnancy-associated plasma protein-A and asthma," *Advances in Therapy*, vol. 24, no. 2, pp. 362–367, 2007.

[18] E. Guclu, A. Coskun, A. Tokmak et al., "Does pregnancy-associated plasma protein A have a role in allergic rhinitis?," *American Journal of Rhinology*, vol. 22, no. 3, pp. 219–222, 2008.

[19] F. Talay, M. Tosun, Z. A. Yasar et al., "Evaluation of pregnancy-associated plasma protein-A levels in patients with chronic

obstructive pulmonary disease and associations with disease severity," *Inflammation*, vol. 39, pp. 1130–1133, 2016.

[20] P. Gururajan, P. Gurumurthy, P. Nayar et al., "Pregnancy associated plasma protein-A (PAPP-A) as an early marker for the diagnosis of acute coronary syndrome," *Indian Heart Journal*, vol. 64, no. 2, pp. 141–145, 2012.

[21] P. Sargento, V. Perea, V. Ladera, P. Lopes, and J. Oliveira, "The Epworth Sleepiness Scale in Portuguese adults: from classical measurement theory to Rasch model analysis," *Sleep and Breathing*, vol. 19, no. 2, pp. 693–701, 2015.

[22] M. W. Johns, "A new method for measuring daytime sleepiness: the Epworth Sleepiness Scale," *Sleep*, vol. 14, no. 6, pp. 540–545, 1991.

[23] M. W. Johns, "Sleepiness in different situations measured by the Epworth Sleepiness Scale," *Sleep*, vol. 17, no. 8, pp. 703–710, 1994.

[24] M. W. Johns, "Daytime sleepiness, snoring, and obstructive sleep apnea. The Epworth Sleepiness Scale," *Chest*, vol. 103, no. 1, pp. 30–36, 1993.

[25] A. Bayes-Genis, C. A. Conover, M. T. Overgaard et al., "Pregnancy-associated plasma protein A as a marker of acute coronary syndromes," *New England Journal of Medicine*, vol. 345, no. 14, pp. 1022–1029, 2001.

[26] E. Conti, M. Volpe, C. Carrozza et al., "Pregnancy-associated plasma protein-A and acute coronary syndromes: cause or consequence?," *Journal of the American College of Cardiology*, vol. 46, no. 8, pp. 1583-1584, 2005.

[27] P. Eickhoff, A. Valipour, D. Kiss et al., "Determinants of systemic vascular function in patients with stable chronic obstructive pulmonary disease," *American Journal of Respiratory and Critical Care Medicine*, vol. 178, no. 12, pp. 1211–1218, 2008.

[28] D. A. McAllister, J. D. Maclay, N. L. Mills et al., "Arterial stiffness is independently associated with emphysema severity in patients with chronic obstructive pulmonary disease," *American Journal of Respiratory and Critical Care Medicine*, vol. 176, no. 12, pp. 1208–1214, 2007.

[29] O. Zakiyanov, M. Kalousova, M. Kratochvilova, V. Kriha, T. Zima, and V. Tesar, "Determinants of circulating matrix metalloproteinase-2 and pregnancy-associated plasma protein-A in patients with chronic kidney disease," *Clinical Laboratory*, vol. 58, pp. 471–480, 2012.

[30] L. Fialova, M. Kalousova, J. Soukupova et al., "Relationship of pregnancy-associated plasma protein-A to renal function and dialysis modalities," *Kidney and Blood Pressure Research*, vol. 27, no. 2, pp. 88–95, 2004.

[31] G. E. Carpagnano, S. A. Kharitonov, O. M. P. Resta FoschinoBarbaro, E. Gramiccioni, and P. J. Barnes, "Increased 8-isoprostane and interleukin-6 in breath condensate of obstructive sleep apnea patients," *Chest*, vol. 122, no. 4, pp. 1162–1167, 2002.

[32] M. Korkmaz, H. Korkmaz, F. Kucuker, S. N. Ayyıldız, and S. Çankaya, "Evaluation of the association of sleep apnea-related systemic inflammation with CRP, ESR, and neutrophil-to-lymphocyte ratio," *Medical Science Monitor*, vol. 21, pp. 477–481, 2015.

Tiotropium for the Treatment of Asthma: Patient Selection and Perspectives

V. Madhu Chari and Robert Andrew McIvor

McMaster University, Firestone Institute for Respiratory Health, Hamilton, ON, Canada

Correspondence should be addressed to Robert Andrew McIvor; amcivor1@cogeco.ca

Academic Editor: Fulvio Braido

Asthma is a chronic disease of airway inflammation with a large global burden. Despite established, guideline-based stepwise therapy, a significant proportion of patients remain symptomatic and poorly controlled. As such, there is a need for additional safe, effective, convenient, and cost-effective therapies that can be broadly applied across a range of asthma phenotypes. Tiotropium is a long-acting muscarinic antagonist (LAMA) that leads to bronchodilation by blocking endogenous acetylcholine receptors in the airways. Tiotropium has long been approved for the treatment of chronic obstructive pulmonary disease, and it has recently been recognized for its safety and efficacy in improving lung function and controlling asthma. Evidence from several Phase III trials in the adult and paediatric population has shown that tiotropium is well tolerated and significantly improves a range of endpoints as an add-on treatment to ICS therapy, regardless of baseline characteristics and clinical phenotypes. Consequently, regulatory authorities worldwide have recently licensed tiotropium as the only LAMA approved for the treatment of asthma. This review provides an overview of safety and efficacy data and discusses the use of tiotropium in patients across the range of asthma severities, ages, and phenotypes.

1. Introduction

Asthma is a heterogeneous condition that is usually characterized by chronic airway inflammation and defined by symptoms including wheeze, shortness of breath, chest tightness, and cough that vary with time and intensity, along with variable expiratory airflow limitation [1]. This chronic disease is estimated to have a global prevalence of up to 18%, and it is estimated that 400 million people worldwide will be affected by 2025 [1, 2]. Asthma is the most common chronic childhood disease [3] and continues to impose a substantial burden on healthcare systems, society, and families across developing as well as high-income countries [1]. The broad aims of treating asthma are to (1) maintain normal activity levels via symptom control and (2) minimize exacerbations, medication side effects, and the development of fixed airflow limitation.

The Global Initiative for Asthma (GINA) strategy recommends a stepwise approach to the pharmacologic management of asthma, building on a base of inhaled corticosteroids (ICSs) [1]. Data from the UK estimate that approximately 65% of the patients being treated with at least a combination of an ICS and a long-acting β_2-agonist (LABA) (i.e., GINA Step 3) remain uncontrolled [4]. This places patients at increased risk of exacerbations, which, along with greater disease severity, is associated with increased costs of asthma care, both direct (related to provision of health services) and indirect (lost productivity) [5]. GINA Step 5 options are limited, and their application can be further constrained by access (bronchial thermoplasty), specific biomarker profiles (biologics) [6], or systemic side effects (oral corticosteroids). Thus, there is an ongoing unmet need for additional cost-effective and safe add-ons to ICS-LABA in the optimization of those with persistent asthma at GINA Steps 3–5.

In asthma, adherence to treatment can be quite poor, ranging from <50% in children to 30–70% in adults; this is disconcerting as poor adherence has been associated with not only worse symptoms and quality of life but also exacerbation frequency and mortality [7]. Controller medications with longer half-lives and once-daily administration are not only more convenient but may also improve treatment adherence. Tiotropium is a once-daily, long-acting muscarinic antagonist (LAMA) that has established effectiveness in chronic obstructive pulmonary disease (COPD), improving lung function, quality of life, and exacerbation frequency [8–10]. Recent and emerging data from the tiotropium clinical program (Phase II and III studies) in recent years are demonstrating that tiotropium may have a role as an effective long-acting bronchodilator in asthma as well. In fact, since 2015, tiotropium add-on therapy has been incorporated into the GINA guidelines in the stepwise management of asthma, starting at Step 4.

This review discusses the use of tiotropium in patients across a range of ages and asthma severities and provides an overview of the safety and efficacy data, patient selection considerations, and future perspectives.

2. Mechanism of Tiotropium

The bronchial tree in humans is largely innervated by the parasympathetic cholinergic system, and it is the muscarinic receptor subtypes (M1, M2, and M3) which are the predominant functional acetylcholine receptors expressed in the lung [11]. Through the effector tissues of the airway smooth muscle and mucous glands, cholinergic drive and dysfunction of muscarinic receptors contribute to bronchial smooth muscle contraction, airway hyperresponsiveness, and mucus secretion in airway diseases [12]. Furthermore, acetylcholine is thought to exert proinflammatory effects through chemoattraction and subsequent cytokine release [13]. As such, the utility of muscarinic antagonists is facilitating bronchodilation in a means that is complementary to LABAs [2]. The role of short-acting anticholinergics in asthma was evaluated in the beginning of 1980s, with ipratropium bromide—a nonselective M1-, M2-, and M3-receptor antagonist with a duration of action ranging from 4 to 8 hours—being the most widely studied. A meta-analysis demonstrated that, in the acute setting, the early administration of inhaled anticholinergics to short-acting β2-agonist (SABA) therapy particularly benefits children and adults with moderate-to-severe obstruction and also reduces admission rates by 30% [14]. For chronic asthma, a Cochrane review found that short-acting anticholinergics (including ipratropium bromide, oxitropium bromide, and nebulised atropine methonitrate) provided an incremental benefit in peak flow versus placebo and no added benefit to SABAs; however, the authors acknowledge that some patient subgroups may derive some benefit from short-acting anticholinergics, including those intolerant to SABAs and those with nocturnal asthma, concurrent fixed airway obstruction, and asthma of a longer duration [15].

The LAMA tiotropium more selectively antagonizes M1 and M3 receptor subtypes and does so with an up to 20-fold higher affinity than does ipratropium; this along with its slow dissociation from the M3 receptor in particular confers a half-life of approximately 35 hours and thus permits once-daily dosing [16]. In addition to bronchodilation and reduction of secretions and mucus gland hypertrophy, LAMAs have also demonstrated anti-inflammatory effects (e.g., inhibition of alveolar neutrophil migration and decreased levels of IL-6, TNF-α, and leukotriene B4) in vitro and in bronchoalveolar lavages [16].

3. Tiotropium in Asthma: The Evidence Base

A number of Phase II studies initially established the efficacy and safety of tiotropium delivered by a Respimat® Soft Mist inhaler (hereafter referred to as tiotropium Respimat; Boehringer Ingelheim, Ingelheim am Rhein, Germany) in adult patients with symptomatic asthma; all of these were randomized, double-blind, placebo-controlled studies and had treatment durations ranging from 4 to 16 weeks. In a crossover study of 107 patients with uncontrolled, severe asthma on a background treatment of (at minimum) high-dose ICSs and LABAs, the add-on of tiotropium Respimat at 5 μg once daily for 8 weeks significantly improved peak FEV1 (difference from placebo 139 mL, $p < 0.001$); the higher dose of 10 μg once daily did not confer any additional bronchodilator benefit [17]. The role of tiotropium as an add-on therapy to ICSs in moderate asthma was then assessed in a dose-ranging, four-way crossover study comparing once-daily tiotropium Respimat at doses of 5, 2.5, and 1 μg to placebo; patients were not permitted to be on an LABA at the time of enrollment [18]. All doses of tiotropium Respimat were found to improve peak FEV1 at 4 weeks compared to placebo, with the 5 μg dose resulting in the largest adjusted mean difference (188 mL, 95% CI: 140–236 mL). With the abovementioned studies establishing the 5 μg dose of tiotropium Respimat as a safe and effective add-on therapy in moderate-to-severe asthma, Timmer et al. sought to investigate whether this would be affected by dosing regimen, comparing twice-daily tiotropium at 2.5 μg to once-daily tiotropium at 5 μg [19]. After 4 weeks, no significant difference in bronchodilator efficacy was found between either dosing strategy, with both providing improvements in the FEV1 $AUC_{(0-24\,h)}$ response versus placebo (158 mL for 5 μg once daily, 149 mL for 2.5 μg twice daily; both $p < 0.01$). Both the 5 μg once-daily and 2.5 μg twice-daily tiotropium Respimat treatments also had comparable improvements in peak and trough FEV1 recordings, as well as predosing morning and evening PEFs.

A comprehensive Phase III study programme detailed below, and summarized in Table 1 [20], has demonstrated the safety and efficacy of tiotropium in adult patients with mild, moderate, and severe asthma. The majority of the Phase III trials have evaluated tiotropium in the Respimat form, with the Tiotropium Bromide as an Alternative to Increased Inhaled Corticosteroid in Patients Inadequately Controlled on a Lower Dose of Inhaled Corticosteroid study (TALC Study, NCT00565266) being one of the exceptions. In this three-way crossover study, adults with moderate, persistent asthma with confirmed bronchodilator reversibility or hyperresponsiveness received 14-week treatments of doubled ICSs (beclomethasone 160 μg twice daily), tiotropium (18 μg via Spiriva® HandiHaler), or salmeterol (50 μg twice daily) [21]. Here, once-daily tiotropium significantly improved morning and evening PEF ($p < 0.001$),

Table 1: Results of Phase III adult asthma studies with tiotropium Respimat 5 μg.

Study name	Treatment duration (weeks)	N	Primary and key secondary endpoints	Difference from placebo	
PrimoTinA-asthma severe persistent asthma [21]	48	912	Peak FEV1, week 24, mean (CI) mL	86 (20, 152) ($p = 0.01$) trial 1	154 (91, 217) ($p < 0.001$) trial 2
			Trough FEV1, week 24, mean (CI) mL	88 (27, 149) mL ($p = 0.01$) trial 1	111 (53, 169) mL ($p < 0.001$) trial 2
			Time to first severe exacerbation	21% reduction in risk (HR 0.79; 95% CI: 0.62, 1.00; $p = 0.03$)	
			ACQ-7, adjusted mean score	NS	−0.2 ($p = 0.003$) trial 2
MezzoTinA-asthma moderate persistent asthma [22]	24	2103	Peak FEV1, mean (CI) mL	198 (142, 253) mL ($p < 0.0001$) trial 1	169 (116, 222) mL ($p < 0.0001$) trial 2
			Peak FVC, mean (CI) mL	102 (42, 162) mL ($p = 0.0008$) trial 1	89 (30, 147) mL ($p = 0.0031$) trial 2
			ACQ-7, adjusted mean score	−0.12 (SD 0.04; $p = 0.0084$)	
GraziaTinA-asthma mild persistent asthma [23]	12	465	Peak FEV1, week 12, mean (CI) mL	128 mL (95% CI: 57, 199; $p < 0.001$)	
			Trough FEV1, week 12, mean (CI) mL	122 mL (95% CI: 49, 194; $p < 0.001$)	
			ACQ-7 total score, week 12	0.014 (95% CI: −118, 0.146; $p = 0.83$)	

ACQ-7, 7-question Asthma Control Questionnaire; CI, confidence interval; FEV1, forced expiratory volume in 1 second; FVC, forced vital capacity; HR, hazard ratio; ICSs, inhaled corticosteroids; NS, not significant; SD, standard deviation. Table reproduced from E. R. McIvor and R. A. McIvor [20].

FEV1 ($p = 0.004$), and asthma control as determined by the Asthma Control Questionnaire (ACQ; $p < 0.001$) compared to doubling of the ICSs. Tiotropium was found to be noninferior to salmeterol when comparing the effects on PEF, FEV1, asthma control and symptoms, and sputum eosinophils.

The PrimoTinA-asthma® study comprised two replicate, randomized controlled trials (NCT00772538 and NCT00776984) which evaluated the long-term (48 weeks) efficacy and safety of tiotropium Respimat (5 μg) in 912 patients with poorly controlled, severe persistent asthma [22]. Adults enrolled in this study had demonstrated persistent airflow limitation as determined by an FEV1 ≤80% or ≤70% of the FVC post-bronchodilator and ≥1 exacerbation requiring systemic glucocorticoids in the past year. For background treatment, patients were on high-dose ICSs (≥800 μg budesonide or equivalent/day) and LABAs at minimum; stable dosing of theophylline, leukotriene modifiers, anti-IgE therapy, and oral glucocorticoids (≤5 mg prednisone/equivalent per day) was permitted. When compared to placebo, treatment with 5 μg of tiotropium led to an improvement in the primary outcomes of peak and trough FEV1 at 24 weeks ($p \leq 0.01$) and time to first exacerbation (282 days for tiotropium versus 226 days for placebo, $p = 0.03$; corresponding to a risk reduction of 21% (HR 0.79)) [22]. Despite the effect of add-on tiotropium on exacerbations as well as a secondary outcome of time to first worsening (181 days for tiotropium versus 315 days for placebo, $p < 0.001$; 31% risk reduction (HR 0.69)), the minimal clinically important difference in ACQ-7 and Asthma Quality of Life Questionnaire (AQLQ) scores was not achieved. The MezzoTinA-asthma® trials (NCT01172808 and NCT01172821) were two randomized, double-blinded parallel group trials which assessed the safety and efficacy of tiotropium (at 5 and 2.5 μg once daily), with salmeterol as an active comparator as add-on therapy to medium-dose ICSs (400–800 μg/day) in 2103 patients with moderate, symptomatic asthma [23]. In the pooled analyses, tiotropium and salmeterol had similar efficacy on lung function as determined by peak and trough FEV1 ($p < 0.001$ versus placebo) as well as ACQ-7 responder rates (odds ratio (OR) 1.32 for 5 μg tiotropium, $p = 0.035$; 1.33 for 2.5 μg tiotropium, $p = 0.031$; 1.46, $p = 0.0039$ for salmeterol; p values versus placebo) [23], indicating that tiotropium is a safe and effective alternative to salmeterol in this patient population. Due to low event rates, the secondary outcome of the median time to 1st exacerbation could not be calculated. It should be noted that the MezzoTinA-asthma trials were not powered to assess superiority between the different active treatments (tiotropium 2.5 μg and 5 μg, and salmeterol). The GraziaTinA-asthma® study (NCT01316380) then evaluated tiotropium Respimat at 5 and 2.5 μg in 464 patients with mild-to-moderate persistent asthma on only low-to-medium dosing of ICSs (200–400 μg/day) [24]. At 12 weeks, both doses of tiotropium led to a significant increase in the primary outcome of the mean difference in peak FEV1 (5 μg, 128 mL; 2.5 μg, 159 mL; $p < 0.001$) as well as secondary outcomes of trough FEV1, FEV1 $AUC_{(0-3\,h)}$, and PEF (morning and evening) compared to placebo; the trial was not powered to demonstrate differences between the two doses of tiotropium. Across the PrimoTinA-asthma, MezzoTinA-asthma, and GraziaTinA-asthma studies, the rates of adverse events were comparable across all treatment, comparator, and placebo arms.

Recent systematic reviews published by the Cochrane Library further examined the role of LAMAs in three particular capacities: (1) as an add-on to ICSs [25], (2) as an alternative to LABAs as an add-on to ICSs [26], and (3) as an add-on therapy to patients not well controlled on combination therapy with ICS-LABA [27]. While the search strategy of the reviews included LAMAs other than tiotropium (including glycopyrronium and umeclidinium), only studies using tiotropium (both HandiHaler® and Respimat forms) were ultimately included in the analyses. Across four studies with 2277 participants, the addition of tiotropium to ICSs was found to lower the rate of exacerbations requiring oral corticosteroids (OR 0.63, 95% CI: 0.46–0.93), as well as to produce a consistent benefit across a range of lung function measures, when compared to ICSs alone [25]. All-cause severe adverse events and exacerbations requiring admission were rare. Analyses from four studies (a total of 2049 patients) comparing LAMAs to LABAs as add-on therapy to ICSs in asthma found that there was no difference in the rate of exacerbations requiring oral corticosteroids and that the slightly worse quality of life scores (as determined by AQLQ and ACQ) and slightly improved lung function (a mean difference of 50 mL in trough FEV1) conferred by LAMA therapy were of unclear clinical significance [26]. Across three studies with 1197 adult asthma patients on combination ICS-LABA therapy, the addition of tiotropium (studied over 48–52 weeks) led to fewer exacerbations; however the confidence interval did not rule out a lack of difference (OR 0.76, 95% CI: 0.57–1.02, moderate-quality evidence); there was high-quality evidence demonstrating a benefit to lung function with the addition of tiotropium (versus placebo) to ICS-LABA [27]. Overall, these reviews illustrated that tiotropium serves as an effective bronchodilator and a possible means of reducing exacerbations across varying severities of asthma in patients who remain symptomatic on at least ICSs, particularly as add-on therapy to ICS/LABA. This reflects the recommendation in the GINA strategy, where tiotropium is now recommended as an alternative add-on treatment at Steps 4 and 5 in patients ≥ 12 years of age with a history of exacerbations [1].

4. Patient Selection and Safety Considerations

Evidence from the comprehensive clinical trial programme with tiotropium has demonstrated it as a well-tolerated treatment improving lung function and asthma control in adults, regardless of severity [22–24]. In general, patients enrolled in this programme were men and women aged 18–75 (with a mean age of 43 to 53) who were diagnosed with asthma before age 40, had no prior smoking history or were ex-smokers with a total less than 10 pack-years, and were symptomatic at screening and randomization (as defined by a mean ACQ-7 score of ≥1.5). In the studies of mild and moderate asthma, the diagnosis of asthma had to be confirmed at screening via demonstration of bronchodilator reversibility. Main exclusion criteria in these trials were a diagnosis of COPD, serious coexisting illness (e.g., recent acute coronary syndrome or hospitalization for cardiac failure, lung diseases other than asthma, and recently treated malignancy), and concurrent use of other anticholinergic bronchodilators.

Subsequent subgroup analyses of these trials have provided further insight into the patient phenotypes that would also benefit from tiotropium as an add-on bronchodilator. Asthma can conceptually be distinguished into T_H2-asthma (e.g., allergic, eosinophilic, and exercise-induced asthma) and non-T_H2-asthma (e.g., smoking-related, neutrophilic, and obesity-associated). Preplanned analyses of the PrimoTinA-asthma (severe) and MezzoTinA-asthma (moderate) found that ~20%/~15% of severe/moderate patients had elevated IgE (≥430 μg/L) and that ~10%/~5% of severe/moderate patients had blood eosinophilia ($\geq 0.6 \times 10^9$), respectively; analyses were then performed in subgroups of patients with T_H2- and non-T_H2-asthma, the former defined by the presence of both elevated IgE and blood eosinophilia [28, 29]. Independent of the T_H2-status, the addition of once-daily tiotropium (versus placebo) to at least ICSs in adults with moderate-to-severe symptomatic asthma reduced the risk of severe exacerbation and asthma worsening [29] and, furthermore, improved symptom control based on the ACQ-7 responder rates [28]. The link between obesity and asthma is a complex and significant one: obesity is a major risk factor for the development of asthma (possibly through mechanical and proinflammatory changes), and asthma in obese patients tends to be more severe and less treatment responsive [30]. Furthermore, a distinct non-T_H2 phenotype of "obesity-related asthma" which is later onset and less corticosteroid responsive has been proposed [31]. As well, the entity of asthma in the elderly (AIE) presents a diagnostic and management challenge due to a number of factors, including but not limited to underdiagnosis, high rates of morbidity and mortality, nuances in airway remodelling and structural changes of the aging lung, altered immune response, exclusion from clinical trials, and more common medication adverse events [32]. In subgroup analyses of data from the replicate PrimoTinA-asthma trials (i.e., severe, persistent asthma), the influence of various baseline characteristics on tiotropium's improvements in lung function, exacerbation rate, and asthma control was examined. Of note, at week 24, tiotropium 5 μg led to improvements in the coprimary endpoints of peak FEV1 and trough FEV1, along with the secondary endpoints of time to first severe exacerbation and first episode of asthma worsening independent of age (stratified into the age groups <40, 40–60, and >60) and BMI (stratified into the groups <20, 20 to <25, 25 to <30, and ≥30 kg/m^2) [33].

Noneosinophilic asthma represents a large proportion of patients with asthma and falls into the endotype of non-T_H2 asthma. Increased airway neutrophilia—outside of the acute exacerbation setting where neutrophilis can be the dominant inflammatory cell type—has been associated with more clinically severe asthma, lower pre- and postbronchodilator FEV1, thicker airway walls, and more air trapping [31, 34]. Patients with this phenotype also tend to be less corticosteroid sensitive, and biologic agents targeting mediators of noneosinophilic inflammation (e.g., interleukin 17 and tumor necrosis factor-α) have yet to demonstrate clinical efficacy [35]. To date, no large randomized study has evaluated tiotropium or other LAMAs in this particular phenotype. However, a small study (N = 17, no placebo arm) demonstrated that the proportion of neutrophils in induced sputum

Table 2: Phase III studies with tiotropium Respimat in children and adolescents with asthma.

Study name	Patients (asthma severity and age)	Treatment duration (weeks)	Baseline therapy	N (treatment group)	Study drug
RubaTinA-asthma	Moderate persistent 12- to 17-year-olds	48	At least ICSs	259	
PensieTinA-asthma	Severe persistent 12- to 17-year-olds	12	ICSs + ≥1 controller	257	
CanoTinA-asthma	Moderate persistent 6- to 11-year-olds	48	At least ICSs	270	Tiotropium Respimat 2.5 and 5 μg
VivaTinA-asthma	Severe persistent 6- to 11-year-olds	12	At least ICSs/+ ≥1 controller	262	
NinoTinA-asthma	Persistent 1- to 5-year-olds		At least ICSs	67	

ICSs, inhaled corticosteroids; LABA, long-acting β_2-agonist. Table reproduced from E. R. McIvor and R. A. McIvor [20].

positively correlated with the improvement in FEV1 conferred by a 4-week treatment of tiotropium in patients with severe asthma; these patients were on a baseline treatment of high-dose ICSs (equivalent of 800–1600 μg budesonide/day), and 23.5% were additionally on maintenance oral corticosteroids [36]. As such, a noneosinophilic sputum profile may predict a better response to LAMA (e.g., tiotropium) add-ons; however, the proposed mechanism has yet to be elucidated, and this concept has, unfortunately, yet to be studied on a larger clinical scale.

Recent tiotropium trials have also demonstrated its safety and efficacy in paediatric populations. Phase II, randomized, dose-ranging studies of tiotropium Respimat (1.25 μg, 2.5 μg, and 5 μg for 4 weeks) in children aged 6–11 years [37] and adolescents aged 12–17 years [38] with symptomatic, moderate asthma despite maintenance treatment with ICSs demonstrated improvements in lung function (as indicated by mean peak FEV1); no dose-dependent response was found. In both studies, tiotropium Respimat was well tolerated with comparable adverse event rates across treatment and placebo groups [37, 38]. There are further five Phase III clinical trial studies in the paediatric population (Table 2 [20]), which are discussed in detail below.

The RubaTinA-asthma® study (NCT01257230) was conducted to assess the efficacy and safety of once-daily tiotropium added to ICSs (200–800 μg/day) with or without LTRAs in adolescent (12- to 17-year-old) patients with moderate persistent asthma [39]. At week 24, the improvement in peak FEV1 within 3 hours ($FEV1_{(0-3\,h)}$) was statistically significant with both tiotropium doses compared with placebo: 5 μg tiotropium, adjusted mean difference 174 mL (95% CI: 76, 272 mL; $p < 0.001$) and 2.5 μg tiotropium, 134 mL (95% CI: 34, 234 mL; $p < 0.01$) [39]. PensieTinA-asthma® was a double-blind, parallel-group trial (NCT01277523) assessing the effect of once-daily tiotropium Respimat add-on to ICSs (400–1600 μg/day) plus one or more controllers, or ICSs (200–800 μg/day) plus two or more controllers in adolescent (12- to 17-year-old) patients with severe persistent asthma [40]. In this study, tiotropium Respimat 5 μg provided numerical improvements in peak $FEV1_{(0-3\,h)}$ compared with placebo (90 mL; $p = 0.104$); however, significant improvements were seen with the 2.5 μg dose (111 mL; $p = 0.046$). While there were positive trends for improvements in lung function and asthma control, the primary efficacy endpoint was not met—this may have been related to the presence of a pronounced placebo response and the relatively short trial period (12 weeks); in comparison, the Phase III tiotropium studies of adolescents [39] and adults [23] with moderate asthma were analyzed at 24 weeks, while those of adults with severe asthma were analyzed at 48 weeks [22].

VivaTinA-asthma®, a 12-week, double-blind, placebo-controlled trial (NCT01634152) was the first Phase III study of tiotropium Respimat in children with severe symptomatic disease. It was conducted in children aged 6–11 years to assess the safety and efficacy of tiotropium Respimat add-on to high-dose ICSs (>400 μg/day) with one or more controller medications, or medium-dose ICSs (200–400 μg/day) with two or more controller medications in severe persistent asthma [41]. Compared with placebo, tiotropium 5 μg add-on therapy significantly improved the primary endpoint, peak $FEV1_{(0-3\,h)}$ (139 mL (95% CI: 75, 203; $p < 0.001$)). Once-daily tiotropium was also well tolerated as an add-on therapy to ICSs with other maintenance therapies in children with severe symptomatic asthma [41]. The objective of the CanoTinA-asthma® study (NCT01634139) was to examine the efficacy and safety of once-daily tiotropium Respimat as an add-on therapy in children (6–11 years old) with moderate persistent asthma on medium-dose ICSs (200–400 μg/day). Both doses of tiotropium Respimat, 5 μg and 2.5 μg, significantly improved $FEV1_{(0-3\,h)}$ at week 24, with adjusted mean differences of 164 mL and 170 mL versus placebo, respectively ($p < 0.01$). In children with moderate symptomatic asthma, once-daily tiotropium as an add-on to usual maintenance therapy was again considered safe and well tolerated [42].

Finally, NinoTinA-asthma® was the first study (NCT01634113) to evaluate the efficacy and safety of tiotropium in preschool children (1–5 years old) with persistent asthma on a stable dose of ICSs. This study found that tiotropium is a well-tolerated add-on option in this population and suggested that there may be a reduction in risk of asthma exacerbations, which were reported as adverse events in this trial [43]. While the current FDA approval of tiotropium

Respimat in asthma applies to those aged 6 and older, data suggest that this device is easy to use by younger age groups as well. A handling study assessing the use of the Respimat inhaler in children aged 5 years and below concluded that it was suitable for children in this age group, although these younger patients are advised to add a valved holding chamber to facilitate its use [44]. To date, the studies in children and adolescents have only evaluated tiotropium as an add-on therapy to at least ICSs across a range of asthma severities; however, a comparative assessment of LABA versus LAMA add-on therapy in the paediatric population has yet to be published.

In clinical trials, the reported rates of discontinuation of tiotropium were similar to placebo arms and ranged from 1 to 11% [18, 22, 23, 45]. There are limited reported data on tiotropium compliance. In the TALC study, the compliance rate was 93.0% (similar to the salmeterol arm) [21], whereas in BELT—an open-label, randomized, pragmatic study which compared tiotropium versus salmeterol add-on therapy to ICSs in black adults with moderate-to-severe asthma for a mean follow-up period of 10 months—the compliance rate was 60% (also similar to the salmeterol arm) [46]. In a randomized, dose-ranging study evaluating tiotropium in symptomatic adolescents (aged 12–17), median compliance ranged from 85 to 87% across treatment groups [38].

Published prescribing information indicates that the most common adverse reactions of tiotropium (i.e., >5% incidence in the 1-year placebo-controlled trials) include upper respiratory tract infections, rhinitis and sinusitis, pharyngitis, dry mouth, nonspecific chest pain, dyspepsia, and urinary tract infections [47]. Tiotropium bromide is contraindicated in patients with a known hypersensitivity to it, atropine, or its derivatives (including ipratropium), and as per other anticholinergic medications, tiotropium should be used with caution in patients with narrow-angle glaucoma or urinary retention [48]. Tiotropium is predominantly renally excreted, and in patients with a creatinine clearance of <50 mL/min (i.e., moderate-to-severe renal impairment), it is to be used only if the anticipated benefit outweighs potential risk, and they should be monitored for the development of anticholinergic side effects [48].

In the COPD literature, there has been concern with regard to inhaled anticholinergics (including tiotropium) and their link to cardiovascular events and mortality [49], but subsequent data from the 4-year UPLIFT study did not support an association between tiotropium HandiHaler and risk of myocardial infarction, stroke, or death from cardiovascular causes [9]. The safety of tiotropium in the Respimat form in COPD has been debated: two systematic reviews and meta-analyses [50, 51] and a large cohort study [52] suggested that its use is associated with an increase in mortality of ~30–50%, with the association being the strongest for cardiovascular and/or cerebrovascular death; however, a large randomized, double-blind parallel group trial of over 17,000 patients with COPD found that, during a mean follow-up of 2.3 years, tiotropium Respimat was noninferior to HandiHaler in the primary endpoint of risk of death and that causes of death and rates of major adverse cardiovascular events were similar across these devices [53].

The earlier-described Phase II and III trials of tiotropium in asthma have demonstrated a favourable adverse effect profile, with event rates that are comparable across different doses and placebo arms. However, in these trials, the safety and tolerance data resulted from analysis of secondary outcomes. In a randomized, double-blind, placebo-controlled parallel group trial of 285 patients with asthma by Ohta et al., tiotropium Respimat (at doses of 5 and 2.5 μg once daily) use over 52 weeks led to a similar rate of the primary outcome of adverse events (AEs) versus placebo (88.6% for 5 μg, 86.8% for 2.5 μg; 89.5% for placebo); the most commonly reported event in tiotropium Respimat 5 μg, 2.5 μg, and placebo groups, respectively, was "nasopharyngitis" (48.2, 44.7, and 42.1%), followed by "asthma" (28.9, 29.8, and 38.6%), "decreased PEFR" (15.8, 7.9, and 21.1%), "bronchitis" (9.6, 13.2, and 7.0%), "phayngitis" (7.9, 13.2, and 3.5%), and "gastroenteritis" (10.5, 3.5, and 5.3%) [54]. Pooled data from seven Phase II and III adult asthma trials (all randomized and double-blinded)—including the study by Ohta et al.—also found that the percentage of AEs was comparable between treatment tiotropium and placebo groups: the most frequent ones were "asthma," "decreased PEFR," and "nasopharyngitis"; the overall incidence of dry mouth and cardiac disorder AEs was comparable across all groups (<1% and <1.5%, resp.) [55].

Based on the established safety and efficacy data of tiotropium Respimat (Spiriva Respimat, Boehringer Ingelheim International GmbH), in September 2015, the FDA had approved its use in the U.S. as a long-term, once-daily maintenance therapy in asthma patients aged 12 and older; the approval was expanded to ages 6 and older in February 2017. The recommended dose in the U.S. is two inhalations of 1.25 μg once daily [56]. In Canada, tiotropium Respimat has been approved as an add-on maintenance bronchodilator in adult patients with asthma who continue to be symptomatic on a combination of ICSs (at minimum, equivalent to ≥500 μg fluticasone/day or ≥800 μg budesonide/day) plus LABAs and who have experienced ≥1 severe exacerbations in the previous year, at the recommended dose of two inhalations of 2.5 μg once daily, which parallels the approval in the European Union [48, 57]. It is unclear as to why these agencies have different approved doses; however, as reviewed earlier, both the 2.5 and 5 μg doses of tiotropium have been found to have comparable effects when studied together. Tiotropium has also been approved in Japan for patients aged 15 years and over, and it is undergoing review in other countries [58].

5. Further Perspectives

Recent studies have assessed the real-world effectiveness of tiotropium. A retrospective study of 2042 adults with asthma found that, in the first year following the addition of tiotropium (93% via HandiHaler, 7% via Respimat at 5 μg), there was a decrease in the incidence of both primary outcomes of exacerbations (patients experiencing ≥1 exacerbation were decreased from 37 to 27%, $p < 0.001$) and respiratory events requiring antibiotic prescriptions (from 58 to 47%, $p < 0.001$) [59]. Unlike the earlier-presented data from the Phase III randomized trials, no significant changes in lung function were found with the addition of tiotropium; this negative finding may be related to the inclusion of smokers (~50% had an active smoking history, whereas those with >10 pack-year smoking history were excluded from trials) and the limited control on lung function data inherent to a retrospective study including timing of the measurements with regard to time of day, or relative to tiotropium initiation [59]. In a randomized, open-label, parallel-group pragmatic trial of 1070 black adults with moderate-to-severe asthma, the effect of tiotropium HandiHaler as add-on therapy to ICSs on time to first exacerbation was compared with LABAs (salmeterol or formoterol) [46]. Over a follow-up period of up to 18 months, the time to first exacerbation, as well as the mean number of exacerbations per person-year, did not differ between the tiotropium and LABA arms. There was also no difference in the two treatment groups in the secondary outcomes of FEV1, rescue medication use, and other patient-reported outcomes (AQLQ, ACQ, and Symptom Utility Index).

Cost-effectiveness represents an additional factor to consider when determining the real-world application of a medication. In 2014, Willson et al. found tiotropium to be a cost-effective add-on therapy, from the perspective of the UK National Health Service, to adult asthma patients uncontrolled on ICS-LABA combination by analyzing the PrimoTinA-asthma trial database [60]. Using a Markov modelling framework—which included seven mutually exclusive health states (three states of asthma control, three states of exacerbation, and death)—the authors analyzed costs and quality-adjusted life-years (QALYs). The model, utilizing the £20,000–£30,000 per QALY-gained willingness-to-pay threshold that is commonly accepted in the UK, found that the tiotropium add-on therapy generated an incremental 0.19 QALYs and £5389 in costs over a lifetime, resulting in an incremental cost-effectiveness ratio of £28,383 per QALY gained [60, 61]. Essentially, the addition of tiotropium, while increasing drug acquisition costs, was found to reduce exacerbation-related expenditures and also improve patients' quality of life.

The incorporation of tiotropium at Step 4 in recent iterations of the GINA guidelines targets the unmet need for optimal disease control in those with persistent, severe asthma, serving as a well-tolerated add-on therapy to ICS-LABA. However, given the results of director comparator studies between salmeterol and tiotropium as add-on therapies to ICSs, one wonders if LAMAs could serve as an equivalent alternative to LABAs in those with asthma and, as such, be positioned earlier in stepwise therapy. When compared to salmeterol, tiotropium was found to have similar efficacy in improving lung function (AM and PM PEF, FEV1) measured at 14 and 24 weeks in patients with moderate, persistent asthma with confirmed bronchodilator reversibility [21, 23]. In a pragmatic trial conducted over 18 months, tiotropium was found to have similar effects as LABA (salmeterol or formoterol) therapy on time to first exacerbation [46]. However, a Cochrane Library systematic review concluded that current evidence is not strong enough to support LAMAs as a LABA substitute, given that the comparative effects on exacerbations and serious adverse events are unclear based on short trial duration, as well as the larger evidence base supporting LABA versus placebo as an ICS add-on [26]. As such, the decision to favour LAMAs as an add-on versus LABAs would be on an individual patient level. Some studies, including the TALC study comparing tiotropium versus salmeterol, have shown that patients can develop tolerance to LABAs and impaired SABA response [21, 62–64], and thus, tachyphylaxis to LABAs could preferentially favour LAMAs as an ICS add-on therapy. Furthermore, follow-up analyses of the TALC study data found that adult asthma patients with higher cholinergic tone (as indicated by a lower resting heart rate) and the extent of airway obstruction (as indicated by the FEV1/FVC ratio) predicted a positive clinical response to tiotropium (versus salmeterol); ethnicity, gender, atopy, IgE levels, asthma duration, and BMI were not predictors [65]. While that study did not demonstrate sputum eosinophilia as a predictor of tiotropium response, sputum neutrophilia has been shown in another study to correlate positively with the FEV1 improvement at 4 weeks conferred by the addition of tiotropium [36]. It is hoped that future studies will assess these factors in a larger, prospective fashion to provide a practical and potentially guideline-based approach to long-acting bronchodilator choice in the clinical setting.

With regard to direct comparator trials, tiotropium as an add-on therapy to symptomatic asthma patients on at least ICSs has been demonstrated to be superior to doubling of ICSs [21], and comparable to LABA addition in adults [21, 23, 45, 46], across various clinical outcomes. However, the relative place and preference of tiotropium with respect to other potential GINA Step 4 strategies (e.g., theophylline and leukotriene receptor antagonists (LTRAs)) have yet to be addressed directly by large, blinded, randomized trials. Given the availability of other effective and safe treatments and the relatively modest properties on bronchodilation and symptom control [66–69], clinical practice guidelines have not recommended theophylline as a preferred controller therapy. However, its low cost offers an advantage over other add-on therapies added to ICSs, which may favour its use in developing nations [70]. There are controversies in the clinical evidence supporting the efficacy of LTRAs; for example, a meta-analysis of six clinical studies assessing montelukast as an add-on therapy in mild-to-moderate asthma showed significantly improved effectiveness in symptom control and exacerbation risk compared with ICSs [71]. In contrast, in other studies of patients treated with high-dose ICSs ($\geq 1000\,\mu g$), the addition of montelukast showed no improvement in symptoms, lung function, or reduced SABA use [72, 73]. A Cochrane review published this year concluded that the addition of LTRAs reduces moderate and severe exacerbations and improves lung function and asthma control compared with the same dose of ICSs but that the evidence does not support this class of controller therapy as an ICS-sparing agent [74]. LTRAs may be useful in particular situations, including those intolerant of or unwilling to use ICSs and those with allergic rhinitis, aspirin-induced asthma, viral-induced wheezing, and asthma in the elderly [1, 75]. Data from a randomized, but unblinded, study of 297 patients on budesonide (400 μg/day) found that a 6-month trial of add-on montelukast safely improved FEV1, SGRQ, and rescue medication use at a faster rate than add-on doxofylline or tiotropium [76].

6. Summary

Tiotropium has recently been demonstrated as a well-tolerated and effective add-on treatment for adults, adolescents, and children with persistent, symptomatic asthma. The demonstrated efficacy and safety profiles, regardless of baseline characteristics and asthma severity, are encouraging. Furthermore, the effect of tiotropium on various clinical outcomes is consistent across patient subgroups and phenotypes which have historically imposed treatment challenges, including obesity, the elderly, and noneosinphilic asthma, which makes tiotropium a worthy consideration as an add-on bronchodilator in the treatment of asthma patients on, at minimum, inhaled corticosteroids. Future research is needed to investigate the long-term effectiveness of tiotropium, its relative efficacy, and safety compared to alternative treatment options at GINA Step 4 and its role as an alternative maintenance inhaler to LABAs.

Disclosure

Robert Andrew McIvor has received honoraria from AstraZeneca, Boehringer-Ingelheim, Merck, Novartis, Pfizer, Roche, Teva, Takeda, and Trudell for attendance at advisory boards and providing CME.

References

[1] Global Initiative for Asthma (GINA), "Global Strategy for Asthma Management and Prevention," GINA Report, Global Initiative for Asthma, 2017.

[2] M. Masoli, D. Fabian, S. Holt, R. Beasley, and Global Initiative for Asthma Program, "The global burden of asthma: executive summary of the GINA Dissemination Committee report," *Allergy*, vol. 59, no. 5, pp. 469–478, 2004.

[3] World Health Organization, *Asthma*, Fact Sheet No. 307, Updated, vol. 2013, World Health Organization, Geneva, Switzerland, 2016, http://www.who.int/mediacentre/factsheets/fs307/en/.

[4] D. M. N. Price, A. Mulgirigama et al., "P17 the burden of ICS/LABA-treated asthma patients in the UK adult population," *Thorax*, vol. 68, no. 3, p. A82, 2013.

[5] K. Bahadori, M. M. Doyle-Waters, C. Marra et al., "Economic burden of asthma: a systematic review," *BMC Pulmonary Medicine*, vol. 9, no. 1, p. 24, 2009.

[6] A. Chang and Y. Bosse, "Targeting single molecules in asthma benefits few," *Trends in Molecular Medicine*, vol. 22, no. 11, pp. 935–945, 2016.

[7] M. Engelkes, H. M. Janssens, J. C. de Jongste, M. C. Sturkenboom, and K. M. Verhamme, "Medication adherence and the risk of severe asthma exacerbations: a systematic review," *European Respiratory Journal*, vol. 45, no. 2, pp. 396–407, 2015.

[8] C. Vogelmeier, B. Hederer, T. Glaab et al., "Tiotropium versus salmeterol for the prevention of exacerbations of COPD," *New England Journal of Medicine*, vol. 364, no. 12, pp. 1093–1103, 2011.

[9] D. P. Tashkin, B. Celli, S. Senn et al., "A 4-year trial of tiotropium in chronic obstructive pulmonary disease," *New England Journal of Medicine*, vol. 359, no. 15, pp. 1543–1554, 2008.

[10] C. Karner, J. Chong, and P. Poole, "Tiotropium versus placebo for chronic obstructive pulmonary disease," *Cochrane database of systematic reviews*, vol. 7, p. CD009285, 2014.

[11] E. D. Bateman, S. Rennard, P. J. Barnes et al., "Alternative mechanisms for tiotropium," *Pulmonary Pharmacology & Therapeutics*, vol. 22, no. 6, pp. 533–542, 2009.

[12] L. Rogers and N. A. Hanania, "Role of anticholinergics in asthma management: recent evidence and future needs," *Current Opinion in Pulmonary Medicine*, vol. 21, no. 1, pp. 103–108, 2015.

[13] K. Racke and S. Matthiesen, "The airway cholinergic system: physiology and pharmacology," *Pulmonary Pharmacology & Therapeutics*, vol. 17, no. 4, pp. 181–198, 2004.

[14] G. J. Rodrigo and J. A. Castro-Rodriguez, "Anticholinergics in the treatment of children and adults with acute asthma: a systematic review with meta-analysis," *Thorax*, vol. 60, no. 9, pp. 740–746, 2005.

[15] M. Westby, M. Benson, and P. Gibson, "Anticholinergic agents for chronic asthma in adults," *Cochrane Database of Systematic Reviews*, vol. 3, p. CD003269, 2004.

[16] S. Quirce, J. Dominguez-Ortega, and P. Barranco, "Anticholinergics for treatment of asthma," *Journal of investigational allergology & clinical immunology*, vol. 25, no. 2, quiz 84–93, pp. 94–85, 2015.

[17] H. A. Kerstjens, B. Disse, W. Schroder-Babo et al., "Tiotropium improves lung function in patients with severe uncontrolled asthma: a randomized controlled trial," *Journal of Allergy and Clinical Immunology*, vol. 128, no. 2, pp. 308–314, 2011.

[18] K. M. Beeh, P. Moroni-Zentgraf, O. Ablinger et al., "Tiotropium Respimat® in asthma: a double-blind, randomised, dose-ranging study in adult patients with moderate asthma," *Respiratory Research*, vol. 15, no. 1, p. 61, 2014.

[19] W. Timmer, P. Moroni-Zentgraf, P. Cornelissen, A. Unseld, E. Pizzichini, and R. Buhl, "Once-daily tiotropium Respimat® 5 mug is an efficacious 24-h bronchodilator in adults with symptomatic asthma," *Respiratory Medicine*, vol. 109, no. 3, pp. 329–338, 2015.

[20] E. R. McIvor and R. A. McIvor, "The evolving role of tiotropium in asthma," *Journal of Asthma and Allergy*, vol. 10, pp. 231–236, 2017.

[21] S. P. Peters, S. J. Kunselman, N. Icitovic et al., "Tiotropium bromide step-up therapy for adults with uncontrolled asthma," *New England Journal of Medicine*, vol. 363, no. 18, pp. 1715–1726, 2010.

[22] H. A. Kerstjens, M. Engel, R. Dahl et al., "Tiotropium in asthma poorly controlled with standard combination therapy," *New England Journal of Medicine*, vol. 367, no. 13, pp. 1198–1207, 2012.

[23] H. A. Kerstjens, T. B. Casale, E. R. Bleecker et al., "Tiotropium or salmeterol as add-on therapy to inhaled corticosteroids for patients with moderate symptomatic asthma: two replicate, double-blind, placebo-controlled, parallel-group, active-comparator, randomised trials," *Lancet Respiratory Medicine*, vol. 3, no. 5, pp. 367–376, 2015.

[24] P. Paggiaro, D. M. Halpin, R. Buhl et al., "The effect of tiotropium in symptomatic asthma despite low- to medium-dose inhaled corticosteroids: a randomized controlled trial," *Journal of Allergy and Clinical Immunology: In Practice*, vol. 4, no. 1, pp. 104.e2–113.e2, 2016.

[25] D. E. Anderson, K. M. Kew, and A. C. Boyter, "Long-acting muscarinic antagonists (LAMA) added to inhaled corticosteroids (ICS) versus the same dose of ICS alone for adults with asthma," *Cochrane database of systematic reviews*, vol. 8, p. CD011397, 2015.

[26] K. M. Kew, D. J. Evans, D. E. Allison, and A. C. Boyter, "Long-acting muscarinic antagonists (LAMA) added to inhaled corticosteroids (ICS) versus addition of long-acting beta2-agonists (LABA) for adults with asthma," *Cochrane database of systematic reviews*, vol. 6, p. CD011438, 2015.

[27] K. M. Kew and K. Dahri, "Long-acting muscarinic antagonists (LAMA) added to combination long-acting beta2-agonists and inhaled corticosteroids (LABA/ICS) versus LABA/ICS for adults with asthma," *Cochrane Database of Systematic Reviews*, vol. 1, p. CD011721, 2016.

[28] J. M. E. M. Fitzgerald, P. Moroni-Zentgraf, R. Luehmann, and E. R. Bleecker, "Once-daily tiotropium Respimat® add-on therapy improves symptom control across severities of symptomatic asthma, independent of allergic status," *American Journal of Respiratory and Critical Care Medicine*, vol. 191, p. A4263, 2015.

[29] T. B. D. R. Casale, J. C. Virchow, M. Engel, P. Moroni-Zentgraf, R. Luehmann, and H. A. M. Kerstjens, "Tiotropium Respimat® add-on therapy reduces exacerbation risk in patients with symptomatic moderate to severe asthma, independent of T helper 2 status," *American Journal of Respiratory and Critical Care Medicine*, vol. 191, p. A4193, 2015.

[30] A. E. Dixon, F. Holguin, A. Sood et al., "An official American Thoracic Society Workshop report: obesity and asthma," *Proceedings of the American Thoracic Society*, vol. 7, no. 5, pp. 325–335, 2010.

[31] S. E. Wenzel, "Asthma phenotypes: the evolution from clinical to molecular approaches," *Nature Medicine*, vol. 18, no. 5, pp. 716–725, 2012.

[32] G. S. Skloot, P. J. Busse, S. S. Braman et al., "An official American Thoracic Society Workshop report: evaluation and management of asthma in the elderly," *Annals of the American Thoracic Society*, vol. 13, no. 11, pp. 2064–2077, 2016.

[33] H. A. Kerstjens, P. Moroni-Zentgraf, D. P. Tashkin et al., "Tiotropium improves lung function, exacerbation rate, and asthma control, independent of baseline characteristics including age, degree of airway obstruction, and allergic status," *Respiratory Medicine*, vol. 117, pp. 198–206, 2016.

[34] J. V. Fahy, "Eosinophilic and neutrophilic inflammation in asthma: insights from clinical studies," *Proceedings of the American Thoracic Society*, vol. 6, no. 3, pp. 256–259, 2009.

[35] N. C. Thomson, "Novel approaches to the management of noneosinophilic asthma," *Therapeutic Advances in Respiratory Disease*, vol. 10, no. 3, pp. 211–234, 2016.

[36] H. Iwamoto, A. Yokoyama, N. Shiota et al., "Tiotropium bromide is effective for severe asthma with noneosinophilic phenotype," *European Respiratory Journal*, vol. 31, no. 6, pp. 1379-1380, 2008.

[37] C. Vogelberg, P. Moroni-Zentgraf, M. Leonaviciute-Klimantaviciene et al., "A randomised dose-ranging study of tiotropium Respimat® in children with symptomatic asthma despite inhaled corticosteroids," *Respiratory Research*, vol. 16, no. 1, p. 20, 2015.

[38] C. Vogelberg, M. Engel, P. Moroni-Zentgraf et al., "Tiotropium in asthmatic adolescents symptomatic despite inhaled corticosteroids: a randomised dose-ranging study," *Respiratory Medicine*, vol. 108, no. 9, pp. 1268–1276, 2014.

[39] E. Hamelmann, E. D. Bateman, C. Vogelberg et al., "Tiotropium add-on therapy in adolescents with moderate asthma: A 1-year randomized controlled trial," *Journal of Allergy and Clinical Immunology*, vol. 138, no. 2, pp. 441 e448–450 e448, 2016.

[40] E. Hamelmann, J. A. Bernstein, M. Vandewalker et al., "A randomised controlled trial of tiotropium in adolescents with severe symptomatic asthma," *European Respiratory Journal*, vol. 49, no. 1, p. 1601100, 2017.

[41] S. J. Szefler, K. Murphy, T. Harper III et al., "A phase III randomized controlled trial of tiotropium add-on therapy in children with severe symptomatic asthma," *Journal of Allergy and Clinical Immunology*, vol. 140, no. 5, pp. 1277–1287, 2017.

[42] O. Schmidt, E. Hamelmann, C. Vogelberg et al., "Late-breaking abstract: once-daily tiotropium Respimat® add-on therapy improves lung function in children with moderate symptomatic asthma," *European Respiratory Journal*, vol. 48, no. 60, p. PA4398, 2016.

[43] H. Bisgaard, M. Vandewalker, L. Graham et al., "Safety of tiotropium in pre-school children with symptomatic persistent asthma," *European Respiratory Journal*, vol. 48, no. 60, 2016.

[44] W. Kamin, M. Frank, S. Kattenbeck, P. Moroni-Zentgraf, H. Wachtel, and S. Zielen, "A handling study to assess use of the Respimat® soft mist inhaler in children under 5 years old," *Journal of Aerosol Medicine and Pulmonary Drug Delivery*, vol. 28, no. 5, pp. 372–381, 2015.

[45] E. D. Bateman, O. Kornmann, P. Schmidt, A. Pivovarova, M. Engel, and L. M. Fabbri, "Tiotropium is noninferior to salmeterol in maintaining improved lung function in B16-Arg/Arg patients with asthma," *Journal of Allergy and Clinical Immunology*, vol. 128, no. 2, pp. 315–322, 2011.

[46] M. E. Wechsler, B. P. Yawn, A. L. Fuhlbrigge et al., "Anticholinergic vs long-acting beta-agonist in combination with inhaled corticosteroids in black adults with asthma: the BELT randomized clinical trial," *JAMA*, vol. 314, no. 16, pp. 1720–1730, 2015.

[47] Boehringer Ingelheim Pharmaceuticals, Inc., "Highlights of prescribing information, Spiriva® Handihaler® (tiotropium bromide inhalation powder), for oral inhalation use," 2016, http://docs.boehringer-ingelheim.com/Prescribing%20Information/PIs/Spiriva/Spiriva.pdf.

[48] Boehringer Ingelheim (Canada) Ltd., "Product monograph, Spiriva® Respimat®," 2016, https://www.boehringer-ingelheim.ca/sites/ca/files/documents/spirivarespimatpmen.pdf.

[49] S. Singh, Y. K. Loke, and C. D. Furberg, "Inhaled anticholinergics and risk of major adverse cardiovascular events in patients with chronic obstructive pulmonary disease: a systematic review and meta-analysis," *JAMA*, vol. 300, no. 12, pp. 1439–1450, 2008.

[50] S. Singh, Y. K. Loke, P. L. Enright, and C. D. Furberg, "Mortality associated with tiotropium mist inhaler in patients with chronic obstructive pulmonary disease: systematic review and meta-analysis of randomised controlled trials," *BMJ*, vol. 342, p. d3215, 2011.

[51] Y. H. Dong, H. H. Lin, W. Y. Shau, Y. C. Wu, C. H. Chang, and M. S. Lai, "Comparative safety of inhaled medications in patients with chronic obstructive pulmonary disease: systematic review and mixed treatment comparison meta-analysis of

randomised controlled trials," *Thorax*, vol. 68, no. 1, pp. 48–56, 2013.

[52] K. M. Verhamme, A. Afonso, S. Romio, B. C. Stricker, G. G. Brusselle, and M. C. Sturkenboom, "Use of tiotropium Respimat soft mist inhaler versus HandiHaler and mortality in patients with COPD," *European Respiratory Journal*, vol. 42, no. 3, pp. 606–615, 2013.

[53] R. A. Wise, A. Anzueto, D. Cotton et al., "Tiotropium Respimat inhaler and the risk of death in COPD," *New England Journal of Medicine*, vol. 369, no. 16, pp. 1491–1501, 2013.

[54] K. Ohta, M. Ichinose, Y. Tohda et al., "Long-term once-daily tiotropium Respimat® is well tolerated and maintains efficacy over 52 weeks in patients with symptomatic asthma in Japan: a randomised, placebo-controlled study," *PLoS One*, vol. 10, no. 4, article e0124109, 2015.

[55] R. Dahl, M. Engel, D. Dusser et al., "Safety and tolerability of once-daily tiotropium Respimat® as add-on to at least inhaled corticosteroids in adult patients with symptomatic asthma: a pooled safety analysis," *Respiratory Medicine*, vol. 118, pp. 102–111, 2016.

[56] Boehringer Ingelheim Pharmaceuticals, Inc., "Highlights of prescribing information, SPIRIVA® RESPIMAT® (tiotropium bromide) inhalation spray, for oral inhalation," 2017, http://docs.boehringer-ingelheim.com/Prescribing Information/PIs/Spiriva Respimat/spirivarespimat.pdf.

[57] H. A. Kerstjens and P. M. O'Byrne, "Tiotropium for the treatment of asthma: a drug safety evaluation," *Expert Opinion on Drug Safety*, vol. 15, no. 8, pp. 1115–1124, 2016.

[58] W. W. Busse, R. Dahl, C. Jenkins, and A. A. Cruz, "Long-acting muscarinic antagonists: a potential add-on therapy in the treatment of asthma?," *European Respiratory Review*, vol. 25, no. 139, pp. 54–64, 2016.

[59] D. Price, A. Kaplan, R. Jones et al., "Long-acting muscarinic antagonist use in adults with asthma: real-life prescribing and outcomes of add-on therapy with tiotropium bromide," *Journal of Asthma and Allergy*, vol. 8, pp. 1–13, 2015.

[60] J. Willson, E. D. Bateman, I. Pavord, A. Lloyd, T. Krivasi, and D. Esser, "Cost effectiveness of tiotropium in patients with asthma poorly controlled on inhaled glucocorticosteroids and long-acting beta-agonists," *Applied Health Economics and Health Policy*, vol. 12, no. 4, pp. 447–459, 2014.

[61] J. Willson, E. D. Bateman, I. Pavord, A. Lloyd, T. Krivasi, and D. Esser, "Erratum to: cost effectiveness of tiotropium in patients with asthma poorly controlled on inhaled glucocorticosteroids and long-acting beta-agonists," *Applied Health Economics and Health Policy*, vol. 14, no. 1, pp. 119–125, 2016.

[62] K. S. Tan, A. Grove, A. McLean, Y. Gnosspelius, I. P. Hall, and B. J. Lipworth. "Systemic corticosteriod rapidly reverses bronchodilator subsensitivity induced by formoterol in asthmatic patients," *American Journal of Respiratory and Critical Care Medicine*, vol. 156, no. 1, pp. 28–35, 1997.

[63] D. H. Yates, H. S. Sussman, M. J. Shaw, P. J. Barnes, and K. F. Chung, "Regular formoterol treatment in mild asthma. Effect on bronchial responsiveness during and after treatment," *American Journal of Respiratory and Critical Care Medicine*, vol. 152, no. 4, pp. 1170–1174, 1995.

[64] J. Elers, U. Strandbygaard, L. Pedersen, and V. Backer, "Daily use of salmeterol causes tolerance to bronchodilation with terbutaline in asthmatic subjects," *Open Respiratory Medicine Journal*, vol. 4, no. 1, pp. 48–50, 2010.

[65] S. P. Peters, E. R. Bleecker, S. J. Kunselman et al., "Predictors of response to tiotropium versus salmeterol in asthmatic adults," *Journal of Allergy and Clinical Immunology*, vol. 132, no. 5, pp. 1068 e1–1074 e1, 2013.

[66] American Lung Association Asthma Clinical Research C, "Clinical trial of low-dose theophylline and montelukast in patients with poorly controlled asthma," *American Journal of Respiratory and Critical Care Medicine*, vol. 175, no. 3, pp. 235–242, 2007.

[67] R. Dahl, B. B. Larsen, and P. Venge, "Effect of long-term treatment with inhaled budesonide or theophylline on lung function, airway reactivity and asthma symptoms," *Respiratory Medicine*, vol. 96, no. 6, pp. 432–438, 2002.

[68] P. L. Paggiaro, D. Giannini, A. Di Franco, and R. Testi, "Comparison of inhaled salmeterol and individually dose-titrated slow-release theophylline in patients with reversible airway obstruction. European Study Group," *European Respiratory Journal*, vol. 9, no. 8, pp. 1689–1695, 1996.

[69] X. Chen, Y. B. Kang, L. Q. Wang et al., "Addition to inhaled corticosteroids of leukotriene receptor antagonists versus theophylline for symptomatic asthma: a meta-analysis," *Journal of Thoracic Disease*, vol. 7, no. 4, pp. 644–652, 2015.

[70] J. P. Watson and R. A. Lewis, "Is asthma treatment affordable in developing countries?," *Thorax*, vol. 52, no. 7, pp. 605–607, 1997.

[71] S. Joos, A. Miksch, J. Szecsenyi et al., "Montelukast as add-on therapy to inhaled corticosteroids in the treatment of mild to moderate asthma: a systematic review," *Thorax*, vol. 63, no. 5, pp. 453–462, 2008.

[72] D. S. Robinson, D. Campbell, and P. J. Barnes, "Addition of leukotriene antagonists to therapy in chronic persistent asthma: a randomised double-blind placebo-controlled trial," *The Lancet*, vol. 357, no. 9273, pp. 2007–2011, 2001.

[73] M. Tonelli, M. Zingoni, E. Bacci et al., "Short-term effect of the addition of leukotriene receptor antagonists to the current therapy in severe asthmatics," *Pulmonary Pharmacology & Therapeutics*, vol. 16, no. 4, pp. 237–240, 2003.

[74] B. F. Chauhan, M. M. Jeyaraman, A. Singh Mann et al., "Addition of anti-leukotriene agents to inhaled corticosteroids for adults and adolescents with persistent asthma," *The Cochrane database of systematic reviews*, vol. 3, p. CD010347, 2017.

[75] C. Marcello and L. Carlo, "Asthma phenotypes: the intriguing selective intervention with Montelukast," *Asthma Research and Practice*, vol. 2, p. 11, 2016.

[76] M. G. Rajanandh, A. D. Nageswari, and K. Ilango, "Assessment of montelukast, doxofylline, and tiotropium with budesonide for the treatment of asthma: which is the best among the second-line treatment? A randomized trial," *Clinical Therapeutics*, vol. 37, no. 2, pp. 418–426, 2015.

Adrenal Insufficiency in Cystic Fibrosis: A Rare Phenomenon?

Sébastien Préville-Ratelle,[1] Adèle Coriati,[2] Aurélie Ménard,[2] Isabelle Bourdeau,[3,4] François Tremblay,[1,4] and Yves Berthiaume[1,2,4]

[1]*Clinique de fibrose kystique, Centre hospitalier de l'Université de Montréal (CHUM), 1051 rue Sanguinet, Montréal, QC, Canada H2X 0C1*
[2]*Institut de recherches cliniques de Montréal (IRCM), 110 Avenue des Pins, Montréal, QC, Canada H2W 1R7*
[3]*Centre de recherche Centre hospitalier de l'Université de Montréal (CRCHUM), 900 rue Saint-Denis, Montréal, QC, Canada H2X 0A9*
[4]*Département de médecine, Faculté de médecine, Université de Montréal, 2900 boul. Édouard-Montpetit, Montréal, QC, Canada H3T 1J4*

Correspondence should be addressed to Yves Berthiaume; yves.berthiaume@ircm.qc.ca

Academic Editor: Christophe Leroyer

Background. The prevalence of adrenal insufficiency (AI) in cystic fibrosis (CF) is unknown. The frequent use of glucocorticoids (inhaled or systemic) may induce the long-term suppression of the hypothalamic-pituitary-adrenal axis. *Methods.* We reviewed the results of adrenocorticotropic hormone (ACTH) stimulation tests done over a 10-year period to evaluate adrenal function in 69 CF patients of the CHUM CF clinic. Clinical characteristics of AI patients were compared to adrenal-sufficient (AS) patients. *Results.* AI was confirmed in 33 of the 69 CF patients. A higher rate of dysglycemia ($P = 0.022$) and of *Aspergillus* positive culture ($P = 0.006$) was observed in AI patients compared to AS patients. Weight, CFTR genotype, and pulmonary function were comparable between AI and AS patients. The use of systemic corticosteroids (SC) prior to the diagnosis of AI was observed in 42.4% of patients. Compared to AI patients without SC, SC-treated AI patients were older and had a higher rate of allergic bronchopulmonary aspergillosis. *Conclusion.* This study is the first to systematically examine the presence of AI in the largest cohort of CF patients studied to date with a prevalence of 8%. Patients treated with corticosteroids and those colonized with *Aspergillus* have a greater risk of AI.

1. Introduction

Adrenal insufficiency (AI) is the result of decreased hormonal production from the cortex of the adrenal gland. AI may be caused by adrenal failure itself (primary AI) or by disease of the pituitary or hypothalamus (secondary or tertiary AI, resp.). The most common cause of secondary AI, however, results from the chronic therapeutic use of glucocorticoids which can suppress the hypothalamic-pituitary-adrenal axis (HPA) and lead to insufficient cortisol production in response to stress [1]. AI is associated with a potential risk of adrenal crisis and severe complications if the diagnosis is delayed. The short adrenocorticotropic hormone (ACTH) stimulation test (Cortrosyn 250 μg) is the most commonly used dynamic evaluation to confirm the diagnosis of AI [2].

Although AI induced by inhaled corticosteroids (ICSs) has been documented in asthmatic adult populations [3], no studies have evaluated the prevalence of AI in the adult cystic fibrosis (CF) population. Trials on the use of ICSs in CF for the treatment of allergic bronchopulmonary aspergillosis did not systematically evaluate adverse events, although the total daily dose of ICSs was at the threshold of adrenal suppression in most studies [4]. To date, there have been only a few case reports of HPA axis suppression in patients with CF caused by the combination of ICSs (mainly fluticasone) and itraconazole, which inhibits cytochrome P450 consequently decreasing the metabolic clearance of ICSs [5–7].

Our clinical experience at the Centre hospitalier de l'Université de Montréal (CHUM) CF clinic suggests a nonnegligible prevalence of AI among our patients. Therefore, we reviewed the results of the ACTH stimulation test performed over a 10-year period to evaluate adrenal function in 69 CF patients and compared the clinical characteristics of CF patients with AI to those of adrenal-sufficient (AS) patients.

2. Methods

This is a cross-sectional retrospective study approved by the Research Ethics Committee and CHUM Institutional Review Committee. This work was carried out in accordance with the Declaration of Helsinki (1964). The records of 385 patients attending the CF clinic between January 1, 2007, and December 31, 2016, were reviewed. Cases were selected from the CF clinic database and from the computerized laboratory system at CHUM. Inclusion criteria for the study were (1) age 18 or more and (2) a documented ACTH stimulation test (Cortrosyn stimulation test).

Two different ACTH stimulation tests have been performed: the low dose (LDCT, Cortrosyn 1 μg) and the high dose (HDST, Cortrosyn 250 μg). The HDST and the LDCT are the alternative less-invasive methods used in hospitals and clinics to assess adrenal function in patients with suspected chronic AI. However, several meta-analysis studies have demonstrated that the LDCT is more sensitive than the HDST to diagnose secondary AI, such as in patients taking corticosteroids, since the HDST uses supraphysiologic doses of ACTH [8, 9]. For these reasons, the LDCT is now preferred. The LDCT must be done by people well-informed in the preparation and the administration of the 1 μg Cortrosyn [10]. To ensure appropriate testing at our CHUM clinic, the hospital pharmacist is responsible for preparing the Cortrosyn syringe and the nurse uses this preparation to perform the test. In both tests, plasma cortisol levels were measured at baseline as well as 30 and 60 minutes after intravenous injection. Normal adrenal function was defined as a minimum plasma cortisol concentration of 500–550 nmol/L before or after ACTH injection in both low-dose and high-dose tests. When peak cortisol was below this threshold, the diagnosis of AI was confirmed and treatment with hydrocortisone (Cortef) was started. Patients with CF who underwent an organ transplantation were excluded from the study. Of the 69 CF patients that underwent an ACTH functional test, 36 were categorized as AS, whereas 33 were diagnosed with AI. Amongst the 36 patients with AS, 33 underwent the LDCT, 2 did the HDST, and 1 patient did an insulin tolerance test [11]. Between the 33 patients with AI, 28 did the LDCT, 2 underwent the HDST, and 3 were diagnosed with AI because they had undetectable (significantly low concentrations in the laboratory results) plasma cortisol levels. Physicians of the CF clinics will prescribe the ACTH test if the patient has a low blood cortisol concentration in the morning. This screening is done once a year with the routine biochemistry monitoring of the patient's condition. An ACTH test is also prescribed if the patient is experiencing significant fatigue that is unrelated to his clinical status. In other words, the patient feels always tired and does not have a lot of energy, in presence of stable lung function and weight and in absence of significant systemic inflammation.

Demographics (age, sex, weight, and body mass index (BMI)), pulmonary disease characteristics (forced expiratory volume in 1 sec (FEV1), forced vital capacity (FVC), residual volume (RV), oxygen dependence, CFTR genotype, and noninvasive ventilation support), comorbidities (pancreatic and hepatic dysfunction as evidenced by abnormal level of hepatic enzymes or presence of cirrhosis), dysglycemia (diabetes or impaired glucose tolerance), allergic bronchopulmonary aspergillosis (ABPA), microbiological data (bacteria, fungi, and non-TB mycobacteria), biochemical and hematological data (median value over the past year of hemoglobin and white blood cells, and fasting serum cortisol), and results of the functional ACTH test were collected from all of the patients. The total number of intravenous antibiotic treatments and hospitalizations during the two years preceding the diagnosis of AI as well as the use of ICSs, systemic corticosteroids, and chronic antibiotic therapy (inhaled) were also documented.

Values are expressed as median and interval range for each study group (AS versus AI, and AI with or without systemic corticosteroid). Statistical significance of the differences between study groups was determined by Mann-Whitney Student's t-test, as well as by chi-square (chi^2) regression analysis for genotype and hepatic function. All statistical analyses were done with SPSS for Windows software (version 17.0, SPSS Inc., Chicago, IL, USA). A probability value of $P \leq 0.05$ was considered statistically significant.

3. Results

Over the 10-year period, 385 patients diagnosed with CF were seen at the CHUM CF clinic. In this group of CF patients, 69 patients underwent functional tests, of which 36 patients (41.7% men) had normal responses (AS) and 33 patients (48.5% men) had a confirmed diagnosis of AI. From these data, the prevalence of AI in this cohort was calculated to be 8.6%. Their clinical characteristics are detailed in Tables 1 and 2. The median age and BMI of CF patients with AI were comparable to those that had AS (28.0 years and 21.6 kg/m^2 versus 30 years and 20.9 kg/m^2, resp.) (Table 1). The most frequent genotype was the homozygous delta F508 mutation in both AS and AI (58.3% and 60.6%, resp.). Interestingly, the proportion of patients with dysglycemia was statistically higher in AI patients compared to AS patients (87.9% versus 63.9%, $P = 0.022$). Pancreatic insufficiency, hepatic dysfunction, and presence of ABPA were not increased in AI patients. No difference was observed when comparing parameters of the pulmonary function test (FEV1, FVC, and RV) as well as WBC values between both adrenal function groups (Table 2). Patients with AI were more likely to take ICSs and less prone to use chronic inhaled antibiotics ($P = 0.005$, Table 2). However, the number of hospitalization and the number of IV antibiotic treatments 2 years prior to diagnosis were comparable between AS and AI patients. Finally, the sole microorganisms that had a significant difference of proportionality between AS (17.1%) and AI (48.5%) patients were *Aspergillus* and fungi ($P = 0.006$, Table 2).

Table 1: Clinical characteristics of patients with CF according to their adrenal function ($N = 69$).

	Sufficient	Insufficient	P value
Demographic			
Number of patients	36	33	
Sex (% men)	41.7	48.5	0.572
Age (years)	30.0 (19.0–67.0)	28.0 (19.0–55.0)	0.648
Weight (kg)	54.1 (42.3–83.9)	61.0 (41.1–79.1)	0.084
BMI (kg/m^2)	20.9 (17.5–28.6)	21.6 (17.1–27.5)	0.079
Genotype (% yes)			
Homozygote delF508	58.3	60.6	
Heterozygote delF508	38.9	30.3	0.458*
Others	2.8	9.1	
Comorbidities			
Glucose tolerance (% yes)			
Normal	36.1	12.1	0.022
Dysglycemic	63.9	87.9	0.022
Pancreatic insufficiency (% yes)	91.7	87.9	0.605
Hepatic dysfunction (% yes)	30.3	11.1	0.041
Home oxygen therapy (% yes)	5.6	15.2	0.190
Noninvasive ventilation (% yes)	2.8	6.1	0.507
ABPA (% yes)	16.7	27.3	0.290

BMI, body mass index; dysglycemic is presence of either glucose intolerance or diabetes; hepatic dysfunction is either abnormal level of hepatic enzymes or presence of cirrhosis; ABPA, allergic bronchopulmonary aspergillosis. Median and interval range are shown. P value ≤ 0.05 represents Mann-Whitney Student's t-test. *Chi^2 regression analysis.

Systemic corticosteroid therapy prior to the diagnosis of AI was observed in 14 patients with a median duration of administration of 18 months (varying between 1 week and 74 months) (Table 2). Of these 14 patients, all but one received corticosteroids for more than a month in the year prior to the diagnosis. When comparing with AI patients who did not receive systemic corticosteroids, AI patients taking systemic corticosteroids were older (36.0 years versus 26.0 years, $P = 0.019$) (Table 3). Interestingly, the use of systemic corticosteroids was justified by the diagnosis of allergic bronchopulmonary aspergillosis (ABPA) in 9 cases (64.3%). In addition, AI patients with systemic corticosteroid had significantly lower levels of cortisol at 30 minutes during the ACTH stimulation test ($P = 0.047$). Treatment with systemic corticosteroids was not associated with antifungal treatment. The median number of hospitalizations and of intravenous antibiotic treatments in the two years preceding the diagnosis and the profile of bacterial and fungal infection and medication are detailed in Table 4. ICSs were used in 92.9% of AI patients with systemic corticosteroids. In the 19 patients who had no recent exposure (<2 years) to systemic corticosteroids, all but one were using ICSs. The ICSs used were fluticasone or budesonide mainly at high dosage and sometimes in combination with ciclesonide. The detailed clinical findings of these patients are reported in Tables 3 and 4.

The chronic use of opiates was the suspected etiology of AI in 2 cases. The prolonged intake of voriconazole for the treatment of *Scedosporium apiospermum* was observed in 2 patients. Use of other antifungal agents in the Montreal CF cohort has not been identified (data not shown).

4. Discussion

AI is the inability to produce sufficient amount of steroid hormones (primarily cortisol) from the adrenal glands. Until now, only individual case reports relating CF and AI have appeared in the literature. This is the first study that characterizes a large group of adult patients with CF that had developed AI. Our observations show that, compared to the AS subgroup, the AI subgroup of CF patients exhibited a higher frequency of dysglycemia and had a higher percentage of patients colonized with *Aspergillus*/fungi. AI patients on systemic corticosteroids were also older. Finally, the utilization of ICSs or systemic corticosteroids was more frequent in patients with AI. More interestingly, more than half the AI patients on systemic corticosteroids had ABPA compared to none in the subgroup of patients not taking systemic corticosteroids.

We are the first to estimate the prevalence of AI in an adult CF population. Our data, obtained following review of the clinical records of over 385 CF patients, suggest that the prevalence of AI in our CF population is between 8% and 9%. This value may be underestimated due to the difficulty of recognizing AI and the lack of systematic screening. Although significant, this prevalence is much lower than the one that has been observed in non-CF bronchiectasis. Indeed, in a study of 40 consecutive patients with non-CF bronchiectasis, Rajagopala et al. [12] reported that 40% of patients had a reduced response to functional testing. No association with inhaled or oral corticosteroids therapy, or severity of impairment was identified in this study. In a British study of non-CF bronchiectasis, adrenal suppression was found in 23.5% of subjects not receiving ICSs and in 48.5% of patients receiving it [13]. Skov et al. observed AI in 11 out of 25 patients with CF treated both with itraconazole for ABPA and budesonide [14], while one of the 11 patients treated with itraconazole alone (without budesonide) had AI. More recently, Gilchrist et al. found a higher prevalence of HPA axis suppression in 10 out of 12 patients with CF receiving both itraconazole and inhaled fluticasone compared

TABLE 2: Paraclinical characteristics of patients with CF according to their adrenal function ($N = 69$).

	Sufficient	Insufficient	P value
Pulmonary function test			
FEV1 (% pred)	44.6 (22.0–120.0)	52.9 (27.5–82.6)	0.509
FVC (% pred)	69.9 (32.8–113.8)	72.6 (51.0–97.8)	0.885
RV (% pred)	177.0 (80.0–414.0)	197.5 (126.0–406.0)	0.271
Biochemistry			
Fasting cortisol (nmol/L)	421.0 (191.0–954.0)	146.0 (12.0–335.0)	≤0.001
Cortisol (nmol/L)			
1 μg functional cortrosyn test (n)	33	28	
0 minutes	388.0 (113.0–852.0)	139.5 (10.0–382.0)	≤0.001
30 minutes	628.0 (502.0–1079.0)	354.0 (25.0–491.0)	≤0.001
60 minutes	510.0 (210.0–902.0)	300.5 (23.0–457.0)	≤0.001
250 μg functional cortrosyn test (n)	2	2	
0 minutes	426.5 (407.0–446.0)	158.5 (26.0–291.0)	NA
30 minutes	637.5 (606.0–669.0)	325.5 (179.0–472.0)	NA
60 minutes	678.0 (664.0–692.0)	309.5 (238.0–381.0)	NA
Hematology			
WBC (10*9/L)	7.6 (4.1–10.8)	8.0 (2.55–17.5)	0.294
Medication			
Systemic corticosteroids (% yes)	0	42.4	≤0.001
Duration (months)	—	18.0 (0.25–74.0)	—
Inhaled corticosteroids (% yes)	66.7	93.9	0.005
Chronic inhaled antibiotic (% yes)	100.0	78.8	0.005
Medical history			
Number of hospitalizations (2 years prior to diagnosis)	2.0 (0–8.0)	2.0 (0–11.0)	0.593
Number of intravenous antibiotic treatments (2 years prior to diagnosis)	3.0 (0–8.0)	3.0 (0–11.0)	0.565
Colonization/microbiology			
Non-TB mycobacteria (% yes)	8.6	3.0	0.335
Staphylococcus aureus (% yes)	31.4	39.4	0.495
Pseudomonas aeruginosa (% yes)	77.1	81.8	0.636
Aspergillus and fungi (% yes)	17.1	48.5	0.006
Stenotrophomonas maltophilia (% yes)	25.0	30.3	0.625
Others (% yes)	19.4	12.1	0.410

FEV1, forced expiratory volume-one second; FVC, forced vital capacity; RV, residual volume; WBC, white blood cell count; TB, tuberculous; NA, not applicable. Median and interval range are shown. P value < 0.05 represents Mann-Whitney Student's t-test.

to patients with CF receiving inhaled fluticasone alone [15]. In all these studies, there was a selection of patients based on either the therapy administered or their clinical status. This might explain the difference in the prevalence observed. A prospective study will be necessary to determine more precisely the prevalence of this condition in CF.

Dysglycemia and *Aspergillus*/fungi colonization also appear as potential risk factors for AI. Our study showed an increased prevalence of dysglycemia (87.9%) in AI compared to AS patients (63.9%). Although this association could be secondary to the chronic inflammatory response associated with diabetes, it could also be a confounding factor since it is well known that chronic use of corticosteroids can lead to heightened blood glucose levels and diabetes [16]. Chronic inflammatory response associated with CF could also explain the presence of AI in patients who did not take corticosteroids. Indeed, Mastorakos et al. have demonstrated that prolonged inflammatory stress induced by a sustained high level of interleukin- (IL-) 6 decreases the reactivity of the HPA axis over time [17]. Inadequate cortisol production has also been demonstrated in rheumatologic patients. The study by Straub et al. showed that levels of ACTH and cortisol, when related to IL-6 and TNF, were relatively lower in untreated patients with early rheumatoid arthritis and reactive arthritis as compared to healthy subjects [18]. Noni et al. reported an association between *Aspergillus* colonization and duration of ICS treatment [19]. A future case-control study is needed to validate these findings, to more precisely determine the real prevalence of AI and its risk factors, and to evaluate the clinical course and repercussions of AI on the quality of life of CF patients. Our observations suggest that CF patients who have an abnormal glucose status (glucose intolerant or CF-related diabetes) or are colonized with *Aspergillus*/fungi or have received systemic corticosteroids as well as have ABPA might benefit from a systematic screening of adrenal function.

Clearly, the utilization of corticosteroids plays a major role in the suppression of the HPA axis in CF patients. In our study, the majority of patients with AI were treated with ICSs for several years. Although the therapeutic use of ICSs remains controversial in the management of CF [4, 20], it remains widespread. There are multiple factors that might explain the association between ICS use and AI in CF. First, chronic airway inflammation is associated with pathological

TABLE 3: Clinical characteristics of adrenal insufficient patients with CF with and without systemic corticosteroids ($N = 33$).

Systemic corticosteroids	Yes	No	P value
Demographic			
Number of patients	14	19	
Sex (% men)	35.7	57.9	0.215
Age (years)	36.0 (21.0–55.0)	26.0 (19.0–39.0)	0.019
Weight (kg)	58.8 (50.0–79.1)	61.2 (41.1–72.8)	0.913
BMI (kg/m^2)	21.3 (19.1–27.4)	21.7 (17.1–27.5)	0.971
Genotype (% yes)			
Homozygote delF508	57.1	63.2	
Heterozygote delF508	35.7	26.3	0.825*
Others	7.1	10.5	
Comorbidities			
Glucose tolerance (% yes)			
Normal	7.1	15.8	0.459
Dysglycemic	92.9	84.2	0.459
Pancreatic insufficiency (% yes)	71.4	100.0	0.014
Hepatic dysfunction (% yes)	21.4	36.8	0.208
Home oxygen therapy (% yes)	7.1	21.1	0.278
Noninvasive ventilation (% yes)	0	10.5	0.217
ABPA (% yes)	64.3	0	≤0.001

BMI, body mass index; dysglycemic is presence of either glucose intolerance or diabetes; hepatic dysfunction is either abnormal level of hepatic enzymes or presence of cirrhosis; ABPA, allergic bronchopulmonary aspergillosis. Median and interval range are shown. P value < 0.05 represents Mann-Whitney Student's t-test. *Chi^2 regression analysis.

TABLE 4: Paraclinical characteristics of adrenal insufficient patients with CF with and without systemic corticosteroids ($N = 33$).

Systemic corticosteroids	Yes	No	P value
Pulmonary function test			
FEV1 (% pred)	56.9 (28.6–73.7)	44.1 (27.5–82.6)	0.536
FVC (% pred)	75.3 (51.0–96.4)	68.6 (56.4–97.8)	0.466
RV (% pred)	188.5 (128.0–221.0)	238.0 (126.0–406.0)	0.051
Biochemistry			
Fasting cortisol (nmol/L)	134.0 (25.0–254.0)	169.5 (12.0–335.0)	0.323
Cortisol (nmol/L)			
1 μg functional cortrosyn test (n)	10	18	
0 minutes	124.5 (25.0–219.0)	167.0 (10.0–382.0)	0.415
30 minutes	314.0 (86.0–425.0)	398.5 (25.0–491.0)	0.179
60 minutes	279.0 (64.0–457.0)	315.5.0 (23.0–425.0)	0.388
250 μg functional cortrosyn test (n)	1	1	
0 minutes	26.0	291.0	NA
30 minutes	179.0	472.0	NA
60 minutes	238.0	381.0	NA
Hematology			
WBC (10*9/L)	9.4 (4.9–17.5)	7.6 (2.6–15.0)	0.074
Medication			
Inhaled corticosteroids (% yes)	92.9	94.7	0.823
Inhaled chronic antibiotic therapy (% yes)	78.6	78.9	0.979
Medical history			
Number of hospitalizations (2 years prior to diagnosis)	2.0 (0–6.0)	4.0 (0–11)	0.151
Number of intravenous antibiotic treatments (2 years prior to diagnosis)	2.5 (0–7.0)	4.0 (0–11)	0.212
Colonization/microbiology			
Non-TB mycobacteria (% yes)	7.1	0	0.244
Staphylococcus aureus (% yes)	42.9	36.8	0.731
Pseudomonas aeruginosa (% yes)	71.4	89.5	0.191
Aspergillus and fungi (% yes)	50.0	47.4	0.883
Stenotrophomonas maltophilia (% yes)	28.6	31.6	0.826
Others (% yes)	14.3	10.5	0.747

FEV1, forced expiratory volume-one second; FVC, forced vital capacity; RV, residual volume; WBC, white blood cell count; TB, tuberculous; NA, not applicable. Median and interval range are shown. P value < 0.05 represents Mann-Whitney Student's t-test.

angiogenesis in the airway [21, 22]. It is suggested that this increase in vascularization in the airway and lungs might lead to increased absorption of corticosteroids into the systemic circulation. Second, since a significant quantity of inhaled corticosteroid is swallowed into the digestive tract, the use of high doses will lead to increased levels in the systemic circulation [23]. Besides absorption, other factors play an important role in the suppression of the HPA axis by ICSs. Indeed, the bioavailability of inhaled compounds is not uniform [24]. Therefore, the ICS compound that has the lowest oral bioavailability would be the best option to decrease undesired corticosteroid effects [24, 25]. Other factors that can affect corticosteroid availability include systemic clearance, receptor affinity, and protein binding capacity [24]. Finally, plasma cortisol concentration varies significantly during the day, with the highest levels measured early in the morning at around 8 AM and the lowest at midnight [24]. Thus, to minimize the secondary effects of corticosteroids on cortisol suppression, it becomes important to consider the elimination half-life of the inhaled compound as well as the drug administration time so that the peak drug level is in phase with the natural cycle of endogenous cortisol. Additional studies are essential to study the pharmacodynamics of ICSs specifically in CF.

The ACTH stimulation test requires multiple steps for its preparation, and it has to be done by experienced personal and is time consuming. Identifying and proposing a management plan where ACTH stimulation is not the primary test that is done but it should be used only to confirm the diagnosis before beginning therapy would be important [26]. A potential management plan including an easy screening tool that can be done during a routine clinical visit will need to be evaluated in future studies.

5. Conclusion

This study is the first to systematically examine adrenal function in a cohort of CF patients. Our analysis would suggest that the prevalence of AI is at least 8% in our adult CF clinic. Therapeutic use of inhaled and systemic corticosteroids was often identified in patients with adrenal suppression. Considering the lack of clear clinical benefit of ICS therapy in CF, our results show the need for additional studies to reduce both the burden of medication and the potential adverse effects of corticosteroid therapy in CF patients.

Acknowledgments

The authors thank all CF patients who participated in this study. Funding from the Lamarre-Gosselin Chair supported Yves Berthiaume, and a Cystic Fibrosis Canada Postdoctoral Fellowship supported Adèle Coriati.

References

[1] F. Guerrero Perez, A. P. Marengo, and C. Villabona Artero, "The unresolved riddle of glucocorticoid withdrawal," *Journal of Endocrinological Investigation*, vol. 40, no. 11, pp. 1175–1181, 2017.

[2] A. Agha, J. W. Tomlinson, P. M. Clark, G. Holder, and P. M. Stewart, "The long-term predictive accuracy of the short synacthen (corticotropin) stimulation test for assessment of the hypothalamic-pituitary-adrenal axis," *Journal of Clinical Endocrinology and Metabolism*, vol. 91, no. 1, pp. 43–47, 2006.

[3] J. H. Wlodarczyk, P. G. Gibson, and M. Caeser, "Impact of inhaled corticosteroids on cortisol suppression in adults with asthma: a quantitative review," *Annals of Allergy, Asthma & Immunology*, vol. 100, no. 1, pp. 23–30, 2008.

[4] I. M. Balfour-Lynn and K. Welch, "Inhaled corticosteroids for cystic fibrosis," *Cochrane Database of Systematic Reviews*, no. 10, p. CD001915, 2014.

[5] J. S. Parmar, T. Howell, J. Kelly, and D. Bilton, "Profound adrenal suppression secondary to treatment with low dose inhaled steroids and itraconazole in allergic bronchopulmonary aspergillosis in cystic fibrosis," *Thorax*, vol. 57, no. 8, pp. 749-750, 2002.

[6] K. M. Main, M. Skov, I. B. Sillesen et al., "Cushing's syndrome due to pharmacological interaction in a cystic fibrosis patient," *Acta Paediatrica*, vol. 91, no. 9, pp. 1008–1011, 2002.

[7] B. B. Albert, M. Jaksic, J. Ramirez et al., "An unusual cause of growth failure in cystic fibrosis: a salutary reminder of the interaction between glucocorticoids and cytochrome P450 inhibiting medication," *Journal of Cystic Fibrosis*, vol. 14, no. 4, pp. e9–e11, 2015.

[8] M. Magnotti and M. Shimshi, "Diagnosing adrenal insufficiency: which test is best–the 1-microg or the 250-microg cosyntropin stimulation test?," *Endocrine Practice*, vol. 14, no. 2, pp. 233–238, 2008.

[9] S. M. Ng, J. C. Agwu, and K. Dwan, "A systematic review and meta-analysis of Synacthen tests for assessing hypothalamic-pituitary-adrenal insufficiency in children," *Archives of Disease in Childhood*, vol. 101, no. 9, pp. 847–853, 2016.

[10] A. K. Younes and N. K. Younes, "Recovery of steroid induced adrenal insufficiency," *Translational Pediatrics*, vol. 6, no. 4, pp. 269–273, 2017.

[11] V. De Sanctis, A. Soliman, M. Yassin, and P. Garofalo, "Cortisol levels in central adrenal insufficiency: light and shade," *Pediatric Endocrinology Reviews*, vol. 12, no. 3, pp. 283–289, 2015.

[12] S. Rajagopala, A. Ramakrishnan, G. Bantwal et al., "Adrenal insufficiency in patients with stable non-cystic fibrosis bronchiectasis," *Indian Journal of Medical Research*, vol. 139, no. 3, pp. 393–401, 2014.

[13] J. Holme, J. W. Tomlinson, R. A. Stockley, P. M. Stewart, N. Barlow, and A. L. Sullivan, "Adrenal suppression in bronchiectasis and the impact of inhaled corticosteroids," *European Respiratory Journal*, vol. 32, no. 4, pp. 1047–1052, 2008.

[14] M. Skov, K. M. Main, I. B. Sillesen, J. Muller, C. Koch, and S. Lanng, "Iatrogenic adrenal insufficiency as a side-effect of combined treatment of itraconazole and budesonide," *European Respiratory Journal*, vol. 20, no. 1, pp. 127–133, 2002.

[15] F. J. Gilchrist, K. J. Cox, R. Rowe et al., "Itraconazole and inhaled fluticasone causing hypothalamic-pituitary-adrenal axis suppression in adults with cystic fibrosis," *Journal of Cystic Fibrosis*, vol. 12, no. 4, pp. 399–402, 2013.

[16] G. Di Dalmazi, U. Pagotto, R. Pasquali, and V. Vicennati, "Glucocorticoids and type 2 diabetes: from physiology to

pathology," *Journal of Nutrition and Metabolism*, vol. 2012, Article ID 525093, 9 pages, 2012.

[17] G. Mastorakos, G. P. Chrousos, and J. S. Weber, "Recombinant interleukin-6 activates the hypothalamic-pituitary-adrenal axis in humans," *Journal of Clinical Endocrinology and Metabolism*, vol. 77, no. 6, pp. 1690–1694, 1993.

[18] R. H. Straub, L. Paimela, R. Peltomaa, J. Scholmerich, and M. Leirisalo-Repo, "Inadequately low serum levels of steroid hormones in relation to interleukin-6 and tumor necrosis factor in untreated patients with early rheumatoid arthritis and reactive arthritis," *Arthritis & Rheumatism*, vol. 46, no. 3, pp. 654–662, 2002.

[19] M. Noni, A. Katelari, G. Dimopoulos et al., "Inhaled corticosteroids and *Aspergillus fumigatus* isolation in cystic fibrosis," *Medical Mycology*, vol. 52, no. 7, pp. 715–722, 2014.

[20] K. Cheng, D. Ashby, and R. L. Smyth, "Oral steroids for long-term use in cystic fibrosis," *Cochrane Database of Systematic Reviews*, no. 12, p. CD000407, 2015.

[21] E. M. Wagner, J. Jenkins, M. G. Perino, A. Sukkar, and W. Mitzner, "Lung and vascular function during chronic severe pulmonary ischemia," *Journal of Applied Physiology*, vol. 110, no. 2, pp. 538–544, 2011.

[22] S. A. McColley, V. Stellmach, S. R. Boas, M. Jain, and S. E. Crawford, "Serum vascular endothelial growth factor is elevated in cystic fibrosis and decreases with treatment of acute pulmonary exacerbation," *American Journal of Respiratory and Critical Care Medicine*, vol. 161, no. 6, pp. 1877–1880, 2000.

[23] E. H. Bel, S. E. Wenzel, P. J. Thompson et al., "Oral glucocorticoid-sparing effect of mepolizumab in eosinophilic asthma," *New England Journal of Medicine*, vol. 371, no. 13, pp. 1189–1197, 2014.

[24] H. Derendorf, G. Hochhaus, B. Meibohm, H. Mollmann, and J. Barth, "Pharmacokinetics and pharmacodynamics of inhaled corticosteroids," *Journal of Allergy and Clinical Immunology*, vol. 101, no. 4, pp. S440–S446, 1998.

[25] D. B. Allen, "Effects of inhaled steroids on growth, bone metabolism and adrenal function," *Expert Review of Respiratory Medicine*, vol. 1, no. 1, pp. 65–74, 2007.

[26] C. P. Woods, N. Argese, M. Chapman et al., "Adrenal suppression in patients taking inhaled glucocorticoids is highly prevalent and management can be guided by morning cortisol," *European Journal of Endocrinology*, vol. 173, no. 5, pp. 633–642, 2015.

Digital Clubbing Is Associated with Higher Serum KL-6 Levels and Lower Pulmonary Function in Patients with Interstitial Lung Disease

Kazushige Shiraishi,[1] Torahiko Jinta,[1] Naoki Nishimura,[1] Hiroshi Nakaoka,[1] Ryosuke Tsugitomi,[1] Kohei Okafuji,[1] Atsushi Kitamura,[1] Yutaka Tomishima,[1] Gautam A. Deshpande,[2] and Tomohide Tamura[1]

[1]*Department of Pulmonary Medicine, St. Luke's International University, St. Luke's International Hospital, Tokyo, Japan*
[2]*Center for Clinical Epidemiology, St. Luke's International University, St. Luke's International Hospital, Tokyo, Japan*

Correspondence should be addressed to Kazushige Shiraishi; shira0124@m.u-tokyo.ac.jp

Academic Editor: Akiteru Goto

Background. Although digital clubbing is a common presentation in patients with interstitial lung disease (ILD), little has been reported regarding its role in assessing patients with ILD. This study evaluated patients with ILD for the presence of clubbing and investigated its association with clinical data. *Methods.* We evaluated patients with ILD who visited the teaching hospital at which the study was conducted, between October 2014 and January 2015. Clubbing, evaluated using a Vernier caliper for individual patients, was defined as a phalangeal depth ratio > 1. We examined the association of clubbing with clinical data. *Results.* Of 102 patients with ILD, we identified 17 (16.7%) with clubbing. The partial pressure of oxygen in arterial blood was lower (65.2 ± 5.9 mmHg versus 80.2 ± 3.1 mmHg; $p = 0.03$), serum Krebs von den Lugen-6 (KL-6) levels were higher (1495.0 ± 277.4 U/mL versus 839.1 ± 70.2 U/mL; $p = 0.001$), and the percent predicted diffusing capacity of carbon monoxide was lower (50.0 ± 6.0 versus 73.5 ± 3.1; $p = 0.002$) in these patients with clubbing. *Conclusions.* Patients with clubbing had lower oxygen levels, higher serum KL-6 levels, and lower pulmonary function than those without clubbing.

1. Introduction

Interstitial lung disease (ILD) is a heterogeneous cluster of pulmonary disorders characterized by diffuse parenchymal lung damage [1]. Disease activity in ILD is objectively assessed by pulmonary function testing, chest radiography, and high-resolution computed tomography (HRCT) [1]. Serum Krebs von den Lugen-6 (KL-6) is a biomarker for ILD [2] and can be used to evaluate disease activity in ILD and to predict clinical outcomes [3].

Digital clubbing was first recognized as a sign of empyema by Hippocrates in the fifth century BC [4]. Studied for centuries, clubbing has been associated with a variety of pulmonary diseases, including infections, ILD, and neoplasms [5]. In the clinic setting, the skilled primary care physician and pulmonology specialist may search for clubbing to identify patients with underlying chronic lung disease. However, little has been reported regarding the value of clubbing when assessing patients with ILD. As such, we carried out a cross-sectional assessment of patients with ILD for the presence of clubbing and investigated its association with clinical data, including blood oxygenation measurements, serum KL-6 levels, and pulmonary function test results.

2. Methods

2.1. Patients and Study Design. This cross-sectional retrospective study examined adult outpatients with a diagnosis of ILD visiting the Pulmonology Department at St. Luke's

Table 1: Characteristics of patients.

Characteristic	Clubbing (−) $n = 85$	Clubbing (+) $n = 17$	p value
Age, years	70.9 ± 12.87	64.2 ± 13.6	0.06
Male sex, number	48 (65)	9 (64)	0.79
Pack-years	26.4 ± 29.2	28.2 ± 40.5	0.83
sPAP, mmHg[†]	30.9 ± 13.0	33.8 ± 14.6	0.49
LVEF, %[†]	62.0 ± 9.7	60.5 ± 9.5	0.61
HRCT imaging patterns			
NSIP	47 (55.3%)	10 (58.8%)	1.00
UIP	12 (14.1%)	2 (11.8%)	1.00
OP	3 (3.5%)	0 (0%)	1.00
Pattern not specified	23 (27.1%)	5 (29.4%)	0.84

Note. Data are means ± standard deviation or number (%); sPAP = systolic pulmonary arterial pressure; LVEF = left ventricular ejection fraction; [†]data were missing for 33 patients in the clubbing (−) group and four patients in the clubbing (+) group for sPAP and 24 patients in the clubbing (−) group and three patients in the clubbing (+) group for LVEF.

International Hospital (Tokyo, Japan) between October 2014 and January 2015. Patients with a history of diseases shown to be associated with clubbing, including lung carcinoma, asbestosis, active tuberculosis, and sarcoidosis [5], were excluded. Each participant was assessed for clubbing after which the medical charts of participants were reviewed and the following data were extracted: age, sex, pack-years of tobacco smoking, systolic pulmonary arterial pressure (sPAP), and left ventricular ejection fraction (LVEF) estimated by Doppler echocardiography, pulse oximeter oxygen saturation (SpO_2), arterial blood gas analysis results, serum KL-6 levels, pulmonary function test results, etiology of ILD, and HRCT imaging patterns of ILD as assessed by radiologists. ILD-GAP index was calculated using the clinical data [6].

2.2. Definition of Clubbing. The presence of clubbing was assessed by objective measurement of a phalangeal depth ratio, calculated by distal phalangeal finger depth (DPD) divided by interphalangeal finger depth (IPD), with the use of a Vernier caliper [7]. Clubbing was defined as the phalangeal depth ratio greater than 1. While there are many techniques available for assessment of clubbing including profile sign, hyponychial angle, and Schamroth sign [4], Myers and Farquhar recommend in their systematic review that the phalangeal depth ratio be used for the objective and quantitative assessment of clubbing [4]. A phalangeal depth ratio above 1 is rare in disease-free subjects and was reported to be independent of race, age, and sex [4]. Technically, the caliper was gently placed on an index finger, and distal/interphalangeal finger depth was measured without pressing the tissue [7].

2.3. Statistical Analysis. Categorical variables were compared using Fisher's exact test, continuous variables were compared using the unpaired t-test, and binomial variables were compared using Fisher's exact test. All statistical analyses were performed using SPSS version 21.0 (SPSS Inc., Armonk, NY, USA). A p value < 0.05 was considered to be statistically significant.

2.4. Ethical Approval. This study was conducted in accordance with the amended Declaration of Helsinki. Ethical approval was provided by the Ethics Committee of St. Luke's International Hospital, and individual participant consent was obtained.

3. Results

3.1. Study Participants. A total of 102 patients with HRCT-confirmed ILD met the inclusion criteria, of whom 17 (16.7%) patients had clubbing. Table 1 shows the clinical and demographic characteristics of patients with ILD. Age, sex, pack-years of smoking, sPAP, LVEF, and HRCT imaging patterns were not significantly different between the two groups. The diagnostic category of ILD, based on the presence of connective tissue disease (CTD) and the high-resolution CT (HRCT) imaging pattern, is shown in Table 2. All patients with connective tissue disease (CTD) had their diagnoses confirmed by an immunology/rheumatology specialist, and a total of 50 patients with connective tissue disease-associated interstitial lung disease (CTD-ILD) were observed. The HRCT imaging pattern was dependent on the radiologists' clinical decision, in accordance with international guidelines [8]. The prevalence of clubbing in relation to each diagnostic category (Table 2) was as follows: non-CTD-ILD with radiological nonspecific interstitial pneumonia (NSIP) pattern, 20.8% ($N = 5$); CTD-ILD, 12.0% ($N = 6$); rheumatoid arthritis-associated interstitial lung disease (RA-ILD), 6.7% ($N = 1$); and systemic sclerosis-associated interstitial lung disease (SSc-ILD), 25.0% ($N = 5$). No clubbing was observed in patients with dermatomyositis-associated interstitial lung disease (DM-ILD) and Sjogren's syndrome-associated interstitial lung disease (SS-ILD).

3.2. Blood Oxygenation Measurements, Serum KL-6, and Pulmonary Function. Table 3 summarizes SpO_2, arterial blood gas results, serum KL-6 levels, and pulmonary function test results for patients with and without clubbing. The following blood oxygenation measurements were significantly lower in those with clubbing: SpO_2 (92.7 ± 1.2 ($N = 17$) versus 96.0 ± 0.3 ($N = 78$); $p < 0.001$) and the partial pressure of oxygen in arterial blood (PaO_2; 65.2 ± 5.9% ($N = 6$) versus 80.2 ± 3.1 mmHg ($N = 23$); $p = 0.033$). Serum KL-6 was significantly higher in patients with clubbing (1495.0 ± 277.4 U/mL ($N = 14$) versus 839.1 ± 70.2 U/mL ($N = 82$); $p = 0.001$). The following pulmonary function test results were significantly lower in those with clubbing: %FEV_1 (82.2 ± 4.7 ($N = 15$) versus 98.9 ± 2.9 ($N = 63$); $p = 0.01$); %FVC (77.7 ± 3.5 ($N = 15$) versus 94.3 ± 2.7 ($N = 63$); $p = 0.006$); %VC (78.6 ± 3.5 ($N = 15$) versus 96.3 ± 2.7 ($N = 63$); $p = 0.003$); and %DLCO (50.0 ± 6.0 ($N = 12$) versus 73.5 ± 3.1 ($N = 57$); $p = 0.002$). Although the difference was not significant, the ILD-GAP index was higher in

Table 2: Diagnostic category of participants.

Diagnostic category	Clubbing (−) $n = 85$	Clubbing (+) $n = 17$	p value	Prevalence of clubbing
CTD-ILD	44 (51.8%)	6 (35.3%)	0.29	12.0%
RA-ILD	14 (16.5%)	1 (5.9%)	0.46	6.7%
NSIP pattern	7	1	—	—
UIP pattern	3	0	—	—
Pattern not specified	4	0	—	—
DM-ILD	12 (14.1%)	0 (0%)	1	0.0%
NSIP pattern	12	0	—	—
SSc-ILD	15 (17.6%)	5 (29.4%)	0.32	25.0%
NSIP pattern	8	4	—	—
UIP pattern	1	0	—	—
OP pattern	1	0	—	—
Pattern not specified	5	1	—	—
SS-ILD	3 (3.5%)	0 (0%)	1	0.0%
NSIP pattern	1	0	—	—
UIP pattern	1	0	—	—
OP pattern	1	0	—	—
Non-CTD-ILD	41 (48.2%)	11 (64.7%)	0.29	21.1%
NSIP pattern	19 (22.4%)	5 (29.4%)	0.54	20.8%
HP suspected	1	1	—	—
IIP	0	1	—	—
UIP pattern	7 (8.2%)	2 (11.8%)	0.64	22.2%
HP suspected	1	0	—	—
OP pattern	1 (1.2%)	0 (0%)	1	0.0%
Pattern not specified	14 (16.5%)	4 (23.5%)	0.49	22.2%

CTD-ILD = connective tissue disease-associated interstitial lung disease; RA = rheumatoid arthritis; NSIP = nonspecific interstitial pneumonia; UIP = usual interstitial pneumonia; DM = dermatomyositis; SSc = systemic sclerosis; OP = organizing pneumonia; SS = Sjogren's disease; HP = hypersensitivity pneumonia; IIP = idiopathic interstitial pneumonia.

patients with clubbing (2.17 ± 0.5 U/mL ($N = 12$) versus 1.28 ± 0.3 U/mL ($N = 57$); $p = 0.154$).

Similarly, SpO_2 was significantly lower in patients with clubbing in the CTD-ILD group (93 ± 2.5 ($N = 6$) versus 96.6 ± 0.3 ($N = 38$); $p = 0.004$), serum KL-6 was significantly higher (2262 ± 547.4 U/mL ($N = 6$) versus 969.7 ± 108.2 U/mL ($N = 43$); $p = 0.0006$), and pulmonary function test results were significantly lower in those with clubbing (%DLCO: 45.3 ± 4.1 ($N = 6$) versus 73.5 ± 4.2 ($N = 33$); $p = 0.008$). Although not significant, the same trend was observed in the non-CTD-ILD NSIP group. PaO_2 values for the CTD-ILD group and the non-CTD-ILD NSIP group are not shown because the numbers of measurements obtained were very small.

4. Discussion

In this study, we showed that the presence of clubbing in patients with ILD was associated with lower blood oxygenation levels, higher serum KL-6 levels, and lower pulmonary function when compared to those without clubbing, regardless of the underlying etiology of ILD. Because lower blood oxygenation levels and low pulmonary function are seen in patients with advanced ILD, our results suggest that clubbing may be associated with disease progression. Higher serum KL-6 levels in patients with clubbing also suggest that ILD disease activity may also be associated with the presence of clubbing. In concordance with these findings, the ILD-GAP score was higher in patients with clubbing, suggesting that the presence of clubbing could also be associated with poor prognosis.

We also found that the prevalence of clubbing in patients with radiological NSIP pattern, RA-ILD, and SSc-ILD was 20.8%, 6.7%, and 25%, respectively. To our knowledge, this study is the first to report the prevalence of clubbing in SSc-ILD. The prevalence of clubbing in NSIP and RA-ILD was consistent with that in previous reports [9–11]. We did not find any patient with clubbing in those with DM-ILD, which is consistent with previous reports of clubbing being rare in DM-ILD [12]. We confirmed that clubbing is indeed uncommon in DM-ILD; this result would suggest that clubbing in patients with DM-ILD may indicate the presence of an occult pathology, such as lung carcinoma or other CTD. Ishioka et al. reported that four out of 33 patients with CTD-ILD had clubbing, and the prevalence of clubbing in CTD-ILD was significantly lower than in patients with idiopathic interstitial pneumonia (16 out of 44 patients) [13]. Similarly, the prevalence of clubbing in patients with CTD-ILD (12.0%) was lower than in patients with non-CTD-ILD (21.1%) in the

TABLE 3: Clinical data analysis between patients with and without clubbing.

Variable	Clubbing (−)	Clubbing (+)	p value
All patients with ILD[†]	$n = 85$	$n = 17$	—
SpO_2, %	96.0 ± 0.3	92.7 ± 1.2	<0.001
PaO_2, mmHg	80.2 ± 3.1	65.2 ± 5.9	0.033
$PaCO_2$, mmHg	36.8 ± 1.1	39.5 ± 1.6	0.263
KL-6, U/mL	839 ± 70	1495 ± 277	0.001
%FEV1	98.9 ± 2.9	82.2 ± 4.7	0.010
%FVC	94.3 ± 2.7	77.7 ± 3.5	0.006
%VC	96.3 ± 2.7	78.6 ± 3.5	0.003
%DLCO	73.5 ± 3.1	50.0 ± 6.0	0.002
ILD-GAP index	1.28 ± 0.3	2.17 ± 0.5	0.154
CTD-ILD[‡]	$n = 44$	$n = 6$	—
SpO_2, %	96.6 ± 0.3	93 ± 2.5	0.004
KL-6, U/mL	970 ± 108	2262 ± 547	0.001
%FEV1	94.8 ± 3.5	78.7 ± 9.9	0.09
%FVC	91.3 ± 3.0	73.8 ± 8.3	0.04
%VC	94.0 ± 2.9	75.5 ± 8.3	0.02
%DLCO	73.5 ± 4.2	45.3 ± 4.1	0.008
ILD-GAP index	0.03 ± 0.2	0.83 ± 0.6	0.208
Non-CTD-ILD, NSIP pattern[§]	$n = 19$	$n = 5$	—
SpO_2, %	96.0 ± 0.3	95 ± 0.5	0.173
KL-6, U/mL	669 ± 66	1078 ± 390	0.078
%FEV1	101.7 ± 4.7	82.8 ± 8.6	0.083
%FVC	94.3 ± 2.7	77.7 ± 3.5	0.006
%VC	95.4 ± 6.8	80.9 ± 3.1	0.297
%DLCO	77.0 ± 6.5	53.0 ± 14.8	0.129
ILD-GAP index	3.00 ± 0.3	3.00 ± 0.6	1.000

Note. Data are means ± standard error; SpO_2 = pulse oximeter oxygen saturation; PaO_2 = partial pressure of oxygen in arterial blood; $PaCO_2$ = partial pressure of carbon dioxide in arterial blood; ILD = interstitial lung disease; KL-6 = Krebs von den Lugen-6; FEV1 = forced expiratory volume in 1 second; FVC = forced vital capacity; VC = vital capacity; DLCO = diffusing capacity of carbon monoxide; NSIP = nonspecific interstitial pneumonia; CTD-ILD = connective tissue disease-associated interstitial lung disease; [†]data were missing for eight patients in the clubbing (−) group for SpO_2; 62 patients in the clubbing (−) group and 11 patients in the clubbing (−) group for PaO_2 and $PaCO_2$, respectively; three patients in the clubbing (−) group and one patient in the clubbing (+) group for KL-6; 22 patients in the clubbing (−) group and two patients in the clubbing (+) group for %FEV1, %FVC, and %VC; 28 patients in the clubbing (−) group and five patients in the clubbing (+) group for %DLCO and ILD-GAP index; [‡]data were missing for six patients in the clubbing (−) group for SpO_2; one patient in the clubbing (−) group for KL-6; nine patients in the clubbing (−) group for %FEV1, %FVC, and %VC; and 11 patients in the clubbing (−) group for %DLCO and ILD-GAP index; [§]data were missing for one patient in the clubbing (−) group for KL-6; four patients in the clubbing (−) group for %FEV1, %FVC, and %VC; and one patient in the clubbing (−) group for %DLCO and ILD-GAP index.

current study. There may be specific cellular or molecular mechanisms underlying CTD-ILD that suppress the emergence of clubbing, or there may be mechanisms in non-CTD-ILD that promote the emergence of clubbing. Further research on the pathophysiology of clubbing is needed to explain the difference.

We found that hypoxia is associated with clubbing in patients with ILD, and we presume from this that hypoxia could be responsible, to some extent, for clubbing in the study population. Several mechanisms including hypoxia and growth factors have been proposed for the pathogenesis of clubbing; however, the true mechanism of pathogenesis remains elusive [5]. Uppal et al. found that 15-hydroxyprostaglandin dehydrogenase, the enzyme-mediating prostaglandin degradation, is responsible for familial cases of clubbing and hypertrophic osteoarthropathy [14]. They also showed that elevated prostaglandin E2 (PGE2) levels were found in homozygous familial cases [14]. Their report suggests that clubbing may be mediated by PGE2. In accordance with that theory, Kozak et al. reported that clubbing in patients with lung cancer was associated with elevated urinary levels of PGE2 [15]. Cyclooxygenase-derived prostanoids are reported to be important mediators that regulate pulmonary function in normal and pathological conditions, and with regard to the relationship between PGE2 and ILD, PGE2 has been shown to be a key factor that controls fibroblast differentiation and proliferation in mouse models of pulmonary fibrosis [16]. In addition, cyclooxygenase-2, which induces PGE2, is reported to be widely expressed in the epithelium of patients with idiopathic pulmonary fibrosis (IPF), asbestosis, or cryptogenic organizing pneumonia [17]. Given these findings, measuring serum PGE2 levels in patients with ILD who have clubbing might be an interesting area of future research, although other factors, including hypoxia, growth hormones, platelet-derived growth factor, and vascular endothelial growth factor, have also been discussed in relation to the pathogenesis of clubbing [5].

This study has some limitations. First, many data were missing in the pulmonary function tests, which could have biased the results. However, missing data were mostly in the clubbing (−) population, and the patients without pulmonary function test data were clinically stable. That is, the results might have favored the clubbing (+) population. Second, radiographic quantification and histopathological assessment of ILD were not performed. In addition, although 52 non-CTD-ILD patients were identified in the study, patients with IPF or hypersensitivity pneumonitis were not included. This was due to difficulties in the diagnosis of interstitial pneumonia, the short study period, and the retrospective nature of the study. Lastly, the present study was a single-center, cross-sectional study, and the number of outcomes was not enough for adequate power in some analyses.

5. Conclusions

In conclusion, patients with clubbing showed lower blood oxygenation levels, higher serum KL-6 levels, and lower pulmonary function when compared with patients without clubbing, regardless of the underlying etiology of ILD. The results suggest that clubbing may be associated with disease progression, disease activity, and prognosis in ILD.

Disclosure

An earlier version of this work was presented as a poster at the American Thoracic Society International Conference, 2016 [18].

Acknowledgments

The authors thank the staff of the Department of Pulmonary Medicine for their encouragement during the study and the staff of the Center for Information Systems for patient identification.

References

[1] S. C. Mathai and S. K. Danoff, "Management of interstitial lung disease associated with connective tissue disease," *BMJ*, vol. 352, p. h6819, 2016.

[2] J. Kobayashi and S. Kitamura, "KL-6: a serum marker for interstitial pneumonia," *Chest*, vol. 108, no. 2, pp. 311–315, 1995.

[3] N. Ishikawa, N. Hattori, A. Yokoyama, and N. Kohno, "Utility of KL-6/MUC1 in the clinical management of interstitial lung diseases," *Respiratory Investigation*, vol. 50, no. 1, pp. 3–13, 2012.

[4] K. A. Myers and D. R. Farquhar, "The rational clinical examination. Does this patient have clubbing?," *JAMA*, vol. 286, no. 3, pp. 341–347, 2001.

[5] K. E. Spicknall, M. J. Zirwas, and J. C. English III, "Clubbing: an update on diagnosis, differential diagnosis, pathophysiology, and clinical relevance," *Journal of the American Academy of Dermatology*, vol. 52, no. 6, pp. 1020–1028, 2005.

[6] C. J. Ryerson, E. Vittinghoff, B. Ley et al., "Predicting survival across chronic interstitial lung disease: the ILD-GAP model," *Chest*, vol. 145, no. 4, pp. 723–728, 2014.

[7] R. P. Baughman, K. L. Gunther, J. A. Buchsbaum, and E. E. Lower, "Prevalence of digital clubbing in bronchogenic carcinoma by a new digital index," *Clinical and Experimental Rheumatology*, vol. 16, no. 1, pp. 21–26, 1998.

[8] G. Raghu, H. R. Collard, J. J. Egan et al., "An official ATS/ERS/JRS/ALAT statement: idiopathic pulmonary fibrosis: evidence-based guidelines for diagnosis and management," *American Journal of Respiratory and Critical Care Medicine*, vol. 183, no. 6, pp. 788–824, 2011.

[9] J. McDonagh, M. Greaves, A. R. Wright, C. Heycock, J. P. Owen, and C. Kelly, "High resolution computed tomography of the lungs in patients with rheumatoid arthritis and interstitial lung disease," *British Journal of Rheumatology*, vol. 33, no. 2, pp. 118–122, 1994.

[10] B. A. Rajasekaran, D. Shovlin, P. Lord, and C. A. Kelly, "Interstitial lung disease in patients with rheumatoid arthritis: a comparison with cryptogenic fibrosing alveolitis," *Rheumatology*, vol. 40, no. 9, pp. 1022–1025, 2001.

[11] X. Li, C. Chen, J. Xu et al., "Nonspecific interstitial pneumonia and usual interstitial pneumonia: comparison of the clinicopathologic features and prognosis," *Journal of Thoracic Disease*, vol. 6, no. 10, pp. 1476–1481, 2014.

[12] B. Bradley, H. M. Branley, J. J. Egan et al., "Interstitial lung disease guideline: the British Thoracic Society in collaboration with the Thoracic Society of Australia and New Zealand and the Irish Thoracic Society," *Thorax*, vol. 63, no. 5, pp. v1–v58, 2008.

[13] S. Ishioka, K. Nakamura, A. Maeda et al., "Clinical evaluation of idiopathic interstitial pneumonia and interstitial pneumonia associated with collagen vascular disease using logistic regression analysis," *Internal Medicine*, vol. 39, no. 3, pp. 213–219, 2000.

[14] S. Uppal, C. P. Diggle, I. M. Carr et al., "Mutations in 15-hydroxyprostaglandin dehydrogenase cause primary hypertrophic osteoarthropathy," *Nature Genetics*, vol. 40, no. 6, pp. 789–793, 2008.

[15] K. R. Kozak, G. L. Milne, S. M. Bentzen, and T. I. Yock, "Elevation of prostaglandin E_2 in lung cancer patients with digital clubbing," *Journal of Thoracic Oncology*, vol. 7, no. 12, pp. 1877-1878, 2012.

[16] R. T. Dackor, J. Cheng, J. W. Voltz et al., "Prostaglandin E_2 protects murine lungs from bleomycin-induced pulmonary fibrosis and lung dysfunction," *American Journal of Physiology–Lung Cellular and Molecular Physiology*, vol. 301, no. 5, pp. L645–L655, 2011.

[17] E. Lappi-Blanco, R. Kaarteenaho-Wiik, P. K. Maasilta, S. Anttila, P. Pääkkö, and H. J. Wolff, "COX-2 is widely expressed in metaplastic epithelium in pulmonary fibrous disorders," *American Journal of Clinical Pathology*, vol. 126, no. 5, pp. 717–724, 2006.

[18] K. Shiraishi, T. Jinta, N. Nishimura et al., "Digital clubbing is associated with higher serum KL-6 levels and lower pulmonary function in patients with interstitial lung disease," in *Proceedings of the poster presented at the American Thoracic Society International Conference*, San Francisco, CA, USA, May 2016, http://www.atsjournals.org/doi/pdf/10.1164/ajrccm-conference.2016.193.1_MeetingAbstracts.A5006.

8

Endobronchial Ultrasound Transbronchial Needle Aspiration in Thoracic Diseases: Much More than Mediastinal Staging

Juliana Guarize,[1] **Monica Casiraghi**,[1] **Stefano Donghi**,[1] **Cristina Diotti**,[1] **Nicolo Vanoni**,[1] **Rosalia Romano**,[1] **Chiara Casadio**,[2] **Daniela Brambilla**,[1] **Patrick Maisonneuve**,[3] **Francesco Petrella**,[1,4] **and Lorenzo Spaggiari**[1,4]

[1]*Division of Thoracic Surgery, European Institute of Oncology, Milan, Italy*
[2]*Division of Pathology, European Institute of Oncology, Milan, Italy*
[3]*Division of Epidemiology and Biostatistics, European Institute of Oncology, Milan, Italy*
[4]*Department of Oncology and Hemato-Oncology, University of Milan, Milan, Italy*

Correspondence should be addressed to Juliana Guarize; juliana.guarize@ieo.it

Academic Editor: Hisao Imai

Background and Objective. EBUS-TBNA has revolutionized the diagnostic approach to thoracic diseases from a surgical to minimally invasive procedure. In non small-cell lung cancer (NCSLC) patients, EBUS-TBNA is able to dictate the consecutive therapy both for early and advanced stages, providing pathological diagnosis, mediastinal staging, and even adequate specimens for molecular analysis. This study reports on the ability of EBUS-TBNA to make different diagnoses and dictates the consecutive therapy in a large cohort of patients presenting different thoracic diseases. *Methods.* All procedures performed from January 2012 to September 2016 were reviewed. Five groups of patients were created according to the main indications for the procedure. Group 1: lung cancer staging; Group 2: pathological diagnosis in advanced stage lung cancer; Group 3: lymphadenopathy in previous malignancies; Group 4: pulmonary lesions; Group 5: unknown origin lymphadenopathy. In each group, the diagnostic yield of the procedure was analysed. Non malignant diagnosis at EBUS-TBNA was confirmed by a surgical procedure or clinical and radiological follow-up. *Results.* 1891 patients were included in the analysis. Sensitivity, negative predictive value, and diagnostic accuracy in each group were 90.7%, 79.4%, and 93.1% in Group 1; 98.5%, 50%, and 98.5% in Group 2; 92.4%, 85.1%, and 94.7% in Group 3; 90.9%, 51.0%, and 91.7% in Group 4; and 25%, 83.3%, and 84.2% in Group 5. Overall sensitivity, negative predictive value, and accuracy were 91.7%, 78.5%, and 93.6%, respectively. *Conclusions.* EBUS-TBNA is the best approach for invasive mediastinal investigation, confirming its strategic role and high accuracy in thoracic oncology.

1. Introduction

Mediastinal adenopathy has always been assessed by radiological imaging such as computed tomography (CT) and positron emission tomography (PET), with high sensitivity but a low diagnostic accuracy for the purposes of correct clinical decision-making [1]. To date, mediastinoscopy has been considered the gold standard for diagnosis and mediastinal staging with high sensitivity and accuracy, but the procedure has been progressively underused due to its high invasiveness, risk of complications, and the need to be performed in experienced centres [2].

In the early 2000's, a minimally invasive convex probe endobronchial ultrasound (EBUS) procedure able to perform real-time transbronchial needle aspiration (TBNA) was described with high accuracy for mediastinal and hilar lymph node staging [3]. Since then, EBUS-TBNA has gradually changed the way mediastinal staging is performed and rapidly improved its value with new indications in lung cancer management, becoming the standard of care [4].

In thoracic oncology, EBUS-TBNA has revolutionized the diagnostic approach to lung cancer and other neoplasms from a surgical to minimally invasive procedure. Especially in non small-cell lung cancer (NCSLC), EBUS-TBNA is able to dictate the consecutive therapy both for early and advanced stages, providing pathological diagnosis, mediastinal staging, and even adequate specimens for molecular analysis [5]. In addition, EBUS-TBNA has been described in different clinical scenarios, particularly for the diagnosis and definition of granulomatosis such as sarcoidosis [6] and tuberculosis [7] and for pathological assessment of mediastinal and hilar recurrences from previous malignancies [8, 9].

This study reports the largest published experience in the use of EBUS-TBNA in a high-volume thoracic oncology institution. We aimed to describe the utility and diagnostic yield of EBUS-TBNA in different clinical scenarios in thoracic diseases, dividing our series into five different groups according to the main indication for the procedure (Group 1: lung cancer staging, Group 2: pathological diagnosis in advanced stage lung cancer, Group 3: lymphadenopathy in previous malignancies, Group 4: pulmonary lesions, and Group 5: unknown origin lymphadenopathy) and reporting our results in terms of sensitivity, negative predictive value, and diagnostic accuracy.

2. Methods

This single-centre retrospective study with a prospective follow-up was approved by the Institutional Review Board and the individual consent was obtained.

From January 2012 to September 2016, 1958 EBUS-TBNA procedures were performed at our institution. The indications for EBUS-TBNA, lymph node stations, number of lymph nodes sampled, cytological results, and cancer cell type were obtained for the analysis. To better standardize the series, different groups of patients were defined according to the indication for the procedure.

Group 1 included patients referred for EBUS-TBNA for mediastinal staging in potentially operable lung cancer and patients with mediastinal involvement but no evidence of distant metastasis. Patients with proven or suspected NSCLC were included, and pathological cell type was performed in the same procedure. According to our institutional protocol, suspect lymph nodes were defined as lymph nodes with a pathological PET scan uptake and/or enlarged lymph nodes with more than 1 cm in the short axis at the CT scan.

Group 2 included patients with metastatic and/or bulky mediastinal disease referred for EBUS-TBNA for pathological diagnosis and molecular mutational analysis for targeted therapy; Group 3 included patients with a previous (thoracic or extrathoracic) malignancy who developed mediastinal and hilar lymphadenopathies suspected for recurrence; Group 4 included patients who underwent EBUS-TBNA for primary tissue sampling in pulmonary lesions (paratracheal or peribronchial); and Group 5 included patients with mediastinal and hilar lymphadenopathy of unknown origin with no history of malignancy. Diagnostic sensitivity, accuracy, and negative predictive value were calculated according to standard definitions. Sensitivity was calculated for the diagnosis of malignancy.

EBUS-TBNA samples were considered diagnostic when a definitive diagnosis was obtained. Lymph node samples negative for malignancy underwent surgical confirmation (mediastinoscopy or VATS) or clinical and radiological follow-up (at least 12 months of follow-up). Patients with loss of follow-up were excluded.

EBUS-TBNA samples were considered false negative when surgery changed the final diagnosis, or there was clinical and radiological progression of the disease during follow-up. EBUS-TBNA samples insufficient or inadequate for diagnosis were considered false negative in the calculation of diagnostic accuracy. Patients without a specific diagnosis at EBUS-TBNA (benign or malignant) but a definitive non-malignant diagnosis at mediastinoscopy were considered false negative.

During EBUS-TBNA procedures, all lymphadenopathies with increased PET scan pathological uptake were sampled in patients with a non-malignant diagnosis at rapid on-site evaluation (ROSE), and at least one mediastinal and two hilar stations were sampled when ROSE was negative for tumour cells and suspected for lymphadenitis granulomatosis.

Patients with negative EBUS-TBNA samples were referred for confirmatory surgical procedures after a multidisciplinary team discussion with thoracic surgeons, pulmonologists, radiologists, oncologists, and radiotherapists when lymphadenopathies were considered highly suspicious for recurrence based on CT and/or PET scan characteristics.

2.1. EBUS-TBNA Technical Aspects. EBUS-TBNA procedures were performed under local anaesthesia (1% lidocaine), and moderate sedation was provided by an anaesthesiologist with spontaneous ventilation. The same team of interventional pulmonologists using a convex probe (EBUS Convex Probe BF-UC180F; Olympus) and a dedicated ultrasound processor (EU-ME1; Olympus) performed all procedures. All EBUS-TBNA specimens were collected with a 22 gauge dedicated needle (Vizishot NA-201SX-4022; Olympus).

A very small amount of the aspirated material was pushed out by the internal stylet and smeared onto glass slides for immediate on-site evaluation (ROSE). Mirror slides were alcohol-fixed for posterior evaluation. Air-dried smears were immediately stained with a modified May-Grünwald Giemsa stain (MGG Quick Stain; Bio-Optica, Milan, Italy) and evaluated by the cytopathologist to confirm adequate tumour cells and/or lymph node material. The remaining aspirate and other needle passages (at least three needle passages each station) were fixed in a formalin solution for cell block processing and histological evaluation. Alcohol-fixed smears were stained with Papanicolaou and haematoxylin-eosin stains.

3. Results

Out of 1958 patients, 1891 were included in the study. Sixty-seven patients were excluded from statistical analysis due to loss of follow-up with the impossibility to confirm the negativity of lymph node samples. Patients' mean age was 65 years (range: 20–92), 1197 (63.3%) were men.

The leading indication for EBUS-TBNA at our institution was lung cancer staging in 728 (38.5%) patients

Table 1: Patient characteristics and indications for EBUS-TBNA.

Variable	N° or median (range)
Patients (total)	1891
Sex	
Male	1197
Female	694
Age (years)	65 (20–92)
Indications for EBUS-TBNA	
Lung cancer staging	728
Pathological diagnosis and mutational status in advanced stage lung cancer	401
Lymphadenopathy in previous malignancy	320
Diagnosis of pulmonary lesions	290
Unknown origin lymphadenopathy	152

Table 2: Lymph node stations sampled by EBUS-TBNA in 1569 patients*.

Stations	Right		Left
Total		**2298**	
Superior mediastinal		**1003**	
Highest mediastinal (station 1)	1		1
Upper paratracheal (2R/2L)	56		8
Lower paratracheal (4R/4L)	740		197
Inferior mediastinal			
Subcarinal (7)		789	
N1 nodes		**506**	
Hilar (10R/10L)	37		20
Interlobar (11R/11L)	191		174
Lobar (12R/12L)	53		30
Segmental (13R/13L)	0		1

*Tissue sampling of pulmonary lesions in 322 cases.

followed by pathological diagnosis and mutational status in advanced stage lung cancer in 401 (21.2%) patients, lymphadenopathy in previous malignancies in 320 (17%) cases, diagnosis of pulmonary lesions in 290 (15.3%), and diagnosis of unknown origin lymphadenopathy in 152 (8%) patients. Patient characteristics and indications for the procedures are reported in Table 1.

A total of 2298 lymph node stations were sampled: 1003 superior mediastinal: 2 high upper station #1, 56 station #2R, 8 station #2L, 740 station #4R, and 197 station #4L; 789 subcarinal station #7; 506 N1 nodes: 57 hilar (37 station #10R and 20 station #10L), 365 interlobar (191 station #11R and 174 station #11L), 83 lobar (53 station #12R and 30 station #12L), and 1 segmental station #13L. Lymph node sampled locations and number of lymph nodes are listed in Table 2.

Cytological diagnoses were adenocarcinoma in 692 patients, squamous cell carcinoma in 216, neuroendocrine tumours in 143 (102 small-cell lung cancer (SCLC), 19 large-cell neuroendocrine tumours, 9 mixed large- and small-cell neuroendocrine tumours, 10 typical carcinoids, 3 atypical carcinoids), 154 metastases from extrathoracic malignancy, 65 poorly differentiated NSCLC, 24 lymphoproliferative disorders, 34 other malignancies (1 thymoma, 8 mesothelioma, 3 adenoid cystic carcinoma, 6 mixed tumours, 9 poorly differentiated epithelial tumours of unknown origin, 1 sarcoma, and 3 sarcomatoid carcinomas), 100 lymphadenitis granulomatosis (97 sarcoid-like reaction and 3 tuberculosis), 316 normal/reactive lymph nodes, and 28 other non-neoplastic diagnoses (Table 3).

Overall sensitivity, negative predictive value, and diagnostic accuracy were 91.7% (95% CI: 90.1–93.0), 78.5% (95% CI: 74.9–81.7), and 93.6% (95% CI: 92.4–94.6), respectively.

3.1. Group 1: Lung Cancer Staging. Out of 728 (60.2%) patients, 438 underwent EBUS-TBNA for mediastinal staging and the diagnosis of the cell-type tumour in the same procedure, and 244 (33.5%) had a previous pathological diagnosis of NSCLC, and EBUS-TBNA was performed for complete mediastinal staging, and in 46 (6.3%) patients, EBUS-TBNA was performed for restaging the mediastinum after induction chemotherapy for stage IIIA (pN2) NSCLC. In this group, EBUS-TBNA was diagnostic for malignancy in 485 (66.6%) patients, and a mean of 1, 5 lymph nodes per patient was biopsied. In 187 (25.7%) cases, EBUS-TBNA revealed normal or reactive lymph node samples, and in six (0.8%), EBUS-TBNA revealed a granulomatous reaction in five cases of sarcoid-like reaction compatible with sarcoidosis and one case of necrotizing granulomatosis with a positive culture for *Mycobacterium tuberculosis*.

Malignant diagnoses included 278 adenocarcinoma, 102 squamous cell carcinoma, 55 neuroendocrine, 27 poorly differentiated nonsmall-cell lung cancer, and 23 other malignancies (6 metastasis from a nonthoracic malignancy, 5 lymphoma, 4 mesothelioma, 1 carcinosarcoma, 1 mixed squamous cell and adenocarcinoma, and 6 undifferentiated epithelioid neoplasms).

Fourty-six patients underwent EBUS-TBNA for restaging the mediastinum after neoadjuvant chemotherapy. There were 16 out of 46 (34.8%) positive for malignancy and 6 (13%) false negative cases. From false negative cases, four patients received chemotherapy and mediastinal radiotherapy and two patients' neoadjuvant chemotherapy. Sensitivity, negative predictive value, and diagnostic accuracy in this subgroup of patients were 66.7% (95% CI: 45.4–82.8), 78.1% (95% CI: 61.2–89), and 84.8% (95% CI: 71.8–92.4), respectively.

Among 193 patients with a nonmalignant diagnosis at EBUS-TBNA, 146 underwent surgical procedures for primary tumours confirming the negativity of lymph node samples, and 47 patients were excluded from surgery for clinical reasons and underwent a mean of 17.9 month's clinical and radiological follow-up. In this group, there were 50 (6.9%) false-negative samples. Sensitivity, negative predictive value, and diagnostic accuracy in the staging group were 90.7% (95% CI: 87.9–92.8), 79.4% (95% CI: 73.9–84.0), and 93.1% (95% CI: 91.1–94.8), respectively.

3.2. Group 2: Pathological Diagnosis and Mutational Status in Advanced Stage Lung Cancer. This group comprised 401 patients. In 344 (85.8%) patients, EBUS-TBNA was performed

Table 3: Cytological results of EBUS-TBNA.

Cytological results	Number of patients
Adenocarcinoma	692
Squamous cell carcinoma	216
Neuroendocrine tumour	143
SCLC	102
Large-cell neuroendocrine tumour	19
Mixed large- and small-cell neuroendocrine	9
Typical carcinoid	10
Atypical carcinoid	3
Metastasis from extrathoracic malignancy	154
NSCLC poorly differentiated (NAS)	65
Lymphoproliferative disorders	24
Other nonneoplastic diagnosis	28
Lymphadenitis granulomatosis	100
Sarcoid-like granulomas	97
Tuberculosis	3
Other malignancies*	34
Reactive/normal lymph nodes	316

*Other malignancies included 1 thymoma, 8 mesothelioma, 3 adenoid cystic carcinoma, 6 mixed tumours, 9 poorly differentiated epithelial tumours of unknown origin, 1 sarcoma, and 3 sarcomatoid carcinoma.

for the first cell type diagnosis in stages IIIB and IV lung cancer, and in 57 (14.2%) patients, the procedure was performed after an initial established pathological diagnosis for tissue sampling for molecular analysis including the epidermal growth factor (EGFR) mutational profile, anaplastic lymphoma kinase (ALK) fusion genes, and mesenchymal-epithelial transition (MET) protooncogene amplification. Sensitivity, negative predictive value, and diagnostic accuracy in this group were 98.5% (95% CI: 96.7–99.3), 50% (95% CI: 25.4–74.6), and 98.5% (95% CI: 96.8–99.3), respectively.

3.3. Group 3: Lymphadenopathy in Previous Malignancy. Out of 320 (59.4%) patients, 190 had a diagnosis of a recurrence of a previous tumour and 113 (35.3%) had a different diagnosis from the previous tumour. There were 17 (5.3%) false negative cases. In 97 patients, EBUS-TBNA revealed a definitive nonmalignant diagnosis, and 35 patients had evidence of a granulomatosis disease. Twenty-two out of 114 (19.3%) patients with nonmalignant diagnoses at EBUS-TBNA underwent mediastinoscopy or other surgical procedures to confirm the negativity of EBUS-TBNA diagnosis, and 92 (80.7%) patients underwent clinical and radiological median follow-up of 17 months. Sensitivity, negative predictive value, and diagnostic accuracy were 92.4% (95% CI: 88.1–95.2), 85.1% (95% CI: 77.4–90.5), and 94.7% (95% CI: 91.7–96.7), respectively.

3.4. Group 4: Pulmonary Lesions. EBUS-TBNA was diagnostic for malignancy in 241 out of 290 (83.1%) cases. Cytological diagnoses were 10 lymphoproliferative disorders, 95 adenocarcinomas, 55 squamous cell carcinoma, 25 neuroendocrine tumours, 29 metastasis from other neoplasms, 14 poorly differentiated nonsmall-cell lung cancer, and 13 other malignancies (2 mixed adenocarcinomas and neuroendocrine, 2 adenoid cystic carcinomas, 1 pleomorphic carcinoma, 1 sarcomatoid carcinoma, 1 nonspecific CTM, 3 epithelioid mesotheliomas, 1 poorly differentiated epithelioid neoplasm, 1 mesenchymal neuron neoplasm, and 1 sarcoma). EBUS-TBNA revealed a nonmalignant diagnosis in 25 cases: 5 hamartomas, 4 fibrotic lesions after radiotherapy, 6 bronchogenic cyst, 1 pericardial cyst, 1 benign leiomyoma, 5 pneumonias, 1 mycetoma and 2 cases of granulomatosis (1sarcoidosis and 1 tuberculosis). In this group of patients, sensitivity, negative predictive value, and diagnostic accuracy were 90.9% (95% CI: 86.9–93.8), 51.0% (95% CI: 37.5–64.4), and 91.7% (95% CI: 88.0–94.4), respectively.

3.5. Group 5: Unknown Origin Lymphadenopathy. This group included 152 patients: 59 granulomatosis lymphadenitis, 60 reactive lymph nodes, 3 lymphoproliferative disorders, 2 adenocarcinomas, 2 metastasis from other sites (thyroid and breast), 1 small-cell lung cancer, 1 ectopic thymus tissue, and 24 false negative samples. Sensitivity, negative predicted value, and diagnostic accuracy were 25% (95% CI: 13.3–42.1), 83.3% (95% CI: 76.4–88.5), and 84.2% (95% CI: 77.6–89.2), respectively. The diagnostic performance of EBUS-TBNA in the different groups of patients according to clinical indication for the procedure is shown in Table 4.

4. Discussion

Many literature studies have reported on EBUS-TBNA experience for mediastinal staging in lung cancer patients and some have described the utility of EBUS-TBNA in other pathologies with mediastinal lymphadenopathies such as sarcoidosis, tuberculosis, and lymphoma [10, 11].

During the last decade, EBUS-TBNA has become an essential diagnostic procedure in thoracic disease, revolutionizing the approach to diagnosis and treatment and guiding the best treatment option in a large number of patients. To date, the procedure has been widely used to perform mediastinal staging and has been included in almost all guidelines as the preferred first approach for invasive mediastinal staging in lung cancer patients [4, 12].

A recent meta-analysis showed a sensitivity of EBUS-TBNA for mediastinal staging ranging from 81 to 95% [13]. Likewise, an Italian multicentre trial published in 2017 analysed 485 patients showing a sensitivity of 90% with a diagnostic accuracy of 93% [14]. In agreement with these publications, our study showed an EBUS-TBNA sensitivity for malignant disease of 90.7% and a diagnostic accuracy of 93.1% in 728 patients in our Group 1 patients (lung cancer staging). Surprisingly, the final EBUS-TBNA diagnosis was lymphoma in five patients with a single pulmonary lesion and mediastinal lymphadenopathies highly suspected for lung cancer. EBUS-TBNA samples were able to subtype the lymphoma in three of the five (60%) cases achieving a definitive diagnosis of Hodgkin's lymphoma, classic variation, showing the feasibility of lymphoma diagnosis and subclassification by EBUS-TBNA

TABLE 4: Diagnostic performance of EBUS in the different groups.

EBUS	Overall	Group 1	Group 2	Group 3	Group 4	Group 5
Total	1891	728	401	320	290	152
True negative	441	193	6	97	25	120
False negative	121	50	6	17	24	24
True positive	1329	485	389	206	241	8
Performance	% (95% CI)	% (95% CI)	% (95% CI)	% (95% CI)	% (95% CI)	% (95% CI)
Sensitivity	91.7 (90.1–93.0)	90.7 (87.9–92.8)	98.5 (96.7–99.3)	92.4 (88.1–95.2)	90.9 (86.9–93.8)	25.0 (13.3–42.1)
Specificity	100 (99.1–100)	100 (98.0–100)	100 (61.0–100)	100 (96.2–100)	100 (86.7–100)	100 (96.9–100)
PPV	100 (99.7–100)	100 (99.2–100)	100 (99.0–100.)	100 (98.2–100)	100 (98.4–100)	100 (67.6–100)
NPV	78.5 (74.9–81.7)	79.4 (73.9–84.0)	50.0 (25.4–74.6)	85.1 (77.4–90.5)	51.0 (37.5–64.4)	83.3 (76.4–88.5)
Accuracy	93.6 (92.4–94.6)	93.1 (91.1–94.8)	98.5 (96.8–99.3)	94.7 (91.7–96.7)	91.7 (88.0–94.4)	84.2 (77.6–89.2)

samples even if the need for further histological evaluation remains essential in many cases [15, 16]. In the subgroup of patients who underwent EBUS-TBNA for restaging the mediastinum after neoadjuvant chemotherapy, there were a relative higher incidence of inadequate samples due to the presence of fibrosis in the mediastinum and the difficulty of the procedure specially after chemoradiotherapy.

Considering our Group 2 (pathological diagnosis and mutational status in advanced stage lung cancer), EBUS-TBNA sensitivity and diagnostic accuracy were both 98.5%. EBUS-TBNA also provided adequate material for molecular analysis whenever requested in advanced stage adenocarcinomas in 98% of cases. This datum confirms our previous published experience of molecular analysis with EBUS-TBNA specimens where we showed a sensitivity of 96.9% [17]. Our previous study also demonstrated that molecular analysis obtained from EBUS-TBNA specimens was equivalent to that obtained from surgical specimens, with no differences in terms of sensitivity and diagnostic accuracy [17].

Due to the low invasive and the feasibility of repeated procedures, EBUS-TBNA is the ideal procedure to establish a cell-type diagnosis and to provide adequate specimens for molecular assay in advanced lung cancer patients. The procedure's high accuracy and low risk of complications make it suitable for low performance status patients who could still benefit from targeted therapy [18].

In Group 3 (lymphadenopathy in previous malignancy), EBUS-TBNA showed a sensitivity and diagnostic accuracy of 92.4% and 94.7%, respectively, in agreement with a previous similar study published by Navani et al. and also with our previous reported experience in this subset of patients [8, 9]. In this group of patients, EBUS-TBNA was a crucial diagnostic approach. The results of this study showed that 35.3% of patients with lymphadenopathy suspected for a recurrence did not really have a recurrence, and EBUS-TBNA revealed a different diagnosis. From all nonmalignant diagnoses, lymphadenitis granulomatosis was found in 36% of patients. EBUS-TBNA specimens provided adequate diagnosis avoiding unnecessary treatments in cases of nonmalignant disease and guiding therapy in cases of recurrence.

In the diagnosis of Group 4 patients (pulmonary lesions), EBUS-TBNA demonstrated a sensitivity and accuracy of 90.9% and 91.7%, respectively, in line with Nakajima et al.'s published data (sensitivity of 94.1% and diagnostic accuracy of 94.3% in the diagnosis of peribronchial and peritracheal lesions) [19]. Clinical presentations vary widely in this group, and EBUS-TBNA was able to establish a correct diagnosis in the vast majority of cases also in nonmalignant intrapulmonary lesions. Some interesting findings in this group included the diagnosis of a benign leiomyoma, a mycetoma, and ectopic thymus tissue.

In the investigation of Group 5 (unknown origin lymphadenopathy), EBUS-TBNA presented a diagnostic accuracy of 84.2%. Due to the very low prevalence of malignancy in this group of patients, sensitivity was not surprisingly very low (25%). The vast majority of patients in this group had an inflammatory disease with the most frequent diagnosis of granulomatous lymphadenitis compatible with sarcoidosis.

Our results refer to the largest published series in EBUS-TBNA, in a high-volume thoracic oncology institution, demonstrating the utility and high accuracy of EBUS-TBNA in different clinical scenarios in daily clinical practice.

Some additional findings have also emerged from this study. First, our study showed a wide use of EBUS-TBNA in elderly patients (732 patients over 70 years old and 120 over 80 years old), with a very low rate (0.74%) of postprocedure minor complications and no major events. Other interesting findings included the possibility to repeat biopsies easily and safely, obtaining tumour specimens for genetic assessment in stage IV NSCLC patients and in other tumour recurrences without the need for further more invasive procedures. These aspects highlight the importance of EBUS-TBNA as a diagnostic approach in different thoracic oncology scenarios, underpinning modern oncological strategy also for fragile patients and thereby avoiding more invasive and demanding procedures.

An essential aspect to achieve optimal results is the specimen handling in EBUS-TBNA [5]. The use of ROSE and synergy with the pathologist is crucial during the procedure both to obtain the best specimen collection and to achieve all pathological, immunohistochemistry, and molecular analyses. Despite some different previous points of view regarding ROSE [20–22], a recent metaexpert panel review showed that ROSE is necessary to reach all molecular analyses and to prevent invasive surgical procedures after EBUS-TBNA [23].

Our study has some limitations. The first is its retrospective nature, which probably limits and influences all of the variables included in the analysis. Another bias is that not all patients underwent a surgical procedure (mediastinoscopy or VATS) to confirm negative EBUS-TBNA samples but all patients had a clinical and radiological follow-up longer than 15 months.

In our experience, EBUS-TBNA is not just a technique, but a philosophy for the investigation of thoracic disease. EBUS-TBNA feasibility and optimal results largely depend on the cytopathology and pulmonologists' experience but also the way the procedure is performed. Adequate sedation and ROSE are crucial and should always be used. In experienced hands, EBUS-TBNA offers everything chest physicians need for the best medical practice without further invasive procedures. Surgical procedures are still required in highly suspicious NSCLC cases when EBUS-TBNA is negative for malignancy and in some cases for lymphoma subtyping.

In conclusion, EBUS-TBNA represents the best diagnostic approach in many different clinical scenarios in high-volume thoracic oncology centres and dictates the consecutive treatment option in the vast majority of patients. EBUS-TBNA is useful and accurate in a high percentage of cases underpinning modern oncological therapy, guiding the best treatment options in lung cancer and avoiding useless and invasive procedures in case of benign disease.

Based on our previous expertise, we are developing new applications for EBUS-TBNA such as a new protocol for EBUS-TBNA primary lung cancer cell culture and microRNA profile in stage IIIA (pN2) NSCLC patients, testing the feasibility of a microRNA profile obtained from EBUS-TBNA [24] and the correlation with the prediction of chemotherapy response. In addition, new molecular analyses are being developed, and the correlation between PDL-1 expression and tumour histology is under evaluation.

Abbreviations

EBUS-TBNA: Endobronchial ultrasound transbronchial needle aspiration
NSCLC: Nonsmall-cell lung cancer
ROSE: Rapid on-site evaluation
VATS: Video-assisted thoracoscopy.

References

[1] P. De Leyn, D. Lardinois, P. E. Van Schil et al., "ESTS guidelines for preoperative lymph node staging for non-small cell lung cancer," *European Journal of Cardio-Thoracic Surgery*, vol. 32, no. 1, pp. 1–8, 2007.

[2] Z. T. Hammound, R. C. Anderson, B. F. Meyers et al., "The current role of mediastinoscopy in the evaluation of thoracic disease," *Journal of Thoracic and Cardiovascular Surgery*, vol. 118, no. 5, pp. 894–899, 1999.

[3] K. Yasufuku, M. Chiyo, Y. Sekine et al., "Real-time endobronchial ultrasound-guided transbronchial needle aspiration of mediastinal and hilar lymph nodes," *Chest*, vol. 126, no. 1, pp. 122–128, 2004.

[4] F. C. Detterbeck, M. A. Jantz, M. Wallace, J. Vansteenkiste, and G. A. Silvestri, "Invasive mediastinal staging of lung cancer," *Chest*, vol. 132, no. 3, pp. 202S–220S, 2007.

[5] T. Nakajima and K. Yasufuku, "How I do it–optimal methodology for multidirectional analysis of endobronchial ultrasound-guided transbronchial needle aspiration samples," *Journal of Thoracic Oncology*, vol. 6, no. 1, pp. 203–206, 2011.

[6] S. Garwood, M. A. Judson, R. Hoda, M. Fraig, and P. Doelken, "Endobronchial ultrasound for the diagnosis of pulmonary sarcoidosis," *Chest*, vol. 132, no. 4, pp. 1298–1304, 2007.

[7] S. Dhooria, R. Agarwal, A. N. Aggarwal, A. Bal, N. Gupta, and D. Gupta, "Differentiating tuberculosis from sarcoidosis by sonographic characteristics of lymph nodes on endobronchial ultrasonography: a study of 165 patients," *Journal of Thoracic and Cardiovascular Surgery*, vol. 148, no. 2, pp. 662–667, 2014.

[8] N. Navani, M. Nankivell, I. Woolhouse et al., "Endobronchial ultrasound-guided transbronchial needle aspiration for the diagnosis of intrathoracic lymphadenopathy in patients with extrathoracic malignancy: a multicenter study," *Journal of Thoracic Oncology*, vol. 6, no. 9, pp. 1505–1509, 2011.

[9] J. Guarize, M. Casiraghi, S. Donghi et al., "EBUS-TBNA in PET-positive lymphadenopathies in treated cancer patients," *ERJ Open Research*, vol. 3, no. 4, p. 00009-2017, 2017.

[10] J. Geake, G. Hammerschlag, P. Nguyen et al., "Utility of EBUS-TBNA for diagnosis of mediastinal tuberculous lymphadenitis: a multicentre Australian experience," *Journal of Thoracic Disease*, vol. 7, no. 3, pp. 439–448, 2015.

[11] C. B. Marshall, B. Jacob, S. Patel et al., "The utility of endobronchial ultrasound-guided transbronchial needle aspiration biopsy in the diagnosis of mediastinal lymphoproliferative disorders," *Cancer Cytopathology*, vol. 119, no. 2, pp. 118–126, 2011.

[12] P. De Leyn, D. Lardinois, P. E. Van Schil et al., "ESTS guidelines for preoperative lymph node staging for non-small cell lung cancer," *European Journal of Cardio-Thoracic Surgery*, vol. 32, no. 1, pp. 1–8, 2007.

[13] C. M. Kinsey and D. A. Arenberg, "Endobronchial ultrasound-guided transbronchial needle aspiration for non-small cell lung cancer staging," *American Journal of Respiratory and Critical Care Medicine*, vol. 189, no. 6, pp. 640–649, 2014.

[14] N. Rotolo, A. Imperatori, M. Nosotti et al., "Multicentric study of endobronchial ultrasound-transbronchial needle aspiration for lung cancer staging in Italy," *Journal of Thoracic Disease*, vol. 9, no. S5, pp. S370–S375, 2017.

[15] H. M. Ko, G. da Cunha Santos, G. Darling et al., "Diagnosis and subclassification of lymphomas and non-neoplastic lesions involving mediastinal lymph nodes using endobronchial ultrasound-guided transbronchial needle aspiration," *Diagnostic Cytopathology*, vol. 41, no. 12, pp. 1023–1030, 2013.

[16] V. W. Rusch, "Mediastinoscopy: an obsolete procedure?," *Journal of Thoracic and Cardiovascular Surgery*, vol. 142, no. 6, pp. 1400–1402, 2011.

[17] C. Casadio, J. Guarize, S. Donghi et al., "Molecular testing for targeted therapy in advanced non-small cell lung cancer: suitability of endobronchial ultrasound transbronchial needle aspiration," *American Journal of Clinical Pathology*, vol. 144, no. 4, pp. 629–634, 2015.

[18] G. A. Masters, S. Temin, C. G. Azzoli et al., "Systemic therapy for stage IV non-small-cell lung cancer: American Society of Clinical Oncology Clinical Practice Guideline Update," *Journal of Clinical Oncology*, vol. 33, no. 30, pp. 3488–3515, 2015.

[19] T. Nakajima, K. Yasufuku, T. Fujiwara et al., "Endobronchial ultrasound-guided transbronchial needle aspiration for the

diagnosis of intrapulmonary lesions," *Journal of Thoracic Oncology*, vol. 3, no. 9, pp. 985–988, 2008.

[20] T. Nakajima, K. Yasufuku, F. Saegusa et al., "Rapid on-site cytologic evaluation during endobronchial ultrasound-guided transbronchial needle aspiration for nodal staging in patients with lung cancer," *Annals of Thoracic Surgery*, vol. 95, no. 5, pp. 1695–1699, 2013.

[21] M. Joseph, T. Jones, Y. Lutterbie et al., "Rapid on-site pathologic evaluation does not increase the efficacy of endobronchial ultrasonographic biopsy for mediastinal staging," *Annals of Thoracic Surgery*, vol. 96, no. 2, pp. 403–410, 2013.

[22] M. Oki, H. Saka, C. Kitagawa et al., "Rapid on-site cytologic evaluation during endobronchial ultrasound-guided transbronchial needle aspiration for diagnosing lung cancer: a randomized study," *Respiration*, vol. 85, no. 6, pp. 486–492, 2013.

[23] D. Jain, T. C. Allen, D. L. Aisner et al., "Rapid on-site evaluation of endobronchial ultrasound-guided transbronchial needle aspirations for the diagnosis of lung cancer: a perspective from members of the Pulmonary Pathology Society," *Archives of Pathology & Laboratory Medicine*, vol. 142, no. 2, pp. 253–262, 2017.

[24] J. Guarize, F. Bianchi, E. Marino et al., "MicroRNA expression profile in primary lung cancer cells lines obtained by endobronchial ultrasound transbronchial needle aspiration," *Journal of Thoracic Disease*, vol. 10, no. 1, pp. 408–415, 2017.

Burden of Respiratory Syncytial Virus Hospitalizations

Ian Mitchell,[1] Isabelle Defoy,[2] and ElizaBeth Grubb[3]

[1]*Alberta Children's Hospital, 2888 Shaganappi Trail NW, Calgary, AB, Canada T6B 6A8*
[2]*AbbVie Corporation, 8401 Trans-Canada Highway, Saint-Laurent, QC, Canada H4S 1Z1*
[3]*AbbVie, Inc., 1 N. Waukegan Road, North Chicago, IL 60064, USA*

Correspondence should be addressed to ElizaBeth Grubb; elizabeth.grubb@abbvie.com

Academic Editor: Christophe Leroyer

Objective. To examine the socioeconomic burden of respiratory syncytial virus (RSV) disease for Canadian infants hospitalized for the condition. *Data and Methods.* The descriptive study used data collected in Alberta, Canada, during 2 consecutive RSV seasons. Infants (<1 year of age) were included if they had not received palivizumab and were hospitalized with a confirmed diagnosis of RSV. Hospitalization resource use and parental time burden, out-of-pocket costs, lost work productivity, and stress and anxiety were assessed. *Results.* 13.4% of all infants ($n = 67$) had intensive care unit (ICU) admission, and average ICU stay for these infants was 6.5 days. Families had average out-of-pocket expenses of 736.69 Canadian dollars (CAD $), and the average time both parents spent in hospital was nearly 7 days (164.0 hours). For working parents ($n = 43$), average absenteeism was 49% and overall work impairment was 77.8%. Parents also exhibited significant parental stress (3.6 on the Parental Stressor Scale: 43.9 state anxiety and 36.9 trait anxiety scores). *Conclusions.* Results indicate a high burden associated with the hospitalization of an infant due to RSV disease in terms of resource use, time, productivity, costs, and stress, even among a population of infants not considered to be at risk for the condition.

1. Introduction

Respiratory syncytial virus (RSV) is the most common cause of lower respiratory tract infections (LRTIs) in children worldwide [1] and is the leading cause of infant hospital admissions in developed countries [2, 3]. While nearly all children are affected by RSV by the time they are 2 years old [4], those less than 1 year of age have more severe RSV disease [5]. For example, in British Columbia between 2008 and 2010, 77% of all pediatric (<19 years of age) patients hospitalized with a confirmed diagnosis of RSV disease were age 1 or younger [6]. Overall, RSV was found to be a major viral cause of hospital admissions in Canada, with an estimated rate of 130 per 100,000 [7]. Infants with certain comorbid conditions, including prematurity, bronchopulmonary dysplasia, and congenital heart disease (CHD) are more likely to have severe RSV disease [8]. Only symptomatic treatment is available for these infants and may include a stay in the pediatric intensive care unit (ICU). While there is no effective vaccine, prophylaxis with a monoclonal antibody targeted at the RSV (palivizumab) may be administered by monthly injections throughout the RSV season. Palivizumab prophylaxis is generally reserved for vulnerable infants at the highest risk of severe disease [8].

Although only a small percentage of children in Canada require hospitalization for RSV [9, 10], a United States (US) study has indicated that inpatient care accounts for the majority of the total disease medical costs [11]. In addition to this evidence of high direct costs, studies from other countries have demonstrated that RSV hospitalizations are associated with significant indirect costs [12, 13]. Building on this previous research, the present study descriptively analyzed a sample of Canadian infants hospitalized with RSV disease with 2 goals. One of these goals was to identify possible risk factors for RSV hospitalization in Canada for patients under 1 year of age who were not eligible for and therefore did not receive palivizumab prophylaxis. The other was to provide a more complete and current picture of the socioeconomic burden of RSV hospitalization. This study examined both the direct costs associated with RSV hospitalizations and the indirect costs, including out-of-pocket (OOP) payments, lost productivity, and parental stress and anxiety.

2. Materials and Methods

This publication reports on data collected in Alberta Children's Hospital, Calgary, Alberta, Canada, for a study conducted during 2 consecutive RSV seasons (2010/2011 and 2011/2012). This was the only Canadian site in the Multinational Parent Burden Study, a prospective, observational survey-based analysis designed and implemented to quantify the humanistic burden that infant RSV/LRTI-associated hospitalizations have on parents and caregivers [14, 15].

Infants included in the study were < 1 year of age, had not received palivizumab prophylaxis, and were hospitalized with a confirmed diagnosis of RSV/LRTI, which was identified by a rapid direct fluorescent-antibody assay (DFA) test. Premature infants were 33–35 weeks of gestational age and were identified as having a low risk of RSV disease using the Canadian Risk-Scoring Tool (RST) [16]. The study was approved by the Conjoint Health Research Ethics Board, University of Calgary. Informed parental consent was obtained for all participants, and parent screening, consent, and enrollment occurred at the time of infant discharge. Parents completed a discharge survey and a follow-up survey, with data collected regarding parental characteristics, productivity, and parental stress and anxiety. Information on infant characteristics (severity of illness, comorbidities, and hospitalization) was obtained from chart reviews.

Measures of the burden associated with RSV were captured by hospitalization resource use and length of stay (LOS), as well as by the parental time burden and OOP costs associated with RSV hospitalizations (reported in Canadian dollars (CAD \$)). In addition, lost work productivity was assessed via a Work Productivity and Activity Impairment questionnaire that was specific to and validated for caregivers of children hospitalized with respiratory illness (WPAI: CHRI) [17]. The WPAI: CHRI assessed absenteeism, presenteeism, overall work impairment, and activity impairment. Absenteeism was defined as time away from work, presenteeism was defined as impaired productivity while at work, overall work impairment was defined as a weighted sum of absenteeism and presenteeism, and activity impairment was defined as impairment in activities performed outside of work. WPAI: CHRI outcomes are expressed as impairment percentages, with higher numbers indicating greater impairment and less productivity [17].

The study also included patient-reported outcome (PRO) assessments of stress and anxiety for parents of infants with RSV. In addition to capturing resource utilization associated with infant RSV disease, stress levels were assessed by the Parental Stressor Scale: Infant Hospitalization (PSS: IH), while anxiety was assessed using the State-Trait Anxiety Inventory (STAI). The PSS: IH is a validated measure, scored on a 5-point scale that assesses stress experienced by parents when an infant is admitted to the hospital environment. The scale accounts for the stress induced by the appearance and behavior of the sick infant, the alterations in the parental role that occur as a result of the infant's hospitalization and treatment for acute illness, and the sights and sounds of the setting in which nursing occurs [18, 19]. The STAI comprises validated scales for state (S-anxiety) and trait (T-anxiety) anxiety. State anxiety evaluates past, present, and future feelings of apprehension, tension, nervousness, and worry and is an indicator of changes in transitory anxiety. The trait anxiety scale evaluates how people generally feel and determines feelings of anxiety as a long-standing general personality trait. Both the S-anxiety and T-anxiety scales are based upon the parent's responses to questions each of which requires a ranking from 1 to 4, with cumulative scores ranging from 20 to 80 and with higher scores indicating higher perceived levels of anxiety [20, 21].

This study was designed to describe the burden of the disease, with no a priori identified hypotheses. As such, there was no specific sample size required for the study. However, to obtain adequate data to inform results, the study set a goal of enrolling a minimum of 50 infants. All analyses were conducted using SAS, version 9.3 (SAS Institute, Inc., Cary, NC).

3. Results

Sixty-seven infants residing in Alberta, Canada (Table 1) met the study inclusion criteria. A slight majority were male (52.2% male versus 47.8% female), and a large majority were breastfed (86.6%), while about 1/5 (19.4%) were identified as having been born prematurely (mean gestational age = 34.5 weeks). With the exception of RSV, the infants appeared to be relatively healthy, with only a very small percentage having a comorbid diagnosis. The most frequently diagnosed comorbid conditions were chronic congenital heart disease (10.5%), a skin condition (6.0%), and chronic wheezing or asthma (4.5%). In a majority of the infant's families, the parents were married (97.0%) and had at least 1 child in day care (98.5%). A large proportion (43.3%) of the mothers ($n = 67$) and 29.5% of the fathers ($n = 44$) were self-identified as smokers (Table 2). Most of the parents in this study were employed, with 84.1% of the fathers and 9% of the mothers employed and currently working and with another 49.3% of the mothers employed but on parental leave.

Figures 1 and 2 illustrate the in-hospital resource use of all of the infants and compare the resource use of the premature and full-term infants. Results revealed that 95.5% of all infants received supplemental oxygen and 13.4% had an ICU admission. The average hospital LOS was 5.7 days overall and 5.1 days in the pediatric ward. Among patients who went to the ICU ($N = 9$), the average LOS was 6.5 days. While no tests of statistical significance were performed, results revealed that preterm infants were less likely than full-term infants to use supplemental oxygen (92.3% versus 96.3%) but more likely to have an ICU admission (15.4% versus 13.0%). The premature infants also had a longer mean ICU LOS (8.1 days versus 6.2 days).

TABLE 1: Demographic characteristics of infants hospitalized and families of infants hospitalized.

Infants hospitalized ($n = 67$)		
Variable	Mean or N	SD or %
Sex		
Male	35	52.2%
Female	32	47.8%
Gestational age at birth, weeks (mean; SD)	37.3	1.7
Infant chronological age, months (mean; SD)	2.7	2.5
Breastfed		
Yes	58	86.6%
No	9	13.4%
Length of time child was breastfed, months[a]	1.8	1.8
Comorbidities[b]		
Allergies	2	3.0%
Chronic lung disease	1	1.5%
Chronic congenital heart disease	7	10.5%
Chronic wheezing or asthma	3	4.5%
Down's syndrome	2	3.0%
Severely immunocompromised	1	1.5%
Skin condition	4	6.0%
Maturity status		
Mature	54	80.6%
Premature	13	19.4%
Gestational age for premature infants, weeks (mean; SD)	34.5	2.1
Families of infants hospitalized ($n = 67$)		
Married		
Yes	65	97.0%
No	2	3.0%
At least 1 child in day care		
Yes	66	98.5%
No	1	1.5%
Number of children attending day care (mean; SD)	1.7	0.5
Number of siblings (mean; SD)	1.6	1.6

SD = standard deviation; [a]among those who were breastfed; [b]rates of cystic fibrosis and organ transplants were also examined although no infant received either diagnosis.

In addition to hospital resource utilization, the study also gathered information about parental time lost, including work time, time at the hospital, and travel time to and from the hospital, as well as OOP costs associated with infant hospitalizations for RSV (Table 3). The average time both parents spent in the hospital was nearly 7 full days (164.0 hours), suggesting that each set of parents missed more than 3 days of work (24.7 hours/8 hours of work per day) when their infant was hospitalized. In addition to the time burden, the mean OOP expenses associated with an RSV hospitalization totaled CAD $736.69 and consisted of CAD $151.50 in transportation costs to/from the hospital, CAD $273.33 in costs for child care and home health, and CAD $311.86 in other OOP costs such as over-the-counter medications or medical equipment purchases, meals and lodging expenses, and any other nontransportation or home expenses, the parent classified as "other." Parents of premature infants had lower transportation costs than parents of full-term infants (CAD $107.60 versus CAD $160.85), consistent with the hypothesis that their spending more time in the hospital was associated with fewer trips between the hospital and home.

Figure 3 illustrates the lost work productivity for both parents associated with their infant's hospitalization. Results revealed that average absenteeism was 49.0%, presenteeism was 51.4%, overall work impairment was 77.8%, and activity impairment was 81.7%. While working fathers experienced more absenteeism (51.3% versus 27.8%), presenteeism (62.7% versus 21.4%), and overall work impairment (78.4% versus 73.0%) compared to working mothers, working mothers reported more activity impairment than working fathers (88.0% versus 74.2%). In addition to lost work productivity experienced by working fathers and mothers, Figure 4 examines additional disease burden associated with the psychological health of the parents. The PRO

Table 2: Demographic characteristics of parents of infants hospitalized.

Variable	Fathers ($n = 44$)		Mothers ($n = 67$)	
	Mean or N	SD or %	Mean or N	SD or %
Age, years (mean; SD)	34.6	4.7	32.5	5.9
Education				
Degree/associate/bachelor/post grad/other	35	79.5%	48	71.6%
Attended some and/or completed high school	9	20.5%	19	28.4%
Employed status				
No	5	11.4%	28	41.8%
Parental leave	2	4.5%	33	49.3%
Yes	37	84.1%	6	9.0%
Smoker				
No	31	70.5%	38	56.7%
Yes	13	29.5%	29	43.3%

SD = standard deviation.

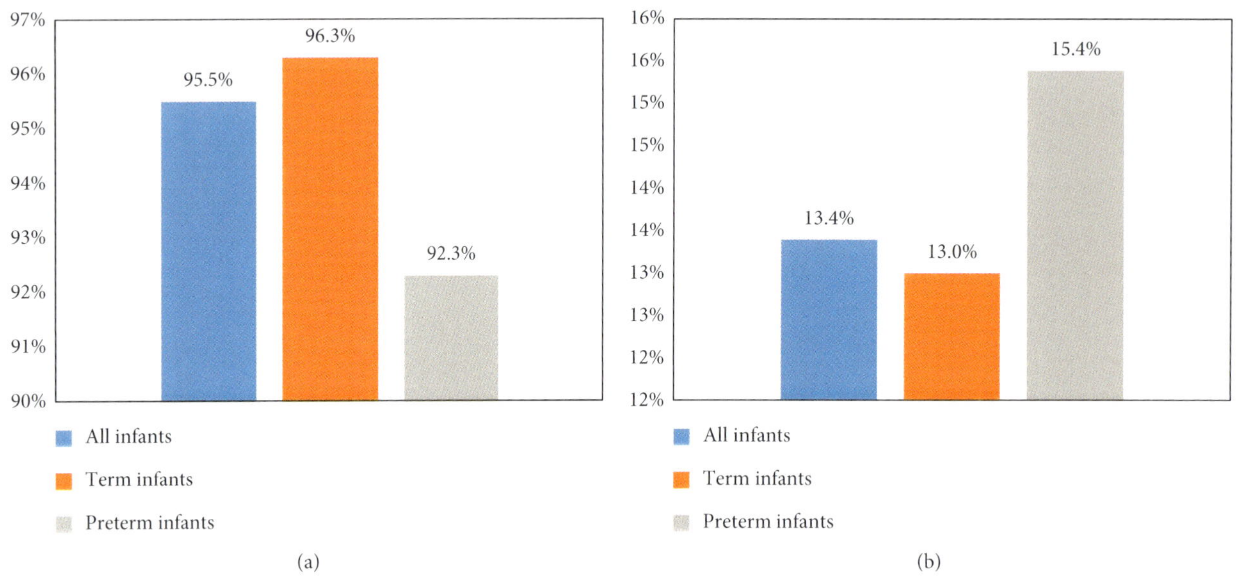

Figure 1: Healthcare resource utilization—by term status. (a) Use of supplemental oxygen. (b) Intensive care admission. Sample size: all infants ($N = 67$), term infants ($N = 54$), and preterm infants ($N = 13$).

instruments revealed that working parents, on average, scored 3.6 out of 5 on the Parental Stressor Scale, with mothers having a higher average score than fathers (3.9 versus 3.5). For all working parents, the average scores on the STAI were 43.9 S-anxiety and 36.9 T-anxiety, and as with the PSS: IH, working mothers had a higher score than working fathers (50.5 versus 42.8 for S-anxiety and 40.0 versus 36.5 for T-anxiety).

4. Discussion

This study examined the burden of hospitalization due to RSV disease for infants who were not considered to be at risk of RSV hospitalization. Results indicate that the burden is substantial in terms of hospital resources, parental costs, lost productivity, and psychological health. The following sections discuss and contextualize RSV risk factors and treatment costs revealed through this analysis of a population of infants residing across Canada.

4.1. Infant Characteristics. Consistent with a wide range of literature [22, 23], this study found a strong association between preterm birth and hospitalization for RSV. Specifically, preterm infants were overrepresented in this study, as they comprised 19.4% of the study population, compared to the estimated < 10% rate of preterm live births in Canada overall [24]. This overrepresentation of preterm infants was especially noteworthy given that, at the time the study was conducted, all pre-term infants < 32 weeks' gestational age, as well as all those who were 33–35 weeks' gestational age and identified as being at high risk of hospitalization, were protected from severe RSV disease with palivizumab and hence were ineligible for this study. Most of the children in the present study were < 6 months old, male, living with siblings, and either in day care themselves or the sibling of a child in day care, while a large minority had a mother (43.3%) and/or a father (29.5%) who smoked. These findings are consistent with a previous comprehensive review of the research, which reported these factors to be the ones most commonly associated with RSV hospitalization among both premature and full-term infants [23]. Finally, the majority (86.6%) of the infants in this study were breastfed, which is consistent with research which has identified breastfeeding as protective for RSV [23, 25, 26].

4.2. Hospital Resource Utilization. National healthcare statistics have shown that the largest share (29.2%) of Canadian healthcare spending is associated with hospitalizations [27]. Consistent with these data, the findings of the present study suggest that when children are hospitalized for RSV, they require inpatient resources at a very high rate. For instance, 13.4% of the infants were admitted to the ICU, with an average ICU LOS of nearly 1 week (mean ICU LOS = 6.5 days), while the preterm infants had even greater odds of an ICU admission, at 15.4%, as well as a higher mean ICU LOS of 8.1 days. Furthermore, the mean pediatric ward LOS in this study was 5.0 days, a finding roughly consistent with the Ontario Case Costing Initiative report of a mean hospital LOS of 3.91 days for pediatric RSV patients [28]. These observed associations between RSV hospitalization, ICU admission, and substantial ICU and hospital LOS are in concert with a number of previous studies, including a UK investigation which reported that RSV accounted for 15.6% of all admissions to intensive therapy units due to respiratory disease [29], a Mexican analysis which reported that 5.2% of infants hospitalized for RSV disease were admitted to the ICU [30], and a French examination which revealed that RSV patients in the pediatric ICU had a median ICU LOS of 8 days [31]. In addition to the significant direct costs, which have been reported in previous research [32], hospitalizations and ICU admissions for RSV disease represent a substantial humanistic burden. For instance, research has documented the dangers of pediatric hospitalization, with medication errors the most common adverse event [33]. In addition to medication errors, which have been shown to be associated with higher death rates in a pediatric population than in the adult population [34], pediatric hospitalizations are associated with other unique challenges, such as the inability of infant patients to convey information verbally to healthcare providers [35]. Moreover, the vast majority (95.5%) of the hospitalized infants in this study were given supplemental oxygen, likely based on pulse oximetry values. It has been shown that pulse oximetry use may lead to lengthening of the hospital stay [36], although acceptance of lower oximetry levels does not compromise the child's care [37].

4.3. Time Burden and Out-of-Pocket Costs. In addition to the burden on hospitals and patients, the families of the RSV-hospitalized infants in this study bore other substantial costs. These costs included the time spent visiting the child in the hospital and the travel time associated with such visits, as well as the related OOP costs for transportation, child care, and paid home help. On average, the family of each patient spent a total of nearly 1 week's time (6.8 days) in the hospital as well as 10.6 hours traveling to and from the hospital. Furthermore, these families incurred OOP costs for transportation (CAD $151.50), home costs (CAD $273.33), and other expenses, such as over-the-counter medications, medical equipment, meals, lodging, and other nontransportation or home costs (CAD $311.86). These findings are generally consistent with a previous investigation which reported that each RSV hospitalization in the US was associated with 218 hours of travel and visit time, as well as $827 (year 2000, US $) in average OOP costs, including travel, parking, visiting, meals, child care, and other expenses [13].

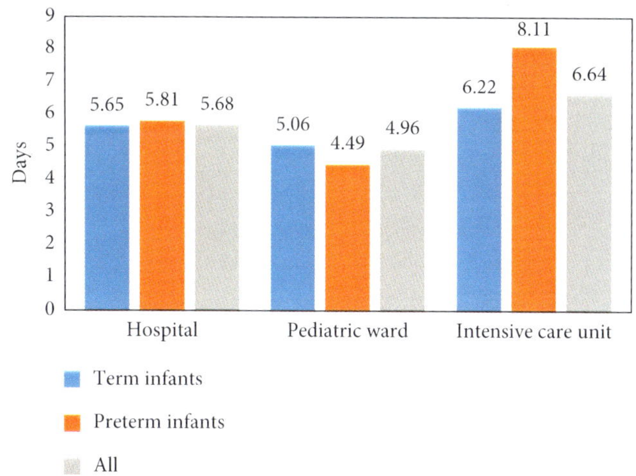

FIGURE 2: Hospital length of stay (LOS)—by term status. Sample size: hospital ($N = 67$): 54 term infants and 13 preterm infants. Pediatric ward ($N = 66$): 54 term infants and 12 preterm infants. Intensive care unit ($N = 9$): 7 term infants and 2 preterm infants.

4.4. Work, Productivity, and Activity Impairment. Each set of parents in this study missed an average of 24.7 hours from work (absenteeism) because of their child's RSV hospitalization. It is hypothesized that this burden may be larger in other countries, such as the US, which do not have as generous a maternity leave policy as Alberta [38]. Furthermore, when a parent in the present investigation went to work during the hospitalization, he or she was, on average, 51.4% less productive than normal (presenteeism). Overall, parents reported an average work impairment of 77.8% due to RSV disease. The functional impairment of the parents also extended outside of work, as an average of 81.7% of each parent's regular, daily activities were prevented (activity impairment) due to the child's RSV hospitalization. Compared to previous reports from caregivers of older children with uncontrolled asthma [39], the parents of the infants with RSV disease in the present study reported much higher levels of absenteeism (49.0% versus 4.5%), presenteeism (51.4% versus 12.7%), overall work impairment (81.7% versus 15.9%), and activity impairment (78.4% versus 19.1%). While patients with uncontrolled asthma were significantly older than those in the current study and not all were hospitalized [39], the results

TABLE 3: Resource use and out-of-pocket costs associated with current hospitalization.

	All patients ($n = 67$)		Term infants ($n = 54$)		Premature infants ($n = 13$)	
	Mean	Range	Mean	Range	Mean	Range
Time burden during hospitalization (hours)						
Average time 1st parent spent in hospital	115.2	20–1,368	117.9	24.5–1,368	103.8	20–200
Average time 2nd parent spent in hospital	48.8	4–200	41.0	4–192	82.6	7–200
Parent time missed work during last 7 days	24.7	0–90	20.5	0–75	42.8	8–90
1st parent travel time to/from hospital	3.7	1–36	3.5	0.1–36	4.4	0.7–30
2nd parent travel time to/from hospital	6.9	2–30	7.6	2–30	3.9	3–8
Out-of-pocket costs associated with hospitalization (Canadian dollars)						
Transportation costs for 1st parent	55.26	2–400	56.76	5–400	50.60	2–80
Transportation costs for 2nd parent	96.24	10–760	104.09	10–760	57.00	20–79
Home costs						
Child care	185.83	25–700	203.00	25–700	100.00	100
Paid home health	87.50	75–100	87.50	75–100	—	—
Other out-of-pocket costs for 1st parent[a]	151.08	10–2,755	148.98	10–2,755	162.31	20–600
Other out-of-pocket costs for 2nd parent[a]	160.78	20–1,600	167.91	20–1,600	132.25	20–450

[a]Other out-of-pocket costs included costs for over-the-counter medications, medical equipment, meals, lodging, and any nontransportation or home costs listed by the parent as "other."

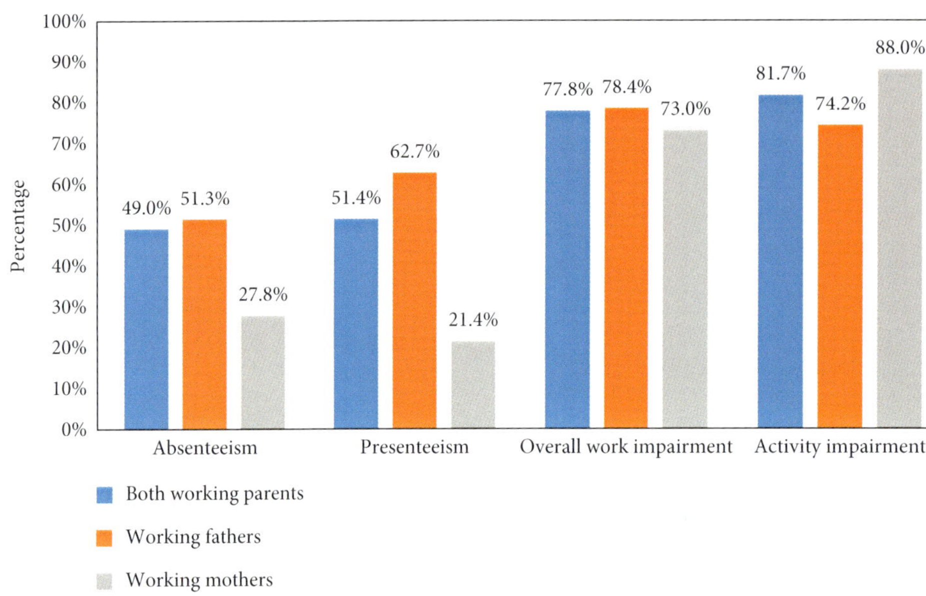

FIGURE 3: WPAI-CHRI. Sample size: both working parents ($N = 43$), working fathers ($N = 37$), and working mothers ($N = 6$).

appear to indicate a significant societal burden associated with RSV disease.

4.5. Parental Anxiety and Stress. The PSS: IH scale of parental stress showed that, in general, mothers experienced more stress than fathers (3.9 versus 3.5). This finding is consistent with research which examined premature infants in the neonatal ICU and found that mothers showed more trauma-related symptoms, were more stressed, anxious, depressed, and angry, and responded more negatively to the situation than fathers [40]. In contrast, other research which examined parents' stress both before and after congenital heart surgery, as well as a study of Chinese-American parents whose child spent 1–3 days in an ICU, found that fathers experienced more stress than mothers [41, 42]. However, both the mothers and the fathers of the infants hospitalized with RSV disease in this study had higher stress levels than did the parents in either of those earlier studies [41, 42]. For example, the examination of Chinese-American parents found average parental stress scores of 2.8 for mothers and 2.9 for fathers [42], compared to the average scores of 3.9 for mothers and 3.6 for fathers found in this study. Furthermore, the present

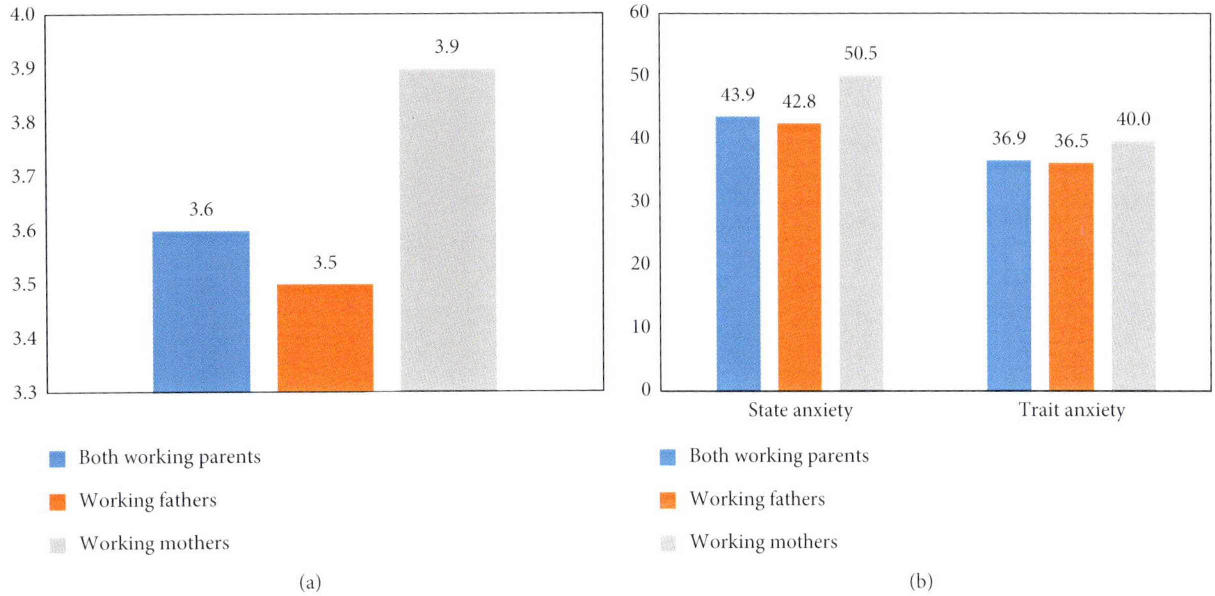

FIGURE 4: Parental stress and anxiety. (a) Parental stressor scale. (b) State-trait anxiety inventory. Sample size: both working parents ($N = 43$), working fathers ($N = 37$), and working mothers ($N = 6$).

study found a higher transitory stress level than that reported previously for mothers whose children were genetically at risk for type 1 diabetes (S-anxiety of 37.0) [43]. Given the large economic costs, marital instability, impaired functioning, and other adverse effects commonly linked to parental stress [44], the increased stress and anxiety of the parents in this study may represent additional economic and humanistic costs associated with RSV disease.

4.6. Limitations. This analysis was conducted using observational data collected from surveys of parents of infants with RSV disease in a pediatric hospital in Canada. Nonrandomization, recruitment bias, and the limited geographical catchment area are all factors that may have influenced the results and may therefore preclude generalization to broader populations. The limited geographical scope of the study is of particular note, since previous research has shown that RSV risk factors vary by region [23]. Further, given the small sample size, the study is purely descriptive in nature. As such, no comparisons between this cohort and a control group or between subgroups of infants, such as preterm and full term, were conducted. Further, the study is unable to statistically compare results across geographic regions and did not collect information on the use of palivizumab prophylaxis. Recall bias may have influenced the participants' responses regarding the amount of time spent away from work and the OOP costs incurred. However, much of the information was obtained at the time of infant discharge from hospital, and the PRO tools used in the study have been shown to have reasonably good psychometric properties [17, 18].

5. Conclusions

In conclusion, this descriptive analysis of Canadian survey data showed a number of key risk factors and a substantial burden associated with the hospitalizations of infants with RSV disease. Almost all (95%) of the hospitalized infants required supplemental oxygen, and 13.4% were admitted to the ICU. For those admitted to the ICU, the mean ICU LOS was approximately 1 week, while the mean pediatric ward LOS was also substantial, at approximately 5 days (mean). The adults who cared for these infants also had a significant time burden associated with visiting their child in the hospital, and they incurred additional burdens in terms of OOP expenses, absenteeism, presenteeism, daily impairment, and significant psychological stress. These findings extend the literature by analyzing the indirect costs of RSV hospitalizations in Canada, where parents will not face the additional burden of paying directly for physician care or costs of hospitalization.

Authors' Contributions

All authors contributed to the development of the publication and maintained control over the final content.

Acknowledgments

The authors wish to thank Monica Ruff, BSc, research assistant at the University of Calgary for her assistance with study recruitment and enrollment, Dominic Falconi, PhD, a former employee of AbbVie, for his assistance with interpretation of the data, and Shivaji Manthena, an employee of AbbVie, for conducting the statistical analysis of the data collected in the study. The authors also wish to thank all parents who participated in this study. Financial support for the study was provided by AbbVie Inc.; design and study conduct were shared by Ian Mitchell and AbbVie

Inc. AbbVie participated in the interpretation of data, review, and approval of the manuscript. HealthMetrics Outcomes Research, LLC, provided medical writing and editing services in the development of this manuscript.

References

[1] E. A. F. Simoes, "Respiratory syncytial virus infection," *Lancet*, vol. 354, no. 9181, pp. 847–852, 1999.

[2] S. Leader and K. Kohlhase, "Respiratory syncytial virus-coded pediatric hospitalizations, 1997 to 1999," *Pediatric Infectious Disease Journal*, vol. 21, no. 7, pp. 629–632, 2002.

[3] R. O'Donnell and M. Roe, "Respiratory syncytial virus bronchiolitis," in *Case Studies in Pediatric Critical Care*, pp. 1–12, Cambridge University Press, Cambridge, UK, 2009.

[4] W. P. Glezen, L. H. Taber, A. L. Frank, and J. A. Kasel, "Risk of primary infection and reinfection with respiratory syncytial virus," *American Journal of Diseases of Children*, vol. 140, no. 6, pp. 543–546, 1986.

[5] M. Lanari, S. Vandini, M. G. Capretti, T. Lazzarotto, and G. Faldella, "Respiratory syncytial virus infections in infants affected by primary immunodeficiency," *Journal of Immunology Research*, vol. 2014, Article ID 850831, 6 pages, 2014.

[6] P. Santibanez, K. Gooch, P. Vo, M. Lorimer, and Y. Sandino, "Acute care utilization due to hospitalizations for pediatric lower respiratory tract infections in British Columbia, Canada," *BMC Health Services Research*, vol. 12, p. 451, 2012.

[7] D. L. Schanzer, J. M. Langley, and T. W. S. Tam, "Hospitalization attributable to influenza and other viral respiratory illnesses in Canadian children," *Pediatric Infectious Disease Journal*, vol. 25, no. 9, pp. 795–800, 2006.

[8] B. Resch, "Respiratory syncytial virus infection in high-risk infants—an update on palivizumab prophylaxis," *Open Microbiology Journal*, vol. 8, pp. 71–77, 2014.

[9] T. Moraes, "Are we too passive in our attempts to prevent respiratory syncytial virus infection in Northern Canada?," *Canadian Respiratory Journal*, vol. 21, no. 3, pp. 163–164, 2014.

[10] B. A. Paes, I. Mitchell, A. Banerji, K. L. Lanctôt, and J. M. Langley, "A decade of respiratory syncytial virus epidemiology and prophylaxis: translating evidence into everyday clinical practice," *Canadian Respiratory Journal*, vol. 18, no. 2, pp. e10–e19, 2011.

[11] L. C. Paramore, V. Ciuryla, G. Ciesla, and L. Liu, "Economic impact of respiratory syncytial virus-related illness in the US: an analysis of national databases," *PharmacoEconomics*, vol. 22, no. 5, pp. 275–284, 2004.

[12] C. J. Miedema, A. W. Kors, W. E. Tjon A Ten, and J. L. Kimpen, "Medical consumption and socioeconomic effects of infection with respiratory syncytial virus in the Netherlands," *Pediatric Infectious Disease Journal*, vol. 20, no. 2, pp. 160–163, 2001.

[13] S. Leader, H. Yang, J. DeVincenzo, P. Jacobson, J. P. Marcin, and D. L. Murray, "Time and out-of-pocket costs associated with respiratory syncytial virus hospitalization of infants," *Value in Health*, vol. 6, no. 2, pp. 100–106, 2003.

[14] P. Vo, K. Gooch, M. Lorimer et al., "Parental awareness of respiratory syncytial virus (RSV) during infancy: a multinational survey assessment," *Presented at the 31st meeting of the Eurppean Society for Paediatric Infectious Diseases (ESPID 2013)*, 2013, http://w3.kenes-group.com/apps/espid2013/abstracts/pdf/78.pdf.

[15] P. Vo, I. Mitchell, K. L. Gooch, S. Manthena, M. J. Holton, and M. Ruff, "The disease burden associated with infant hospitalization for a lower respiratory tract infection (LRTI) in Canada," *Value in Health*, vol. 17, no. 3, p. A179, 2014.

[16] B. Paes, S. Steele, M. Janes, and J. Pinelli, "Risk-Scoring Tool for respiratory syncytial virus prophylaxis in premature infants born at 33–35 completed weeks' gestational age in Canada," *Current Medical Research and Opinion*, vol. 25, no. 7, pp. 1585–1591, 2009.

[17] M. Reilly, I. Mitchell, K. Gooch et al., "Preliminary validation of the work productivity activity impairment (WPAI) in caregivers of children hospitalized for respiratory illness (WPAI: CHRI) in Germany and Canada," *Value in Health*, vol. 15, no. 7, p. A650, 2012.

[18] M. S. Miles and S. H. Brunssen, "Psychometric properties of the parental stressor scale: infant hospitalization," *Advances in Neonatal Care*, vol. 3, no. 4, pp. 189–196, 2003.

[19] S. L. Docherty, M. S. Miles, and D. Holditch-Davis, "Worry about child health in mothers of hospitalized medically fragile infants," *Advances in Neonatal Care*, vol. 2, no. 2, pp. 84–92, 2002.

[20] C. Spielberger, R. Gorsuch, R. Lushene, R. Vagg, and G. Jacobs, *Manual for the State-Trait Anxiety Inventory*, Consulting Psychologists Press, Palo Alto, CA, USA, 1983.

[21] J. S. Needle, M. O'Riordan, and P. G. Smith, "Parental anxiety and medical comprehension within 24 hrs of a child's admission to the pediatric intensive care unit," *Pediatric Critical Care Medicine*, vol. 10, no. 6, pp. 668–674, 2009.

[22] J. L. Robinson, N. Le Saux, Canadian Paediatric Society, and Infectious Diseases and Immunization Committee, "Preventing hospitalizations for respiratory syncytial virus infection," *Paediatrics and Child Health*, vol. 20, no. 6, pp. 321–333, 2015.

[23] A. T. Borchers, C. Chang, M. E. Gershwin, and L. J. Gershwin, "Respiratory syncytial virus—a comprehensive review," *Clinical Reviews in Allergy and Immunology*, vol. 45, no. 3, pp. 331–379, 2013.

[24] March of Dimes, "Born too soon global map," *March of Dimes: A fighting chance for every baby*, 2016, http://www.marchofdimes.org/mission/global-preterm.aspx.

[25] L. R. Bulkow, R. J. Singleton, R. A. Karron, L. H. Harrison, and Alaska RSV Study Group, "Risk factors for severe respiratory syncytial virus infection among Alaska native children," *Pediatrics*, vol. 109, no. 2, pp. 210–216, 2002.

[26] E. A. F. Simões, X. Carbonell-Estrany, J. R. Fullarton et al., "European risk factors' model to predict hospitalization of premature infants born 33–35 weeks' gestational age with respiratory syncytial virus: validation with Italian data," *Journal of Maternal-Fetal and Neonatal Medicine*, vol. 24, no. 1, pp. 152–157, 2011.

[27] Canadian Institute for Health Information, "Canada's health care spending growth slows | CIHI," 2015, https://www.cihi.ca/en/spending-and-health-workforce/spending/canadas-health-care-spending-growth-slows.

[28] K. L. Lanctôt, S. T. Masoud, B. A. Paes et al., "The cost-effectiveness of palivizumab for respiratory syncytial virus prophylaxis in premature infants with a gestational age of 32–35 weeks: a Canadian-based analysis," *Current Medical Research and Opinion*, vol. 24, no. 11, pp. 3223–3237, 2008.

[29] E. R. Gaunt, H. Harvala, C. McIntyre, K. E. Templeton, and P. Simmonds, "Disease burden of the most commonly detected respiratory viruses in hospitalized patients calculated using the disability adjusted life year (DALY) model," *Journal of Clinical Virology*, vol. 52, no. 3, pp. 215–221, 2011.

[30] S. Vizcarra-Ugalde, M. Rico-Hernández, C. Monjaras-Ávila et al., "Intensive care unit admission and death rates of infants admitted with respiratory syncytial virus lower respiratory

tract infection in Mexico," *Pediatric Infectious Disease Journal*, vol. 35, no. 11, pp. 1199–1203, 2016.

[31] A.-L. Soilly, C. Ferdynus, O. Desplanches, M. Grimaldi, and J. B. Gouyon, "Paediatric intensive care admissions for respiratory syncytial virus bronchiolitis in France: results of a retrospective survey and evaluation of the validity of a medical information system programme," *Epidemiology and Infection*, vol. 140, no. 4, pp. 608–616, 2012.

[32] J. F. Dasta, T. P. McLaughlin, S. H. Mody, and C. T. Piech, "Daily cost of an intensive care unit day: the contribution of mechanical ventilation," *Critical Care Medicine*, vol. 33, no. 6, pp. 1266–1271, 2005.

[33] S. Lacey, J. B. Smith, and K. Cox, "Pediatric safety and quality," *in Patient Safety and Quality: An Evidence-Based Handbook for Nurses*, R. G. Hughes, Ed., Agency for Healthcare Research and Quality (US), Rockville, MD, USA, 2008.

[34] J. Phillips, S. Beam, A. Brinker et al., "Retrospective analysis of mortalities associated with medication errors," *American Journal of Health-System Pharmacy*, vol. 58, no. 19, pp. 1835–1841, 2001.

[35] A. C. Beal, J. P. T. Co, D. Dougherty et al., "Quality measures for children's health care," *Pediatrics*, vol. 113, no. 1, pp. 199–209, 2004.

[36] A. R. Schroeder, A. K. Marmor, R. H. Pantell, and T. B. Newman, "Impact of pulse oximetry and oxygen therapy on length of stay in bronchiolitis hospitalizations," *Archives of Pediatrics and Adolescent Medicine*, vol. 158, no. 6, pp. 527–530, 2004.

[37] S. Cunningham, A. Rodriguez, K. A. Boyd, E. McIntosh, S. C. Lewis, and BIDS Collaborators Group, "Bronchiolitis of Infancy Discharge Study (BIDS): a multicentre, parallel-group, double-blind, randomised controlled, equivalence trial with economic evaluation," *Health Technology Assessment*, vol. 19, no. 71, pp. 1–172, 2015.

[38] Alberta Government, "Employment standards code: maternity leave and parental leave," 2014. https://work.alberta.ca/documents/Maternity-Leave-and-Parental-Leave.pdf.

[39] B. B. Dean, B. C. Calimlim, P. Sacco, D. Aguilar, R. Maykut, and D. Tinkelman, "Uncontrolled asthma: assessing quality of life and productivity of children and their caregivers using a cross-sectional internet-based survey," *Health and Quality of Life Outcomes*, vol. 8, p. 96, 2010.

[40] C. Ionio, C. Colombo, V. Brazzoduro et al., "Mothers and fathers in NICU: the impact of preterm birth on parental distress," *Europe's Journal of Psychology*, vol. 12, no. 4, pp. 604–621, 2016.

[41] L. S. Franck, A. McQuillan, J. Wray, M. P. W. Grocott, and A. Goldman, "Parent stress levels during children's hospital recovery after congenital heart surgery," *Pediatric Cardiology*, vol. 31, no. 7, pp. 961–968, 2010.

[42] S.-Y. S. Lee, K. A. Lee, S. H. Rankin, A. Alkon, and S. J. Weiss, "Acculturation and stress in Chinese-American parents of infants cared for in the intensive care unit," *Advances Neonatal Care*, vol. 5, no. 6, pp. 315–328, 2005.

[43] S. B. Johnson, A. E. Baughcum, S. K. Carmichael, J.-X. She, and D. A. Schatz, "Maternal anxiety associated with newborn genetic screening for type 1 diabetes," *Diabetes Care*, vol. 27, no. 2, pp. 392–397, 2004.

[44] R. C. Kessler and P. E. Greenberg, "The economic burden of anxiety and stress disorders," *in Neuropsychopharmacology: The Fifth Generation of Progress*, K. L. Davis, D. Charney, J. T. Coyle, and C. Nemeroff, Ed., pp. 982–992, American College of Neuropsychopharmacology, Brentwood, TN, USA, 2002.

10

Asthma Control and Asthma Medication Use among Swedish Elite Endurance Athletes

Hampus Persson, Anne Lindberg, and Nikolai Stenfors

Department of Public Health and Clinical Medicine, Division of Medicine, Umeå University, Östersund, Umeå, Sweden

Correspondence should be addressed to Nikolai Stenfors; nikolai.stenfors@umu.se

Academic Editor: David Halpin

Background. Asthma is common in elite athletes. In this study, we examined the use of asthma medication and asthma control in endurance athletes in Sweden and compared the findings with those in a reference group of patients with asthma. *Methods.* The Asthma Control Test (ACT) and a questionnaire on asthma, respiratory symptoms, and medication use were posted to endurance athletes ($n = 711$) and the reference group of patients with asthma ($n = 1026$). Four hundred and sixty-nine athletes (66%) responded, of whom 141 (20%) reported physician-diagnosed asthma. In the reference group, 397 (39%) responded. *Results.* Seventy-seven percent of the athletes with asthma reported using asthma medication during the previous year; 39% used short/long-acting β2-agonists, 31% used inhaled corticosteroids, and 31% used both daily. According to the ACT scores, 19%, 24%, and 58% of athletes with asthma had uncontrolled, partially controlled, or well-controlled asthma, respectively. After adjustment, there was no difference in ACT scores or daily use of asthma medication between the study groups. *Conclusions.* Many endurance athletes had uncontrolled or partially controlled asthma, and one-third used inhaled corticosteroids and long-acting β2-agonists daily. Their adjusted ACT scores and use of asthma medication were similar to the values in the reference population.

1. Introduction

The prevalence of asthma in Sweden is estimated to be 10% in the population aged 16–35 years [1]. However, the prevalence of asthma is higher in athletes, especially those participating in sports associated with high ventilation rates [2–5]. Recently, the prevalence of physician-diagnosed asthma among Swedish elite cross-country skiers was estimated at 35% [6].

The reason for the increased prevalence of asthma in winter endurance athletes is believed to be a consequence of repeated and prolonged inhalation of dry air, leading to heat loss, dehydration, and airway damage. In addition, the cooling process seems to induce bronchoconstriction via the parasympathetic nervous system, and subsequent rewarming leads to mucosal edema and further narrowing of the airways [7, 8].

According to the guidelines, the first step in the treatment of asthma is a short-acting β2-agonist (SABA), as required. Step 2 is the addition of regular daily inhalation of corticosteroids (ICS). In Step 3, the dose of ICS can be increased and/or a daily long-acting β2-agonist (LABA) can be added [9]. A recent population-based study in Sweden showed that 19% of patients with asthma regularly used the third step of asthma treatment, that is, a fixed combination of ICS + LABA [10]. In the western parts of Sweden, the use of pharmacotherapy for asthma increased by 54% between 1992 and 2010, and the proportion of subjects with asthma using ICS increased by fivefold during that time [10].

A significant increase in use of asthma medication was documented among Finnish Olympic athletes between 2002 and 2009, even though there was no significant increase in the prevalence of either asthma or asthma symptoms, and 4% used ICS + LABA [11]. It was reported that 7% of Danish elite athletes used asthma medication in 2005 and that 79% used ICS alone or in combination with SABA or LABA [12]. Another study from Australia found no difference in the prevalence of asthma or use of β2-agonists between athletes and an age-matched control group [13]. In contrast, Finnish athletes competing in endurance and team sports were reported to use significantly more asthma medication than an age-matched control group [14]. However, none of these studies reported on the use of asthma medication in relation to asthma control in athletes.

Selection of appropriate asthma medication is a key to disease control, and there is a lack of data on asthma control in elite endurance athletes. The primary aims of this study were to examine the level of asthma control and to determine the use of asthma medication in detail, specifically SABA/LABA, ICS, and ICS + LABA, among elite endurance athletes with current asthma. A secondary aim was to compare these findings with those in a reference population of patients with asthma recruited from health care registers.

2. Materials and Methods

2.1. Study Design. This cross-sectional survey was part of a 5-year prospective postal questionnaire study on the prevalence, incidence, and remission of airway symptoms and asthma in Swedish elite endurance athletes. The study has been described in detail previously [6] and was approved by the Regional Ethical Review Board at Umeå University, 2011-186-31M (2011-06-07) and 2016/146-32 (2016-05-03).

2.2. Settings and Participants. Two study populations were included. One study group included Swedish elite athletes participating in cross-country skiing, biathlons, ski-orienteering, or orienteering at international or highest national levels. These athletes consisted of students at seven National Elite Sports Schools, Swedish junior and senior national team members, students at the three Swedish Ski Universities where elite athletes combine an elite career with higher education, and the top 80 Swedish orienteers aged 20–30 years according to the national ranking in 2011. A total of 711 eligible athletes were invited to participate in a postal questionnaire survey in September 2014 and 2015. The other study (reference) group included patients who were identified through primary and specialist health care records to have been born between 1985 and 1999 in the region of Jämtland-Härjedalen and to have a diagnosis of asthma (ICD code J45) in 2011–2015. Patients with asthma who were already included in the group of athletes were excluded. In total, 1026 eligible reference subjects were invited to participate in the postal questionnaire survey in September 2016. To match the smoking habits of the athletes, ex-smokers and current smokers were excluded from the analyses.

2.3. Study Variables. The postal questionnaire was a shortened version of the European Community Respiratory Health Survey II, which includes questions on asthma, drug utilization, airway symptoms, smoking history, family history of asthma, and health care contacts [15], and included an additional question regarding physical training. Subjects with physician-diagnosed asthma were also asked to complete the Asthma Control Test (ACT). The ACT is a well-validated questionnaire consisting of 5 questions on activity limitations, shortness of breath, awakenings with asthma, use of rescue medication, and general asthma control [16]. One reminder was sent out to all nonresponders.

The key variables investigated in the study are outlined below, along with an explanation of how each variable was assessed:

(1) "Physician-diagnosed asthma" was identified by the responses to the questions "Have you ever had asthma?" and "Was it diagnosed by a doctor?"

(2) "Medication" was identified by the responses to the question, "Have you used any asthma medication, including inhalers, sprays, or pills, during the last 12 months?" Asthma medication was categorized as SABA/LABA, ICS, or ICS + LABA. Montelukast was used by a small proportion in both study groups and is not presented in the results. The frequency of use of asthma medication was categorized as "never," "sometimes," "for more/less than 2 months per year," or "daily."

(3) "Current asthma" was defined as physician-diagnosed asthma and use of asthma medication during the previous 12 months.

(4) "Age of asthma onset" was determined by the response to the question, "How old were you when you had your first asthma attack?"

(5) "Smoking status" was determined by the responses to the questions, "Have you been smoking one or more cigarettes per day for at least one year?" and "Have you been smoking during the last month?"

(6) "Training" was assessed by the response to the question, "On average, during the last 12 months, for how many hours/week did you exercise so much that you got out of breath or became sweaty?"

(7) "Family history of asthma" was determined by the response to the question, "Do any of your parents or siblings have asthma?"

(8) "Allergy" was identified from the response to the question, "Do you have any nasal allergies, including hay fever?"

(9) "Health care contact" was assessed by the response to the question, "Have you had any health care contacts due to airway problems in the last 12 months?"

(10) "Asthma control" was assessed using the ACT and was reported both as a continuous variable ranging from 5 to 25 points and was categorized as "uncontrolled" (≤19 points), "partially controlled" (20–21 points), or "well controlled" (≥22 points) [16].

2.4. Statistical Analysis. The assumption was made a priori that 25% of the athletes and 15% of the reference subjects would be using ICS + LABA daily. We calculated that inclusion of 146 athletes would require 294 reference subjects to reach a power of 80% with an α level of 5%. A reference group of 1000 patients with a response rate of 30% was thus expected to be sufficient to detect a difference in daily use of ICS + LABA between the study groups.

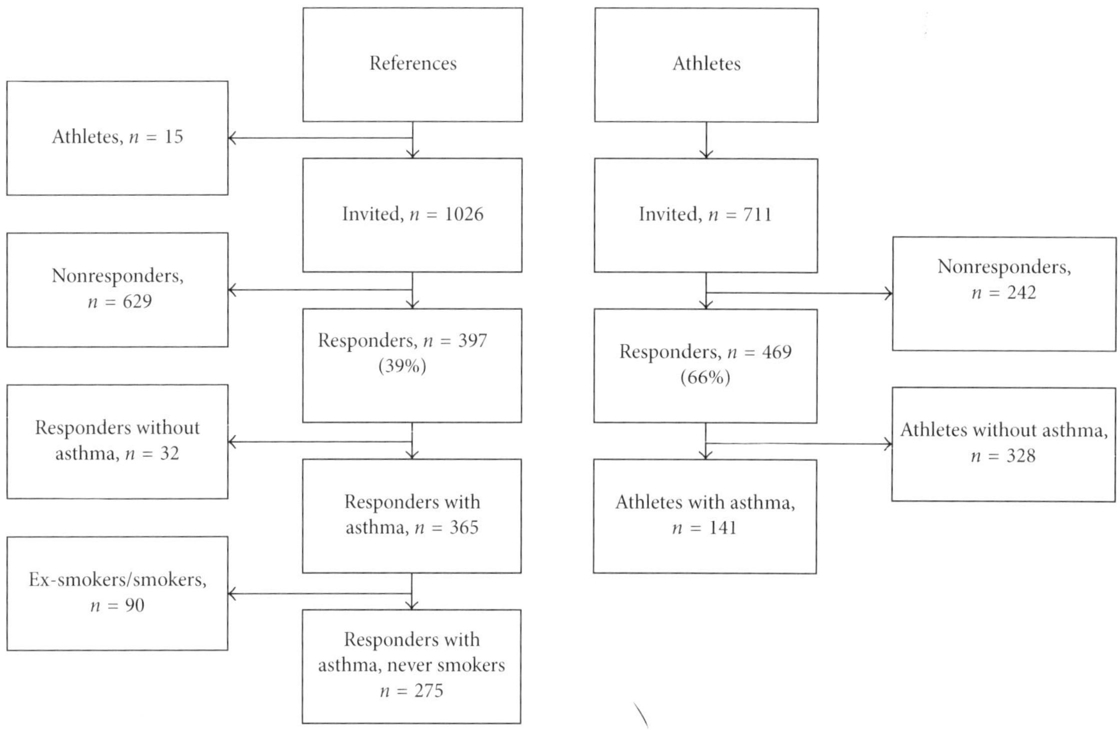

FIGURE 1: Flowchart of study participants.

Reference subjects who answered "No" ($n = 11$) or had no medication recorded or missing data regarding "physician-diagnosed asthma" ($n = 21$) were excluded. The two groups were matched with regard to smoking habits in order to exclude smoking as a source of bias in the reference group; ex-smokers and current smokers ($n = 90$) were excluded from the reference group. Use of asthma medication and the ACT score data are presented only for subjects with current asthma.

Continuous variables were compared between the study groups using Student's t-test and categorical variables using Pearson's chi-squared test. To compare the use of asthma medication between the study groups, the subjects were dichotomized, respectively, into those who did and did not use SABA/LABA, ICS, or ICS + LABA on a daily basis. Similarly, the proportions of subjects with "uncontrolled," "partially controlled," or "well-controlled" asthma were compared between the study groups on the basis of the dichotomized responses on the ACT. A p value < 0.05 was considered to be statistically significant.

After the bivariate analysis, multivariate Poisson regression analyses were performed in each group, and the data for the two study groups were then pooled to test for an independent association between the ACT score and being an elite athlete. Subject's age, age at asthma onset, allergy, shortness of breath after exercise, and respiratory-related health care contacts during the previous 12 months were included as covariates in the model.

3. Results

3.1. Subject Characteristics. Four hundred and sixty-nine (66%) of the 711 athletes invited to participate in the survey responded, and all were nonsmokers. Of these, 141 (20%) reported having physician-diagnosed asthma. Three hundred and ninety-seven (39%) of the 1026 eligible reference subjects responded. Of these, 122 were excluded either because they did not have physician-diagnosed asthma ($n = 32$) or were ex-smokers or current smokers ($n = 90$), leaving 275 reference subjects for inclusion in the analysis (Figure 1). Among the athletes with asthma, 82 (58%) were cross-country skiers, 26 (18%) were biathletes, and 19 (13%) were orienteers. Eighty-six (54%) were or had been national team members, and 55 (39%) were secondary school students.

A detailed description of the two study populations is presented in Table 1. The athletes had a lower mean age and a higher mean number of training hours per week when compared with the reference group. The reported age of asthma onset was older in the athletes than in the reference subjects. The prevalence of current physician-diagnosed asthma, determined by the use of asthma medication during the previous 12 months, was lower in the athlete group than in the reference group (77% versus 88%, $p = 0.002$).

3.2. Asthma Control. When classified by ACT scores, 58% of the athletes with current asthma reported that their asthma was well controlled, whereas 23% reported partially controlled asthma and 19% reported uncontrolled asthma (Table 2). These three subgroups of athletes, based on the level of asthma control, differed in their number of health care contacts during the previous 12 months, daily use of asthma medication, and use of SABA/LABA and ICS + LABA; the highest numbers in all categories were for athletes reporting uncontrolled asthma (Table 3).

TABLE 1: Demographic and clinical characteristics of a group of Swedish elite endurance athletes and a health care-based reference population of patients with asthma.

	Athletes ($n = 141$)	References ($n = 275$)	p value
Age (years), mean (SD)	21.5 (4.5)	25.6 (6.4)	**<0.001**
Women	79 (56)	181 (66)	0.051
Training (hours/week), mean (SD)	11.7 (4.4)	4.9 (4.5)	**<0.001**
Current asthma	108 (77)	243 (88)	**0.002**
Age of asthma onset (years), mean (SD)	13.3 (4.5)	9.8 (6.7)	**<0.001**
Allergy	54 (50)	203 (74)	**<0.001**
Family history of asthma	78 (59)	149 (58)	0.866
Health care contacts[1]	25 (18)	75 (27)	**0.031**
Shortness of breath[2]	27 (19)	95 (35)	**0.001**

The data are presented as n (%) unless otherwise stated; significant p values are shown in bold; [1]respiratory-related health care contacts in the previous 12 months; [2]shortness of breath following strenuous activity in the previous 12 months; SD, standard deviation.

TABLE 2: Level and distribution of asthma control in Swedish endurance athletes with current asthma.

	Uncontrolled ($n = 19$)	Partially controlled ($n = 24$)	Well controlled ($n = 59$)	p value*
Female sex	11 (58)	17 (71)	32 (54)	0.378
Age (years), mean (SD)	19.8 (3.7)	21.3 (4.2)	22.2 (4.8)	0.174
Age of asthma onset (years), mean (SD)	13.4 (4.3)	16.5 (4.0)	12.1 (4.8)	**0.009**
Allergy	9 (47)	14 (58)	23 (44)	0.517
Training (hours/week), mean (SD)	12.9 (2.7)	13.1 (3.8)	11.1 (4.8)	0.855
Shortness of breath[1]	8 (42)	7 (29)	10 (17)	0.079
Health care contacts[2]	9 (47)	8 (33)	7 (12)	**0.003**
Family history of asthma	12 (63)	13 (62)	37 (69)	0.828
Daily SABA/LABA	14 (74)	12 (50)	15 (25)	**<0.001**
Daily ICS	9 (47)	7 (29)	18 (31)	0.353
Daily ICS + LABA	10 (53)	8 (33)	13 (22)	**0.039**

The data are presented as n (%) unless otherwise stated; significant p values are shown in bold; [1]shortness of breath following strenuous exercise in the previous 12 months; [2]respiratory-related health care contacts in the previous 12 months; ICS, inhaled corticosteroids; SABA/LABA, short-acting $\beta 2$-agonists/long-acting $\beta 2$-agonists; SD, standard deviation; *Pearson's chi-squared test.

TABLE 3: Level and distribution of asthma control in a health care-based reference group of patients with current asthma who have never smoked.

	Uncontrolled ($n = 82$)	Partially controlled ($n = 57$)	Well controlled ($n = 102$)	p value*
Females	55 (67)	35 (61)	67 (66)	0.779
Age (years), mean (SD)	24.1 (4.2)	25.6 (4.7)	26.7 (7.8)	**0.006**
Age of asthma onset (years), mean (SD)	7.9 (6.2)	9.7 (7.6)	11.3 (6.3)	**0.003**
Allergy	69 (84)	42 (74)	74 (73)	0.148
Training (hours/week), mean (SD)	5.0 (5.5)	5.3 (4.4)	4.7 (3.7)	0.827
Shortness of breath[1]	48 (59)	21 (38)	24 (24)	**<0.001**
Health care contacts[2]	39 (48)	15 (26)	20 (20)	**<0.001**
Family history of asthma	46 (61)	32 (62)	54 (56)	0.739
Daily SABA/LABA	50 (61)	14 (25)	8 (8)	**<0.001**
Daily ICS	26 (32)	13 (23)	17 (17)	**0.056**
Daily ICS + LABA	36 (44)	13 (23)	38 (37)	**0.037**

The data are presented as n (%) unless otherwise stated; significant p values are shown in bold; [1]shortness of breath following strenuous exercise in the previous 12 months; [2]respiratory-related health care contacts in the previous 12 months; ICS, inhaled corticosteroids; SABA/LABA, short-acting $\beta 2$-agonists/long-acting $\beta 2$-agonists; SD, standard deviation; *Pearson's chi-squared test.

In the reference group, 102 patients (42%) reported well-controlled asthma (Table 3). Those with uncontrolled asthma had more shortness of breath, used more daily asthma medication, and had had more health care contacts during the previous 12 months.

Athletes whose ACT scores indicated well-controlled asthma reported no or little limitation in daily activities (Figure 2(a)), seldom experiencing shortness of breath (Figure 2(b)), and few awakenings with asthma (Figure 2(c)), and considered their asthma to be well or completely controlled (Figure 2(e)). Many athletes with well-controlled asthma reported use of rescue medication once or twice daily or 2-3 times per week (Figure 2(d)), whereas the athletes with uncontrolled asthma used SABA at least 2-3 times per week (Figure 2(b)).

The athletes had a significantly higher mean ACT score than the reference subjects (Table 4) but included a smaller proportion of subjects with uncontrolled asthma and a larger proportion of subjects with well-controlled asthma (Table 4).

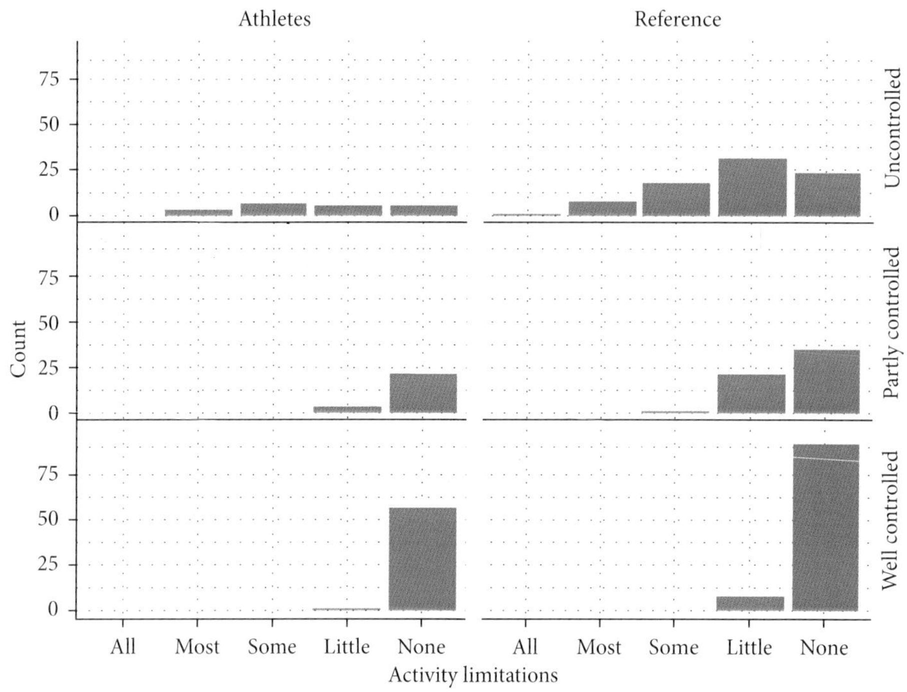

(a)

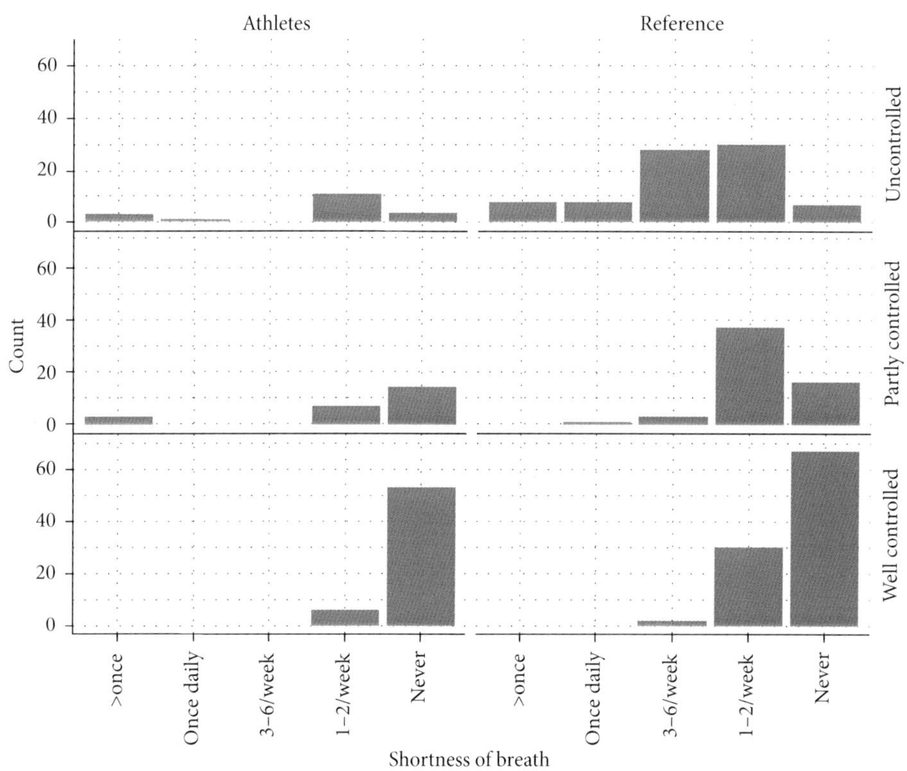

(b)

FIGURE 2: Continued.

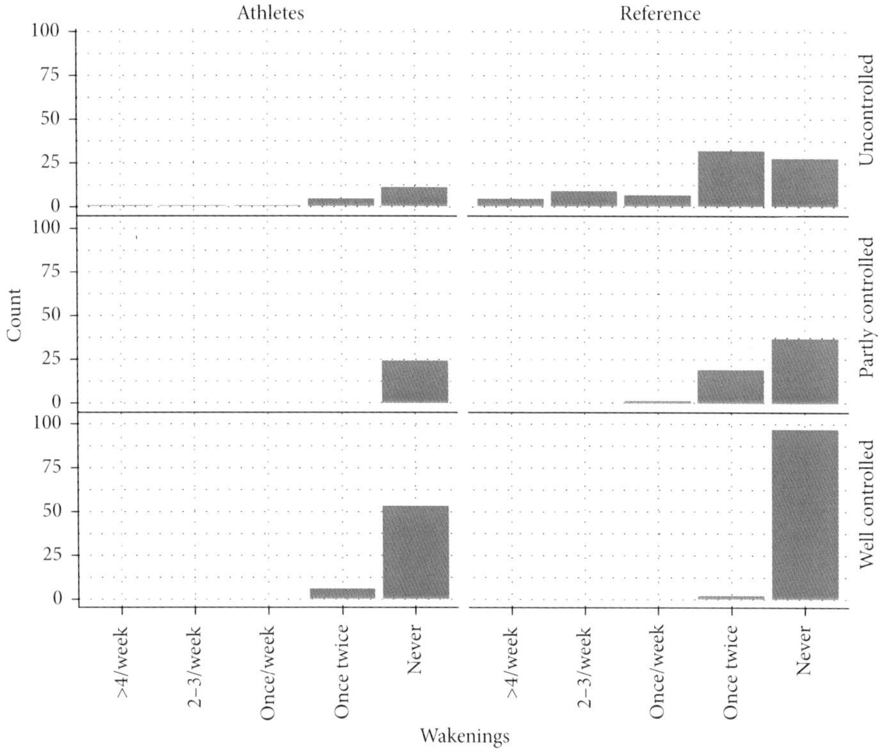

(c)

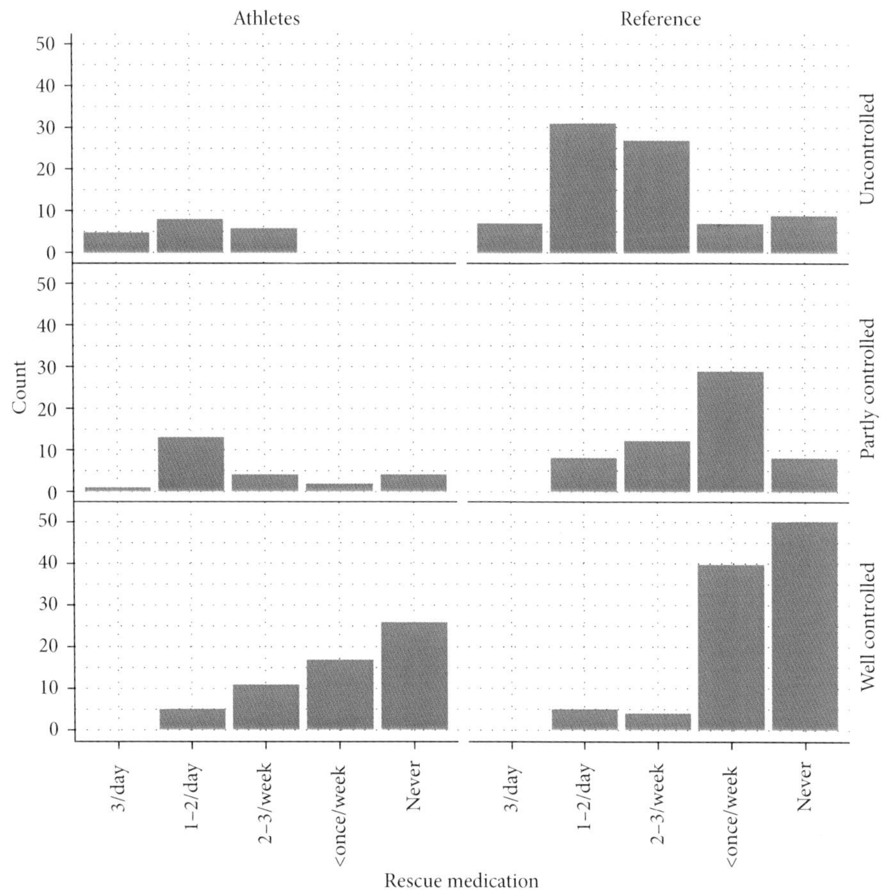

(d)

Figure 2: Continued.

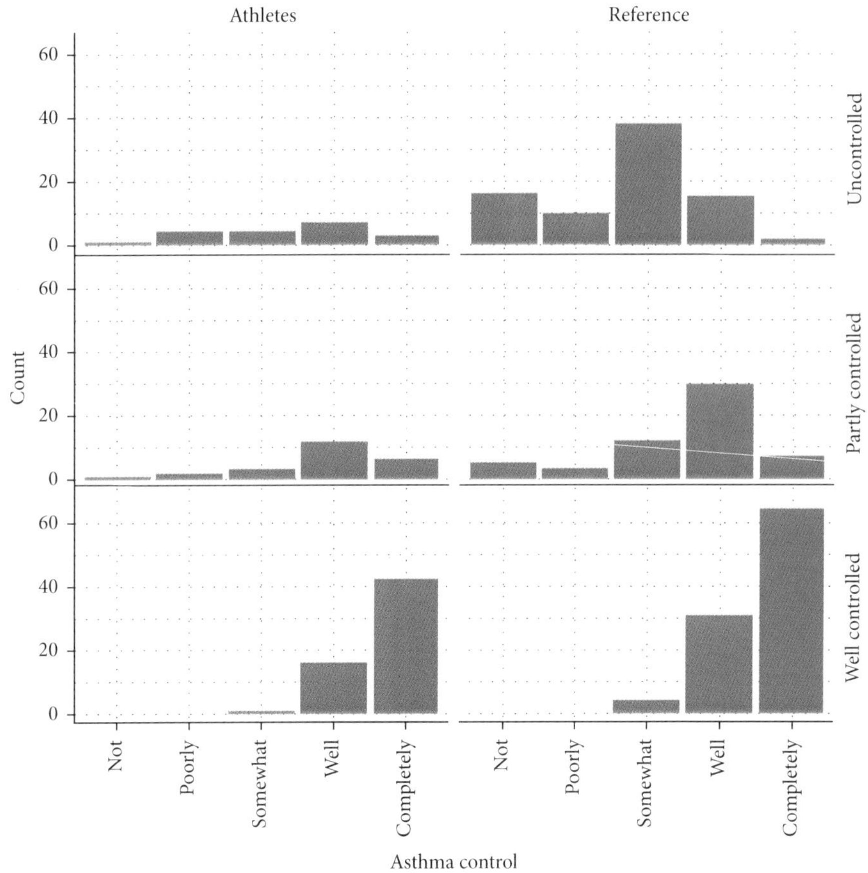

(e)

Figure 2: Results for each ACT question. The results are stratified by study population and ACT category. (a) "In the past 4 weeks, how much of the time did your asthma keep you from getting as much done at work, school or at home?" (all of the time, most of the time, some of the time, a little of the time, or none of the time). (b) "During the past 4 weeks, how often have you had shortness of breath?" (more than once a day, once a day, 3 to 6 times a week, once or twice a week, or not at all). (c) "During the past 4 weeks, how often did your asthma symptoms (wheezing, coughing, shortness of breath, chest tightness, or pain) wake you up at night, or earlier than usual in the morning?" (4 or more nights a week, 2 to 3 nights a week, once a week, once or twice, or not at all). (d) "During the past 4 weeks, how often have you used your rescue inhaler or nebulizer medication?" (3 or more times per day, 1 or 2 times per day, 2 or 3 times per week, once a week or less, or not at all). (e) "How would you rate your asthma control during the past weeks?" (not controlled at all, poorly controlled, somewhat controlled, well controlled, or completely controlled).

There were no significant sex-related differences in ACT scores within any of the groups. In the multivariate Poisson regression model, there were no associations between ACT score and age, age at asthma onset, allergy, shortness of breath after exercise, or respiratory-related health care contacts during the previous 12 months. However, in the reference group, there was an independent positive association between the ACT score and the age at asthma onset ($p = 0.020$) and an independent negative association between the ACT score and exercise-induced shortness of breath ($p = 0.002$) and the number of health care contacts ($p = 0.001$). When the data for the athletes and reference subjects were pooled, there was no independent association between the study group and ACT score ($p = 0.165$).

3.3. Asthma Medication. Of the athletes with current asthma, 39% used SABA/LABA daily, 31% used ICS daily, and 31% used ICS + LABA daily. Overall, 43% of the athletes used ICS or ICS + LABA daily. Athletes with an ACT score indicating uncontrolled asthma reported more daily use of $\beta 2$-agonists and ICS + LABA (Table 2). There were no statistically significant differences in the proportions of subjects who used SABA/LABA, ICS, or ICS + LABA daily between the study groups (Table 5). There were also no significant sex-related differences in the use of asthma medication between the groups.

4. Discussion

This postal questionnaire survey evaluated disease control and use of asthma medication in 141 elite endurance athletes with asthma and a reference population of 275 nonathletic patients with asthma. Among the elite athletes, 108 (77%) had current asthma, that is, had used asthma medication during the previous 12 months; 39% used SABA/LABA, 31% used ICS, and 31% used ICS + LABA on a regular daily basis.

TABLE 4: Bivariate analyses comparing ACT scores and levels of the control based on ACT scores between Swedish elite endurance athletes and a reference group of patients with current asthma who have never smoked.

	Athletes (n = 108)	References (n = 242)	p value
ACT score, mean (SD)	22.2 (2.9)	21.0 (4.0)	**0.004**
Uncontrolled[1]	19 (19)	81 (34)	**0.005**
Partially controlled[2]	24 (24)	57 (23)	0.965
Well controlled[3]	59 (58)	102 (42)	**0.009**

The data are presented as n (%); significant p values are shown in bold; [1]ACT score ≤ 19; [2]ACT score 20–21; [3]ACT score ≥ 22; ACT, Asthma Control Test; SD, standard deviation.

TABLE 5: Use of asthma medication by Swedish elite endurance athletes and a reference group of patients with current asthma and a statistical comparison between the two groups.

	Athletes (n = 108)	References (n = 242)	p value*
SABA/LABA			
Never	32 (30)	40 (17)	
Sometimes	30 (28)	101 (42)	
Less than 2 months	0 (0)	12 (5)	
More than 2 months	4 (4)	16 (7)	
Daily	42 (39)	73 (30)	0.101
ICS			
Never	56 (52)	135 (56)	
Sometimes	14 (13)	34 (14)	
Less than 2 months	1 (1)	8 (3)	
More than 2 months	3 (3)	9 (4)	
Daily	34 (31)	56 (23)	0.099
ICS + LABA			
Never	64 (59)	126 (52)	
Sometimes	5 (5)	17 (7)	
Less than 2 months	3 (3)	5 (2)	
More than 2 months	3 (3)	7 (3)	
Daily	33 (31)	87 (36)	0.326

To compare the two groups with regard to use of asthma medication, the subjects were dichotomized into those who did and did not use SABA/LABA, ICS, or ICS + LABA daily; *comparison of proportions of daily users of SABA/LABA, ICS, and ICS + LABA between the study groups; ICS, inhaled corticosteroids; SABA/LABA, short-acting β2-agonists/long-acting β2-agonists.

According to the ACT scores, 19% of athletes had current asthma that was uncontrolled, 25% had partly controlled asthma, and 58% had well-controlled asthma. Athletes with uncontrolled asthma reported frequent use of SABA/LABA; after adjustment for confounding factors, their ACT scores and daily use of asthma medication did not differ significantly from the values observed in the reference population of patients with asthma who had never smoked.

To the best of our knowledge, this is the first study to compare asthma control and use of asthma medication between elite athletes with asthma and nonathletic patients with asthma. In order to perform at their best, athletes should not be limited by respiratory problems. This is especially true for those with high ventilation rates, such as endurance athletes. Hence, it was not unexpected that the majority (almost 60%) of the endurance athletes in the present study had well-controlled asthma. However, we were surprised to find that up to one-quarter of the elite endurance athletes were classified as having partly controlled asthma and nearly one-fifth as having uncontrolled asthma, which suggests that it is possible to pursue endurance sports at an elite level without well-controlled asthma. Another explanation could be that ACT is an inadequate tool for assessment of asthma control in elite athletes. Depending on how the athletes interpret the questionnaire, both over- and underestimation of asthma control may occur. Although well validated, ACT may have poor accuracy for assessment of uncontrolled asthma [16], and some of the ACT questions might be poorly adapted for elite athletes. The question "During the past 4 weeks, how often have you had shortness of breath?" might lead to a falsely low score among elite athletes training once or twice a day, whereas "shortness of breath" for a subject with a limited amount of physical activity might be a better indicator of inadequate treatment. In the present study, surprisingly few athletes with current asthma reported shortness of breath after exercise. It is difficult to find publications reporting prevalence of exercise-induced asthma (EIA) among athletes with asthma. Our findings may have several explanations. Firstly, elite athletes with asthma may thoroughly and consistently prevent EIA by pharmacotherapy and consequently not experience shortness of breath after exercise. Secondly, elite endurance athletes training 10–20 hours/week may have a different interpretation of and a high threshold for "shortness of breath post exercise." Further, the question "How often do you use a β2-agonist?" might be misleading because many athletes use these medications before training and/or competitions simply to avoid EIA. SABA may be used in a controlled manner prior to exercise in order to prevent EIA or as unplanned rescue during/after exercise when EIA occurs. From a clinical perspective, the subject/athlete in the latter example could be considered having a poorer level of asthma control. Therefore, athletes might have had misleadingly low ACT scores and subsequently high proportions with uncontrolled and partially controlled asthma.

Several studies have assessed asthma control using ACT in "nonelite athletic" subjects. In those studies, the prevalence of uncontrolled asthma (defined as an ACT score $\leq$ 19 points) varied in the range of 50%–58% [17–19]. In comparison with those results, both the athletes and the reference subjects in our study appeared to have fairly good asthma control. After adjustments, being an elite athlete was not associated with a higher ACT score. Female sex, early asthma onset, increasing age, and a smoking history are well-known risk factors for uncontrolled asthma [17–19]. The group of athletes in our present study contained a significantly smaller proportion of women, had later asthma onset, and were younger than the reference group, which may explain why being an athlete per se was not associated with better asthma control.

Fifty-two (48%) of the 108 athletes with current asthma in our study used a fixed combination of ICS + LABA sometimes to daily, which is similar to observations in Finnish Olympic athletes reported in 2004 [14]. Direct comparison of the studies is difficult because of differences in the study populations: the Finnish athletes were older, a majority were men, and they trained more. Another study reported on the use of asthma medication by 694 Danish elite athletes who had applied for a therapeutic use exemption for their asthma medication in 2005 [20]. Of 445 athletes who were using asthma medication, 140 (32%) used a fixed combination of ICS + LABA. This finding suggests a trend of increasing use of ICS and/or ICS + LABA among Scandinavian athletes, which may be related to the introduction of the fixed-dose combination inhalers, that is, ICS + LABA [10, 21].

The relatively high use of ICS or ICS + LABA in the present study may also explain why the athletes used less SABA/LABA when compared with Australian summer sports athletes [13]. Of 52 Australian athletes with "ever-doctor diagnosed asthma" who used medication for asthma or asthma-like symptoms, 54% used SABA, 25% used LABA, and 44% used ICS. The lower use of SABA/LABA in the present study could indicate better controlled asthma in Swedish (mostly winter) endurance athletes than in summer sports athletes from Australia or perhaps simply different traditions of asthma pharmacotherapy between the two countries.

Athletes who used SABA/LABA frequently tended to have uncontrolled asthma when classified by their ACT scores. However, frequent use of SABA/LABA contributes to a lower ACT score, which may cause asthma to be classified as partially controlled or uncontrolled. We suggest that this particular group of athletes should receive extra medical attention in order to evaluate and optimize their disease control. However, this study was cross-sectional, so we cannot conclude that frequent use of SABA/LABA is a cause or an effect of uncontrolled asthma. It is in line with our clinical experience that a large proportion of elite endurance athletes are/feel controlled on Step 1 treatment with SABA only and seldom need/use controllers (ICS or ICS/LABA).

In our reference group of patients with asthma who had never smoked, 31% used ICS + LABA daily, which is higher than the rate of 19% reported in a population-based cohort of patients with asthma [10]. Again, direct comparison between the two studies is difficult because our reference group was younger than that in the population-based study, which included patients up to 78 years of age and also smokers.

The present study has some limitations in that the diagnosis of asthma, level of asthma control, and use of asthma medication were based on self-reported data and were not confirmed by medical records or prescriptions of medication. The low response rate of 39% in the reference group may represent a degree of selection bias. A nonresponse analysis would be of value, however, was not included in the original study design and ethical approval. Two Scandinavian questionnaire-based studies found that nonresponders were significantly more likely to be men, younger, and current smokers but found no significant differences with regard to the prevalence of asthma-like symptoms or use of asthma medication [22, 23]. However, an earlier questionnaire-based survey conducted in northern Sweden found that respiratory symptoms and use of asthma medication were more common among nonresponders [24], highlighting the risk of underestimating the prevalence of respiratory symptoms using postal surveys. Our reference group was included based on health care records, so we can assume that they had had a recent consultation for their asthma, that is, during 2011–2015. However, the distribution of asthma control in the reference group is almost identical to the findings from primary care in Sweden 2001 and 2005, a survey with 60% response rate [25]. Altogether, it is possible that the reference group was skewed towards patients with symptomatic asthma and frequent use of asthma medication and thus underestimated ACT scores and overestimated use of asthma medication in this group.

The 66% response rate for the athletes in this study can be considered representative of Swedish endurance athletes, who are competing mostly in a cold climate. Given that the Swedish guideline for asthma treatment follows the international guidelines, the results of our study may be generalizable to endurance athletes outside of Sweden.

It has been shown that German elite athletes with high ventilation rates use significantly more asthma medication than those with medium or low ventilation rates, but no significant difference in use was observed between summer and winter athletes [5]. These observations support our present findings regarding asthma medication and suggest that they may also be applicable to summer endurance athletes, such as long-distance runners and racing cyclists.

5. Conclusions

According to our postal questionnaire survey, 39% of Swedish endurance athletes with current asthma used SABA/LABA and 31% used ICS + LABA daily. Most of the athletes had well-controlled asthma (58%), and those with uncontrolled asthma (19%) reported frequent use of SABA/LABA. Their ACT scores and daily use of asthma medication did not significantly differ from the results in the reference population of patients with asthma who had never smoked. Being an elite endurance athlete per se was not associated with either the ACT score or daily use of asthma medication. All patients with asthma should be monitored regularly. Elite endurance athletes using $\beta 2$-agonists several times per week may have uncontrolled asthma and need extra attention in order to minimize the risk of respiratory limitations.

Acknowledgments

The authors wish to thank the coaches at the Swedish National Elite Sport Schools, national teams, and ski universities for recruitment and data collection, and the Swedish Ski Association, Biathlon Association, and Swedish Orienteering Federation for recruitment and general support. This study was financially supported by the Visare Norr Fund, Northern County Council's Regional Federation, and by the Research & Development Unit of the Jämtland County Council, Sweden.

References

[1] J. Lötvall, L. Ekerljung, E. P. Rönmark et al., "West Sweden Asthma Study: prevalence trends over the last 18 years argues no recent increase in asthma," *Respiratory Research*, vol. 10, no. 1, p. 94, 2009.

[2] K. Larsson, P. Ohlsen, L. Larsson, P. Malmberg, P.-O. Rydström, and H. Ulriksen, "High prevalence of asthma in cross country skiers," *BMJ*, vol. 307, no. 6915, pp. 1326–1329, 1993.

[3] T. Heir and S. Oseid, "Self-reported asthma and exercise-induced asthma symptoms in high-level competitive cross-country skiers," *Scandinavian Journal of Medicine & Science in Sports*, vol. 4, no. 2, pp. 128–133, 1994.

[4] I. J. Helenius, H. O. Tikkanen, and T. Haahtela, "Association between type of training and risk of asthma in elite athletes," *Thorax*, vol. 52, no. 2, pp. 157–160, 1997.

[5] C. Selge, S. Thomas, D. Nowak, K. Radon, and B. Wolfarth, "Asthma prevalence in German Olympic athletes: A comparison of winter and summer sport disciplines," *Respiratory Medicine*, vol. 118, pp. 15–21, 2016.

[6] J. Norqvist, L. Eriksson, L. Söderström, A. Lindberg, and N. Stenfors, "Self-reported physician-diagnosed asthma among Swedish adolescent, adult and former elite endurance athletes," *Journal of Asthma*, vol. 52, no. 10, pp. 1046–1053, 2015.

[7] K. H. Carlsen, S. D. Anderson, L. Bjermer et al., "Exercise-induced asthma, respiratory and allergic disorders in elite athletes: epidemiology, mechanisms and diagnosis: Part I of the report from the Joint Task Force of the European Respiratory Society (ERS) and the European Academy of Allergy and Clinical Immunology (EAACI) in cooperation with GA2LEN," *Allergy*, vol. 63, no. 4, pp. 387–403, 2008.

[8] S. R. Del Giacco, D. Firinu, L. Bjermer, and K.-H. Carlsen, "Exercise and asthma: an overview," *European Clinical Respiratory Journal*, vol. 2, no. 1, pp. 279–284, 2015.

[9] S. Hurd and R. Decker, *2016 Gina Report: Global Strategy for Asthma Management and Prevention*, Global Initiative for Asthma (GINA), 2016, http://www.ginasthma.org.

[10] L. Ekerljung, A. Bjerg, A. Bossios et al., "Five-fold increase in use of inhaled corticosteroids over 18 years in the general adult population in West Sweden," *Respiratory Medicine*, vol. 108, no. 5, pp. 685–693, 2014.

[11] A. Aavikko, I. Helenius, A. Alaranta, T. Vasankari, and T. Haahtela, "Asthma medication is increasingly prescribed for Finnish Olympic athletes—for a reason?," *Journal of Asthma*, vol. 49, no. 7, pp. 744–749, 2012.

[12] T. Lund, L. Pedersen, B. Larsson, and V. Backer, "Prevalence of asthma-like symptoms, asthma and its treatment in elite athletes: asthma and its treatment in elite athletes," *Scandinavian Journal of Medicine & Science in Sports*, vol. 19, no. 2, pp. 174–178, 2008.

[13] S. Locke and G. Marks, "Are the prevalence and treatment of asthma similar in elite athletes and the aged-matched non-athlete population?: Prevalence and treatment of asthma in elite athletes," *Scandinavian Journal of Medicine & Science in Sports*, vol. 17, no. 6, pp. 623–627, 2007.

[14] A. Alaranta, H. Alaranta, P. Palmu et al., "Asthma medication in Finnish Olympic athletes: no signs of inhaled $\beta 2$-agonist overuse," *Medicine & Science in Sports & Exercise*, vol. 36, no. 6, pp. 919–924, 2004.

[15] The European Community Respiratory Health Survey II Steering Committee, "The European Community Respiratory Health Survey II," *European Respiratory Journal*, vol. 20, no. 5, pp. 1071–1079, 2002.

[16] R. A. Nathan, C. A. Sorkness, M. Kosinski et al., "Development of the asthma control test: a survey for assessing asthma control," *Journal of Allergy and Clinical Immunology*, vol. 113, no. 1, pp. 59–65, 2004.

[17] A. Corrado, T. Renda, G. Polese, and A. Rossi, "Assessment of asthma control: the SERENA study," *Respiratory Medicine*, vol. 107, no. 11, pp. 1659–1666, 2013.

[18] R. H. Stanford, A. W. Gilsenan, R. Ziemiecki, X. Zhou, W. R. Lincourt, and H. Ortega, "Predictors of uncontrolled asthma in adult and pediatric patients: analysis of the Asthma Control Characteristics and Prevalence Survey Studies (ACCESS)," *Journal of Asthma*, vol. 47, no. 3, pp. 257–262, 2010.

[19] P. Demoly, P. Paggiaro, V. Plaza et al., "Prevalence of asthma control among adults in France, Germany, Italy, Spain and the UK," *European Respiratory Review*, vol. 18, no. 112, pp. 105–112, 2009.

[20] T. K. Lund, L. Pedersen, and V. Backer, "The use of anti-asthmatic medication among Danish elite athletes," *Ugeskrift for Laeger*, vol. 169, no. 50, pp. 4355–4359, 2007.

[21] J. R. Davidsen, J. Søndergaard, J. Hallas, H. C. Siersted, J. Lykkegaard, and M. Andersen, "Increased use of inhaled corticosteroids among young Danish adult asthmatics: an observational study," *Respiratory Medicine*, vol. 104, no. 12, pp. 1817–1824, 2010.

[22] E. P. Rönmark, L. Ekerljung, J. Lötvall, K. Torén, E. Rönmark, and B. Lundbäck, "Large scale questionnaire survey on respiratory health in Sweden: effects of late- and non-response," *Respiratory Medicine*, vol. 103, no. 12, pp. 1807–1815, 2009.

[23] P. Bakke, A. Gulsvik, P. Lilleng, O. Overå, R. Hanoa, and G. E. Eide, "Postal survey on airborne occupational exposure and respiratory disorders in Norway: causes and consequences of non-response," *Journal of Epidemiology & Community Health*, vol. 44, no. 4, pp. 316–320, 1990.

11

Optimizing the Delivery of Inhaled Medication for Respiratory Patients: The Role of Valved Holding Chambers

R. Andrew McIvor,[1] Hollie M. Devlin,[2] and Alan Kaplan[3,4,5]

[1]*St. Joseph's Healthcare Hamilton, McMaster University, Hamilton, ON, Canada*
[2]*Hollie Devlin Consulting, Toronto, ON, Canada*
[3]*Family Physician Airways Group of Canada, Richmond Hill, ON, Canada*
[4]*Department of Family and Community Medicine, University of Toronto, Toronto, ON, Canada*
[5]*Health Quality Ontario COPD Community Standards Project, Toronto, ON, Canada*

Correspondence should be addressed to R. Andrew McIvor; amcivor1@cogeco.ca

Academic Editor: Massimo Pistolesi

Valved holding chambers (VHCs) have been used with pressurized metered-dose inhalers since the early 1980s. They have been shown to increase fine particle delivery to the lungs, decrease oropharyngeal deposition, and reduce side effects such as throat irritation, dysphonia, and oral candidiasis that are common with use of pressurized metered-dose inhalers (pMDIs) alone. VHCs act as aerosol reservoirs, allowing the user to actuate the pMDI device and then inhale the medication in a two-step process that helps users overcome challenges in coordinating pMDI actuation with inhalation. The design of VHC devices can have an impact on performance. Features such as antistatic properties, effective face-to-facemask seal feedback whistles indicating correct inhalation speed, and inhalation indicators all help improve function and performance, and have been demonstrated to improve asthma control, reduce the rate of exacerbations, and improve quality of life. Not all VHCs are the same, and they are not interchangeable. Each pairing of a pMDI device plus VHC should be considered as a unique delivery system.

1. Introduction

Inhaled therapy is the gold standard for treatment of asthma [1] and chronic obstructive pulmonary disease (COPD) [2] in patients treated with pressurized metered-dose inhalers (pMDIs). The first pMDI was introduced in 1956 by Riker Laboratories Inc. and constituted a significant advancement in the delivery of aerosol medication [3]. pMDIs are now the most widely used devices for the delivery of aerosol medication because of their low cost, effectiveness, and relative simplicity of use [4]. However, despite instruction, many patients are unable to use their pMDIs correctly, with the most common error being the inability to synchronize actuation with inhalation [5].

Spacer devices were introduced in 1958 to improve medication delivery into the lungs and reduce deposition in the mouth and throat [3]. Spacers have undergone a significant transformation since their origin as simple home-made tubes such as toilet paper tubes, plastic cups, and empty vinegar bottles [3]. In 1981, both cone and tube spacers were proven to improve medication deposition on the conducting airways without changing alveolar deposition [6]. Around the same time, the valved holding chamber (VHC) was introduced. The VHC built on the spacer design by adding a one-way inhalation valve at the exit of the chamber which traps the aerosolized medication within the chamber until the user inhales. VHCs improve pMDI medication delivery, reduce oropharyngeal deposition of medication, and help users overcome challenges in coordinating pMDI actuation with inhalation [7–9]. In 1994, Holzer and Muller [10] showed that valve construction had an impact on the delivery of medication. Subsequent to 1994, VHCs were further improved with respect to facemask design in order to obtain a better face-to-facemask seal, incorporation of antistatic materials to reduce attraction of medication to the chamber walls, and feedback features such as whistles which indicate correct inhalation speed and inhalation indicators (Figure 1).

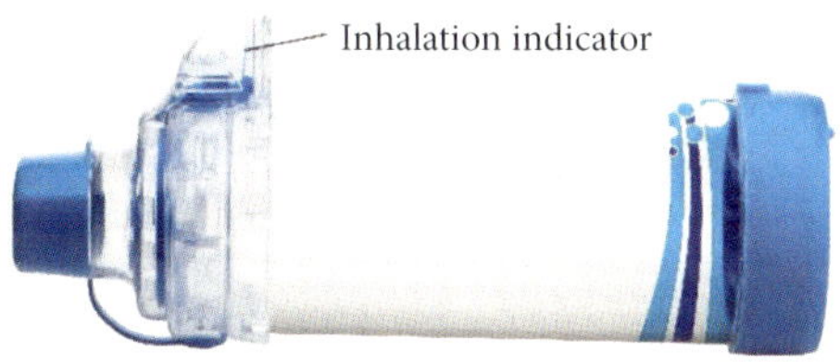

Figure 1: Valved holding chamber featuring an inhalation indicator.

In 2009, the European Medicines Agency recognized the significant role of the VHC in drug delivery when they recommended that the development of drug products using a pMDI include testing with at least one named VHC. In addition, they recommended that if a VHC was to be substituted or added, appropriate equivalency data for the alternative VHC must be presented [11].

Current guidelines for asthma [1, 9] and chronic obstructive pulmonary disease (COPD) [2] mention the use of a spacer in conjunction with pMDIs but do not discuss VHCs in great detail or provide much guidance on their use for health-care providers or caregivers. The American Academy of Allergy Asthma and Immunology (AAAAI) states that VHCs with whistles and one-way valves are preferable to spacers [12].

2. pMDIs and the Challenges of Inhaler Technique

Inhaled therapies can be very effective treatment for lung diseases. However, they must be used correctly for patients to obtain their full benefit. Poor inhaler technique is common with all types of inhalers and has been examined extensively [5, 13, 14]. A review of 2123 asthma patients by the National Services for Health Improvement found that without training, 86% failed to properly use their inhaler [15]. Another study showed that only 1 out of 10 patients using an MDI were able to perform all essential steps correctly [16]. Even with inhaler training, some people will revert back to bad technique, and some will not benefit from training [17]. The most common errors associated with pMDIs are the lack of coordination between actuation and inhalation; halting inhalation when the cool spray hits the back of the throat; not holding the breath long enough (>5 seconds) after inhalation; no exhalation prior to actuation; and not shaking the suspension prior to use [13, 18]. A recent literature review indicates that inhaler technique has not improved over the past 40 years [19].

Implications of poor technique include unintentional noncompliance (patient is compliant but has poor inhaler technique) [14], significantly reduced efficacy of the medications [5, 13, 18], increased risk of hospitalizations and emergency room visits, and poor disease control [13]. Giraud and Roche [18] showed that 71% of adult asthmatic patients are unable to use their inhaler devices effectively, resulting in decreased control of asthma symptoms. All of these lead to increased health-care expenditure [20]. Factors that impact the ability of patients to correctly use inhalers include age, coordination, inhaler technique training, choice of inhaler type, and use of multiple inhalers [2].

Additional challenges arise when patients are prescribed multiple inhaler devices that require different inhalation techniques. While pMDIs require a slow and deep breath, dry powder inhalers (PDIs), and breath-actuated metered-dose inhalers (BA-MDI) require a fast and deep inhalation [20, 21]. Multiple inhaler users compared to single inhaler users have been shown to experience significantly more exacerbations, have a higher risk of exacerbations, higher rates of inpatient admissions, inpatient days, urgent care visits, and outpatient visits [22].

Patients using two or more inhaler types that require different inhaler techniques are prone to a higher frequency of errors and have impaired outcomes. Bosnic-Anticevich et al. [23] showed lower rates of exacerbation and reduced use of high doses of short-acting beta agonists in COPD patients requiring more than one inhaler when the inhalers require similar inhalation techniques compared to inhalers that require different inhaler techniques.

Challenges resulting from poor inhaler technique often start at the point of prescription. The clinicians responsible for teaching inhaler technique, including nurses, doctors, and respiratory therapists, are often unable to describe or perform the critical steps for using inhalers [24, 25]. One study showed that only 14.2% of >1500 physicians who frequently prescribe medications delivered by inhaled devices had adequate knowledge of inhaled therapy, including correct use of inhalers [26].

3. Valved Holding Chambers (VHCs)

A key challenge with pMDIs is the potential for unwanted deposition of drug and excipients in the mouth and the back of the throat. This remains an issue with hydrofluoroalkane (HFA) formulations and to some extent with slower, finer spray products [27, 28]. Spacer devices and VHCs were initially designed to increase delivery of aerosol medications to the lungs while reducing the oropharyngeal deposition [3]. The space between the pMDI and the user's mouth allows for a reduction of aerosol velocity and particle size through both evaporation and particle impaction on the spacer wall. Together, this leads to an increase in the proportion of fine particles delivered to the lungs, a decrease in large particle deposition in the mouth and throat [29] (Figure 2) and reduction of associated side effects such as throat irritation, dysphonia, and oral candidiasis that are common with use of pMDIs alone [4, 29]. VHCs act as aerosol reservoirs, allowing the user to actuate the pMDI device and then inhale the medication in a two-step process that reduces the need to coordinate actuation and inhalation at the same time [30]. This is a particularly important advantage of using VHCs with pMDI devices.

The design of the device can have an impact on its performance. Throughout the development of VHCs, it was recognized that while large-volume holding chambers increase lung deposition to a greater degree than tube spacers or small holding chambers, they could be cumbersome for patients. Currently available devices range in volume from 50–750 ml [4]. Larger VHCs may be less portable and appealing, especially among children and teens, which may

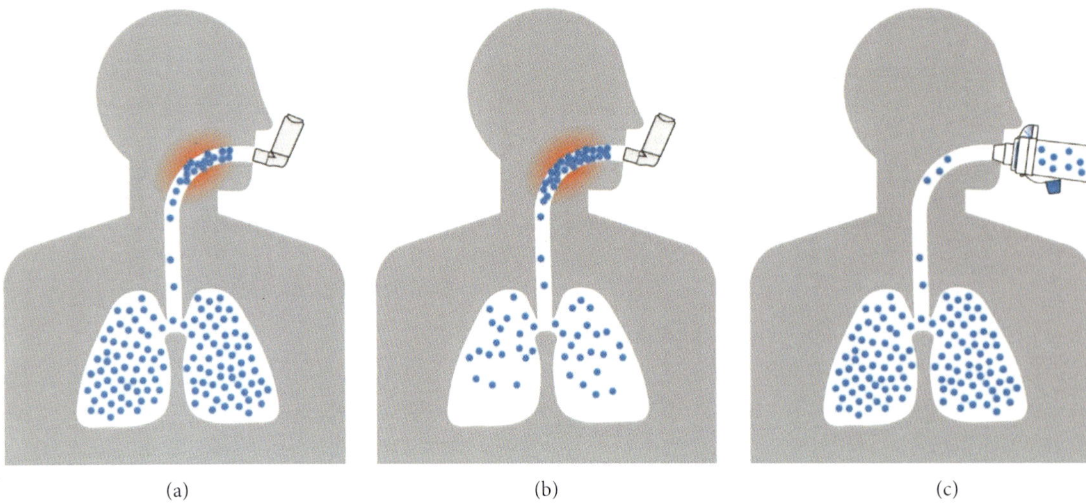

FIGURE 2: Lung deposition of inhaled medication is improved with perfect pMDI technique and with valved holding chamber. (a) Inhaler alone with perfect technique. (b) Inhaler alone with poor technique. (c) Inhaler with valved holding chamber.

impair adherence [4]. Chambers with volumes from 150 to 250 ml have been shown to be as effective as those with volumes of 750 ml [31]. Smaller chamber sizes are generally more effective for infants and small children as they require fewer tidal breaths to empty. One brand introduced in 1983 was the result of a design study to determine the optimal size of chamber, focusing on minimizing the size of the chamber without significantly reducing fine particle output [8].

Roller et al. [32] found that specifically for children (to ages 17 years) using VHCs with pMDI devices, slow inhalation and breath hold (5–10 seconds) may be more effective than tidal breaths for lung deposition of extra-fine aerosols for users who are capable of this type of breathing. For younger children or individuals with less ability to control their breathing (e.g., delayed or impaired development), tidal breathing is appropriate. Oropharyngeal and gastrointestinal deposition is reduced using VHCs regardless of inhalation technique.

VHCs fitted with facemasks are useful for infants, young children [1], and elderly patients [4, 31, 33]. There are various facemask designs available. The most important features for optimum aerosol delivery are a tight but comfortable facemask fit and reduced facemask dead space [30]. Esposito-Festen et al. [34] demonstrated that the efficiency of a pMDI-spacer facemask strongly depends on the size and location of facemask leaks. Minor leaks can reduce the lung dose by half compared to lung dose received with a facemask with a perfect seal, and leaks near the nose result in more rapidly decreased lung dose compared to leaks near the chin. A flexible facemask that conforms to the user's face to prevent leakage is optimal [31].

The valves of VHCs ideally allow the aerosolized medication to remain in the chamber until inhalation and the patient to exhale to the atmosphere without blowing the aerosol out of the chamber. Valve design and placement impact the rebreathed volume of the device, which is especially critical for use with infants and young children [20]. Valves are usually the only moving part of a VHC and are made from flexible components. Users should be taught to inspect the valve integrity when cleaning their VHC devices.

Some plastic VHC devices have an inherent electrostatic charge or may build up electrostatic charge within the chamber, which attracts drug particles to the chamber walls and may reduce drug delivery to the lungs [29]. Electrostatic charges may also result in inconsistent delivery of the medication [30]. Drug delivery through the use of antistatic chambers can provide clinically relevant improvement in bronchodilator response during acute, reversible bronchospasm such as nocturnal bronchospasm [35]. Researchers found that forced expiratory volume in 1 second (FEV1) increased by 21–25% when using an antistatic chamber and concluded that delivery of albuterol through an antistatic chamber provides a clinically relevant improvement in bronchodilator response during acute, reversible bronchospasm [35]. More recently, Burudpakdee et al. [36] examined a retrospective study database and identified 9325 patients with asthma in each of two groups: those using a pMDI with the AeroChamber Plus® Flow-Vu® Antistatic Valved Holding Chamber (AC-FV AVHC) and those using pMDI with any nonantistatic VHC (control group). The use of the AC-FV AVHC was associated with lower exacerbation rates, delayed time to first exacerbation, and lower exacerbation-related costs when compared to control nonantistatic VHCs. Further, the proportion of patients visiting the emergency department (ED) was significantly lower in the AC-FV AVHC group than the control cohort (10.8% versus 12.4%; $p < 0.05$), and the number of ED visits per patient was also significantly lower (0.15 visits versus 0.18 visits for the control VHC; $p < 0.05$).

Electrostatic charge within a VHC can also be reduced somewhat by priming the device with multiple actuations of the aerosol medication, but the number of actuations depends on the content of the aerosol and can be wasteful of medication. Alternately, washing the chamber with a mild detergent without rinsing and then allowing it to drip dry has proven more effective. The charge may reaccumulate after about 30 days [20, 31, 37].

Both for hygiene reasons and to prevent deterioration in valve function, spacers should be washed on a regular basis [38]. Each spacer has its own particular recommended washing and use procedures, and so it is important to follow the instructions in the Patient Information Leaflet (PIL). Spacers made of antistatic materials or metals such as steel or aluminum are less subject to this problem and therefore, with the incorporation of an effective antistatic material, remove the need for washing with detergent prior to first use [31].

4. Use of pMDIs with and without VHCs

Many studies have assessed disease control and oropharyngeal deposition using pMDIs with and without spacers or VHCs. Leach and Colice [28] conducted a small pilot study which showed that both the AeroChamber™ and Volumatic™ devices used in the study reduced oropharyngeal deposition of HFA-134a-beclomethasone dipropionate (BDP) and CFC-BDP. They found that oropharyngeal deposition of HFA-BDP was reduced from approximately 28% to 4% with the AeroChamber. Roller et al. [32] demonstrated a higher lung deposition and marked reduction in oropharyngeal deposition of BDP extra-fine particles when delivered via an HFA-driven inhaler with an attached VHC compared with delivery via the HFA-driven inhaler alone. Levy et al. [5] found better asthma control in significantly more patients using BDP through a breath-actuated pMDI device ($p < 0.0001$) or a spacer ($p < 0.0001$) compared with those using pMDIs alone.

Several studies have assessed the efficacy and cost-effectiveness of treating moderate and acute asthma exacerbations in children and adults in the ED setting. The use of pMDI plus spacer delivers equal or better clinical outcomes than nebulizers, with significant savings in costs and health-care provider time compared to nebulizers [39–43].

The majority of studies assessing the effectiveness of using VHCs with pMDIs are conducted under clinical trial settings, with careful training of participants in the devices used, and monitoring to ensure adherence of both medication use and correct use of devices. Guilbert et al. [44] reviewed anonymous medical record data from UK databases of patients with asthma prescribed fine and extra-fine particle ICS with and without spacers. They found no difference in rate of severe exacerbations and acute respiratory events. The authors recognize that the real-life nature of this study data means that the patients were not chosen through highly selective processes that are normally included in clinical trial designs. They were unable to determine if patients had been taught to use their devices correctly, whether or not they used them correctly, or in fact if the patients were adherent to treatment (i.e., did they use medications as prescribed, and did they use the spacers).

5. VHCs Are Not Interchangeable

VHCs are available in various sizes (Table 1) and, as has been described earlier, incorporate attributes such as valving, chamber shape/material, and facemask size and seal, each can have an impact upon drug delivery. Each pairing of a pMDI device plus VHC should be considered as a unique delivery system. Suggett et al. [45] assessed six VHCs and their associated facemasks for their ability to deliver fine particles in an *in vitro* simulated child model. They demonstrated significantly more medication delivery from the AeroChamber Plus* Flow-Vu* VHC compared with any of the other antistatic devices evaluated, and regardless of device pretreatment modality. Blake et al. [46] examined the lung bioavailability of fluticasone propionate pMDI administered through AeroChamber Plus with facemask and Babyhaler® VHCs in children from 1 to 4 years of age. Clinically significant differences in lung bioavailability were observed between the devices. Based on the study results, the authors recommend that parents, clinicians, and pharmacists should be educated not to interchange VHCs once a child is stable on a particular ICS dose and VHC combination and that VHC prescriptions should include a no substitutions statement. A recent study [47] reported an *in vitro* statistical equivalence study comparing a number of different, similarly sized VHCs in terms of particle size distribution of the medication delivered. The study demonstrated that only the two AeroChamber Plus VHC variants were equivalent; all the other VHCs tested were both statistically and likely clinically different (i.e., lower fine particle mass).

Suggett et al. [48] used an *in vitro* model to assess the difference between two antistatic and three nonconducting VHCs that look similar, using the AeroChamber Plus* Flow-Vu* as the reference. Devices were tested before and after following manufacturer-recommended washing procedures. The influence of wash on the fine particle mass delivered from the antistatic devices AeroChamber Plus* Flow-Vu* and Pocket Chamber was minimal but was significant on the three nonconducting VHCs for which a prewash was required to mitigate the effect of static charge and resultant reduced fine particle mass. Fine particle mass and total emitted mass (under simulated coordinated and uncoordinated use) were examined and statistically compared. All devices showed significantly different (reduced) results compared to reference.

6. VHC Approval Process

The European Medicines Agency (EMA) recommends that the development and registration process for new pMDIs includes testing and supporting data (*in vitro* and *in vivo*) of the pMDIs when used with specific VHC devices [49]. A separate communication stated that patients whose asthma is well controlled and who are using a spacer should always use the same type of spacer and not switch between spacers [50]. The EU registration documentation for pMDIs (Summary of Product Characteristics and Patient Information Leaflet) specifically note the VHC to be used should be based upon the device used in the product development/registration studies. For example, in Europe, the following pMDI products recommend the AeroChamber Plus brand of VHCs: Airomir, AirSalb, Alvesco, Atrovent, Flutiform, Fostair, Qvar, Seretide, and Sirdupla. The EMA is

Table 1: Valved holding chambers available in Canada.

Device	Manufacturer	Material	Antistatic	Volume
A2A Spacer	Clement Clarke, UK	Plastic	Low static	210 ml
AeroChamber Plus Flow-Vu	Trudell Medical International, Canada	Plastic	√	149 ml
Aerochamber Plus Z STAT®	Trudell Medical International, Canada	Plastic	√	149 ml
InspiraChamber®	InspirRx Inc., USA	Plastic	√	Not available
Leverhaler™	BirdSong Medical	Plastic	—	Not available
Life Brand Inhalation Chamber	ProtecSom, France	Plastic	—	Not available
LiteAire®	Thayer Medical	Cardboard	—	160 ml
OptiChamber Diamond®	Philips Respironics, USA	Plastic	√	140 ml
ProChamber™	Philips Respironics, USA	Plastic	—	145 ml
RespiChamber®	Trudell Medical International, Canada	Plastic	Static resistant	149 ml
Space Chamber Plus™ compact	Medical Developments International	Plastic	√	160 ml

alone in requiring data for a "*specific named spacer*" in order to support pMDI approval generally. The US Food and Drug Administration (FDA), Health Canada, and Japan's Pharmaceuticals and Medical Devices Agency are silent on this issue. As was stated by Dissanayake and Suggett [47], the FDA's position is perhaps the most surprising in view of the agency's zealous approach to dose selection for novel inhaled products and stringent "weight of evidence" approach for generic inhalers which requires the demonstration of in vitro, pharmacokinetic, and clinical equivalence between test and reference devices to support generic product approval. In relation to the equivalence study they performed, the authors go on to state that "in this context, ignoring a two-fold difference in respirable dose between VHCs, as in the present study, is difficult to rationalise. Harmonisation of regulatory guidelines across regions would seem desirable."

It is interesting to note that the regulatory review process for devices occurs through a different body than the pMDI drug products they are to be used with. A medical device should be developed following design controls and applicable regional and International Organization for Standardization (ISO) standards. Depending upon the device classification in a given market, approval is requested or self-certification provided. Although, for example, in Canada, there is a standard for the testing and performance of VHCs [51]; it is not known to what extent all commercially available chambers satisfy the standard as such data are not required in order to gain a registration. This may lead to substandard VHCs being available for patient use without meeting minimal quality and performance standards.

7. Education

Ongoing patient education is a critical factor of correct inhaler technique, adherence, and disease control. A single event of instruction with the prescription of an inhaled medication and/or spacer or VHC is not sufficient to ensure correct inhaler technique. For example, Kamps et al. [52] demonstrated that three comprehensive instruction sessions increased the number of patients demonstrating correct inhalation technique of pMDI plus spacer from 57.4% to 97.9%. Amin et al. [53] assessed patient and physician confidence in the usage of inhalers used to treat COPD. They found that approximately 30% of patients had low confidence in their ability to use their inhalers and that low confidence was associated with lower adherence and poor COPD-related health status.

Education on the correct use of VHCs with pMDIs is important to avoid the potential for new errors introduced with the VHC. These may include as incorrect device assembly, incorrect inhalation after actuation (e.g., waiting too long to inhale), and actuating more puffs than required. [4].

Each VHC device comes with directions for use [31, 38]. Generally, spacers should be positioned before actuating the pMDI, and movement of the spacer should also be avoided, as this will reduce the drug available for inhalation due to impaction on the sides of the spacer wall. Patient education must be specific to the pMDI and the VHC used [4].

Clinicians can support patients in several ways:

(i) Check inhaler technique often.

(ii) Keep devices consistent when changing or adding medications, that is, try not to mix pMDI and DPI devices. Each new pairing of pMDI and VHC requires instruction specific to the devices being used.

(iii) Use appropriate training aids for encouraging slow inhalation with pMDI devices [14].

(iv) Ensure that VHCs are used with pMDIs by infants and children and by patients with poor coordination or inhaler technique.

(v) Ensure that VHCs are used when prescribing corticosteroids with pMDI to reduce oropharyngeal side effects and absorption via the gut.

(vi) Ensure that an appropriate antistatic VHC is prescribed to prevent losses of medication to chamber walls.

(vii) Instruct patients and caregivers to clean and use VHCs according to the PIL [31, 38].

(viii) Ensure that VHCs with facemasks for infants and young children fit correctly with a good seal to the face, and that parents/caregivers understand the importance of no leaks [31].

(ix) A dedicated inhalation indicator is available in one brand of VHC (AeroChamber Plus Flow-Vu). This can help provide visual feedback with respect to correct inhalation and facemask seal. *In vivo* studies show that the use of a chamber with the Flow-Vu

Inhalation Indicator was associated with improved satisfaction and caregiver quality of life [54].

8. Summary

Inhaled aerosol therapy remains the cornerstone of effective treatment of asthma and COPD. While the medications themselves have not changed dramatically over the past decades, the delivery devices have changed. Technology has allowed the development of more efficient and user-friendly inhalers. Nevertheless, incorrect inhaler technique remains a significant barrier to many users of inhaled medications. The most common errors reported for the use of pMDIs are lack of coordination between actuation and inhalation, halting inhalation when the cool spray hits the back of the throat, not holding the breath long enough (>5 seconds) after inhalation, no exhalation prior to actuation, and not shaking the suspension prior to use. Valved holding chambers confer distinct advantages to the first two challenges. VHCs allow users to approach inhalation of aerosol medication as a two-step process: actuation into to chamber, followed by inhalation from the VHC mouthpiece. Technology has also allowed the development of more effective VHCs. There are now antistatic chambers, better valves, more effective facemasks, and other innovations that help deliver the intended dose of medication. VHCs have been proven to improve pMDI medication delivery to the lungs, reduce oropharyngeal deposition, and help users overcome challenges in coordinating pMDI actuation with inhalation [8]. Moreover, newer VHCs with multiple advances (antistatic chamber and inhalation indicators) have been reported to improve asthma control, reduce the rate of exacerbations, and improve quality of life [36, 54]. VHCs are not all the same, and also are not interchangeable. Ongoing education is critical to ensure that users are consistently able to use their inhalers.

Disclosure

Alan Kaplan is a member of the Advisory Board or Speakers Bureau for AstraZeneca, Benton Dickinson, Boehringer Ingelheim, Grifols GSK, Johnson & Johnson, Mylan, Merck, Novartis, Novo Nordisk, Paladdin, Pfizer, Purdue, Sanofi, Takeda, and Trudell. Hollie Devlin received honoraria from Trudell Medical International. Andrew McIvor received honoraria for providing CME and attending Advisory Boards and Clinical trials for AstraZeneca, Boehringer Ingelheim, GSK, Merck, Novartis, Takeda, Teva, and Trudell and also is an employee of McMaster University and St. Joseph's Healthcare, Hamilton Ontario.

References

[1] Global Initiative for Asthma (GINA), *Global Strategy for Asthma Management and Prevention*, September 2017, http://ginasthma.org/2017-gina-report-global-strategy-for-asthma-management-and-prevention/.

[2] Global Strategy for the Diagnosis, *Management and Prevention of COPD, Global Initiative for Chronic Obstructive Lung Disease (GOLD) 2017*, September 2017, http://goldcopd.org.

[3] S. W. Stein and C. G. Thiel, "The history of therapeutic aerosols: a chronological review," *Journal of Aerosol Medicine and Pulmonary Drug Delivery*, vol. 30, no. 1, pp. 20–41, 2017.

[4] F. Lavorini and G. A. Fontana, "Targeting drugs to the airways: the role of spacer devices," *Expert Opinion on Drug Delivery*, vol. 6, no. 1, pp. 91–102, 2009.

[5] M. L. Levy, A. Hardwell, E. McKnight, and J. Holmes, "Asthma patients' inability to use a pressurized metered-dose inhaler (pMDI) correctly correlates with poor asthma control as defined by the Global Initiative for Asthma (GINA) strategy: a retrospective analysis," *Primary Care Respiratory Journal*, vol. 22, no. 4, pp. 406–411, 2013.

[6] S. P. Newman, F. Moren, D. Pavia, F. Little, and S. W. Clarke, "Deposition of pressurized suspension aerosols inhaled through extension devices," *American Review of Respiratory Disease*, vol. 124, no. 3, pp. 317–320, 1981.

[7] S. P. Newman, A. B. Millar, T. R. Lennard-Jones, F. Moren, and S. W. Clarke, "Improvement of pressurised aerosol deposition with Nebuhaler spacer device," *Thorax*, vol. 39, no. 12, pp. 935–941, 1984.

[8] D. Corr, M. Dolovich, D. McCormack, R. Ruffin, G. Obminski, and M. Newhouse, "Design and characteristics of a portable breath actuated, particle size selective medical aerosol inhaler," *Journal of Aerosol Science*, vol. 13, no. 1, pp. 1–7, 1982.

[9] M. D. Lougheed, C. Lemiere, S. D. Dell et al., "Canadian Thoracic Society Asthma Management Continuum—2010 Consensus Summary for children six years of age and over, and adults," *Canadian Respiratory Journal*, vol. 17, no. 1, pp. 15–24, 2010.

[10] P. M. Holzner and B. W. Muller, "An in vitro evaluation of various spacer devices for metered-dose inhalers using the Twin Impinger," *International Journal of Pharmaceutics*, vol. 106, no. 1, pp. 69–75, 1994.

[11] European Medicines Agency, *Guideline on the Requirements for Clinical Documentation for Orally Inhaled Products (OIP) Including the Requirements for Demonstration of Therapeutic Equivalence between Two Inhaled Products for Use in the Treatment of Asthma and Chronic Obstructive Pulmonary Disease (COPD) in Adults and for Use in the Treatment of Asthma in Children and Adolescents*, September 2017, http://www.ema.europa.eu/docs/en_GB/document_library/Scientific_guideline/2009/09/WC500003504.pdf.

[12] American Academy of Allergy Asthma and Immunology, *Spacers and Valved Holding Chambers (VHCs) for Use with Metered Dose Inhalers (MDIs)*, October 2017, https://www.aaaai.org/conditions-and-treatments/library/asthma-library/spacers-asthma.

[13] A. S. Melani, M. Bonavia, V. Cilenti et al., "Inhaler mishandling remains common in real life and is associated with reduced disease control," *Respiratory Medicine*, vol. 105, no. 6, pp. 930–938, 2011.

[14] D. Price, S. Bosnic-Anticevich, A. Briggs et al., "Inhaler competence in asthma: Common errors, barriers to use and recommended solutions," *Respiratory Medicine*, vol. 107, no. 1, pp. 37–46, 2013.

[15] A. Hardwell, V. Barber, T. Hargadon, E. McKnight, J. Holmes, and M. L. Levy, "Technique training does not improve the ability of most patients to use pressurised metered-dose inhalers (pMDIs)," *Primary Care Respiratory Journal*, vol. 20, no. 1, pp. 92–96, 2011.

[16] R. D. Restrepo, M. T. Alvarez, L. D. Wittnebel et al., "Medication adherence issues in patients treated for COPD," *International Journal of Chronic Obstructive Pulmonary Disease*, vol. 3, no. 3, pp. 371–384, 2008.

[17] E. R. McFadden Jr., "Improper patient techniques with metered dose inhalers: clinical consequences and solutions to misuse," *Journal of Allergy and Clinical Immunology*, vol. 96, no. 2, pp. 278-283, 1995.

[18] V. Giraud and N. Roche, "Misuse of corticosteroid metered-dose inhaler is associated with decreased asthma stability," *European Respiratory Journal*, vol. 19, no. 2, pp. 246–251, 2002.

[19] J. Sanchis, I. Gich, and S. Pefersen, "Systemic review of errors in inhaler use: has patient technique improved over time?," *Chest*, vol. 150, no. 2, pp. 394–406, 2016.

[20] J. B. Fink and B. K. Rubin, "Problems with inhaler use: a call for improved clinician and patient education," *Respiratory Care*, vol. 50, no. 10, pp. 1360–1375, 2005.

[21] T. Capstick and I. Clifton, "Inhaler technique and training in people with chronic obstructive pulmonary disease and asthma," *Expert Review of Respiratory Medicine*, vol. 6, no. 1, pp. 92–101, 2012.

[22] A. P. Yu, A. Guerin, D. P. de Leon et al., "Clinical and economic outcomes of multiple versus single long-acting inhalers in COPD," *Respiratory Medicine*, vol. 105, no. 12, pp. 1861–1871, 2011.

[23] S. Bosnic-Anticevich, H. Chrystyn, R. Costello et al., "The use of multiple respiratory inhalers requiring different inhalation techniques has an adverse effect on COPD outcomes," *International Journal of Chronic Obstructive Pulmonary Disease*, vol. 12, pp. 59–71, 2017.

[24] M. Lee-Wong and P. H. Mayo, "Results of a programme to improve house staff use of metered dose inhalers and spacers," *Postgraduate Medical Journal*, vol. 79, no. 930, pp. 221–225, 2003.

[25] N. A. Hanania, R. Wittman, S. Kesten, and K. R. Chapman, "Medical personnel's knowledge of and ability to use inhaling devices: metered-dose inhalers, spacing chambers and breath-actuated dry powder inhalers," *Chest*, vol. 105, no. 1, pp. 111–116, 1994.

[26] V. Plaza, J. Sanchis, P. Roura et al., "Physician's knowledge of inhaler devices and inhalation techniques remains poor in Spain," *Journal of Aerosol Medicine and Pulmonary Drug Delivery*, vol. 25, no. 1, pp. 16–22, 2012.

[27] Y. S. Cheng, C. S. Fu, D. Yazzie, and Y. Zhou, "Respiratory deposition patterns of salbutamol pMDI with CFC and HFA-134a formulations in a human airway replica," *Journal of Aerosol Medicine*, vol. 14, no. 2, pp. 255–266, 2001.

[28] C. L. Leach and G. L. Colice, "A pilot study to assess lung deposition of HFA-beclomethasone and CFC-beclomethasone from a pressurized metered dose inhaler with and without add-on spacers and using varying breathold times," *Journal of Aerosol Medicine and Pulmonary Drug Delivery*, vol. 23, no. 6, pp. 355–361, 2010.

[29] A. Nair, D. Menzies, M. Barnes, M. Burns, L. McFarlane, and B. J. Lipworth, "Respirable dose delivery of fluticasone propionate from a small valved holding chamber, a compact breath actuated integrated vortex device and a metered dose inhaler," *British Journal of Clinical Pharmacology*, vol. 66, no. 1, pp. 20–26, 2008.

[30] F. Lavorini, "The challenge of delivering therapeutic aerosols to asthma patients," *ISRN Allergy*, vol. 2013, Article ID 102418, 17 pages, 2013.

[31] J. P. Mitchell and M. W. Nagel, "Valved holding chambers (VHCs) for use with pressurized metered-dose inhalers (pMDIs): a review of causes of inconsistent medication delivery," *Primary Care Respiratory Journal*, vol. 16, no. 4, pp. 207–214, 2007.

[32] C. M. Roller, G. Zhang, R. G. Troedson, C. L. Leach, P. N. Le Souëf, and S. G. Devadason, "Spacer inhalation technique and deposition of extrafine aerosol in asthmatic children," *European Respiratory Journal*, vol. 29, no. 2, pp. 299–306, 2007.

[33] R. W. Morton and J. P. Mitchell, "Design of facemasks for delivery of aerosol-based medication via pressurized metered dose inhaler with valved holding chamber: key issues that affect performance," *Journal of Aerosol Medicine*, vol. 20, no. 1, pp. S29–S45, 2007.

[34] J. E. Esposito-Festen, B. Ates, F. J. M. van Vliet, A. F. M. Verbraak, J. C. de Jongste, and H. A. W. M. Todden, "Effect of a facemask leak on aerosol delivery from a pMDI-spacer system," *Journal of Aerosol Medicine*, vol. 17, no. 1, pp. 7–14, 2004.

[35] S. Prabhakaran, J. Shuster, S. Chesrown, and L. Hendeles, "Response to albuterol MDI delivered through an anti-static chamber during nocturnal bronchospasm," *Respiratory Care*, vol. 57, no. 8, pp. 1291–1296, 2012.

[36] C. Burudpakdee, V. Kushnarev, D. Coppolo, and J. Suggett, "A retrospective study of the effectiveness of AeroChamber Plus® Flow-Vu® antistatic valved holding chamber for asthma control," *Pulmonary Therapy*, vol. 3, no. 2, pp. 283–296, 2017.

[37] F. Pierart, J. H. Wildhaber, I. Vrancken, S. G. Devadason, and P. N. Le Souef, "Washing plastic spacers in household detergent reduces electrostatic charge and greatly improves delivery," *European Respiratory Journal*, vol. 13, no. 3, pp. 673–678, 1999.

[38] L. B. Laube, H. M. Janssens, F. H. C. de Jongh et al., "What the pulmonary specialist should know about the new inhalation therapies," *European Respiratory Journal*, vol. 37, no. 6, pp. 1308–1417, 2011.

[39] Q. Doan, A. Shefrin, and D. Johnson, "Cost-effectiveness of metered-dose inhalers for asthma exacerbations in the pediatric emergency department," *Pediatrics*, vol. 127, no. 5, pp. E1105–E1111, 2011.

[40] K. B. Newman, S. Milne, C. Hamilton, and K. Hall, "A comparison of albuterol administered by metered-dose inhaler and spacer with albuterol by nebulizer in adults presenting to an urban emergency department with acute asthma," *Chest*, vol. 121, no. 4, pp. 1036–1041, 2002.

[41] A. M. Leversha, S. G. Campanella, and R. P. Aickin, "Asher MI costs and effectiveness of spacer versus nebulizer in young children with moderate and severe acute asthma," *Journal of Pediatrics*, vol. 136, no. 4, pp. 497–502, 2000.

[42] N. Mason, N. Roberts, N. Yard, and M. R. Partridge, "Nebulisers or spacers for the administration of bronchodilators to those with asthma attending emergency departments?," *Respiratory Medicine*, vol. 102, no. 7, pp. 993–998, 2008.

[43] J. A. Castro-Rodriguez and G. J. Rodrigo, "β-agonists through metered-dose inhaler with valved holding chamber versus nebulizer for acute exacerbation of wheezing or asthma in children under 5 years of age: a systematic review with meta-analysis," *Journal of Pediatrics*, vol. 145, no. 2, pp. 172–177, 2004.

[44] T. W. Guilbert, G. Colice, J. Grigg et al., "Real-life outcomes for patients with asthma prescribed spacers for use with either extrafine- or fine-particle inhaled corticosteroids," *Journal of Allergy and Clinical Immunology. In Practice*, vol. 5, no. 4, pp. 1040.e4–1049.e4, 2017.

[45] J. Suggett, M. Nagel, H. Shcneider, and J. Mitchell, "Clinically appropriate testing of different valved holding chamber facemask combinations investigating simulated delivered mass to

the carina," *European Respiratory Journal*, vol. 46, p. PA 1805, 2015.

[46] K. Blake, R. Mehta, T. Spencer, R. L. Kunka, and L. Hendeles, "Bioavailability of inhaled fluticasone propionate via chambers/masks in young children," *European Respiratory Journal*, vol. 39, no. 1, pp. 97–103, 2012.

[47] S. Dissanayake and J. Suggett, "A review of the *in vitro* and *in vivo* valved holding chamber (VHC) literature with a focus on the AeroChamber Plus Flow-Vu Anti-static VHC," *Therapeutic Advances in Respiratory Disease*, vol. 12, 2018.

[48] J. A. Suggett, M. W. Nagel, C. Doyle, V. Avvakoumova, and J. P. Mitchell, "Statistical performance evaluation of similar looking valved holding chambers: if it looks the same, does it perform the same?," in *Proceedings of the Respiratory Drug Delivery 2016*, pp. 539–542, Scottsdale, Arizona, April 2016.

[49] S. Dissanayake, "Application of the EU guidelines for pharmacokinetic studies of locally acting orally inhaled drug products," in *Respiratory Drug Delivery 2010*, R. N. Dalby, P. R. Byron, J. Peart, J. D. Suman, S. J. Farr, and P. M. Young, Eds., vol. 1, pp. 293–304, DHI Publishing, River Grove, IL, USA, 2010.

[50] *Drug Safety Update: Inhaled Medicines Containing Corticosteroids*, UK Government, 2008, https://www.gov.uk/drug-safety-update/inhaled-medicines-containing-corticosteroid.

[51] M. B. Dolovich and J. P. Mitchell, "Canadian Standards Association standard CAN/CSA/Z264.1-02:2002: a new voluntary standard for spacers and holding chambers used with pressurized metered-dose inhalers," *Canadian Respiratory Journal*, vol. 11, no. 7, pp. 489–495, 2004.

[52] A. W. A. Kamps, P. L. P. Brand, and R. J. Roorda, "Determinants of correct inhalation technique in children attending a hospital-based asthma clinic," *Acta Paediatrica*, vol. 91, no. 2, pp. 159–163, 2002.

[53] A. N. Amin, V. Ganapathy, A. Roughley, and M. Small, "Confidence in correct inhaler technique and its association with treatment adherence and health status among US patients with chronic obstructive pulmonary disease," *Patient Preference and Adherence*, vol. 11, pp. 1205–1212, 2017.

[54] W. G. Ammari, S. Toor, P. Chetcuti, J. Stephenson, and H. Chrystyn, "Evaluation of asthma control, parents' quality of life and preference between AeroChamber Plus and AeroChamber Plus Flow-Vu spacers in young children with asthma," *Journal of Asthma*, vol. 52, no. 3, pp. 301–307, 2015.

ADRB2 Arg16Gly Polymorphism and Pulmonary Function Response of Inhaled Corticosteroids plus Long-Acting Beta Agonists for Asthma Treatment

Xi Wang, Qian Li, Ruming Liu, Jin He, Di Wu, Yun Wang, and Jun Zhang

The Department of Clinical Pharmacy, The First Affiliated Hospital of Kunming Medical University, Kunming, China

Correspondence should be addressed to Jun Zhang; zhangjun_pharmacy@163.com

Academic Editor: Jörg D. Leuppi

Background. The beta-2 adrenergic receptor (ADRB2) Arg16Gly polymorphism may alter the bronchodilation response to long-acting beta2-agonists, thereby influencing the clinical effectiveness of LABAs plus corticosteroids (ICS) treatment. But the results of individual studies are inconclusive. *Methods.* A systematic search was conducted in PubMed, Embase, the Cochrane Database, WHO International Clinical Trials Registry Platform, Chinese National Knowledge Infrastructure, Wanfang, Chinese BioMedical Literature Database, and VIP databases. The meta-analysis was performed with RevMan statistical software (version 5.2), and potential publication bias was estimated by Egger's test using STATA (version 12.0), with $p < 0.05$ indicating significant publication bias. *Results.* We found 5 cohort studies with a total of 632 patients and included them in the meta-analysis. There are no significant differences in pulmonary function response between patients with the Arg/Arg and Arg/Gly phenotype (SMD −0.04, 95% CI −0.45 to 0.37; $p = 0.84$). There were also no significant differences in the pulmonary function response between patients with the Arg/Arg and Gly/Gly phenotype (MD −0.03, 95% CI −0.07 to 0.02; $p = 0.28$). *Conclusions.* Our systematic review and meta-analysis suggest that ADRB2 Arg16Gly polymorphism is not associated with pulmonary response to asthma treatment with ICS plus LABAs.

1. Introduction

According to the World Health Organization (WHO), asthma is an important noncommunicable disease with 235 million patients worldwide in 2013. The combination of inhaled corticosteroids (ICS) and long-acting beta2-agonists (LABAs) is a widely used maintenance therapy for asthma. Recent studies have revealed that beta-2 adrenergic receptor (ADRB2) polymorphism may mediate the bronchodilation response to LABA, thereby influencing the clinical effectiveness of combination treatment [1]. However, reports of the effect of Arg16Gly polymorphism on ADRB2 function are not conclusive [2, 3]. Some found no significant differences in the improvement of pulmonary function in asthmatic patients with different ADRB2 genotypes [4, 5]. Others found that the effectiveness of ICS and LABAs treatment was increased in asthma patients with the Arg/Arg phenotype [6]. We performed a systematic review and meta-analysis to investigate the association of Arg16Gly polymorphism of ADRB2 and pulmonary function response of LABAs plus ICS combination treatment in asthma patients.

2. Methods

We followed the STREGA (Strengthening the REporting of Genetic Association) guidelines to review the methods and results of studies reporting on the influence of ADRB2 Arg16Gly polymorphism on the pulmonary function response of ICS and LABAs treatment of asthma patients.

2.1. Literature Search. Two investigators (Wang and Li) independently searched PubMed, Embase, the Cochrane Database, WHO International Clinical Trials Registry

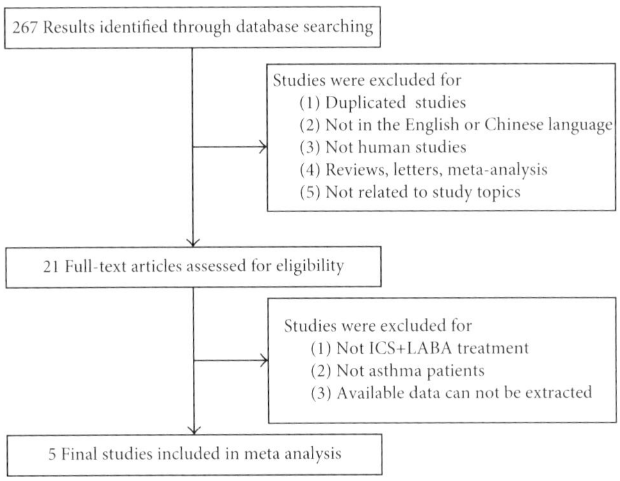

Figure 1: Flow chart of article selection.

Platform, Chinese National Knowledge Infrastructure, Wanfang, Chinese BioMedical Literature Database, and VIP databases. The last search was conducted on June 31, 2016. The searches followed the following strategy: (salmeterol OR formoterol OR LABAs OR long-acting beta 2 agonists) AND (adrenergic receptor OR ADRB2 OR adrenoceptor beta 2) AND (polymorphism OR SNP* OR variant OR mutation) AND asthma.

2.2. Study Selection. A flow chart of study selection is presented in Figure 1. Studies were selected independently by two investigators (Wang and Li) and were included if they met the following criteria:

(1) If they evaluated the relationship between ADRB2 Arg16Gly polymorphism and fixed dose ICS-LABAs combination treatment in asthma
(2) If they included data on dosage and duration of treatment, genotype distribution, and measurement of pulmonary function
(3) If they were cohort or case-control studies in humans

Studies were excluded if they met any of the following criteria:

(1) If they were reviews, comments, letters, or editorials
(2) If they were duplicated or overlapping studies
(3) If they were not published in the English or Chinese language

2.3. Data Extraction and Quality Assessment. Data on first author's name, year of publication, ethnicity of participants, number of participants, sex ratio, age, asthma treatment, pulmonary function measurements, and genotyping measurements were extracted from the included study.

The primary outcomes were changes in pulmonary function from baseline, including forced expiratory volume in the first second (FEV1), peak expiratory flow (PEF), and forced vital capacity (FVC).

A quality assessment of the studies was performed independently by two observers using the Newcastle-Ottawa Scale (NOS) criteria, which include scoring of the method of group selection, comparability of participants, and clinical outcomes. The highest score is 9, and a score ≥ 6 indicates high methodological quality. Differences were resolved by discussion.

2.4. Statistical Analysis. The meta-analysis was performed with RevMan statistical software (version 5.2), and potential publication bias was estimated by Egger's test using STATA (version 12.0), with $p < 0.05$ indicating significant publication bias. The mean difference (MD) was calculated if the studies being compared used the same pulmonary function measurements, otherwise the standardized mean difference (SMD) was calculated, both with 95% confidence intervals (CIs). Study heterogeneity was assessed by the Cochran's Q and I^2 tests.

3. Results

3.1. Studies Selection and Characteristics. 267 articles were identified by electronic and manual searches from the databases mentioned, and 246 articles were excluded based on the titles and abstracts, then 16 articles were excluded after reviewing the full text. Finally, 5 cohort studies were included in the meta-analysis, ranging from 2006 to 2015 [4, 5, 7–9]. A total of 632 patients were included: 176 patients were with ArgArg phenotype, 265 patients were with ArgGly phenotype, and 184 patients were with GlyGly phenotype.

Two studies were carried out among Chinese Han people [7, 9], one study was carried out among Iranian [8], and other studies were carried out among mixed population or population without specification [4, 5].

In three studies, the subjects were entered two or sixteen weeks run-in period, only using albuterol or ipratropium bromide as needed to relieve asthma symptoms, then entered to the treatment of FSC period [4, 5, 7]. In two studies, the subjects were directly entered to the treatment of FSC period [8, 9].

One study examined the changes of morning PEF and FEV1 from baseline at the end of 12 weeks of treatment with FSC, 250/50 μg diskus twice daily.

One study examined the changes of FEV1% predicted and FEV1/FVC from baseline at the end of 4 weeks of treatment with FSC, 250/50 μg diskus twice daily. One study examined the changes of morning PEF, afternoon PEF, and predose FEV1 from baseline at the end of 16 weeks of treatment with FSC, 100/50 μg diskus twice daily. One study examined the changes of morning PEF and FEV1 from baseline at the end of 12 weeks of treatment with FSC, 100/50 μg diskus twice daily. One study examined the changes of PEF, FEV1, and FVC from baseline at the end of 16 weeks of treatment with FSC, 100/25 μg diskus twice daily and albuterol as needed. There were no significant differences in baseline pulmonary function characteristics across the Arg16Gly genotypes in these 5 studies.

Table 1: Characteristics and methodological quality of included studies.

	First author	Year	Ethnicity	Case number	Age (year)	Gender (male/female)	Main drugs and dose (μg, bid)	Follow-up (week)	Outcome measure	Genotyping measurement	HWE	NOS score
1	Qiu et al. [7]	2014	Chinese Han	68	>18	no data	FSC (250/50)	12	AM PEF and FEV1	Sequencing	Yes	7
2	Soleimani et al. [8]	2013	Iranian	28	27–65	8/18	FSC (250/50)	4	FEV1% predicted and FEV1/FVC	PCR-RFLP	Yes	6
3	Bleecker et al. [5]	2009	Mixed population	270	>12	106/194	FSC (100/50)	16	AM PEF, PM PEF, and FEV1	Tag man	—	7
4	Bleecker et al. [4]	2006	Mixed population	183	>15	81/102	FSC (100/50)	12	AM PEF, FEV1	Not mentioned	Yes	7
5	Wu et al. [9]	2015	Chinese Han	83	>5	48/35	FSC (100/25)	16	FVC, FEV1, PEF	PCR-RFLP	Yes	7

Study or subgroup	Arg/Arg Mean	Arg/Arg SD	Arg/Arg Total	Arg/Gly Mean	Arg/Gly SD	Arg/Gly Total	Weight	Std. mean difference IV, random, 95% CI
Bleecker et al.	0.53	0.07	29	0.59	0.06	65	24.9%	−0.94 (−1.40, −0.48)
Bleecker et al.	0.22	0.03	87	0.21	0.03	91	27.4%	0.33 (0.04, 0.63)
Qiu et al.	0.44	0.09	21	0.45	0.11	26	22.9%	−0.10 (−0.67, 0.48)
Wu et al.	0.42	0.11	31	0.39	0.19	39	24.7%	0.19 (−0.29, 0.66)
Total (95% CI)			168			221	100.0%	−0.12 (−0.71, 0.47)

Heterogeneity: $\tau^2 = 0.30$; $\chi^2 = 21.71$, df = 3 ($p < 0.0001$); $I^2 = 86\%$

Test for overall effect: $Z = 0.40$ ($p = 0.69$)

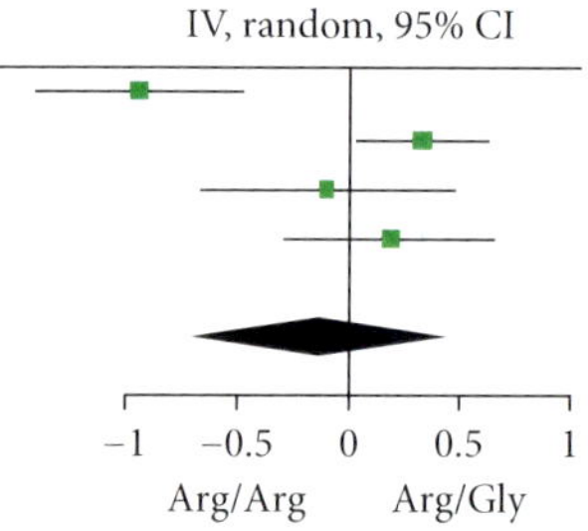

Figure 2: Forest plots of the association between the ADRB2 Arg16Gly polymorphism and pulmonary function response of inhaled ICS plus LABAs for asthma treatment (Arg/Arg or Arg/Gly) with 4 studies included.

Four studies include the patients with ArgArg, ArgGly, or GlyGly phenotypes, and one study include the patients with ArgArg or ArgGly phenotypes.

Direct sequencing was conducted in one study [7], PCR-RFLP (polymerase chain reaction-restriction fragment length polymorphism) was conducted in the other two studies [8, 9], and TaqMan SNP Genotyping was conducted in one study [5]. No specific genotyping method was mentioned in one study [4]. The distribution of the Arg16Gly phenotypes in all included studies was in Hardy–Weinberg equilibrium (HWE), except one study chose ninety subjects per Arg16Gly phenotype [5].

The characteristics and methodological quality of studies are summarized in Table 1, with the first author's name, year of publication, characteristics of patients, asthma treatment, genotyping measurements, and outcome measurements. All the studies were validated by NOS quality assessment.

3.2. ADRB2 Arg16Gly Polymorphism and Pulmonary Function Response of Inhaled ICS plus LABAs for Asthma Treatment. The differences of pulmonary function in patients with the Arg/Arg or Arg/Gly phenotype were investigated in 5 cohort studies with a total 417 participants. The changes of FEV1(L) were the outcome measure in the 4 studies [4, 5, 7, 9], The changes of FEV1/FEC were the outcome measure in one study [8]. First, we included the 4 studies which chose FEV1 as the outcome measure to the meta-analysis with a total 389 participants, MD of FEV1 with random-effect model was performed. As shown in Figure 2, no difference of pulmonary function was found between the two phenotypes (MD −0.01, 95% CI −0.05 to 0.03; $p = 0.63$). Then, we included the 5 studies to the meta-analysis with a total 417 participants, SMD with random-effect model was performed since different pulmonary functions were measured. As shown in Figure 3, no difference of pulmonary function was found between the two phenotypes either (SMD −0.04, 95% CI −0.45 to 0.37; $p = 0.84$). Publication bias was assessed by Egger's test, and no significant publication bias was detected in the included studies (Table 2).

The differences of pulmonary function in patients between the two phenotypes (Arg/Arg and Gly/Gly) were investigated in 4 cohort studies with a total 352 participants. FEV1(L) was the outcome measure, and MD of FEV1 with random-effect model was performed in the analysis. As shown in Figure 4, no difference of pulmonary function was found between the two phenotypes (MD −0.03, 95% CI

Study or subgroup	Arg/Arg Mean	Arg/Arg SD	Arg/Arg Total	Arg/Gly Mean	Arg/Gly SD	Arg/Gly Total	Weight	Std. mean difference IV, random, 95% CI
Bleecker et al.	0.53	0.07	29	0.57	0.06	89	22.1%	−0.64 (−1.06, −0.21)
Bleecker et al.	0.22	0.03	87	0.21	0.03	91	25.2%	0.33 (0.04, 0.63)
Qiu et al.	0.44	0.09	21	0.43	0.07	26	18.4%	0.12 (−0.45, 0.70)
Soleimani et al.	1.28	6.23	8	3.44	5.99	20	13.3%	−0.35 (−1.17, 0.48)
Wu et al.	0.42	0.11	31	0.39	0.19	39	20.9%	0.19 (−0.29, 0.66)
Total (95% CI)			176			265	100.0%	−0.04 (−0.45, 0.37)

Heterogeneity: $\tau^2 = 0.15$; $\chi^2 = 14.63$, df = 4 ($p = 0.006$); $I^2 = 73\%$
Test for overall effect: $Z = 0.20$ ($p = 0.84$)

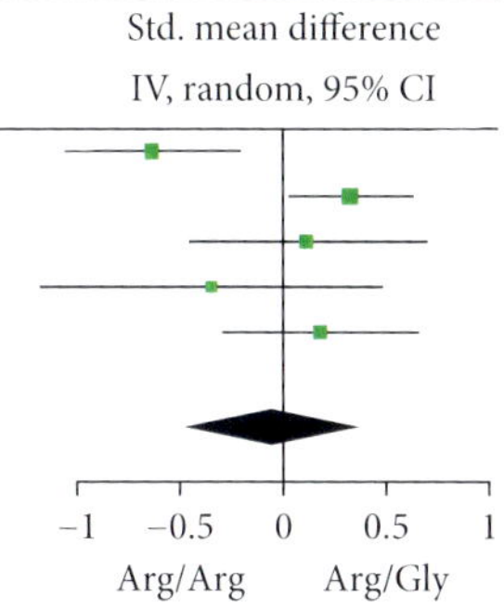

FIGURE 3: Forest plots of the association between the ADRB2 Arg16Gly polymorphism and pulmonary function response of inhaled ICS plus LABAs for asthma treatment (Arg/Arg or Arg/Gly) with 5 studies included.

TABLE 2: Egger's test.

Polymorphism	ArgArg versus ArgGly	ArgArg versus GlyGly
Numbers of studies	417	353
p value	0.398	0.391

$p < 0.05$, statistically significant publication bias.

Study or subgroup	Arg/Arg Mean	Arg/Arg SD	Arg/Arg Total	Gly/Gly Mean	Gly/Gly SD	Gly/Gly Total	Weight	Mean difference IV, random, 95% CI
Bleecker et al.	0.53	0.07	29	0.59	0.06	65	30.0%	−0.06 (−0.09, −0.03)
Bleecker et al.	0.22	0.03	87	0.21	0.03	91	33.3%	0.01 (0.00, 0.02)
Qiu et al.	0.44	0.09	21	0.45	0.11	15	20.3%	−0.01 (−0.08, 0.06)
Wu et al.	0.42	0.11	31	0.48	0.14	13	16.5%	−0.06 (−0.15, 0.03)
Total (95% CI)			168			184	100.0%	−0.03 (−0.07, 0.02)

Heterogeneity: $\tau^2 = 0.00$; $\chi^2 = 22.34$, df = 3 ($p < 0.0001$); $I^2 = 87\%$
Test for overall effect: $Z = 1.07$ ($p = 0.28$)

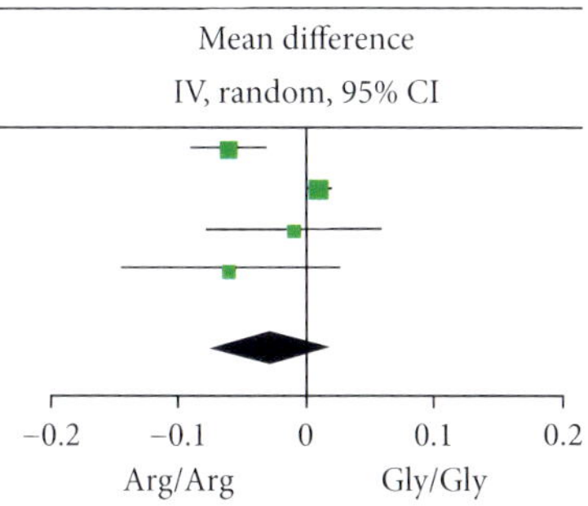

FIGURE 4: Forest plots of the association between the ADRB2 Arg16Gly polymorphism and pulmonary function response of inhaled ICS plus LABAs for asthma treatment (Arg/Arg or Gly/Gly) with 4 studies included.

−0.07 to 0.02; $p = 0.28$). Publication bias was assessed by Egger's test, and no significant publication bias was detected in the included studies (Table 2)

4. Discussion

Beta2 agonist is one kind of inhaled bronchodilators, which relaxed bronchial smooth muscle by activating ADRB2 [10]. It is classified as short-acting beta agonists (SABAs) or as long-acting beta agonists (LABAs). Inhaled SABAs monotherapy is mainly used in mild or intermittent asthma patients. Since LABAs monotherapy may increase the risk of death from asthma, combination of LABAs and ICS is recommended for maintaining treatment in asthma [6]. Among around 80 identified polymorphisms in the beta-2 adrenergic receptor gene, ADRB2 Arg16Gly polymorphism is one of the most common nonsynonymous SNPs [1, 11]. ADRB2 Arg16Gly polymorphism has been shown to have functional effects in vitro. Green et al. found that human airway smooth muscle cells expressing Gly16 homozygotes resulted in enhanced ADRB2 agonist-promoted down-regulation of ADRB2 compared with Arg16 homozygotes [12]. Some studies examined the clinical effect of ADRB2 Arg16Gly polymorphism on the asthmatic patient's response to LABAs plus ICS therapy, but the results were inconsistent [2, 6, 7]. Thus, this is the first systematic review and meta-analysis to estimate the effect of ADRB2 Arg16Gly polymorphism on pulmonary function in asthma patients treated with ICS plus LABAs. We did not find any significant differences of pulmonary function in patients with the Arg/Arg or Arg/Gly phenotype. Patients bearing the Arg/Arg or Gly/Gly phenotype also did not show significant different pulmonary functions. The meta-analysis results suggested that ADRB2 Arg16Gly polymorphism is not associated with pulmonary function response to asthma treatment with ICS plus LABAs.

Our analysis has limitations. Firstly, Egger's test found no significant publication bias in the included studies.

However, useful data may be available in unpublished or unpresented studies and in studies that were not published in English or Chinese. Also, two potentially eligible studies were not included because of incomplete data [13, 14]. Secondly, we found significant heterogeneity among the studies, including different methods for diagnosis of asthma, different patient populations (e.g., sample size, asthma severity, age, ethnicity, and sex ratio), different fluticasone propionate and salmeterol dosage, and different treatment duration. These differences may influence the reliability of the results.

In conclusion, based on the data derived from the included studies, this systematic review and meta-analysis indicated that ArgGly polymorphism of ADRB2 may not be a predictive genetic marker of pulmonary function response to LABAs plus ICS treatment in asthma patients. Although a definitive conclusion is not possible, additional studies with larger sample sizes are warranted to address the question.

Acknowledgments

This study was supported by National Natural Science Foundation of China (Grant nos. 81360108 and 81560252), specialized fund for training of high-level talents in Health and Family Planning in Yunnan Province (Grant no. L-201614), The First Affiliated Hospital of Kunming Medical University Research Fund for the Doctor (Grant no. 2015BS002), Yunnan Applied Basic Research Projects-Joint Special Fund Project (Grant no. 2015FB029), and Health Science and Technology Internal Research Institution Project of Yunnan Province (Grant no. 2014NS190).

References

[1] J. J. Lima, "Do genetic polymorphisms alter patient response to inhaled bronchodilators?," *Expert Opinion on Drug Metabolism and Toxicology*, vol. 10, no. 9, pp. 1231–1240, 2014.

[2] M. E. Wechsler, S. J. Kunselman, V. M. Chinchilli et al., "Effect of β2-adrenergic receptor polymorphism on response to longacting β2 agonist in asthma (LARGE trial): a genotype-stratified, randomised, placebo-controlled, crossover trial," *The Lancet*, vol. 374, no. 9703, pp. 1754–1764, 2009.

[3] D. K. Lee, G. P. Currie, I. P. Hall, J. J. Lima, and B. J. Lipworth, "The arginine-16 beta2-adrenoceptor polymorphism predisposes to bronchoprotective subsensitivity in patients treated with formoterol and salmeterol," *British Journal of Clinical Pharmacology*, vol. 57, no. 1, pp. 68–75, 2004.

[4] E. R. Bleecker, S. W. Yancey, L. A. Baitinger et al., "Salmeterol response is not affected by beta2-adrenergic receptor genotype in subjects with persistent asthma," *Journal of Allergy and Clinical Immunology*, vol. 118, no. 4, pp. 809–816, 2006.

[5] E. R. Bleecker, H. S. Nelson, M. Kraft et al., "2-Receptor polymorphisms in patients receiving salmeterol with or without fluticasone propionate," *American Journal of Respiratory and Critical Care Medicine*, vol. 181, no. 7, pp. 676–687, 2009.

[6] K. Blake and J. Lima, "Pharmacogenomics of long-acting beta2-agonists," *Expert Opinion on Drug Metabolism and Toxicology*, vol. 11, no. 11, pp. 1733–1751, 2015.

[7] Y. Qiu, D. Zhang, Y. Qin et al., "Effect of beta2-adrenergic receptor gene Arg16Gly polymorphisms on response to long-acting beta2-agonist in Chinese Han asthmatic patients," *Multidisciplinary Respiratory Medicine*, vol. 9, no. 1, p. 22, 2014.

[8] F. Soleimani, F. Fahimi, P. Adimi Naghan et al., "The effect of polymorphisms of beta2 adrenoceptors on response to long-acting beta2 agonists in Iranian asthmatic patients," *Iranian Journal of Allergy, Asthma and Immunology*, vol. 12, no. 4, pp. 383–390, 2013.

[9] Q. W. Wu, X. M. Wan, X. Zhu, X. Fu, and C. Pu, "The variation of coding region of ADRB2 gene and asthmatic children's response to LABAs plus ICS therapy," *Pharmacotherapy (in Chinese language)*, vol. 20, pp. 1150–1155, 2015.

[10] R. Aalbers, C. Vogelmeier, and P. Kuna, "Achieving asthma control with ICS/LABA: a review of strategies for asthma management and prevention," *Respiratory Medicine*, vol. 111, pp. 1–7, 2016.

[11] S. B. Liggett, "The pharmacogenetics of beta2-adrenergic receptors: relevance to asthma," *Journal of Allergy and Clinical Immunology*, vol. 105, no. 2, pp. S487–S492, 2000.

[12] S. A. Green, J. Turki, P. Bejarano, I P. Hall, and S B. Liggett, "Influence of beta 2-adrenergic receptor genotypes on signal transduction in human airway smooth muscle cells," *American Journal of Respiratory Cell and Molecular Biology*, vol. 13, no. 1, pp. 25–33, 1995.

[13] S. W. Yancey, M. Klotsman, H. G. Ortega, L. D. Edwards, and W. H. Anderson, "Acute and chronic lung function responses to salmeterol and salmeterol plus fluticasone propionate in relation to Arg16Gly beta(2)-adrenergic polymorphisms," *Current Medical Research and Opinion*, vol. 25, no. 4, pp. 1011–1018, 2009.

[14] S. H. Kim, Y. M. Ye, G. Y. Hur et al., "Effect of beta2-adrenergic receptor polymorphism in asthma control of patients receiving combination treatment," *Yonsei Medical Journal*, vol. 50, no. 2, pp. 182–188, 2009.

13

Intrabullous Adhesion Pexia (IBAP) by Percutaneous Pulmonary Bulla Centesis: An Alternative for the Surgical Treatment of Giant Pulmonary Bulla (GPB)

Wei-Liang Li,[1] Yong-Hua Li,[2] Yu-Bo Yang,[1] and Li-Hui Lv[2]

[1]*Department of Respiratory and Critical Care Medicine, Mingzhou Hospital, Zhejiang University, No. 168 West Taian Road, Ningbo, Zhejiang 315199, China*
[2]*Department of Respiratory and Critical Care Medicine, Donghai Hospital, Ningbo University, No. 377 Zhongshan East Road, Ningbo 315040, China*

Correspondence should be addressed to Wei-Liang Li; ipec2012@126.com

Academic Editor: Franz Stanzel

Background and Objective. Most patients with giant pulmonary bulla (GPB) are treated by surgery; however, there is a subset for whom surgery is not a viable option, such as those with contraindications, or those unwilling to undergo operation. Therefore, an alternative minimally invasive method is desired for this subpopulation. The aim of this study was to explore an alternative procedure for treating GPB. *Methods.* This was a prospective, nonrandomized, single-arm, unblinded study evaluating the efficacy and safety of intrabulla adhesion pexia (IBAP) procedure in GPB patients. The study was conducted between December 2004 and April 2017. *Results.* There were 38 cases in 36 patients (33 males and 3 females) with the target GPB cavities varying in size (range, 10 cm × 7 cm × 5 cm to 15 cm × 8 cm × 30 cm (anteroposterior diameter × medial-lateral diameter × superoinferior diameter)). After IBAP treatment, the closure ratio of GPB in one month was 86.84% (33/38), while the dyspnea index significantly decreased from 4.11 ± 1.11 to 2.24 ± 1.15 ($P < 0.01$). In addition, the mean FEV1 (L) increased from 1.06 ± 0.73 to 1.57 ± 1.13 ($P < 0.01$), while RV (L) decreased from 2.77 ± 0.54 to 2.36 ± 0.38 ($P < 0.01$) and TLC (L) decreased from 6.46 ± 1.21 to 5.86 ± 1.08 ($P < 0.01$). Moreover, PaO_2 (mmHg) increased from 52.18 ± 8.31 to 68.29 ± 12.34, while the 6 MWD increased by 129.36% from 131.58 ± 105.24 to 301.79 ± 197.90 ($P < 0.01$). Collectively, these data indicated significant improvement in pulmonary function and exercise tolerance after IBAP treatment. Furthermore, no deaths occurred during IBAP treatment, and no cases of aggravated GPB relapse were reported during the 12-month follow-up period. *Conclusions.* IBAP is a promising strategy for the treatment of GPB. Our findings demonstrated that IBAP had a noteworthy therapeutic effect, desirable safety, and ideal long-term efficacy for GPB.

1. Introduction

Giant pulmonary bulla (GPB) or giant emphysematous bulla (GEB), a bulla occupying more than one-third of the involved hemithorax, usually requires removal by surgical procedures such as bullectomy or lobectomy. However, surgery is associated with many complications, such as pneumothorax due to prolonged air leak, atrial fibrillation, infection, bleeding and respiratory failure, and even death in severe patients after operation [1–6].

Notably, patients with advanced age or poor cardiopulmonary functional reserves might be not ideal candidates for or may not be willing to undergo surgical procedures [7]. Although great efforts have been made to improve the safety and efficacy of surgical procedures in treating high-risk patients with GPB over the past three decades [8–11], controlling surgical damage, reducing postoperative complications, and improving therapeutic effectiveness are still challenging [12].

In this study, we introduce an alternative convenient procedure named intrabullous adhesion pexia (IBAP)

involving computer tomography (CT)-guided percutaneous pulmonary bulla centesis, IBAP with biomedical fibrin sealant, and closed intracavity drainage under continuous negative pressure. We evaluated the efficacy and safety of IBAP in GPB patients who either had contraindications or were unwilling to undergo surgery.

2. Materials and Methods

2.1. Patient Recruitment and Study Design. All of the GPB patients were enrolled based on CT diagnosis and symptomatic dyspnea, and they were admitted to hospital from the outpatient department. These consecutive patients were unsuitable for or unwilling to accept surgical resection but willing to accept IBAP treatment.

According to underlying comorbidities, such as acute exacerbation of COPD, pulmonary infection, bronchial asthma, or bronchiectasis, patients received necessary treatments, such as anti-inflammatories, anti-infectives, or antihistamines, prior to IBAP procedures. Antibiotics, such as cephazolin or amikacin, were employed as preventive medication. Appropriate antibiotics were used according to the infection.

This was a prospective, nonrandomized, single-arm, unblinded study. Because of insufficient sample, the research period occurred over 13 years; all efforts were made to maintain similar procedures and technical skills of the pulmonologist during this 13-year study. All of the operative procedures were performed by the same pulmonologist and the same fibrin sealant was used in all of the operations.

The primary end point was the closure ratio of the target GPB in one month after the IBAP procedures. The secondary end points were the mortality related to the IBAP procedure, dyspnea scores, pulmonary function, 6 MWT, and the reappearance ratio of the closed GPB or the shrunk GPB in 12 months after the IBAP procedures.

This study was approved by the institutional ethics committee and conducted in compliance with the Declaration of Helsinki. Informed consent was obtained from all of the patients.

2.2. Operative Procedure. All of the operative procedures were performed by the pulmonologist, the professor, and the chief physician of the Department of Respiratory and Critical Care Medicine, Mingzhou Hospital, Zhejiang University. The method did not change and the professional level of the pulmonologist was stable throughout the 13 years.

Intrabullous adhesion pexia (IBAP) procedure was performed under local anesthesia in the CT scan suite, and the vital signs of patients were closely monitored during the perioperative period. Percutaneous pulmonary bulla centesis was performed by omnidirectional injection into the GPB with 10 ml of porcine fibrin sealant such that the biological glue could be distributed evenly within the target bulla. The Porcine Fibrin Sealant kit was produced by Hangzhou Puji Biotechnology Co., Ltd, containing 5 ml of 30.0 mg/ml fibrinogen in 6.0–7.0 mg/ml sodium chloride solution and 5 ml 450–850 IU/ml thrombin in 35.0–45.0 mmol/L calcium chloride solution. Then, the sealant was inserted into the target GPB through a disposable pigtail drainage catheter (14 G) attached to a closed intracavity drainage set under continuous negative pressure (at 14–18 cm H_2O). For secondary pneumothorax caused by the bulla centesis, pleural cavity-closed drainage under continuous negative pressure (at 14–18 cm H_2O) was a routine additional procedure. When the target GPB closed or collapsed to stable cavities without secondary pneumothorax for 72 hours with radiological examination (chest CT scan), the drainage catheters were blocked, and then would be removed 24 hours later after further confirmation.

2.3. Assessment. On the first day of admission and one week after the drainage tube was removed, the severity of patients' condition was evaluated according to the results of objective tests. Arterial oxygen tension (PaO_2) and arterial carbon dioxide tension ($PaCO_2$) were examined by a blood-gas analyzer (GEM Premier 3000, USA). If the patient's condition permitted, pulmonary function including forced expiratory volume in 1 second (FEV1), residual volume (RV), and total lung capacity volume (TLC) was calculated from the flow-volume curve by the qualified technician using spirometry (CHEST AC-8800-D, Japan). Twelve cases in 11 patients did not complete pulmonary function tests because they were unable or unwilling to cooperate. Functional exercise capacity was assessed by using a 6 min walking distance (6 MWD) test. The 6 MWD test results of patients who could not walk initially were marked as 0 meter. The relationship between dyspnea and physical disability was evaluated by dyspnea index (from 1 to 5) based on the Medical Research Council (MRC) scale [13], which classifies this symptom into five grades (on a scale from I to V). The chest CT was performed at the 3rd month, 6th month, and 12th month after the primary end point.

2.4. Clinical Follow-Up. As a routine, clinical follow-up was carried out with outpatient service and chest CT scan. Outcomes assessed were closure time of the target GPB after the IBAP procedures, mortality related to the IBAP procedure, and the reappearance of the closed GPB or progress of the shrunken GPB after the IBAP procedures.

2.5. Statistical Analysis. All of the data were tested for normality and presented as mean ± standard deviation (SD). Differences between the preoperative and postoperative data were tested by paired Student's *t*-test using SPSS 17.0 software. A P value < 0.05 was considered significant.

3. Results

3.1. Patient Characteristics. A total of 38 cases in 36 patients (33 males and 3 females) with the average age of 67.53 years (range: 41–78) were diagnosed as GPB from December 2004 to April 2017 and underwent IBAP treatment. According to CT scan findings, the target GPB cavities varied in size from smallest at 10 cm × 7 cm × 5 cm to the largest cavity at 15 cm × 8 cm × 30 cm (anteroposterior diameter × medial-lateral diameter × superoinferior diameter). Moreover, there were 11 target GPBs located in the left lung and 27 in the right. Two patients had two target GPBs, while the other 34 patients each had a single target GPB. As shown in Table 1, all cases enrolled in this study had various degrees of dyspnea (four patients with grade II, 9 with grade III, four grade IV, and 21 with grade V) before IBAP treatment, and a total of 34 cases with grade III to V were classified as having serious dyspnea. Besides, 31 cases met the criteria of respiratory failure ($PaO_2 < 60$ mmHg) based on arterial blood gas (ABG) analysis. All of the cases except for two cases had underlying pulmonary comorbidities, and 15 other cases were complicated by cor pulmonale. Chronic obstructive pulmonary disease (COPD) was the leading disease diagnosed in 23 cases, followed by asthma (five cases), interstitial lung disease (5 cases), and bronchiectasis (4 cases). One patient (with two GPB cases) had no comorbidities but had a history of spontaneous pneumothorax. Other co-occurring illnesses that may have influenced respiratory function or acid-base balance in blood and survival of the patients included one case each of liver cancer, esophageal cancer, rectal carcinoma and hernia of the ventral wall, prostate cancer, and bilateral hydronephrosis caused by urinary calculi.

3.2. Therapeutic Effectiveness. The target GPB in 29 cases were closed within 7 days and 4 closed within 15 days after IBAP procedure. The GPB in the remaining 5 cases shrank to stable cavities in 10 days (3 cases), 14 days (1 case), and 30 days (1 case), respectively. The outcome indicated high effectiveness in closure of the target GPB, with a closure ratio of 86.84% (33/38) in one month after the IBAP procedures. The time length with chest tube in place was 9.00 ± 5.33 days in this study group. A representative case is shown in Figure 1 to visually demonstrate the therapeutic effect of the IBAP. To ensure patient safety, two patients (patient #1 and patient #7) with two separate target GPBs accepted two rounds of IBAP treatment with an interval between the two procedures. Patient #7 had comorbidities, such as COPD, cor pulmonale, rectal carcinoma, and hernia of ventral wall, and accepted IBAP for the GPB at the right lung in February 2007 and treatment for the left lung in December 2008 as shown in Figure 2. There was no recurrent bulla until the patient died of rectal carcinoma in March 2010.

After treatment, dyspnea in all of the cases was relieved or even disappeared as the index was significantly decreased from 4.11 ± 1.11 to 2.24 ± 1.15 ($P < 0.01$). Patients also showed significant improvement in pulmonary function and exercise tolerance. As shown in Table 2, mean FEV1 (L) increased from 1.06 ± 0.73 to 1.57 ± 1.13 ($P < 0.01$), while RV (L) decreased from 2.77 ± 0.54 to 2.36 ± 0.38 ($P < 0.01$) and TLC (L) decreased from the level of 6.46 ± 1.21 to 5.86 ± 1.08 ($P < 0.01$). Furthermore, PaO_2 (mmHg) increased from 52.18 ± 8.31 to 68.29 ± 12.34 and respiratory failure was reversed in 25 of 31 patients ($P < 0.01$), while $PaCO_2$ declined but without statistical significance ($P > 0.05$). The 6 MWD, which represented exercise tolerance, was also improved after treatment as the mean distance (m) walked in 6 minutes increased 129.36% from 131.58 ± 105.24 to 301.79 ± 197.90 ($P < 0.01$).

Heterogeneity was investigated by subgroup analysis. The study population was further stratified into COPD group and non-COPD group based on history of COPD before GPB treatment. As shown in Table 3, the pulmonary function and exercise tolerance improved in patients with or without history of COPD ($P < 0.01$). Importantly, significant change in the level of $PaCO_2$ was observed, which decreased in the COPD group ($P < 0.01$) but increased in the non-COPD group ($P < 0.01$) after IBAP. It is worth mentioning that three patients (patient #2, 7, and 8), who could barely walk initially before IBAP treatment, had an improved 6 MWD of 42 m, 72 m, and 528 m, respectively.

3.3. Adverse Events. As shown in Table 4, the most common complications were mild noninfective inflammation of the ipsilateral lung reported in all 38 cases (Figure 1(b), Figure 3(b), and Figure 4(b)). In addition, ipsilateral pleural effusion was reported in 32 cases (31 patients) while ipsilateral secondary pneumothorax was reported in 24 cases (22 patients) as common complications. Only 5 cases (5 patients) of pleural effusion required nonroutine additional closed drainage. Ipsilateral secondary pneumothorax was absorbed gradually by pleural cavity closed drainage under continuous negative pressure as a routine additional procedure during IBAP. There were only two cases of tension pneumothorax, both of which were resolved within one month. It is shown in Figure 3 by the third representative case (patient #35) with tension pneumothorax after the IBAP procedure. Subcutaneous emphysema developed in 7 cases (6 patients), which was mild in severity and was self-absorbed later. Asymptomatic ipsilateral pleural thickening was found in 13 cases via CT scan. There were no cases of bronchopleural fistula and no deaths occurred during IBAP treatment.

3.4. Clinical Follow-Up. Thirty-two of 36 patients were clinically followed up until April 30, 2017, with a median follow-up time of 67.53 months (9 to 148 months), and 4 patients were lost at 10, 50, 52, and 56 month, respectively, of follow-up. Over 12 years, 14 patients died of various diseases such as acute exacerbation of COPD in six patients at month 12, 53, 58, 60, 99, and 114 after IBAP, respectively; acute coronary syndrome in four patients at month 73, 62, 26, and 10 after IBAP, respectively; esophageal cancer in one patient at the 42nd month, rectal carcinoma in one patient at the 37th month, sepsis caused by trauma in one patient at the 88th month, and severe pneumonia in one patient at the 17th month after IBAP, respectively. None of these deaths was related to the IBAP treatment. At the conclusion of the follow-up deadline, 18 patients were alive and 4 of them (patient #1, 2, 5, and 30) still had normal indices at the deadline.

The thoracic CT scan showed none of GPB relapsed or aggravated in these patients during clinical follow-up. While

Table 1: Clinical characteristics of patients.

Case no.	Patient no.	Sex	Age	Dyspnea index	ABG analysis (mmHg)		Lung function (L)			6 MWD (m)
					PaO_2	$PaCO_2$	FEV1	RV	TLC	
1	1	M	41	3	61	38	1.95	2.20	6.45	215
2	1	M	42	2	68	40	2.37	1.87	5.35	347
3	2	M	52	5	50	30				0
4	3	M	42	5	46	34	0.59	2.76	6.60	21
5	4	M	62	3	64	34	2.39	1.89	6.33	289
6	5	M	41	3	57	45	0.45	3.58	6.98	286
7	6	M	71	5	56	53	1.10	2.85	6.92	35
8	7	M	64	5	49	40				0
9	8	F	47	5	42	31				0
10	9	M	58	5	45	50				92
11	10	F	43	2	55	36	1.70	2.57	3.61	311
12	11	F	64	5	45	30	0.45	2.91	6.45	125
13	12	M	57	2	74	35	2.18	1.96	6.33	234
14	13	M	63	5	42	67	0.41	3.45	7.51	64
15	14	M	69	5	50	50	0.46	2.82	7.15	56
16	15	M	63	5	45	31	0.40	2.54	2.85	122
17	7	M	65	4	50	36	.			97
18	16	M	61	3	58	37	0.72	3.41	7.31	296
19	17	M	48	5	46	31	.			56
20	18	M	69	5	42	62	0.39	3.25	7.20	64
21	19	M	71	5	45	39	0.63	2.76	6.40	26
22	20	M	65	3	56	53				152
23	21	M	72	5	50	38	0.41	3.21	7.62	125
24	22	M	71	5	42	65				56
25	23	M	61	5	45	52				38
26	24	M	59	3	59	40	0.60	3.65	7.60	296
27	25	M	69	5	44	57	0.43	2.62	7.18	55
28	26	M	61	2	70	32	2.40	1.84	6.33	246
29	27	M	67	3	56	46	0.70	3.47	7.21	280
30	28	M	44	5	50	37				53
31	29	M	58	3	52	39	1.05	2.24	4.15	48
32	30	M	59	4	55	33	0.89	2.55	6.92	135
33	31	M	56	5	45	41				98
34	32	M	68	3	61	45	2.22	3.02	7.55	243
35	33	M	78	5	51	57				14
36	34	M	60	5	45	37	1.08	2.88	6.11	78
37	35	M	75	4	62	46	0.99	3.12	7.02	182
38	36	M	70	4	50	56	0.63	2.67	6.87	165

M: male; F: female; IBAP: intrabullous adhesion pexy; ABG: arterial blood gas; 6 MWD: 6 min walking distance; FEV1: forced expiratory volume in 1 s; RV: residual volume; TLC: total lung capacity volume; PaO_2: arterial partial pressure of oxygen; $PaCO_2$: arterial partial pressure of carbon dioxide. 1 mmHg = 0.133 kPa. Cases 1 and 2 and cases 8 and 17 are the same patients, respectively. Twelve cases in 11 patients (patients 2, 7, 8, 9, 17, 20, 22, 23, 28, 31, and 33) did not test lung function due to their serious conditions or unwillingness. A few patients might give poor cooperation in lung function test because of their serious conditions so that a few values of pulmonary function test might be suspected in their accurateness, but this uncertainty would not affect the statistical conclusion for their own single-arm test values.

an inspiring phenomenon was observed in patient #30, wherein the target GPB, which shrank to a stable cavity in the original IBAP procedure, had closed completely after 3 years (Figure 4).

4. Discussion

It is generally believed that a single small pulmonary bulla, which has negligible influence on lung functions, does not necessarily require treatment. However, for GPB or GEB, especially tension GPB, invasive therapy might be inevitable. Surgical intervention, such as bullectomy or lobectomy, may alleviate symptoms, improve exercise tolerance, and prevent fatal respiratory distress, and it is considered as the routine technique of choice in treating GPB [6, 14]. However, contraindications or complications with the open procedure hamper their clinical application in critical cases, especially for elderly patients [1, 6, 15]. Furthermore, it is highly risky to treat patients with cardiopulmonary insufficiency or other serious underlying conditions by surgical intervention. Damage to the chest wall and postoperative pain would further worsen respiratory function [16]. Therefore, minimally invasive procedures are favorable as alternative methods for the treatment of GPB. Takizawa et al. [9] reported

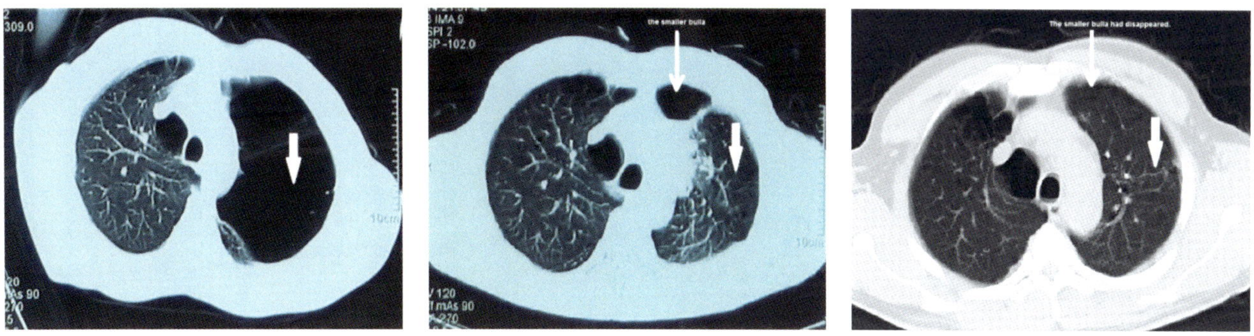

(a) (b) (c)

FIGURE 1: Case 3 (patient 2) of GPB treated by IBAP as shown by CT scan. The 52-year-old male patient with bilateral pulmonary bullae and left GPB (thick arrow) (a). Seven days after IBAP in July 2006, the GPB closed completely (thick arrow), while a smaller bulla in the same side appeared (thin arrow), which may be previously compressed by the target GPB (b). Six years after IBAP, the left GPB did not recur (thick arrow) and the smaller one disappeared (thin arrow) (c).

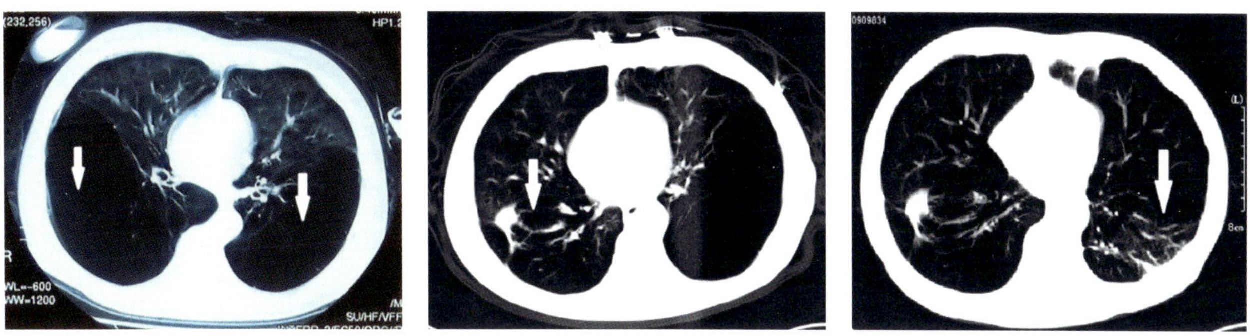

(a) (b) (c)

FIGURE 2: Case 8 and case 17 (patient 7) of GPB. The 65-year-old male patient, who was complicated by COPD, cor pulmonale, hernia of ventral wall, and rectal carcinoma, had two target GPBs in each side of the lung (thick arrows) (a). He accepted the first IBAP for the right GPB in February 2007 (thick arrow) (b) and the second IBAP for the left GPB in December 2008 (thick arrow) (c). No bulla recurred until he died of rectal carcinoma in March 2010.

TABLE 2: Therapeutic effect of IBAP assessed by lung function, ABG analysis, 6 MWD test, and dyspnea index.

Items	*N* (cases)		Before IBAP$^{\$}$	After IBAP$^{\$\$}$
Lung function (L)	26	FEV_1	1.06 ± 0.73	1.57 ± 1.13*
		RV	2.77 ± 0.54	2.36 ± 0.38*
		TLC	6.46 ± 1.21	5.86 ± 1.08*
ABG (mmHg)	38	PaO_2	52.18 ± 8.31	68.29 ± 12.34*
		$PaCO_2$	42.71 ± 10.29	41.05 ± 4.57$^{\#}$
6 MWD (m)	38		131.58 ± 105.24	301.79 ± 197.90*
Dyspnea index	38		4.11 ± 1.11	2.24 ± 1.15*

Data are represented as mean ± standard deviation (SD). As shown in Table 1, 12 of 38 cases did not test lung function due to serious conditions or their unwillingness. IBAP: intrabullous adhesion pexy; ABG: arterial blood gas; 6 MWD: 6 min walking distance; FEV1: forced expiratory volume in 1 s; RV: residual volume; TLC: total lung capacity volume; PaO_2: arterial partial pressure of oxygen; $PaCO_2$: arterial partial pressure of carbon dioxide. 1 mmHg = 0.133 kPa. $^*P < 0.01$; $^{\#}P > 0.05$ (the value of posttreatment compared to before). $^{\$}$On the first day of admission; $^{\$\$}$one week after the drainage tube was removed.

two cases of GPB treated by CT-guided bulla drainage and showed short-term symptomatic improvement. One patient died of pulmonary dsyfunction 21 months later, while the other suffered from prolonged air leak closed with bronchoscopic bronchial occlusion later. Kemp et al. [17] reported one case of GPB who underwent bronchoscopic autologous blood installation in which the patient demonstrated slow improvement in pulmonary function and symptoms. Santini et al. [11] invented a new therapeutic strategy by installing a one-way valve in the segmental bronchi to functionally isolate the airway that supplied the bulla for surgically unfit GPB patients. Except PaO_2 and $PaCO_2$, this strategy showed a significant improvement of respiration in a relatively short-term follow-up. Thus, there is a need to further explore an alternative approach to treat GPB with affirmative safety and long-term effectiveness.

It is hypothesized that stopping one-way aerating manner of pulmonary bulla by injection of fibrin sealant into the target GPB followed by closed intracavity drainage under continuous negative pressure could achieve closure of GPB immediately. Expansion ceaselessly of pulmonary bulla can also compress the surrounding parenchyma, eventually

Table 3: Therapeutic effect in patients stratified by COPD.

Parameter	N (cases)	Items		Before IBAP$^{\$}$	After IBAP$^{\$\$}$
COPD	15	Lung function (L)	FEV_1	0.74 ± 0.47	1.03 ± 0.68*
			RV	3.06 ± 0.32	2.49 ± 0.27*
			TLC	7.04 ± 0.42	6.24 ± 0.53*
	23	ABG (mmHg)	PaO_2	50.09 ± 6.15	62.26 ± 7.71*
			$PaCO_2$	47.91 ± 9.82	41.70 ± 5.46*
		6 MWD (m)		107.74 ± 92.24	263.48 ± 203.84*
		Dyspnea index		4.43 ± 0.84	2.70 ± 1.11*
Non-COPD	11	Lung function (L)	FEV_1	1.49 ± 0.82	2.30 ± 1.24*
			RV	2.38 ± 0.55	2.17 ± 0.43*
			TLC	5.67 ± 1.50	5.33 ± 1.40*
	15	ABG (mmHg)	PaO_2	55.40 ± 10.25	77.53 ± 12.57*
			$PaCO_2$	34.73 ± 3.99	40.07 ± 2.60*
		6 MWD (m)		168.13 ± 116.35	360.53 ± 179.16*
		Dyspnea index		3.60 ± 1.30	1.53 ± 0.83*

Data are expressed as mean ± standard deviation (SD). As shown in Table 1, 12 of 38 cases did not test lung function due to serious conditions or their unwillingness. IBAP: intrabullous adhesion pexy; ABG: arterial blood gas; 6 MWD: 6 min walking distance; FEV1: forced expiratory volume in 1 s; RV: residual volume; TLC: total lung capacity volume; PaO_2: arterial partial pressure of oxygen; $PaCO_2$: arterial partial pressure of carbon dioxide. 1 mmHg = 0.133 kPa. $^{*}P < 0.01$ (the value of posttreatment compared to before). $^{\$}$On the first day of admission; $^{\$\$}$ one week after the drainage tube was removed.

Table 4: The complications in perioperative period in 38 cases.

Perioperative complications	N (cases)	Incidence rates (%)
Noninfective inflammation of the ipsilateral lung	38	100.00
Ipsilateral pleural effusion	32	84.21
In a small amount	27	71.05
In a large amount needing drainage	5	13.16
Ipsilateral secondary pneumothorax	24	63.16
Nontension pneumothorax	22	57.90
Tension pneumothorax	2	5.26
Subcutaneous emphysema	7	18.42
Asymptomatic ipsilateral pleural thickening	13	34.21
Bronchopleural fistula	0	0.00
Mortality	0	0.00

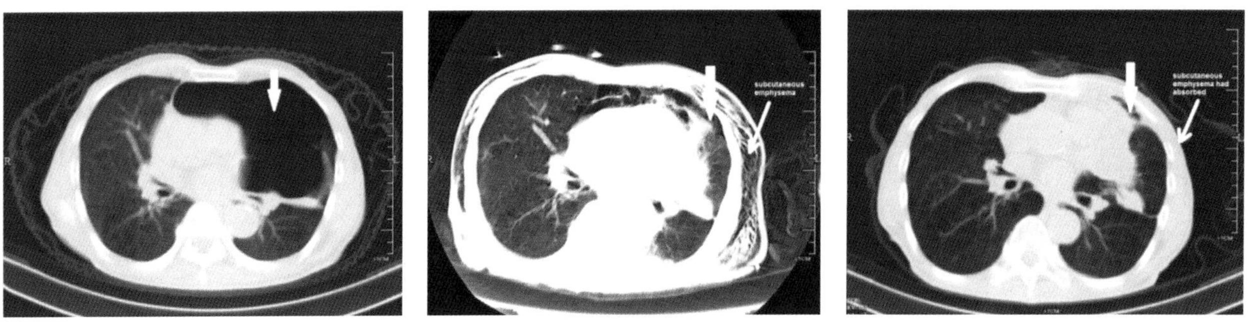

(a) (b) (c)

Figure 3: The patient 35 (case 37), a 75-year-old man, was complicated by COPD, respiratory failure, cor pulmonale, coronary heart disease, hypertension, chronic renal insufficiency, and prostate cancer, had the target GPB in left of the lung (thick arrow) (a). Fourteen days after IBAP in April 2016, the GPB closed completely (thick arrow), while obvious subcutaneous emphysema secondary to tension pneumothorax remained to be absorbed (thin arrow) (b). Three weeks later, the subcutaneous emphysema disappeared (thin arrow) (c), and no bulla recurred (thick arrow) (c) until he died of sudden cardiac death at home in February 2017.

resulting in decreased pulmonary function [18]. On the basis of mechanism of pulmonary bulla formation, an alternative method, the IBAP procedure as mentioned above, was performed under local anesthesia in this study, which achieved high effectiveness in closure of the target GPB with a closure ratio of 86.84% (33/38) in one month after the IBAP procedures, while the other 5 target GPBs shrank to stable cavities, indicating high total effective rate of 100%

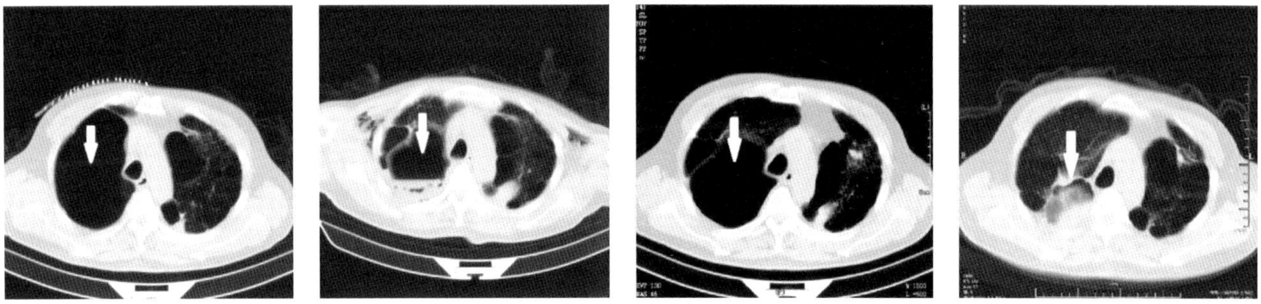

(a) (b) (c) (d)

FIGURE 4: The patient 30 (case 32), a 59-year-old man, was complicated by pneumoconiosis, cor pulmonale, uarthritis, hypertension, and respiratory failure, had the GPB in the right lung (thick arrow) (a). The target GPB shrank to stable cavity in 30 days after the IBAP in March, 2013 (thick arrow) (b) until the second follow-up CT scan in April 2014 (thick arrow) (c). The right GPB closed completely observed at the third follow-up CT scan 3 years after IBAP in March 2016 (thick arrow) (d).

(38/38). Furthermore, IBAP demonstrated a good safety profile; no deaths were related to the IBAP procedure. The intentional procedure of IBAP may have broken the medical traditional taboo of percutaneous pulmonary bulla centesis. Specifically, IBAP treatment resulted in long-term effectiveness with a median follow-up time of 67.53 months (9 to 148 months) accompanied by significant improvement in exercise tolerance and pulmonary function by 6 MWD, FEV1, RV, TLC, PaO_2, and $PaCO_2$ tests (Table 2). Overall, this was a 13-year study of a minimally invasive procedure with reliable safety and encouraging long-term efficacy.

Talcum slurry has been used for decades in pleurodesis to encourage adhesion for recrudescent spontaneous pneumothorax by stimulating exuberant fibrotic response on the surface of visceral and parietal pleura, which is time consuming and may cause unfavorable complications, such as chest pain, fever, nausea, and even respiratory distress [19–21]. In comparison, the porcine fibrin sealant used in the IBAP procedure can be solidified at 37°C and produce intrabullous adhesion within a short time of 3 to 5 minutes by mediating noninfectious inflammation on the surface of the bulla wall, which allows closure of the bulla and reexpansion of collapsed lung parenchyma. Closed intracavity drainage under continuous negative pressure following IBAP can accelerate the process.

Several studies have reported restricted functional improvement after bullectomy in patients with very low FEV1, hypoxaemia, and hypercapnia before surgery [22, 23]. However, most patients in this study who had underlying diseases or poor cardiopulmonary function regarded as surgery contraindications achieved significant improvements in pulmonary function. This difference may be explained as normal or relatively normal pulmonary parenchyma that would have been resected by bullectomy or lobectomy and was reserved by the IBAP procedure. This suggests that IBAP treatment not only reduces dead space effect by closing GPB but also increases the ventilation area by releasing compressed lung tissue. This may be an advantage of IBAP compared with surgical procedures, such as bullectomy and lobectomy.

Although the overall safety profile of this study was promising, there also were complications, such as mild noninfective inflammation of the ipsilateral lung, ipsilateral pleural effusion, and ipsilateral secondary pneumothorax. Ipsilateral pleural effusion and pleural thickening were the major adverse reactions of porcine fibrin sealant, while noninfective inflammation of the ipsilateral lung might have reinforced IBAP. In consideration of the counteraction of anti-inflammation, which might have a negative influence on IBAP, glucocorticoids were not employed in the perioperative period. Ipsilateral secondary pneumothorax was the complication of percutaneous pulmonary bulla centesis. Nevertheless, most of these events were mild and of low frequency, and most were resolved. As a routine procedure and a routine additional procedure of IBAP, intrabullous catheter drainage and pleural cavity catheter drainage under continuous negative pressure might have not only facilitated target bulla closure but also alleviated noninfective inflammation, pleural effusion, pleural thickening, and secondary pneumothorax. In addition, there were five cases that did not completely close but remarkably shrank to stable cavities after IBAP procedure. We posit that bronchobullous fistula, which stalled bulla collapse, may have played an important role in this phenomenon. It may be solved by increasing the dosage of fibrin sealant and/or increasing the frequency of IBAP procedure. Furthermore, the addition of one-way endobronchial valve placement may also shorten the IBAP procedure [24–26].

5. Conclusion

In conclusion, IBAP is a promising strategy for the treatment of GPB, which showed noteworthy therapeutic effect, desirable safety, and remarkable long-term efficacy. IBAP treatment will benefit a wider spectrum of symptomatic GPB patients who are unsuitable for or unwilling to accept surgical resection. However, larger studies are needed to adequately validate the efficacy and safety of IBAP for GPB.

Ethical Approval

This manuscript has obtained approval from the Institutional Review Board (IRB).

Authors' Contributions

Wei-Liang Li conceived the study and was responsible for design, data analysis, and manuscript writing. Yong-Hua Li, Yu-Bo Yang, and Li-Hui Lv were responsible for data acquisition. All authors provided final approval for publication.

Acknowledgments

This study was funded by the Army Medical Innovation Project of PLA (grant no. MS022).

References

[1] P. H. Schipper, B. F. Meyers, R. J. Battafarano, T. J. Guthrie, G. A. Patterson, and J. D. Cooper, "Outcomes after resection of giant emphysematous bullae," *Annals of Thoracic Surgery*, vol. 78, no. 3, pp. 976–982, 2004.

[2] D. Divisi, C. Battaglia, W. D. Francescantonio, G. Torresini, and R. Crisci, "Giant bullous emphysema resection by VATS. Analysis of laser and stapler techniques," *European Journal of Cardio-Thoracic Surgery*, vol. 22, no. 6, pp. 990–994, 2002.

[3] A. Wakabayashi, "Thoracoscopic technique for management of giant bullous lung disease," *Annals of Thoracic Surgery*, vol. 56, no. 3, pp. 708–712, 1993.

[4] J. A. Greenberg, S. Singhal, and L. R. Kaiser, "Giant bullous lung disease: evaluation, selection, techniques, and outcomes," *Chest Surgery Clinics of North America*, vol. 13, no. 4, pp. 631–649, 2003.

[5] G. F. Menconi, F. M. A. Melfi, A. Mussi, A. Palla, M. C. Ambrogi, and C. A. Angeletti, "Treatment by VATS of giant bullous emphysema: results," *European Journal of Cardio-Thoracic Surgery*, vol. 13, no. 1, pp. 66–70, 1998.

[6] A. Palla, M. Desideri, G. Rossi et al., "Elective surgery for giant bullous emphysema: a 5-year clinical and functional follow-up," *Chest*, vol. 128, no. 4, pp. 2043–2050, 2005.

[7] P. Krishnamohan, K. R. Shen, D. A. Wigle et al., "Bullectomy for symptomatic or complicated giant lung bullae," *Annals of Thoracic Surgery*, vol. 97, no. 2, pp. 425–431, 2014.

[8] A. M. Macarthur and S. W. Fountain, "Intracavity suction and drainage in the treatment of emphysematous bullae," *Thorax*, vol. 32, no. 6, pp. 668–672, 1977.

[9] H. Takizawa, K. Kondo, S. Sakiyama, and Y. Monden, "Computed tomography-guided drainage for large pulmonary bullae," *Interactive Cardiovascular and Thoracic Surgery*, vol. 3, no. 2, pp. 283–285, 2004.

[10] M. Noppen, J. C. Tellings, T. Dekeukeleire et al., "Successful treatment of a giant emphysematous bulla by bronchoscopic placement of endobronchial valves," *Chest*, vol. 130, no. 5, pp. 1563–1565, 2006.

[11] M. Santini, A. Fiorelli, G. Vicidomini, V. G. D. Crescenzo, G. Messina, and P. Laperuta, "Endobronchial treatment of giant emphysematous bullae with one-way valves: a new approach for surgically unfit patients," *European Journal of Cardio-Thoracic Surgery*, vol. 40, no. 6, pp. 1425–1431, 2011.

[12] K. H. Lee, S. J. Cho, S. M. Ryu, S. M. Park, K. S. Yie, and S. S. Han, "Fluid-filled giant bulla treated with percutaneous drainage and talc sclerotherapy: a modified brompton technique," *Korean Journal of Thoracic and Cardiovascular Surgery*, vol. 45, no. 2, pp. 134–137, 2012.

[13] J. C. Bestall, E. A. Paul, R. Garrod, R. Garnham, P. W. Jones, and J. A. Wedzicha, "Usefulness of the Medical Research Council (MRC) dyspnea scale as a measure of disability in patients with chronic obstructive pulmonary disease," *Thorax*, vol. 54, no. 7, pp. 581–586, 1999.

[14] K. Van Bael, M. La Meir, and H. Vanoverbeke, "Video-assisted thoracoscopic resection of a giant bulla in vanishing lung syndrome: case report and a short literature review," *Journal of Cardiothoracic Surgery*, vol. 9, no. 1, p. 4, 2014.

[15] S. I. Gunnarsson, K. B. Johannesson, M. Gudjonsdottir, B. Magnusson, S. Jonsson, and T. Gudbjartsson, "Incidence and outcomes of surgical resection for giant pulmonary bullae-a population-based study," *Scandinavian Journal of Surgery*, vol. 101, no. 3, pp. 166–169, 2012.

[16] B. F. Meyers, "Chronic obstructive pulmonary disease * 10: bullectomy, lung volume reduction surgery, and transplantation for patients with chronic obstructive pulmonary disease," *Thorax*, vol. 58, no. 7, pp. 634–638, 2003.

[17] S. V. Kemp, Z. Zoumot, and P. L. Shah, "Three-year follow-up of a patient with a giant bulla treated by bronchoscopic intrabullous autologous blood instillation," *Respiration*, vol. 92, no. 4, pp. 283-284, 2016.

[18] M. E. Ribet, "Cystic and bullous lung disease," *Annals of Thoracic Surgery*, vol. 53, no. 6, p. 1147, 1992.

[19] D. H. Rehse, R. W. Aye, and M. G. Florence, "Respiratory failure following talc pleurodesis," *American Journal of Surgery*, vol. 177, no. 5, pp. 437–440, 1999.

[20] S. Györik, S. Erni, U. Studler, R. Hodek-Wuerz, M. Tamm, and P. N. Chhajed, "Long-term follow-up of thoracoscopic talc pleurodesis for primary spontaneous pneumothorax," *European Respiratory Journal*, vol. 29, no. 4, pp. 757–760, 2007.

[21] P. O. Bridevaux, J. M. Tschopp, G. Cardillo et al., "Short-term safety of thoracoscopic talc pleurodesis for recurrent primary spontaneous pneumothorax: a prospective European multicentre study," *European Respiratory Journal*, vol. 38, no. 4, pp. 770–773, 2011.

[22] K. Nakahara, K. Nakaoka, K. Ohno et al., "Functional indications for bullectomy of giant bulla," *Annals of Thoracic Surgery*, vol. 35, no. 5, pp. 480–487, 1983.

[23] L. Dubois and R. A. Malthaner, "Video-assisted thoracoscopic bullectomy and talc poudrage for spontaneous pneumothoraces: effect on short-term lung function," *Journal of Thoracic and Cardiovascular Surgery*, vol. 140, no. 6, pp. 1272–1275, 2010.

[24] M. Santini, A. Fiorello, V. G. Di Crescenzo, G. Vicidomini, L. Busiello, and P. Laperuta, "Use of unidirectional endobronchial valves for the treatment of giant emphysematous bulla," *Journal of Thoracic and Cardiovascular Surgery*, vol. 139, no. 1, pp. 224–226, 2010.

[25] Q. Tian, Y. An, B. B. Xiao, and L. A. Chen, "Treatment of giant emphysamous bulla with endobronchial valves in patients with chronic obstructive pulmonary disease: a case series," *Journal of Thoracic Disease*, vol. 6, no. 12, pp. 1674–1680, 2014.

[26] C. S. Jeon, J. Kim, and H. Kim, "Successful treatment of a giant emphysematous bulla with an endobronchial valve in a patient with contralateral lung cancer," *Korean Journal of Thoracic and Cardiovascular Surgery*, vol. 50, no. 4, pp. 305–307, 2017.

14

Mechanical Circulatory Support as a Bridge to Lung Transplantation: A Single Canadian Institution Review

Katie Kinaschuk,[1] Sabin J. Bozso,[2] Kieran Halloran,[3] Ali Kapasi,[3] Kathy Jackson,[4] and Jayan Nagendran[2,5,6]

[1] *Faculty of Medicine and Dentistry, University of Alberta, Edmonton, AB, Canada*
[2] *Department of Surgery, Division of Cardiac Surgery, Edmonton, AB, Canada*
[3] *Department of Medicine, University of Alberta, Edmonton, AB, Canada*
[4] *Human Organ Procurement and Exchange Program, Edmonton, AB, Canada*
[5] *Canadian National Transplant Research Program, Edmonton, AB, Canada*
[6] *Alberta Transplant Institute, Edmonton, AB, Canada*

Correspondence should be addressed to Jayan Nagendran; jayan@ualberta.ca

Academic Editor: Antoni Torres

Background. Lung transplant (LTx) waitlists continue to grow internationally. Consequently, more patients are progressing to require mechanical circulatory support (MCS) as a bridge to transplantation (BTT). MCS strategies include interventional lung assist (iLA) and venovenous (VV) and venoarterial (VA) extracorporeal membrane oxygenation (ECMO). We review our series of patients bridged with MCS while listed for LTx. *Methods.* All consecutive patients, listed for LTx requiring MCS as a BTT at the University of Alberta from 2004 to 2015, were included. Patient demographics and outcomes were compared for the 3 groups (iLA, VV-ECMO, and VA-ECMO). *Results.* Of the 24 patients supported with MCS devices, 17 were successfully transplanted and 7 died waiting. In total, 25% ($n = 6$) were bridged with VA-ECMO, 54% ($n = 13$) with VV-ECMO, and 21% ($n = 5$) with iLA. Overall, 71% of patients were bridged successfully to LTx. The 1-year survival posttransplantation was 88%. *Conclusion.* We have demonstrated the feasibility of utilizing the MCS modalities of VA-ECMO, VV-ECMO, and most recently iLA, as a BTT. MCS is a viable strategy for BTT, offering improved survival outcomes for decompensating adult patients awaiting LTx, resulting in excellent survival posttransplantation.

1. Introduction

Over the past several decades, lung transplantation (LTx) has increased significantly as a treatment for end-stage lung disease [1]. As reported by the International Lung Transplant Registry, from 2000 to 2015, a 2.5-fold increase was seen in the number of lung transplants performed internationally. Though incidence of lung transplantation is increasing rapidly, the number of available donor organs has remained an obstacle, with donor organs remaining at a number inconsistent with the growing need. This discrepancy has resulted in long recipient waitlist times, contributing to increased recipient morbidity, and increased waitlist mortality [2]. Presently, waitlist mortality at major North American transplant centres remains at approximately 15–30% [3].

The University of Alberta is the largest tertiary care transplant centre in Western Canada, servicing a catchment size of over 6-million km and approximately 7-million people. Over the past decade, the University of Alberta has seen a significant increase in the number of lung transplantations performed, from 42 in 2010 to 61 in 2015. The average waitlist time at our centre has decreased over the last two decades, with times now comparable with other North American centres at 200 days and an average waitlist mortality of 32%. Survival has been respectable in our experience, with 88% 1-year survival overall posttransplantation.

Mechanical circulatory support (MCS) devices were first introduced in 1950 for cardiac failure, later to be used in pulmonary failure. MCS strategies previously regarded as rescue therapies are more commonly being employed in transplant

Table 1: Patient characteristics.

Characteristics	VV-ECMO ($n = 13$)	VA-ECMO ($n = 6$)	iLA ($n = 5$)
Age in years	44.3	41.1	49.5
Female (%)	46	67	60
BMI	25.7	22.6	22.9
Smoking history (%)	54	33	20
Successfully bridged (%)	53	100	80
Diagnosis			
IPF	5	1	0
PPH	0	1	3
ILD	2	1	1
CF	2	2	0
Sarcoidosis	1	0	0
Others	3	1	1

All numbers provided are means unless otherwise stated.

medicine, specifically in cardiothoracic transplantation as a bridge to transplant (BTT) [4, 5].

It is now recognized that the use of MCS devices can produce satisfactory 1-year survival outcomes for patients requiring MCS bridging prior to their LTx [6, 7]. MCS devices used clinically in transplantation currently include ventricular assist devices, venoarterial and venovenous extracorporeal membrane oxygenation (ECMO), and interventional lung assist (iLA). The iLA is a pumpless low-resistance device that is connected arteriovenously and has been used as a BTT primarily in patients with ventilation-refractory hypercapnic lung failure. This device very effectively removes carbon dioxide while improving oxygenation only marginally. Several studies have demonstrated the feasibility of iLA as a BTT with a variety of cannulation strategies being employed, depending on the etiology of the respiratory failure [8, 9].

Herein, we report our single-centre experience with bridging patients using MCS while listed for LTx.

2. Methods

2.1. Study Design. From January 1, 2004, to December 31, 2015, twenty-four consecutive patients were bridged to double-lung transplantation using MCS with either VV-ECMO, VA-ECMO, or iLA at the UAMHI. The present study involved a single-institution retrospective cohort with the intention of evaluating the overall outcomes of patients bridged to transplant with MCS.

2.2. Donors and Recipients. The lungs used in these cases were all donated after neurological declaration of death. They were provided through the Human Organ Procurement and Exchange (HOPE) program. All recipients were deemed eligible for LTx due to end-stage pulmonary disease. All recipients gave informed consent and the study protocol was approved by the local Research Ethics Board. Recipient charts were evaluated for baseline clinical characteristics and followed for survival.

2.3. MCS Protocol. Allocation of MCS strategy was based on institutional evidence and best practice. The decision to institute MCS was based on institutional knowledge in patients with end-stage respiratory failure refractory to maximal medical therapy. Modality selection was based on a multidisciplinary team conference involving transplant respirologist, transplant surgeons, critical care extracorporeal life support (ECLS) team, social work team, dietary team, and the infectious disease team.

3. Results

3.1. Baseline Characteristics. The study sample included 24 consecutive patients undergoing MCS bridging while awaiting double LTx from January 1, 2004, to December 31, 2015. Baseline demographic data is summarized in Table 1, stratified by MCS modality.

Of the patients bridged with MCS, the distribution of modality of MCS was VV-ECMO 54% ($n = 13$), VA-ECMO 25% ($n = 6$), and ILA 21% ($n = 5$). Based on the small sample size, there were not any significant differences in age or gender, though females were more likely to be bridged compared to patients undergoing transplantation over the same time-period ($p < 0.05$). Further demographics, including diagnosis and rates of successful bridge to transplant, are described in Table 1.

3.2. Outcomes. Outcomes for patients who had MCS bridging instituted are summarized in Table 2. Patients bridged with iLA had the longest mean waitlist time (830 days) and the longest mean bridge time (45 days), compared to VV-ECMO and VA-ECMO ($p < 0.05$). Donor age was greatest in the VA-ECMO recipients (43.2-years) compared to VV-ECMO (29.1-years) and iLA (36.8-years). Actuarial survival to transplantation is shown in Figure 1. Overall, 53% of VV-ECMO, 100% of VA-ECMO, and 80% of iLA patients survived to transplantation. Posttransplantation ICU length of stay did not differ significantly between groups ($p > 0.05$). Primary

TABLE 2: Peri- and posttransplantation characteristics.

Characteristics	VV-ECMO ($n = 7$)	VA-ECMO ($n = 6$)	iLA ($n = 4$)
Waiting list time (d)	95	36	830
Donor age (y)	29.1	43.2	36.8
Cold ischemic time			
Right lung (min)	321	406	262
Left lung (min)	342	454	305
ICU LOS (d)	13.1	14.7	16.5
Hospital LOS (d)	49.7	41	61.5
CPB use (%)	78	100	100
Intubation (d)	12.9	14.7	10.2
PGD 3 at T72	2 (29%)	1 (25%)*	0 (0%)
Bridge time (d)	17.9	19.2	44.8
Survival at 1 year (%)	100	67	100
Overall causes of death			
Sepsis	1	—	—
BOS	1	—	—
Gastrointestinal	—	1	—
Others	—	1	—

*PGD 3 missing in 2 VA-ECMO. All numbers provided are means unless otherwise stated.

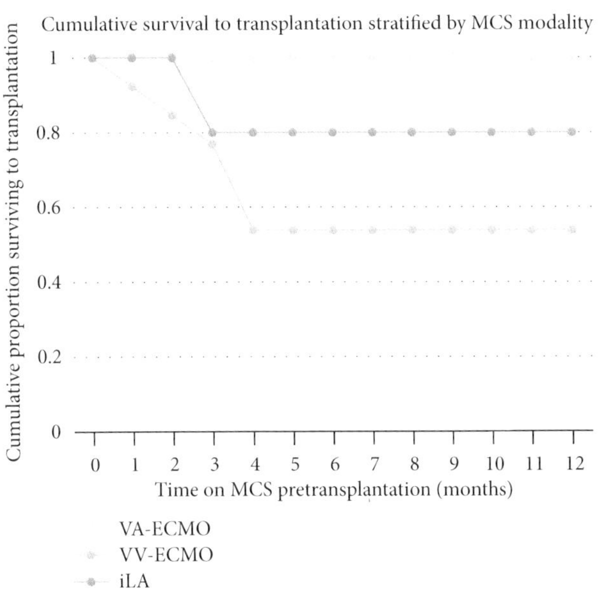

FIGURE 1

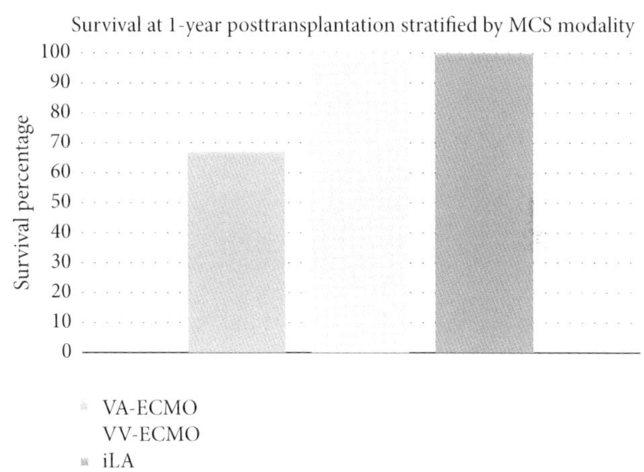

FIGURE 2

graft dysfunction (PGD) Grade 3 occurred in 29% ($n = 2$) of VV-ECMO recipients, 25% of VA-ECMO recipients, and none of the iLA recipients at 72-hour posttransplantation. Survival at 1-year posttransplantation is shown in Figure 2 and was 100% in both the VV-ECMO and iLA groups and 67% in the VA-ECMO group. Overall survival at 1-year posttransplantation was 88%. Causes of death are described in Table 2.

4. Discussion

As there is a growing population of potential recipients that may benefit from lung transplantation, there is an increasing need for bridging strategies in patients that develop end-stage respiratory failure while awaiting lung transplantation. The use of mechanical circulatory support (MCS) bridging remains controversial with limited reported outcomes in the literature. Our experience has also been limited, though similar in size to current reported results [6, 7]. Mason et al. described that there was decreased survival in patients undergoing MCS bridging that is attributed to the perioperative phase; however, patients surviving past 6 months have comparable survival to those patients not requiring pretransplantation MCS [6]. It is important to recognize that this finding may likely be attributed to the acute nature and care of patients requiring BTT, as opposed to the use of MCS devices themselves [10].

The outcomes from the use of MCS as a BTT have improved over time from prior reports. Our results lend support to the feasibility of MCS bridging with an excellent overall 1-year survival of 88% in those patients requiring MCS bridging. This study provides a contemporary analysis of data at a centre with lung transplant volumes within the top 10% of the ISHLT registry database [11] and significant experience utilizing the MCS modalities described. We believe that the improvement in outcomes after MCS bridging is likely due to increased experience and confidence with this approach, advancements in both medical and surgical care, and the development of an experienced multidisciplinary team including transplant respirologists, transplant surgeons, critical care teams, social workers, dieticians, and infectious disease specialists. Furthermore, in our series of bridging patients, rates of PGD at 72 hours (12.5%) were very acceptable in our cohort.

The consideration for the use of MCS strategies as BTT has evolved over time. In recent guidelines, initiation of MCS in hemodynamically marginal patients is recommended to prevent posttransplant outcomes that may be adversely affected by the development of irreversible end-organ dysfunction [12]. Patient selection is determined based on a multidisciplinary discussion as aforementioned. The criteria for MCS modality are also reached by multidisciplinary consensus. VA and VV-ECMO are dependent on cardiac function with VA-ECMO being indicated in combined cardiac and pulmonary failure and VV-ECMO being indicated in isolated respiratory failure. iLA bridging is primarily indicated in patients with ventilation-refractory hypercapnic lung failure. However, due to the pumpless nature of this device, sufficient system perfusion pressure must be maintained. Thus, indications for iLA institution have traditionally been in patients with respiratory failure secondary to pulmonary hypertension. There is potential for extended use beyond these indications, including patients with secondary pulmonary hypertension from other pulmonary diseases including idiopathic pulmonary fibrosis and cystic fibrosis. The outcomes of this study suggest that, in appropriately screened potential recipients, initiation of MCS can lead to acceptable rates of both bridging to transplantation and survival posttransplantation.

There were differences in rates of successful BTT based on type of MCS modality. VV-ECMO portended the worst likelihood of a successful bridge ($n = 7$; 53%) despite providing 100% posttransplantation 1-year survival. By comparison, all patients bridged with VA-ECMO underwent LTx; however, only 67% of recipients were alive at 1 year. This finding likely reflects the acute, poor functional status of those patients requiring VA-ECMO support, leading to variability in organ allocation. The poor survival posttransplantation of those bridged with VA-ECMO highlights the importance of ensuring appropriate organ allocation to recipients with the greatest chance of a good outcome. This may require further reevaluation of suitability for transplantation with weekly discussions of the multidisciplinary team. This approach has now been developed at our program for patients bridged on MCS.

Patients undergoing BTT with the iLA device endured the longest amount of time on the waitlist (mean 830 days) and underwent the longest bridge time (mean 44.8 days). This is likely due to the prevalence of PPH in these patients and difficulty in finding suitable donor organs, especially when combined heart-lung transplantation is indicated. In fact, our centre has recently reported the longest such successful bridge using iLA in a PPH recipient undergoing combined heart-lung transplantation [13]. We anticipate future increased utilization and success for BTT with iLA resulting from prolonged bridge support capability and notable transplant survival outcomes, with 100% of those transplanted following iLA bridging at our institution being alive to date.

The previously described pumpless iLA has the potential for expanded use, potentially in patients with secondary pulmonary hypertension, as well as its indicated use in patients with specified primary pulmonary hypertension. We believe that the shift towards iLA use over ECMO may improve pre-, peri-, and posttransplant outcomes, as the pumpless iLA theoretically eliminates some of the consequences associated with pump-dependent ECMO systems.

This study is not with limitations. Weaknesses include the modest sample population size of 24. These moderate numbers can be attributed to the select population of patients awaiting transplant who are eligible based on device inclusion criteria, to be initiated on one of the previously described MCS modalities. As well, our results represent the retrospective Western-Canadian experience of the past decade. However, with improved technologies, the potential for expansion of indications for different modalities of MCS may improve outcomes with further experience and refinement within the field. We expect this to be particularly true for the iLA device, which offers a pumpless system, theoretically ameliorating some of the drawbacks of the pump-dependent ECMO systems.

5. Conclusion

In the University of Alberta experience, MCS as a BTT offers a viable strategy for improving survival outcomes of decompensating adult patients awaiting lung transplantation. The use of MCS technologies at this institute over the past decade has led to a reduction in waitlist mortality, with very good 1-year posttransplant survival rate of 88%, for those who underwent pretransplant MCS. We believe the utilization of MCS bridging devices, based on our institutional evidence, to be a viable strategy to decrease waitlist mortality in high acuity patients awaiting LTx.

Acknowledgments

This work was supported by Human Organ Procurement and Exchange Program.

References

[1] R. D. Yusen, L. B. Edwards, A. Y. Kucheryavaya et al., "The Registry of the International Society for Heart and Lung Transplantation: thirty-second official adult lung and heart-lung transplantation report—2015; focus theme: early graft failure," *Journal of Heart and Lung Transplantation*, vol. 34, no. 10, pp. 1264–1277, 2015.

[2] J. Gottlieb, "Update on lung transplantation," *Therapeutic Advances in Respiratory Disease*, vol. 2, no. 4, pp. 237–247, 2008.

[3] M. Valapour, M. A. Skeans, B. M. Heubner et al., "OPTN/SRTR 2012 annual data report: lung," *American Journal of Transplantation*, vol. 14, no. 1, pp. 139–165, 2014.

[4] M. Anile, D. Diso, E. Russo et al., "Extracorporeal membrane oxygenation as bridge to lung transplantation," *Transplantation Proceedings*, vol. 45, no. 7, pp. 2621–2623, 2013.

[5] S. David, L. C. Napp, C. Kühn, and M. M. Hoeper, "Extracorporeal membrane oxygenation: principles and medical indications," *Internist*, vol. 57, no. 9, pp. 856–863, 2016.

[6] D. P. Mason, L. Thuita, E. R. Nowicki, S. C. Murthy, G. B. Pettersson, and E. H. Blackstone, "Should lung transplantation be performed for patients on mechanical respiratory support? The US experience," *Journal of Thoracic and Cardiovascular Surgery*, vol. 139, no. 3, pp. 765–773.e1, 2010.

[7] S. Collaud, C. Benden, C. Ganter et al., "Extracorporeal life support as bridge to lung retransplantation: a multicenter pooled data analysis," *Annals of Thoracic Surgery*, vol. 102, no. 5, pp. 1680–1686, 2016.

[8] M. Strueber, M. M. Hoeper, S. Fischer et al., "Bridge to thoracic organ transplantation in patients with pulmonary arterial hypertension using a pumpless lung assist device," *American Journal of Transplantation*, vol. 9, no. 4, pp. 853–857, 2009.

[9] W. Bartosik, J. J. Egan, and A. E. Wood, "The novalung interventional lung assist as bridge to lung transplantation for self-ventilating patients—initial experience," *Interactive Cardiovascular and Thoracic Surgery*, vol. 13, no. 2, pp. 198–200, 2011.

[10] Y. Toyoda, J. K. Bhama, N. Shigemura et al., "Efficacy of extracorporeal membrane oxygenation as a bridge to lung transplantation," *Journal of Thoracic and Cardiovascular Surgery*, vol. 145, no. 4, pp. 1065–1071, 2013.

[11] R. D. Yusen, L. B. Edwards, A. Y. Kucheryavaya et al., "The registry of the international society for heart and lung transplantation: thirty-first adult lung and heart-lung transplant report—2014; focus theme: retransplantation," *Journal of Heart and Lung Transplantation*, vol. 33, no. 10, pp. 1009–1024, 2014.

[12] D. Feldman, Ã. Salpy Pamboukian V, Ã. J. Jeffrey Teuteberg, E. Birks, K. Lietz, S. A. Moore et al., "International society for heart and lung transplantation guidelines for mechanical circulatory support: executive summary," *The Journal of Heart and Lung Transplantation*, vol. 32, no. 2, pp. 157–187, 2013.

[13] V. Vasanthan, M. Garg, M. Maruyama, E. Michelakis, D. H. Freed, and J. Nagendran, "Extended bridge to heart and lung transplantation using pumpless extracorporeal lung assist," *Canadian Journal of Cardiology*, vol. 33, no. 7, pp. 950.e11–950.e13, 2017.

15

The Function of *Ophiocordyceps sinensis* in Airway Epithelial Cell Senescence in a Rat COPD Model

Xiaohui Ma,[1,2] Xingai Jiao,[1] Jinxiang Wu,[1] Jiping Zhao,[1] Yurong Xu,[2] Tian Liu,[1] Jiawei Xu,[1] Lei Yang,[2] and Liang Dong[1]

[1]*Department of Respiratory Medicine, Qilu Hospital of Shandong University, Jinan, Shandong, China*
[2]*Department of Respiratory Medicine, Shandong Chest Hospital, Jinan, Shandong, China*

Correspondence should be addressed to Liang Dong; dl5506@126.com

Academic Editor: Frederik Trinkmann

Ophiocordyceps sinensis (*O. sinensis*) seems to be able to alleviate airway epithelial cell senescence in chronic obstructive pulmonary disease (COPD). The objective of the study is to evaluate the effect of *O. sinensis* on airway epithelial senescence in the COPD model both in vitro and in vivo. We observed the expression of P16 and P21 in the airway epithelia of 30 patients with COPD. The optimal concentration of *O. sinensis* and exposure time of the cigarette smoke extract (CSE) were determined in vitro, and senescence-associated β-galactosidase (SA-β-gal) and 5-bromodeoxyuridine (BrdU) were used to evaluate the senescence and proliferation of human bronchial epithelial (16HBE) cells pretreated with *O. sinensis* by staining kits. COPD model rats were treated with *O. sinensis* at various concentrations to determine the changes in P16 and P21 expression in airway epithelial tissues. It was found that the expression levels of P16 and P21 were higher in the airway epithelia of COPD patients than those in the control group based on immunohistochemical staining, real-time quantitative PCR, and western blotting. The CSE could induce 16HBE cell senescence, and *O. sinensis* could alleviate CSE-induced senescence and promote the proliferation of 16HBE cells. The expression levels of P16 and P21 were also higher in the airway epithelia of COPD model rats; however, the levels of P16 and P21 in the groups treated with all concentrations of *O. sinensis* were obviously lower than those in the COPD model group based on real-time quantitative PCR and western blotting. In conclusion, the CSE can induce airway epithelium senescence, and *O. sinensis* can inhibit CSE-induced cellular senescence, both in vitro and in vivo.

1. Introduction

Chronic obstructive pulmonary disease (COPD) is characterized by an expiratory airflow limitation that is not fully reversible and is associated with an anomalous inflammatory reaction, mainly in response to tobacco smoke. Chronic inflammation is a major histological characteristic of COPD patients [1]. At the same time, senescence plays an important role in the pathogenesis of chronic lung diseases including COPD and lung fibrosis as well [2]. Previous reports have demonstrated the critical role of cellular senescence in respiratory diseases, such as asthma, pulmonary fibrosis, and lung cancer, especially in COPD [3–5].

Cellular senescence is a fundamental property of all cells in which cell growth is arrested under conditions of cellular stress [6]. In general, cellular senescence can be viewed as a protective mechanism against cancer. However, aging and cellular senescence underlie chronic diseases, involving, for instance, the brain (e.g., Alzheimer's disease), the cardiovascular system (e.g., atherosclerosis), and the musculoskeletal system (e.g., osteoporosis), and COPD [4]. Cellular senescence is associated with decreased physiological function and protein degradation and is irreversible [7]. In particular, cellular senescence affects regeneration ability by reducing the amount of hematopoietic stem cells, and aging cells release cytokines to further enhance the inflammatory response, which leads to airway inflammation and airway remodeling in COPD patients [8, 9]. It is not surprising that cellular senescence is induced in the airway epithelial cells of COPD patients. However, the mechanism of cell senescence in COPD is not clear. Therefore, we demonstrated that cellular senescence is required in COPD.

Ophiocordyceps sinensis (*O. sinensis*) has been used in traditional Chinese medicine for a long history. Many bioactive constituents, such as polysaccharides, cordycepin, mannitol, aminophenol, and ergosterol, have been found in *O. sinensis* [10]. Chemical constituents extracted from *O. sinensis* have various pharmacological actions, including nephroprotective, hepatoprotective, anti-inflammatory, antioxidative, and antiapoptotic effects [10]. In COPD patients, artificially cultivated *O. sinensis* can inhibit airway inflammation, improve lung function, correct airway Th1/Th2 ratio imbalance and two-way immune regulation, alleviate respiratory muscle fatigue, and increase exercise tolerance [11]. However, the effects of *O. sinensis* on cell senescence in COPD have not been reported although its functional roles have been widely documented. Based on these previous studies, we hypothesize that the cigarette smoke extract (CSE) can induce airway epithelial senescence in COPD, and *O. sinensis* can alleviate CSE-induced cellular senescence. Therefore, this study investigates how *O. sinensis* regulates cellular senescence in COPD airway epithelium in vivo and in vitro.

2. Materials and Methods

2.1. Ethics Statement. The research was approved by the ethics review committee for human studies at Qilu Hospital, Shandong University, Jinan City, China. All biopsy specimens were obtained from the participants after informed consent was obtained.

2.2. Patients. All biopsy tissues were obtained from the Qilu Hospital of Shandong University (Jinan, Shandong, China) between September 2013 and December 2015. Thirty COPD specimens were obtained from lung cancer resections, and nontumor lung tissues were collected when patients were diagnosed with COPD. Thirty normal lung tissues were obtained from body donations because of trauma or death; these individuals had no obvious pulmonary disease, and the samples were used as a control group.

As shown in Table 1, the age and gender of patients in the COPD group and the control group were similar. Pulmonary function tests were performed based on the predicted forced expiratory volume (FEV1%), the predicted forced vital capacity (FVC%), and the ratio FEV1/FVC (%). The predicted FEV1% and the FEV1/FVC (%) were significantly lower in patients with COPD than those in non-COPD subjects ($p < 0.05$).

2.3. Cells and Reagents. *O. sinensis* liquid was obtained from Hangzhou Sino-US East China Pharmaceutical Co., Ltd (Hangzhou, China). Artificially cultured *O. sinensis* powder was dissolved in normal saline (500 mg/ml) to prepare the turbid liquid suspension. Septwolves cigarettes (tobacco type, tar: 14 mg, nicotine content: 1.2 mg, and carbon monoxide fumes: 15 mg) were obtained from Longyan Tobacco Industry LLC (Longyan, China). Lipopolysaccharides (LPS, L3129) were purchased from Sigma Company (Los Angeles, USA). The 16HBE (human bronchial epithelioid) cell line was purchased from CHI Scientific, Inc. (Shanghai, China).

The 16HBE cells were cultured for six days in high-glucose Dulbecco's modified Eagle's medium (H-DMEM) in 48-well plates (Invitrogen, Life Technologies, New Zealand) containing 10% Gibco® fetal bovine serum (FBS, Invitrogen) at 37°C in a 5% CO_2 atmosphere. Each day, 100 μl of the medium per well was removed and was replaced with fresh medium. The preparation of the CSE was previously described [3, 5]. When cell density was 75%, a CSE solution was added to the 48-well plates at various concentrations (0, 0.5%, 1.0%, 2.0%, and 5.0%; 0.05 ml), and the cells were cultured for an additional 24 hours. Total proteins were extracted for western blotting to the optimal CSE solution concentration screening. When the optimal concentration of the CSE solution (0.05 ml) was added to the cells for durations of 0, 3, 6, and 12 hours (Supplementary Figure 1), the total extracted protein was used to detect P16 and P21 expression by western blotting to determine the best reaction time. To determine the effect of *O. sinensis* on cells, 16HBE cells were pretreated with *O. sinensis* (100 μg/ml) [5] for 2 hours, and the cells were then cultured with the optimal concentration of the CSE solution for 6 hours. The cells of different treatment groups (control group, CSE group, and CSE + *O. sinensis* group) were collected. In the preliminary experiment, we have found that *O. sinensis* (100 μg/ml) does not affect the gross cell morphology, proliferation rate, and apoptosis rate.

Table 1: Clinical characteristics of normal subjects and COPD patients.

	Normal subjects	COPD patients
Male/female	14/16	15/15
Age (years)	58.65 ± 4.72	60.54 ± 5.68
FEV1 (% predicted)	88.21 ± 10.54	56.42 ± 17.43*
FVC (% predicted)	85.73 ± 7.54	78.68 ± 17.92
FEV1/FVC (%)	85.43 ± 11.62	50.86 ± 16.43*

Values are presented as means ± SEM. *$p < 0.05$ versus controls. FEV1, forced expiratory volume in one second; FVC, forced vital capacity; SEM, standard error of the mean.

2.4. Animals and COPD Models. Male Wistar rats (200 ± 20 g) were purchased from the Shandong University Experimental Animal Center. The animals were housed in a temperature of −37°C and humidity-controlled conditions and kept on a 12 h/12 h light/dark cycle, with free access to regular chow and water. The rats were randomly divided into five groups with fifteen rats per group, as described below: control group (CON), COPD group, COPD + low dose of the *O. sinensis* group (LOW, 2.5 g/kg/day), COPD + intermediate dose of the *O. sinensis* group (MID, 5.0 g/kg/day), and COPD + high dose of the *O. sinensis* group (HIG, 7.5 g/kg/day).

The experimental protocol was approved by the Experimental Animal Care and Ethics Committee at the Qilu Hospital of Shandong University, Jinan, China. The detailed procedures for the COPD model rats were described in

Table 2: The sequences of PCR primers used in this study.

Primer	Forward (5′–3′)	Reverse (5′–3′)
P16		
Rat	CTACTCTCCTCCGCTGGGAA	GGCCTAACTTAGCGCTGCTT
Human	CTTGGTGACCCTCCGGATTC	CCACGAGATGTGAACCACGA
P21		
Rat	CAGGCTCAGGAGTTAGCAAGG	TCAACACCCTGTCTTGTCTTCG
Human	AGTACCCTCTCAGCTCCAGG	TGTCTGACTCCTTGTTCCGC
β-actin		
Rat	ATGATTCATCCCACGGCAAG	CTGGAAGATGGTGATGGGTT
Human	CCGTTGCCCTGAGGCTCTTT	CCTTCTGCATCCTGTCAGCAA

a previous report [12, 13]. Briefly, the rats were anesthetized with intraperitoneal ketamine (35 mg/kg) and were administered LPS twice using intratracheal instillation on day 1 (0.2 ml, 1 mg/ml) and day 14 (0.1 ml, 1 mg/ml). The rats were exposed to tobacco smoke from 8 cigarettes for each treatment twice per day during the first two weeks and were then exposed to fifteen cigarettes per treatment three times per day from week 3 to week 12. The rats were placed in a special sealed box connected to a smoke source to receive two or three 30-minute exposures per day at an interval of one to two hours. The control rats were exposed to the air following similar procedures. Different doses of the *O. sinensis* liquid were given by intragastric administration for 14 days to the COPD rats three times a day after 12 weeks of exposure to tobacco smoke. The control group and COPD group rats were administrated by the same amount of normal saline.

2.5. Histological Analysis. The lung tissue blocks from COPD patients, control humans, and each rat group were immersed in 4% paraformaldehyde, embedded in paraffin, and cut into 5 μm thick sections. Lung tissue paraffin sections were prepared for HE staining and immunohistochemical assays. The following primary antibodies were used: anti-p16 (f-12, SC-1661), anti-p21 (C-19, SC397), and β-actin (C4, SC47778). All antibodies were purchased from Santa Cruz Biotechnology, Inc. (Santa Cruz, CA, USA). The dilution rate for both of the primary antibodies used in the immunohistochemical assay was 1 : 150. We count the optical density (OD) of every group's immunohistochemical sections with the software Image-Pro Plus. Briefly, all the pictures were equalized by the "the best equalization" function of the software firstly, and then, the OD values were counted. The details can be seen in the operation manual for the software.

2.6. Western Blotting Analysis. Lung tissues from every group and the human airway epithelial cell line (16HBE) were preserved at −80°C and thawed on ice before use. Total proteins in lung tissue samples and 16HBE cells were extracted prior to western blotting. P16 and P21 antibodies were prepared for the western blotting analysis. The dilution rate for both of the primary antibodies was 1 : 1000.

2.7. Real-Time Fluorescence Quantitative PCR. RNAiso plus, RT reagent kit, Premix Ex Taq Version 2.0, and SYBR Green real-time PCR master mix were purchased from Takara Company (Dalian, China) and were used to perform the real-time quantitative PCR assay. Briefly, total RNA was extracted with RNAiso plus, precipitated with isopropyl alcohol, washed in ethanol, and resuspended in RNase-free water. RNA quantity and quality were determined by spectrophotometry. Two micrograms of total RNA were used for reverse transcription (RT) and the RT reagent kit method as the instruction book described. cDNA was used for quantitative polymerase chain reaction (PCR) and repeated three times. Quantitative PCR products were synthesized. Each 20 μl SYBR Green reaction system contained 1.0 μl cDNA, forward primer 0.75 μl, and reverse primer 0.75 μl, and the primer concentration is 0.1 μmol/l. The following PCR protocol was applied: 95°C for 60 s, 40 cycles of 95°C for 5 s, and 55°C for 30 s. The results were analyzed by the double ΔC_t method, which reflects the expression difference based on the cycle threshold of the target gene relative to that of beta-actin (reference gene) in each sample. The specific PCR primers used for all target genes are shown in Table 2.

2.8. Staining for SA-β-Galactosidase and the BrdU Analysis. The specific protocol was performed as previously described [3]. X-gal was purchased from Sigma-Aldrich Company (USA), and the BrdU Cell Proliferation Assay Kit was purchased from Chemicon International (Temecula, CA, USA) and used following the manufacturer's protocol.

2.9. Statistical Analysis. The statistical analysis was performed using the SPSS 16.0 software package (SPSS Inc., Chicago, IL, USA). Data are expressed as the means ± SEM. To determine significant differences between the COPD patient group and the control group, *t*-tests were used, and to evaluate differences among the three rat groups, one-way ANOVA (analysis of variance) followed by post hoc multiple comparison LSD tests was used. Significance was defined as $p < 0.05$.

3. Results

3.1. The Expression Levels of P16 and P21 Increased in the Airway Epithelia of COPD Patients. In the lung tissue from COPD patients, pathological changes in the airway epithelium, including an injured epithelium structure, goblet cell hyperplasia, cilia falling off, and thickened basement membranes, were observed (Figure 1(a)). The lung tissue

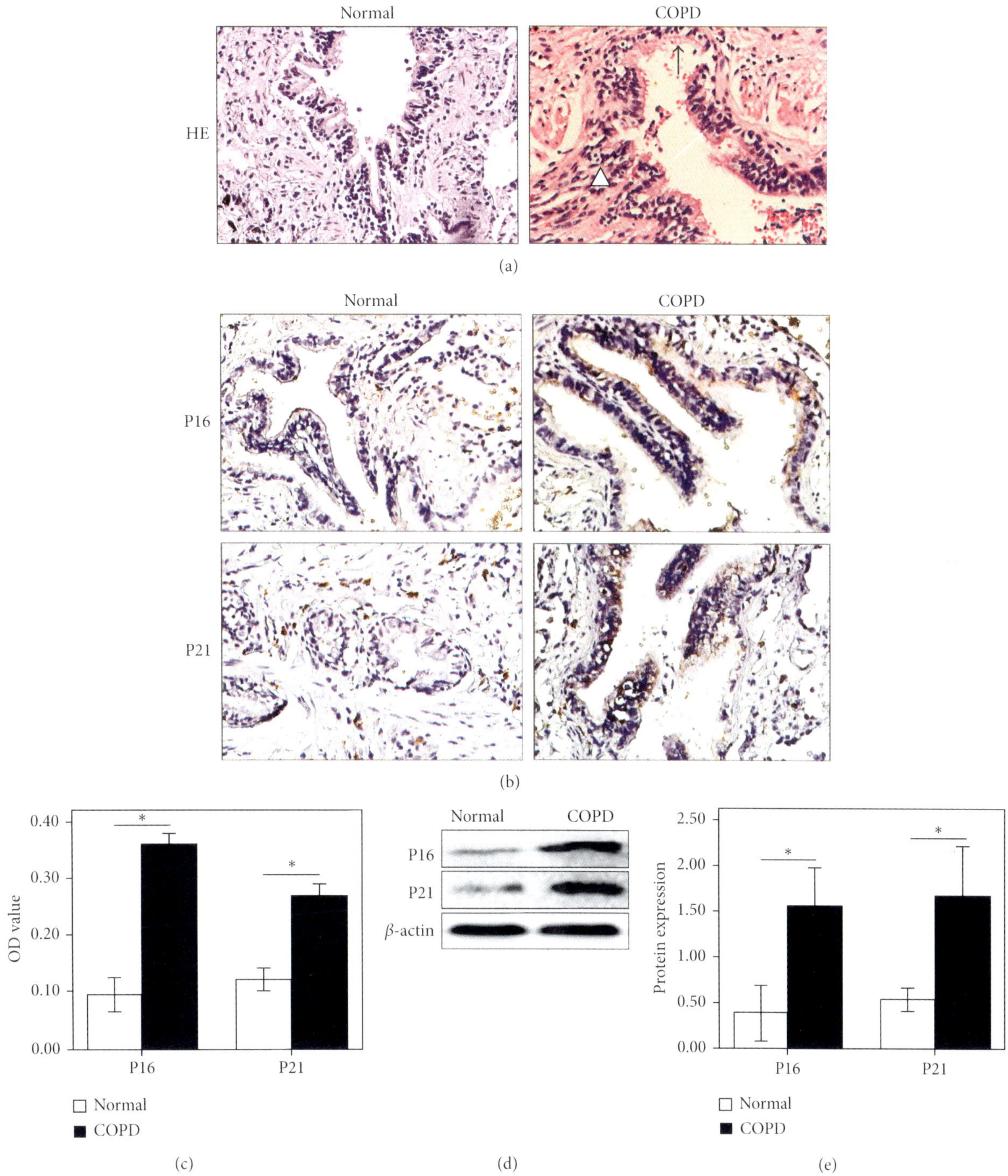

FIGURE 1: The production of P16 and P21 in the airway epithelium of COPD patients. (a) Micrographs of histological sections of the COPD patients' airway showed the loss of epithelial integrity, apparent deciduous epithelial cells (black arrow), cilia lodging (white arrow), and submucosal and bronchial surrounding fibrous tissue hyperplasia (triangle) by HE staining (HE, 400x). (b) The expression of P16 and P21 in the airway epithelium of patients with COPD and control subjects were detected by IHC (200x). (c) Semiquantitative analysis of P16 and P21 expression in COPD and control groups was conducted by the optical density (OD). (d, e) The expression of P16 and P21 in the airway epithelium of patients with COPD and control subjects were determined by western blotting. $^{*}p < 0.05$.

from non-COPD subjects exhibited a normal pulmonary architecture (Figure 1(a)). The P16 and P21 proteins were expressed in both cytoplasm and nuclei of airway epithelial cells by histological analysis (Figure 1(b)), and the expression levels were significantly higher in patients with COPD than those in non-COPD subjects through semiquantitative analysis (Figure 1(c), $p < 0.05$). It was further found that the protein levels of both P16 and P21 were obviously higher in the COPD patient group than those in the control group (Figures 1(d) and 1(e), $p < 0.05$).

3.2. CSE Can Induce Human Bronchial Epithelial Cellular Senescence. To detect the effect of the CSE on airway epithelial cells, we treated 16HBE cells with increasing concentrations of the CSE for different durations. In this study, we found that the expression levels of P16 and P21 increased as the CSE concentration increased. In addition, the CSE at a concentration of 2.0% can efficiently increase the protein expression levels of P16 and P21, but there was no significant difference between the 2.0% and 5.0% treatments. Therefore, the optimal CSE concentration was chosen as 2.0% in this study (Supplementary Figures 2A–2C). 16HBE cells were immersed in 2.0% CSE for the indicated time periods (0 h, 3 h, 6 h, and 12 h), and the expression levels of P16 and P21 were detected. The levels of the two proteins reached a maximum at 6 h, and the expression of these markers was prolonged after stimulation for 12 h; accordingly, the best reaction time was 6 h (Supplementary Figures 2D–2F). To further analyze cellular senescence induced by the CSE, SA-β-gal was stained in 16HBE cells. It was observed that the percent of SA-β-gal-positive cells in the control group (18.25% ± 0.96%) was significantly lower than that in the CSE group (32.25% ± 2.63%) ($p < 0.05$; Supplementary Figures 3A and 3B). In addition, BrdU was used to detect cell proliferation, and the percent of BrdU-positive cells in the control group (30.24% ± 0.89%) was significantly higher than that in the CSE group (19.49% ± 0.62%) ($p < 0.05$; Supplementary Figure 3C). These results suggested that the CSE could promote cellular senescence in bronchial epithelial cells.

3.3. O. sinensis Can Inhibit CSE-Induced Cellular Senescence in Bronchial Epithelial Cells. As shown above, the CSE can induce cellular senescence by increasing the production of P16 and P21. To detect the effect of *O. sinensis* on CSE-induced cellular senescence, 16HBE cells were pretreated with *O. sinensis* for 2 h before stimulation with the CSE, and then, P16 and P21 expression levels were examined. The results showed that *O. sinensis* can reduce the increased P16 and P21 expression induced by the CSE at both the protein and mRNA levels, but the levels were still higher than those of the control group (Supplementary Figures 4A–4C). In addition, the percent of SA-β-gal-positive cells was 25.25% ± 1.70% in cells pretreated with *O. sinensis*, and there was a significant difference compared with CSE-treated cells (32.25% ± 2.63%), indicating that *O. sinensis* can delay CSE-induced cellular senescence (Supplementary Figures 3A and 3B). The percent of BrdU-positive cells in the cells pretreated with *O. sinensis* (25.48% ± 0.78%) was increased, and there was a statistically significant difference comparison with the CSE group, indicating that *O. sinensis* can improve the proliferation of 16HBE cells (Supplementary Figure 3C). These data suggested that *O. sinensis* could inhibit CSE-induced senescence in bronchial epithelial cells, which are consistent with the results of our previous experiments [5].

3.4. O. sinensis Can Inhibit Airway Epithelial Cell Senescence in COPD Rat Models. The lung sections in human COPD patients showed pathological structural changes, including airway epithelial cells that partially fell off, mucosal hyperemia, cilium adhesion or lodging, goblet cell hyperplasia, mucus secretion exuberant and large amounts of mucus retention, and fibrous tissue hyperplasia around the trachea and submucosa. The COPD rat model was successfully constructed based on HE staining of the lung tissue sections (Figure 2(a)). Higher P16 and P21 protein expression levels were observed in both the cytoplasm and nuclei of airway epithelial cells in the COPD model group than in the control group or the *O. sinensis* pretreated group based on IHC staining (Figures 2(b) and 2(c)). For groups treated with different *O. sinensis* concentrations, the protein and mRNA expression levels of P16 and P21 were remarkably lower in rats treated with a moderate dose and high dose of *O. sinensis* than those in rats treated with a low dose of *O. sinensis* (Figures 3(a)–3(e)). These results indicate that *O. sinensis* could inhibit the expression of P16 and P21 in the airway epithelial cells of COPD rats, indicating that *O. sinensis* may play a protective role in airway epithelial cellular senescence.

4. Discussion

Cellular senescence is an important fail-safe mechanism that mainly occurs in response to stress and telomere erosion [14], and senescence can be observed in tumors and loss-of-function disorders, such as Alzheimer's disease, atherosclerosis, osteoporosis, asthma, and COPD. P16 and P21 are involved in cell senescence by inhibiting cyclin-dependent kinases and thereby negatively regulate cell proliferation [9, 15]. As a deeper understanding of COPD pathogenesis is obtained, more and more scholars recognize that cellular senescence not only is present in the COPD lungs but also can explain several key features of the disease. There is a growing realization that COPD involves several processes observed in aging and cellular senescence [8, 16]. In this study, we found increased levels of P16 and P21 expression in the airway epithelial cells of COPD patients; our finding was in accordance with those of our previous study [5]. These proteins have multiple roles in the pathogenesis of the main COPD manifestations, particularly in the propagation of a proinflammatory phenotype, the loss of reparative potential, and the amplification of oxidative stress, which all ultimately lead to tissue damages [17, 18]. A pathophysiological role for cellular senescence in COPD has not been conclusively shown.

Although the mechanism of cellular senescence involved in COPD is not clear in clinical settings, a natural drug could be a good choice for treatment. *O. sinensis* is a fungus endemic to Himalayan alpine habitats at an elevation of 3600–5000 m [19]. *O. sinensis* preserves the intestinal mucosal barrier and may be an adjunct therapy in an endotoxin-induced sepsis rat model based on a pilot study [20, 21]. In this study, we found that *O. sinensis* could indeed inhibit CSE-induced cellular senescence in vitro and in COPD rat models by reducing the expression of P16 and P21. Unfortunately, its mechanism of action is not clear. Perhaps, the most important pathogenic contribution of cellular senescence to the disease process is the enhancement of the inflammatory phenotype by cytokines released from senescent cells, which may underlie self-propagating processes in the COPD lung. A clear implication is that senescent cells,

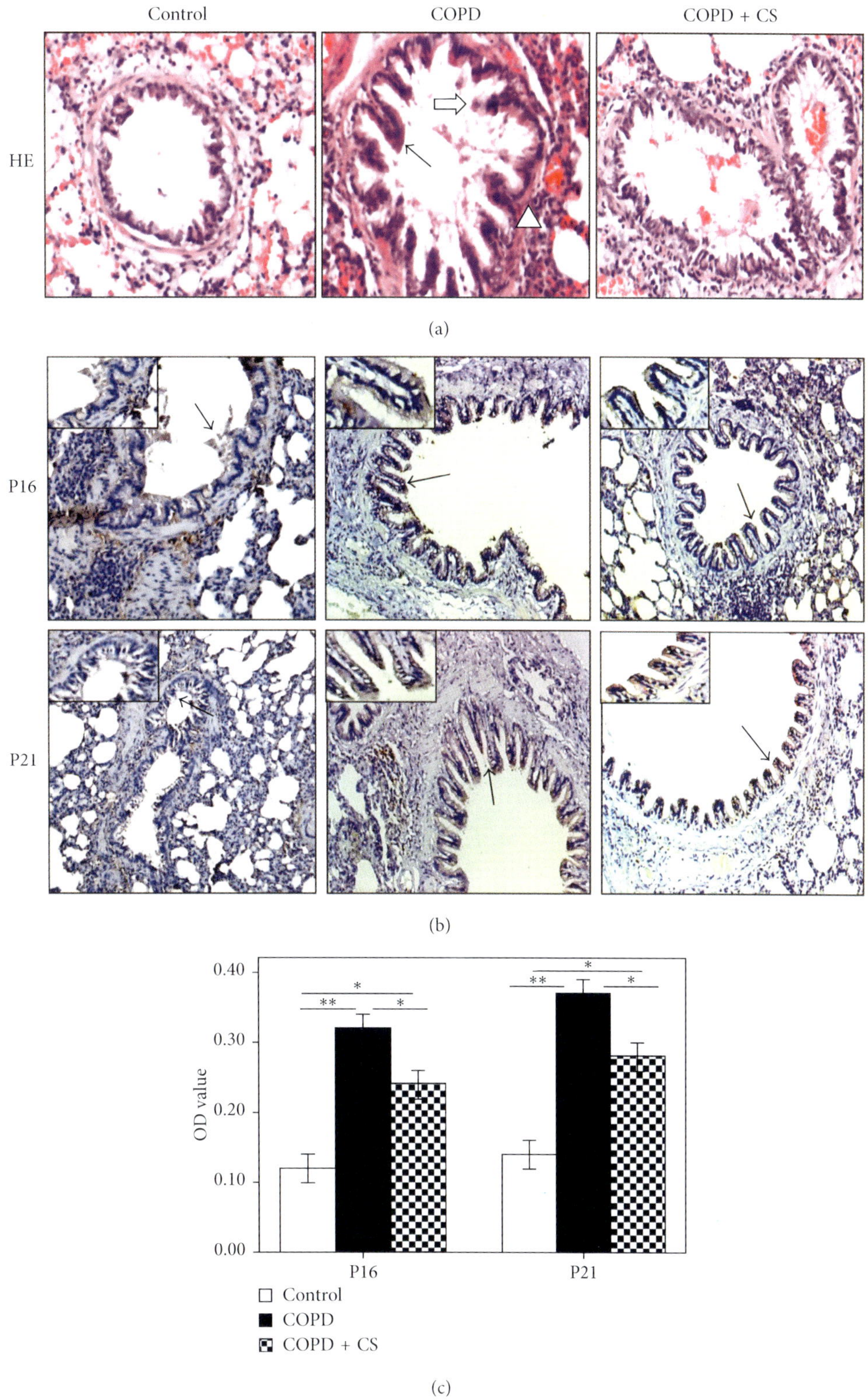

FIGURE 2: The expression of P16 and P21 in the airway epithelial cells of COPD rat models. (a) The pathological structure changes of airway in COPD rats were observed by HE staining (HE, 200x). In the control group, the airway epithelium structure was complete, and cell fall off, cilia lodging, goblet cell hyperplasia, and phlegm retention were not obvious. In the COPD group, airway epithelial cells fall off partly, and mucosal hyperemia, cilium adhesion or lodging, goblet cell hyperplasia (black arrow), mucus secretion exuberant and large amounts of mucus retention (white arrow), and fibrous tissue hyperplasia (triangle) around the trachea and submucosa were obvious. In the COPD + CS group (*O. sinensis* treatment group), in the airway epithelium, cilia lodging, hyperplasia of goblet cells, mucus gland secretion, and submucosal fibrous tissue hyperplasia were also reduced. (b) The expression of P16 and P21 in the airway epithelium of the COPD group and COPD + CS group were detected by IHC (200x). (c) Quantitative analysis of P16 and P21 expression in the COPD group and COPD + CS group. $^{*}p < 0.05$; $^{**}p < 0.01$.

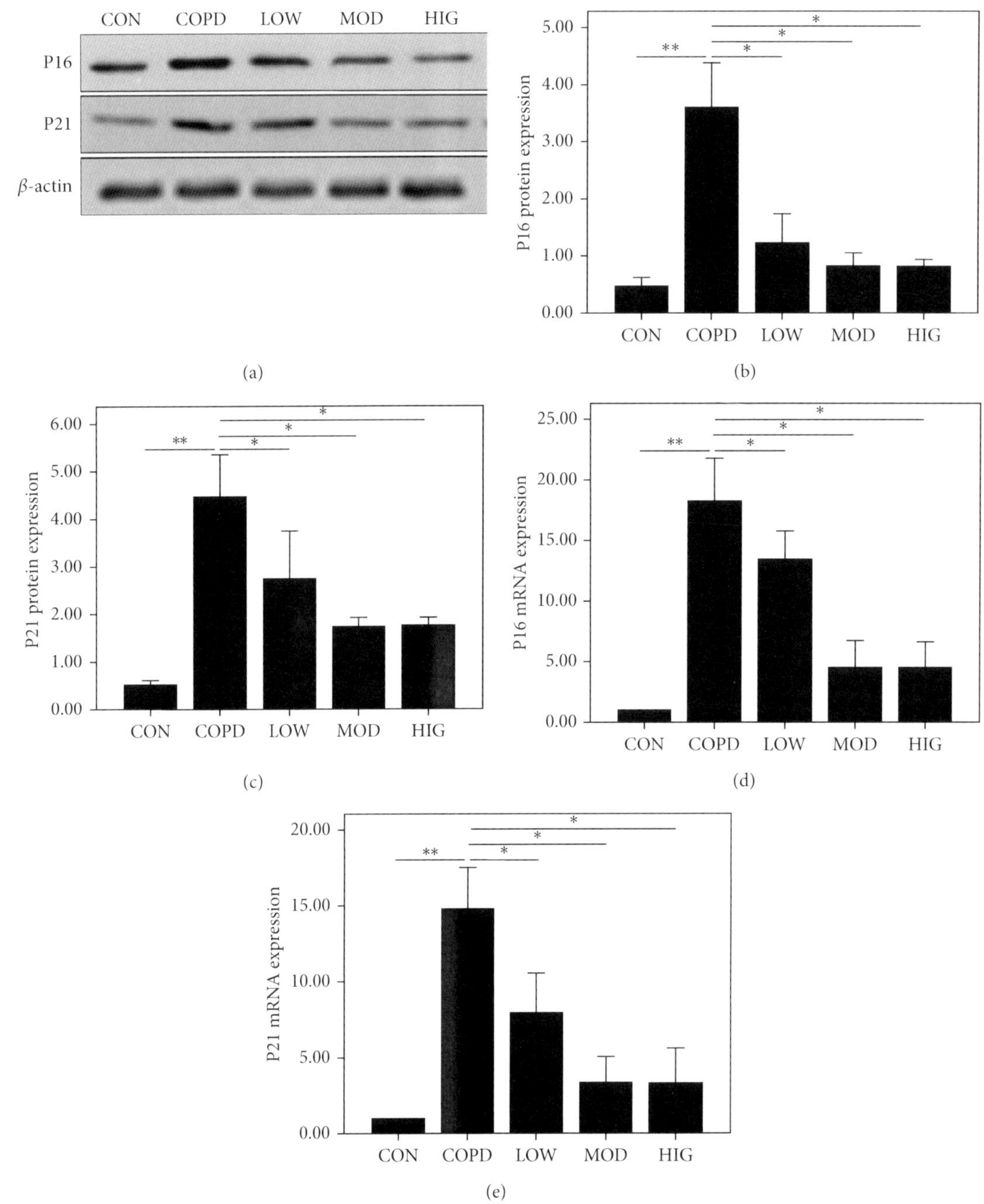

FIGURE 3: The expression of P16 and P21 in lung tissue of COPD rat models were inhibited by *O. sinensis*. (a) The expression of P16 and P21 in lung tissue of all the groups were detected by western blotting. The quantitative analysis of P16 (b) and P21 (c) in lung tissue of the COPD group and COPD + CS group was conducted. The mRNA expression of P16 (d) and P21 (e) in lung tissue of the COPD group and COPD + CS group was analyzed by qPCR. $^{*}p < 0.05$; $^{**}p < 0.01$.

notably progenitor cells, have decreased regenerative properties [22], potentially limiting the ability of the lungs to recover after decades of injury caused by cigarette smoke. Our previous study demonstrated that the CSE could induce cellular senescence in human bronchial epithelial cells, and the ROS/PI3K/AKT/mTOR signaling pathway may play an important role in this process [5]. In a cellular model of hypoxia, cells treated with *O. sinensis* (250 μg/ml) significantly attenuated oxidative stress in hypoxia [19]. This attenuation was attributed to Nrf2-ARE pathway activation, reduced NFκB activity, and increased oxygen availability via HIF1 signaling mechanisms. Furthermore, higher levels of antioxidants and anti-inflammatory mediators, for example, TGF-beta, HO1, and MT, in *O. sinensis*-treated cells might also be responsible for the tolerance of cells to hypoxia [19]. An additional study has shown that *O. sinensis* extracts are highly cytotoxic to human colorectal carcinoma RKO cells and inhibit the growth of tumors in a xenograft model.

The antitumor effect of *O. sinensis* has been associated with the induction of cell cycle arrest and mitochondrial-mediated apoptosis [23]. Our research suggests that the CSE could induce cell senescence in vitro and in COPD rats. Therefore, we speculate that *O. sinensis* may delay cellular senescence via several biological processes by inhibiting P16 and P21 protein expression.

In conclusion, the CSE can induce cellular senescence, and *O. sinensis* can alleviate CSE-induced cellular senescence. This study indicates that *O. sinensis* could be the basis for new therapeutic strategies in COPD. However, the specific mechanism underlying the effects of *O. sinensis* needs further research.

Authors' Contributions

Xiaohui Ma and Xingai Jiao contributed equally to this work.

Acknowledgments

This work was supported by grants from the National Natural Science Foundation of China (Grant nos. 81070016, 81270072, and 2017GSF218056).

References

[1] M. Schuliga, "NF-kappaB signaling in chronic inflammatory airway disease," *Biomolecules*, vol. 5, no. 3, pp. 1266–1283, 2015.

[2] L. Yue and H. Yao, "Mitochondrial dysfunction in inflammatory responses and cellular senescence: pathogenesis and pharmacological targets for chronic lung diseases," *British Journal of Pharmacology*, vol. 173, no. 15, pp. 2305–2318, 2016.

[3] J. Wu, F. Dong, R. A. Wang et al., "Central role of cellular senescence in TSLP-induced airway remodeling in asthma," *PLoS One*, vol. 8, no. 10, article e77795, 2013.

[4] R. M. Tuder, J. A. Kern, and Y. E. Miller, "Senescence in chronic obstructive pulmonary disease," *Proceedings of the American Thoracic Society*, vol. 9, no. 2, pp. 62-63, 2012.

[5] A. Liu, J. Wu, A. Li et al., "The inhibitory mechanism of *Cordyceps sinensis* on cigarette smoke extract-induced senescence in human bronchial epithelial cells," *International Journal of Chronic Obstructive Pulmonary Disease*, vol. 11, pp. 1721–1731, 2016.

[6] J. Campisi, J. K. Andersen, P. Kapahi, and S. Melov, "Cellular senescence: a link between cancer and age-related degenerative disease?," *Seminars in Cancer Biology*, vol. 21, pp. 354–359, 2011.

[7] D. V. Ziegler, C. D. Wiley, and M. C. Velarde, "Mitochondrial effectors of cellular senescence: beyond the free radical theory of aging," *Aging Cell*, vol. 14, no. 1, pp. 1–7, 2015.

[8] P. J. Barnes, "Mechanisms of development of multimorbidity in the elderly," *European Respiratory Journal*, vol. 45, no. 3, pp. 790–806, 2015.

[9] E. Bagdonas, J. Raudoniute, I. Bruzauskaite, and R. Aldonyte, "Novel aspects of pathogenesis and regeneration mechanisms in COPD," *International Journal of Chronic Obstructive Pulmonary Disease*, vol. 10, pp. 995–1013, 2015.

[10] Y. Liu, J. Wang, W. Wang, H. Zhang, X. Zhang, and C. Han, "The chemical constituents and pharmacological actions of *Cordyceps sinensis*," *Evidence-Based Complementary and Alternative Medicine*, vol. 2015, Article ID 575063, 12 pages, 2015.

[11] R. Shaykhiev and R. G. Crystal, "Early events in the pathogenesis of chronic obstructive pulmonary disease: smoking-induced reprogramming of airway epithelial basal progenitor cells," *Annals of the American Thoracic Society*, vol. 11, no. 5, pp. S252–S258, 2014.

[12] A. Al Faraj, A. Sultana Shaik, M. A. Pureza, M. Alnafea, and R. Halwani, "Preferential macrophage recruitment and polarization in LPS-induced animal model for COPD: non-invasive tracking using MRI," *PLoS One*, vol. 9, no. 3, article e90829, 2014.

[13] M. Ji, Y. Wang, X. Li, and Z. Qian, "Up-regulation of ICAM-1mRNA and IL-1βmRNA in lung tissues of a rat model of COPD," *International Journal of Clinical and Experimental Medicine*, vol. 8, no. 11, pp. 21956–21963, 2015.

[14] A. Bernadotte, V. M. Mikhelson, and I. M. Spivak, "Markers of cellular senescence: telomere shortening as a marker of cellular senescence," *Aging*, vol. 8, no. 1, pp. 3–11, 2016.

[15] H. H. Al-Khalaf and A. Aboussekhra, "p16 (INK4A) induces senescence and inhibits EMT through microRNA-141/microRNA-146b-5p-dependent repression of AUF1," *Molecular Carcinogenesis*, vol. 56, no. 3, pp. 985–999, 2016.

[16] W. I. De Boer, H. Yao, and I. Rahman, "Future therapeutic treatment of COPD: struggle between oxidants and cytokines," *International Journal of Chronic Obstructive Pulmonary Disease*, vol. 2, no. 3, pp. 205–228, 2007.

[17] V. Conti, G. Corbi, V. Manzo, G. Pelaia, A. Filippelli, and A. Vatrella, "Sirtuin 1 and aging theory for chronic obstructive pulmonary disease," *Analytical Cellular Pathology*, vol. 2015, Article ID 897327, 8 pages, 2015.

[18] J. M. Park, J. S. Lee, K. R. Lee, S. J. Ha, and E. K. Hong, "*Cordyceps militaris* extract protects human dermal fibroblasts against oxidative stress-induced apoptosis and premature senescence," *Nutrients*, vol. 6, no. 9, pp. 3711–3726, 2014.

[19] M. Singh, R. Tulsawani, P. Koganti, A. Chauhan, M. Manickam, and K. Misra, "*Cordyceps sinensis* increases hypoxia tolerance by inducing heme oxygenase-1 and metallothionein via Nrf2 activation in human lung epithelial cells," *BioMed Research International*, vol. 2013, Article ID 569206, 13 pages, 2013.

[20] L. Gu, H. Johno, S. Nakajima, T. Yoshitomi, S. Takahashi, and M. Kitamura, "Intervention in genotoxic stress-induced senescence by cordycepin through activation of eIF2α and suppression of Sp1," *Toxicological Sciences*, vol. 134, no. 2, pp. 345–354, 2013.

[21] G. S. Gu, J. A. Ren, G. W. Li, Y. J. Yuan, N. Li, and J. S. Li, "*Cordyceps sinensis* preserves intestinal mucosal barrier and may be an adjunct therapy in endotoxin-induced sepsis rat model: a pilot study," *International Journal of Clinical and Experimental Medicine*, vol. 8, no. 5, pp. 7333–7341, 2015.

[22] Y. S. Prakash, "Airway smooth muscle in airway reactivity and remodeling: what have we learned?," *American Journal of Physiology-Lung Cellular and Molecular Physiology*, vol. 305, no. 12, pp. L912–L933, 2013.

[23] S. S. Sohal, C. Ward, W. Danial, R. Wood-Baker, and E. H. Walters, "Recent advances in understanding inflammation and remodeling in the airways in chronic obstructive pulmonary disease," *Expert Review of Respiratory Medicine*, vol. 7, no. 3, pp. 275–288, 2013.

16

Pretreatment Hemoglobin Level Is an Independent Prognostic Factor in Patients with Lung Adenocarcinoma

Yue-Hua Zhang,[1,2] Yuquan Lu,[3] Hong Lu,[1] Meng-Wei Zhang,[1] Yue-Min Zhou,[3,4] and Xiang-Lei Li[1]

[1]*Department of Oncology, Huaihe Hospital of Henan University, Kaifeng 475001, China*
[2]*Department of Oncology, The First Affiliated Hospital of Henan University, Kaifeng 475001, China*
[3]*International Joint Research Laboratory for Cell Medical Engineering of Henan, Huaihe Hospital of Henan University, Kaifeng 475001, China*
[4]*Center of Translational Medicine Center, Huaihe Hospital of Henan University, Kaifeng 475001, China*

Correspondence should be addressed to Yuquan Lu; lll3923@gmail.com and Hong Lu; hhyyluhong@126.com

Academic Editor: Alberto Ruano-Ravina

Background/Aim. Few studies have reported the prognostic value of pretreatment hemoglobin levels in patients with lung adenocarcinoma (LA). In the present study, we retrospectively reviewed 306 LA patients for their prognosis associated with the pretreatment hemoglobin levels. *Methods.* Person-years and case fatality rate (CFR) were calculated from May 2010 to June 2017. Hazard ratio (HR) and 95% confidence intervals (CIs) were estimated using the Cox proportional hazards regression analysis. Survival curves were generated using the Kaplan–Meier analysis. *Results.* Patients with low pretreatment hemoglobin (LPHb) levels had a higher CFR than did patients with normal pretreatment hemoglobin (NPHb) levels (HR = 1.48, 95% CI = 1.06–2.08, and $P = 0.023$). Overall survival of NPHb patients was significantly higher than that of LPHb patients ($P < 0.05$). *Conclusion.* Low pretreatment hemoglobin level was demonstrated to be an independent biomarker for poor prognosis in patients with LA.

1. Introduction

Lung cancer is a common cause of mortality for both men and women [1]. Despite advances in treatment, the five-year overall survival (OS) rate is only 16.3% [2]. In the majority of cases, >80% of lung cancer diagnoses are of the non-small cell lung cancer (NSCLC) type [3], and there are more and more evidences to associate low level of pretreatment hemoglobin with poor survival in patients with NSCLC [4–6]; however, there was no report to associate pretreatment hemoglobin level with the prognosis of adenocarcinoma, a major subtype of NSCLC.

In the present study, we aim to investigate the prognostic value of pretreatment hemoglobin levels for the survival of patients with LA.

2. Materials and Methods

From May 2010 to June 2017, 736 patients with lung cancer were diagnosed at the Henan University Huaihe Hospital (Henan, China). The clinical data were retrospectively collected. After excluding 430 ineligible subjects, a total of 306 patients with LA (152 men and 154 women) were selected as subjects for the present study. All cases of LA were pathologically confirmed. The survival period for each subject was defined as the number of days from the date of diagnosis to the date of mortality. Person-years were calculated for each subject. Patients were included in this study if they had a verified diagnosis of LA, regardless of whether they had received prior lung lobectomy, chemotherapy, or radiotherapy treatments.

The clinical stage was assigned on the basis of the 8th Edition of the TNM Classification for Lung Cancer [7]. Anonymous data regarding age, sex, histological cancer type, TNM stage, Karnofsky performance status (KPS) [8], lung lobectomy, chemotherapy, radiotherapy, smoking status, alcohol consumption, family history, diagnosis date, hemoglobin levels, and date of mortality were obtained retrospectively from the patients' medical records, local death registration departments and telephone follow-ups.

The study was approved by the Medical Ethics Committee of the Henan University Huaihe Hospital.

The pretreatment hemoglobin levels of the patients were obtained. The LPHb level was defined as <120 g/l of hemoglobin in men, and as <110 g/l in women. All patients were dichotomized into an LPHb group (n = 53) and a normal pretreatment hemoglobin (NPHb) group (n = 253). Comparisons of clinical characteristics between the LPHb and NPHb groups were conducted using the chi-squared (χ^2) test. For univariate Cox proportional hazards regression, age, sex, TNM stages, KPS scores, lung lobectomy status, chemotherapy, radiotherapy, smoking status, alcohol consumption, family history, and hemoglobin levels were dichotomized into a favorable group and an unfavorable group. Hazards ratios (HRs) and 95% confidence intervals (CIs) were calculated to estimate associations between the observed factors and case fatality rate (CFR) of patients with LA. A subsequent multivariate analysis using the Cox proportional hazards model estimated the prognostic influence of age, sex, TNM stage, KPS, lung lobectomy, chemotherapy, radiotherapy, and hemoglobin levels on the CFR of patients with LA.

Survival curves were generated using the Kaplan–Meier analysis method, and the log-rank test was used to examine differences in survival between the various hemoglobin groups. All statistical analyses were performed using Stata software version 13 (Stata Corporation, College Station, TX, USA). $P < 0.05$ was considered statistically significant for all analyses.

3. Results

As shown in Table 1, of the 306 patients, 118 (38.6%) were smokers and 38 (12.4%) were alcohol drinkers. In total, 172 (56.2%) patients were at TNM stage IV and 134 (43.8%) were at stage I–III including those unidentified.

Statistical analysis showed that there were significant differences in hemoglobin levels between men and women (P = 0.020), KPS scores (P = 0.003), smokers and non-smokers (P = 0.008), alcohol drinkers and non-drinkers (P = 0.043), and survival time (P = 0.005).

The univariate Cox proportional hazards regression analysis showed that patients who were older than 65 years of age (HR = 1.37 and 95% CI = 1.05–1.78), were at TNM stage IV (HR = 2.16 and 95% CI = 1.65–2.82), had KPS scores < 80 (HR = 1.88 and 95% CI = 1.45–2.43), had not received lung lobectomy (HR = 2.78 and 95% CI = 2.02–3.83), had not received chemotherapy (HR = 1.48 and 95% CI = 1.14–1.91), drank alcohol (HR = 1.69 and 95% CI = 1.17–2.45), or had LPHb levels (HR = 1.61 and 95% CI = 1.16–2.24) had a significantly increased CFR. However, sex, radiotherapy, smoking status, and family history did not have any significant associations with the CFR of patients with LA (Table 2).

The multivariate Cox proportional hazards regression analysis showed that LPHb levels were independently associated with an increased CFR (HR = 1.48 and 95% CI = 1.06–2.08). In addition, lung lobectomy (HR = 2.01, 95% CI = 1.32–3.05), chemotherapy (HR = 1.47 and 95% CI = 1.10–1.95), and alcohol drinking (HR = 1.60, 95% CI = 1.06–2.41) were also independent and favorable prognostic factors (Table 3).

Table 1: Pretreatment hemoglobin levels among clinicopathological and lifestyle factors in lung adenocarcinoma patients, Henan, China, 2017.

	NPHb[1]	LPHb[2]	P value[3]
Age (years)			
<65	147	24	0.087
≥65	106	29	
Sex			
Man	118	34	0.020
Women	135	19	
TNM[4] stage			
I–III	115	19	0.200
IV	138	34	
KPS[5]			
≥80	151	20	0.003
<102	33	60	
Lung lobectomy			
Yes	77	11	0.157
No	176	42	
Chemotherapy			
Yes	131	23	0.267
No	122	30	
Radiotherapy			
Yes	36	5	0.351
No	217	48	
Cigarette smoking			
No	164	24	0.008
Yes	89	29	
Alcohol drinking			
No	226	42	0.043
Yes	27	11	
Family history of cancer			
No	234	50	0.636
Yes	19	3	
Survival year			
≥1 year	100	32	0.005
<1 year	153	21	

[1]NPHb (normal pretreatment hemoglobin): men 120–160 g/l and women 110–150 g/l; [2]LPHb (low pretreatment hemoglobin): men < 120 g/l and women ≤ 110 g/l). [3]Chi-squared (χ^2) test. [4]TNM: tumor-node-metastasis. [5]KPS: Karnofsky performance status.

Kaplan–Meier survival curve estimations showed that patients with LPHb had a poorer OS than did patients with NPHb levels (log-rank test, χ^2 = 8.28, and P = 0.004, Figure 1(a)). When the patients were subdivided by lung lobectomy, the LPHb patients had a poorer OS than the NPHb patients in the no-lung lobectomy group (log-rank test, χ^2 = 7.69, and P = 0.006, Figure 1(b)), a difference not observed in the lung lobectomy group (log-rank test, χ^2 = 0.13, and P = 0.7154, Figure 1(b)).

When we subdivided the patients according to chemotherapy, the LPHb group had a poorer OS than the NPHb patients in the no-chemotherapy group (log-rank test, χ^2 = 12.00, and $P < 0.001$, Figure 1(c)) but not in the chemotherapy group (log-rank test, χ^2 = 0.63, and P = 0.427, Figure 1(c)). The subdivision of patients according to alcohol drinking also showed that the LPHb patients had a poorer OS than the NPHb patients among alcohol drinkers (log-rank test, χ^2 = 12.14, and $P < 0.001$, Figure 1(d)), but not

Table 2: Univariate analysis of prognostic factors for patients with lung adenocarcinoma in Henan, China, 2017.

Factor	Person-years	Cases	Case fatality rate (%)	HR[1]	95% CI[2]	P value
Total	421.3	233	55.3			
Age						
<65	263.7	129	48.9	1.00		
≥65	157.7	104	65.9	1.37	1.05–1.78	0.019
Sex						
Man	201.8	120	59.5	1.00		
Women	219.5	113	51.5	0.87	0.67–1.12	0.280
TNM[3] stage						
I–III	228.9	85	37.1	1.00		
IV	192.5	148	76.9	2.16	1.65–2.82	<0.001
KPS[4] scores						
≥80	269.5	115	42.7	1.00		
<80	151.8	118	77.7	1.88	1.45–2.43	<0.001
Lung lobectomy						
Yes	172.2	49	28.5	1.00		
No	249.1	184	73.9	2.78	2.02–3.83	<0.001
Chemotherapy						
Yes	248.4	117	47.1	1.00		
No	173.0	116	67.1	1.48	1.14–1.91	0.003
Radiotherapy						
Yes	71.6	32	44.7	1.00		
No	349.7	201	57.5	1.33	0.92–1.94	0.132
Smoking						
No	260.2	138	53.0	1.00		
Yes	161.1	95	59.0	1.09	0.84–1.42	0.500
Alcohol						
No	382.9	200	52.2	1.00		
Yes	38.5	33	85.7	1.69	1.17–2.45	0.006
Family history						
No	385.9	218	56.5	1.00		
Yes	35.4	15	42.4	0.73	0.43–1.24	0.248
Hemoglobin[5]						
NPHb	367.1	189	51.5	1.00		
LPHb	54.3	44	81.0	1.61	1.16–2.24	0.004

[1]HR: hazard ratio by multivariate Cox proportional hazards regression. [2]CI: confidence interval. [3]TNM: tumor-node-metastasis. [4]KPS: Karnofsky performance status. [5]Hemoglobin: NPHb (normal pretreatment hemoglobin): men 120–160 g/l and women 110–150 g/l; LPHb (low pretreatment hemoglobin): men < 120 g/l and women ≤ 110 g/l.

among alcohol non-drinkers (log-rank test, $\chi^2 = 3.22$, and $P = 0.073$, Figure 1(d)).

4. Discussion

Our data suggest that pretreatment hemoglobin level, measured at the time of diagnosis, may be an independent predictor for the prognosis of patients with LA, as is the case in the no-lung lobectomy and/or no-chemotherapy patients. To the best of our knowledge, this is the first report that associated pretreatment hemoglobin levels with the prognosis of patients with LA.

Low hemoglobin is common in oncological diseases, such as lung [9, 10], breast [10], gastric [11], and ovarian cancer [12]. There is evidence for a correlation between hemoglobin levels and the prognosis of patients with NSCLC. But precise underlying mechanisms are not fully understood. Tumor cells secrete a number of soluble molecules, including interleukin-6 (IL-6) and tumor necrosis factor-α (TNF-α). These molecules could decrease hemoglobin by changing the hematopoietic environment [13, 14], suppressing erythropoiesis and erythropoietin (EPO) [15], and impairing the EPO response in erythroid progenitor cells [16]. Moreover, in patients with bone metastasis, bone marrow involvement may lead to bone morrow failure, which may then cause low-hemoglobin levels [17] and subsequently lead to hypoxia, which could induce genomic changes and enhance the development of malignancy [18]. Hypoxia may also boost tumor angiogenesis and accelerate metastasis [19]. Moreover, hypoxia may enhance tumor cell resistance to chemotherapy and radiotherapy through the development of multidrug resistance [20].

Table 3: Multivariate analysis of prognostic factors for patients with lung adenocarcinoma in Henan, China, 2017.

Factor	HR[1]	95% CI[2]	P value
Age			
<65	1.00		
≥65	1.20	0.90–1.60	0.211
Sex			
Man	1.00		
Women	0.89	0.66–1.19	0.432
TNM[3] stage			
I–III	1.00		
IV	1.39	0.98–1.99	0.067
KPS[4] scores			
≥80	1.00		
<80	1.24	0.93–1.64	0.139
Lung lobectomy			
Yes	1.00		
No	2.01	1.32–3.05	0.001
Chemotherapy			
Yes	1.00		
No	1.47	1.10–1.95	0.008
Radiotherapy			
Yes	1.00		
No	1.00	0.68–1.49	0.981
Alcohol drinking			
No	1.00		
Yes	1.60	1.06–2.41	0.026
Hemoglobin[5]			
NPHb	1.00		
LPHb	1.48	1.06–2.08	0.023

[1]HR: hazard ratio by multivariate Cox proportional hazards regression. [2]CI: confidence interval. [3]TNM: tumor-node-metastasis. [4]KPS: Karnofsky performance status. [5]Hemoglobin: NPHb (normal pretreatment hemoglobin): men 120–160 g/l and women 110–150 g/l; LPHb (low pretreatment hemoglobin): men < 120 g/l and women ≤ 110 g/l.

For associations of hemoglobin level with lung adenocarcinoma, we did not find previous studies and know little about the mechanisms beneath the surface of water. There was no difference in OS for lung lobectomy group based on Hb, and similar result was found in the chemotherapy group. This is not in line with the previous study of LPHb in patients

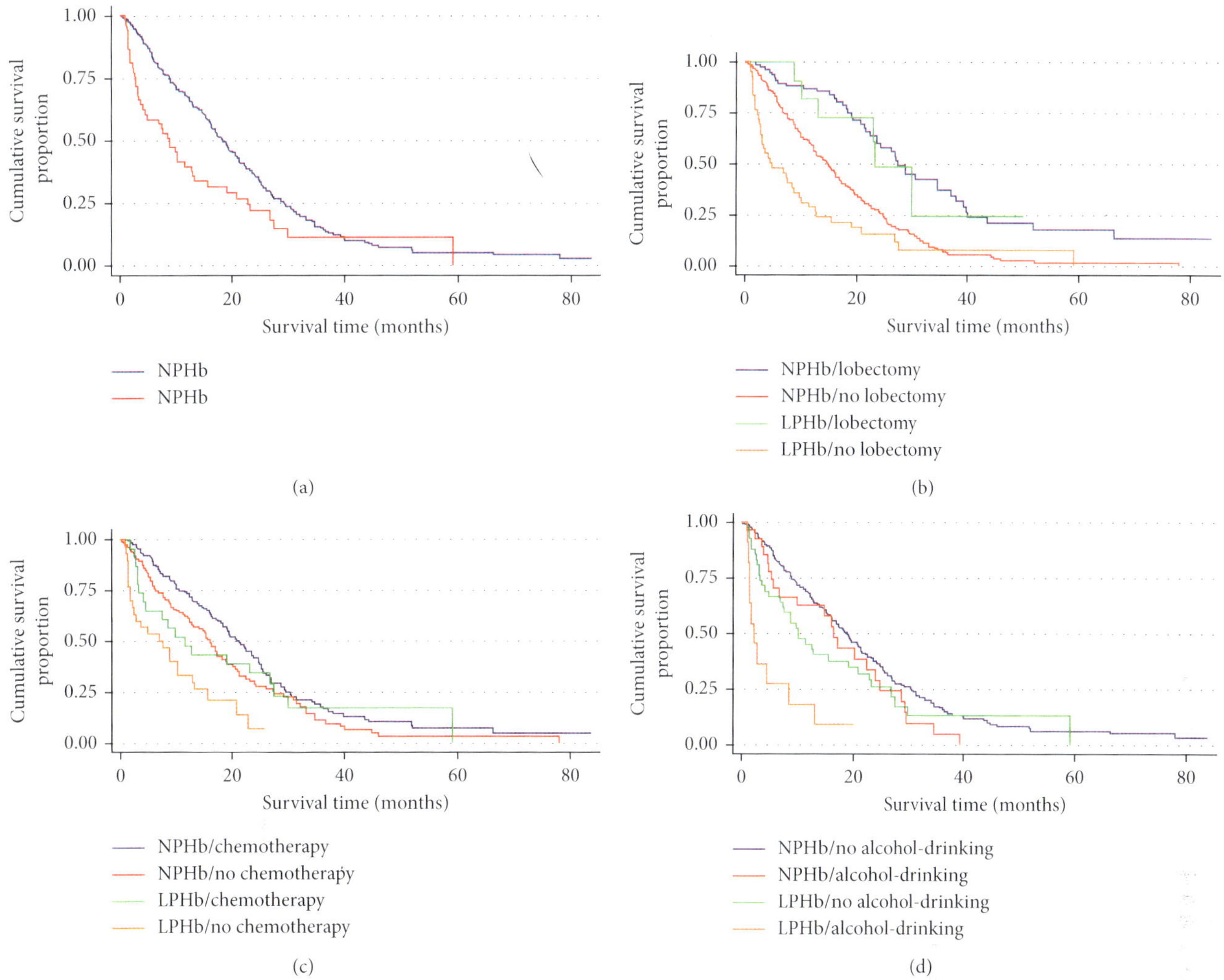

FIGURE 1: Cumulative survival proportion of patients with LA according to their pretreatment hemoglobin levels. Normal pretreatment hemoglobin (NPHb): men 120–160 g/l, women 110–150 g/l; low pretreatment hemoglobin (LPHb): men < 120 g/l and women ≤ 110 g/l). (a) Overall survival (OS) of NPHb and LPHb patients with LA (log-rank test, $\chi^2 = 8.28$, and $P = 0.004$). (b) LPHb patients had a poorer OS than NPHb patients in the no-lung lobectomy group (log-rank test, $\chi^2 = 7.69$, $P = 0.006$) but not among the lung lobectomy group (log-rank test, $\chi^2 = 0.13$, $P = 0.7154$). (c) The LPHb group had a poorer OS than NPHb patients in the no-chemotherapy group (log-rank test, $\chi^2 = 12.00$, and $P < 0.001$) but not among the chemotherapy group (log-rank test, $\chi^2 = 0.63$, and $P = 0.427$). (d) LPHb patients had a poorer OS than NPHb patients among alcohol drinkers (log-rank test, $\chi^2 = 12.14$, and $P < 0.001$), but not among alcohol non-drinkers (log-rank test, $\chi^2 = 3.22$, and $P = 0.073$).

with non-small cell lung cancer [21]. In a previous study of lung adenocarcinoma patients with LPHb, because of lack of data, we could not analyze the reason. In the present study, about half of the patients abandoned clinical treatment (Supplementary Table 1), and their OS was significantly shorter than those who had received clinical treatments (Supplementary Table 2). We thus suggest that it is difficult to exclude possibilities that it is the clinical treatment that had obscured associations of pretreatment hemoglobin with the final OS. Cigarette smoking was not associated with the OS of LA. This is inconsistent with other studies [22, 23]. We think this maybe related to the fact that we only consider cigarette smoking, without considering the detailed smoking index. But alcohol drinking was significantly and independently associated with the OS of LA, which might be supported by previous studies [24, 25]. Those who had LPHb and drank alcohol had a worst OS.

A major strength of our study was the inclusion of a large number of patients with LA, all with a complete set of clinical data, including the pretreatment hemoglobin levels, the complete survival period, records of multiple treatments, and the family history and lifestyle details, including smoking status and alcohol consumption; this enabled us to investigate the prognostic value of pretreatment hemoglobin levels with decreased sample bias and offset heterogeneity. However, there are also limitations to our study. First, our study was retrospective, and the information on posttreatment recurrence was insufficient. Second, we did not follow alterations of hemoglobin level after pretreatment measurement during clinical treatment and afterwards.

Both lung lobectomy and chemotherapy treatments were associated with the prognosis of patients with LA. However, neither significantly affected the prognostic value of the pretreatment hemoglobin levels in the present study. As for associations of alcohol drinking with the prognosis of LA, we suggest further investigations to confirm the finding.

5. Conclusion

Our study suggests that low pretreatment hemoglobin level could be an independent biomarker for poor prognosis in patients with LA. In future clinical studies, the hemoglobin levels should be considered during the work-up of patients with LA in prospective trials, in order to confirm its prognostic significance.

References

[1] R. L. Siegel, K. D. Miller, and A. Jemal, "Cancer Statistics, 2017," *CA: A Cancer Journal for Clinicians*, vol. 67, no. 1, pp. 7–30, 2017.

[2] A. J. Alberg, M. V. Brock, J. G. Ford, J. M. Samet, and S. D. Spivack, "Epidemiology of lung cancer: diagnosis and management of lung cancer, 3rd ed: American College of Chest Physicians evidence-based clinical practice guidelines," *Chest*, vol. 143, no. 5, pp. e1S–e29, 2013.

[3] D. S. Ettinger, D. E. Wood, D. L. Aisner et al., "Non-small cell lung cancer, version 5.2017, NCCN clinical practice guidelines in oncology," *Journal of the National Comprehensive Cancer Network*, vol. 15, no. 4, pp. 504–535, 2017.

[4] M. Tomita, T. Shimizu, M. Hara, T. Ayabe, and T. Onitsuka, "Impact of preoperative hemoglobin level on survival of non-small cell lung cancer patients," *Anticancer Research*, vol. 28, no. 3B, pp. 1947–1950, 2008.

[5] I. Gauthier, K. Ding, T. Winton et al., "Impact of hemoglobin levels on outcomes of adjuvant chemotherapy in resected non-small cell lung cancer: the JBR.10 trial experience," *Lung Cancer*, vol. 55, no. 3, pp. 357–363, 2007.

[6] K. Aoe, A. Hiraki, T. Maeda et al., "Serum hemoglobin level determined at the first presentation is a poor prognostic indicator in patients with lung cancer," *Internal Medicine*, vol. 44, no. 8, pp. 800–804, 2005.

[7] F. U. Kay, A. Kandathil, K. Batra, S. S. Saboo, S. Abbara, and P. Rajiah, "Revisions to the tumor, node, metastasis staging of lung cancer (8th edition): rationale, radiologic findings and clinical implications," *World Journal of Radiology*, vol. 9, no. 6, pp. 269–279, 2017.

[8] C. C. Schag, R. L. Heinrich, and P. A. Ganz, "Karnofsky performance status revisited: reliability, validity, and guidelines," *Journal of Clinical Oncology*, vol. 2, no. 3, pp. 187–193, 1984.

[9] G. Holgersson, M. Sandelin, E. Hoye et al., "Swedish lung cancer radiation study group: the prognostic value of anaemia, thrombocytosis and leukocytosis at time of diagnosis in patients with non-small cell lung cancer," *Medical Oncology*, vol. 29, no. 5, pp. 3176–3182, 2012.

[10] I. Ray-Coquard, J.-F. Morère, F. Scotté, L. Cals, and E.-C. Antoine, "Management of anemia in advanced breast and lung cancer patients in daily practice: results of a French survey," *Advances in Therapy*, vol. 29, no. 2, pp. 124–133, 2012.

[11] L. Vannella, E. Lahner, J. Osborn, and B. Annibale, "Systematic review: gastric cancer incidence in pernicious anaemia," *Alimentary Pharmacology & Therapeutics*, vol. 37, no. 4, pp. 375–382, 2013.

[12] A. D. Altman, X.-Q. Liu, G. Nelson, P. Chu, J. Nation, and P. Ghatage, "The effects of anemia and blood transfusion on patients with stage III-IV ovarian cancer," *International Journal of Gynecological Cancer*, vol. 23, no. 9, pp. 1569–1576, 2013.

[13] S. Banzet, H. Sanchez, R. Chapot, X. Bigard, S. Vaulont, and N. Koulmann, "Interleukin-6 contributes to hepcidin mRNA increase in response to exercise," *Cytokine*, vol. 58, no. 2, pp. 158–161, 2012.

[14] C. C. Sun, V. Vaja, J. L. Babitt, and H. Y. Lin, "Targeting the hepcidin-ferroportin axis to develop new treatment strategies for anemia of chronic disease and anemia of inflammation," *American Journal of Hematology*, vol. 87, no. 4, pp. 392–400, 2012.

[15] Y. Wu, S. Antony, J. L. Meitzler, and J. H. Doroshow, "Molecular mechanisms underlying chronic inflammation-associated cancers," *Cancer Letters*, vol. 345, no. 2, pp. 164–173, 2014.

[16] M. Aapro, W. Jelkmann, S. N. Constantinescu, and B. Leyland-Jones, "Effects of erythropoietin receptors and erythropoiesis-stimulating agents on disease progression in cancer," *British Journal of Cancer*, vol. 106, no. 7, pp. 1249–1258, 2012.

[17] A. Tefferi, S. Hudgens, R. Mesa et al., "Use of the functional assessment of cancer therapy–anemia in persons with myeloproliferative neoplasm-associated myelofibrosis and anemia," *Clinical Therapeutics*, vol. 36, no. 4, pp. 560–566, 2014.

[18] L. P. Schwab, D. L. Peacock, D. Majumdar et al., "Hypoxia-inducible factor 1α promotes primary tumor growth and tumor-initiating cell activity in breast cancer," *Breast Cancer Research*, vol. 14, no. 1, p. R6, 2012.

[19] S. Li, W. Meng, Z. Guan, Y. Guo, and X. Han, "The hypoxia-related signaling pathways of vasculogenic mimicry in tumor treatment," *Biomedicine & Pharmacotherapy*, vol. 80, pp. 127–135, 2016.

[20] L. Milane, Z Duan, and M Amiji, "Role of hypoxia and glycolysis in the development of multi-drug resistance in human tumor cells and the establishment of an orthotopic multi-drug resistant tumor model in nude mice using hypoxic pre-conditioning," *Cancer Cell International*, vol. 11, no. 1, p. 3, 2011.

[21] J. P. Cata, C. Gutierrez, R. J. Mehran et al., "Preoperative anemia, blood transfusion, and neutrophil-to-lymphocyte ratio in patients with stage i non-small cell lung cancer," *Cancer Cell and Microenvironment*, vol. 3, no. 1, p. e1116, 2016.

[22] T. Y. Cheng, S. M. Cramb, P. D. Baade, D. R. Youlden, C. Nwogu, and M. E. Reid, "The international epidemiology of lung cancer: latest trends, disparities, and tumor characteristics," *Journal of Thoracic Oncology*, vol. 11, no. 10, pp. 1653–1671, 2016.

[23] K. J. Jung, C Jeon, and S. H. Jee, "The effect of smoking on lung cancer: ethnic differences and the smoking paradox," *Epidemiology and Health*, vol. 38, p. e2016060, 2016.

[24] J. A. Garcia Lavandeira, A. Ruano-Ravina, K. T. Kelsey et al., "Alcohol consumption and lung cancer risk in never smokers: a pooled analysis of case-control studies," *European Journal of Public Health*, vol. 13, 2017.

[25] J. R. Troche, S. T. Mayne, N. D. Freedman, F. M. Shebl, and C. C. Abnet, "The association between alcohol consumption and lung carcinoma by histological subtype," *American Journal of Epidemiology*, vol. 183, no. 2, pp. 110–121, 2016.

Model for Developing a Health-Related Quality of Life Questionnaire for Chronic Obstructive Pulmonary Disease

Nikolić Emilija,[1] Nikolić Aleksandar,[2] Stević Ruža,[3] Brandmajer Tijana,[1] Mićanović Veselin,[4] and Mašnić Jelena[4]

[1]*Faculty of Medicine, University of Montenegro, 81000 Podgorica, Montenegro*
[2]*D.o.o. "NCG Inzinjering", 81000 Podgorica, Montenegro*
[3]*Faculty of Medicine, University of Belgarde, 11000 Belgrade, Serbia*
[4]*Faculty of Philosophy, University of Montenegro, 81000 Podgorica, Montenegro*

Correspondence should be addressed to Nikolić Emilija; ema.med@t-com.me

Academic Editor: Inmaculada Alfageme

Introduction. The St. George's Respiratory Questionnaire (SGRQ), Modified Medical Research Council (mMRC) Dyspnea Scale, Hospital Anxiety and Depression Scale (HADS), and general health questionnaire (SF-36) are widely used for chronic respiratory diseases such as chronic obstructive pulmonary disease (COPD). *Aim.* We examined the reliability and validity of a modified questionnaire (MQ) to create a model for assessing the health-related quality of life (HRQOL) in COPD. *Method.* In total, 132 COPD patients completed the MQ. Lung function, smoking index, and exacerbation frequency were measured. Cronbach's α coefficient of correlation, standard deviation, and multifactorial nonlinear regression analysis were used to verify the internal validity of the MQ and to develop the mathematical model. *Results.* Female (63) patients had lesser airway obstruction than, and exacerbation frequency similar to that of, male patients. Exacerbation frequency significantly correlated with spirometry parameters in female patients. The MQ total score achieved high internal consistency (Cronbach's $\alpha = 0.89$) and showed significant correlations with exacerbation frequency, smoking habit, and spirometry parameters in male patients ($p < 0.005$). *Conclusion.* The HRQOL questionnaire was shown to be a good indicator of the health status of COPD patients. The mathematical model easily and precisely confirmed the score of HRQOL questionnaire.

1. Introduction

Smoking is the most important cause of chronic obstructive pulmonary disease (COPD), although genes and environmental conditions, such as respiratory infections, air pollution, occupation, diet, and socioeconomic status, are also important aspects [1–3]. The General Guide for Chronic Obstructive Lung Disease (GOLD standard) defines treatment objectives for these patients, which include improving the physical activity and emotional state (quality of life, or QOL). An important clinical aim is preventing further progression and minimizing symptoms [4].

Anxiety and depression often present at later stages (III and IV) of COPD, which indicate a poorer prognosis [5]. The prevalence of depression in COPD patients is approximately 39% [6], and COPD patients have the highest risk of depression among chronic medical illnesses [7]. From a biological perspective, depression, anxiety, and COPD share similar pathological mechanisms. The proinflammatory cytokine interleukin (IL)-6 is increased in depression [8] and COPD [9]. Similarly, neuropeptide Y mediates anxiety and enhances the inflammatory response in bronchi [10]. From a psychological perspective, depression and anxiety predict the health-related quality of life (HRQOL) in COPD patients [11]. From a social perspective, both depression [12] and COPD [13] contribute to significant economic burdens.

The concept of HRQOL is present in medical research to the extent that recent studies have revealed that the measurement of HRQOL is crucial for clinical trials [14–16]. Questionnaires are the main instruments for measuring

HRQOL. In addition to general questionnaires such as short form (SF-36), there are questionnaires for specific diseases [17]. While the St. George's Respiratory Questionnaire (SGRQ) for COPD has proven reliability and sensitivity to clinical changes in the disease, researchers now apply the revised version, the SGRQ-C [18]. Generic and disease-specific measures may capture complementary information, and it may be desirable to incorporate both types of measure in a study, depending on the goal of the study [19].

The Hospital Anxiety and Depression Scale (HADS) is a special questionnaire that identifies the emotional state of a patient. Developed by Zigmond and Snaith in 1983, its purpose is to provide clinicians with a tool for identifying and quantifying depression and anxiety in an acceptable, reliable, and easily applicable form in practice [7].

A recent study has shown that dyspnea can be a strong predictor of mental and physical outcome components in HRQOL questionnaires [20, 21]. Therefore, in this study, we investigated the correlation between the HRQOL of COPD patients and the following parameters: spirometry, smoking habit, and exacerbation frequency. Using multifactorial regression analysis, a mathematical model was developed, which can precisely determine the HRQOL score.

2. Materials and Methods

2.1. Study Population. A total of 132 consecutive COPD patients treated at the Mediterranean Health Centre Igalo and the Public Health Centre Herceg Novi between June 2016 and June 2017 were enrolled. The inclusion criteria included an existing COPD diagnosis and meeting the spirometry criteria for COPD (GOLD 2016) at the initial assessment. The exclusion criterion was a coexisting respiratory disease.

The study was conducted in accordance with the ethical standards of the Committee of Human Experimentation published by the Montenegrins Association of Physiotherapy (Ref. 01-28/08-2/2016), which was performed in accordance with the Declaration of Helsinki.

All patients provided written informed consent.

2.2. Experimental Measures. COPD patients were invited to complete review questionnaires, including items regarding MQ, smoking habits, exacerbation frequency, and pulmonary function test results, at 6-monthly intervals for 1 year.

The SGRQ is a self-administered questionnaire developed by Jones and colleagues in 1991, containing 50 items in three domains. The first 8 items cover the frequency and severity of respiratory symptoms as the symptom domain, the next 16 items concern limitations in activities because of the shortness of breath as the activity domain, and the last 26 items cover the approval, social, and psychological consequence of respiratory diseases as the impact domain. Its results are given as a score ranging from 0 (entirely satisfactory QOL) to 100 (maximally reduced QOL). The questionnaire has been validated for COPD and asthma and is used to assess the health status of other respiratory diseases, such as idiopathic pulmonary fibrosis, bronchiectasis, cystic fibrosis, and pulmonary tuberculosis [22].

Table 1: Descriptive statistics of lung function and exacerbation.

Female	FVC	FEV1	PEF	Exacerbation number
Maximum value	4.6	4.12	10.21	3
Minimum value	1.59	0.58	1.81	0
Range	3.01	3.54	8.4	3
Mean	3.363	2.325	5.652	1.956
Standard deviation	0.948	0.831	1.912	0.864
Male	FVC	FEV1	PEF	Exacerbation number
Maximum value	6.92	5.39	11.29	3
Minimum value	2.25	0.74	1.58	0
Range	4.67	4.65	9.71	3
Mean	4.307	3.001	6.455	2
Standard deviation	1.183	1.238	2.271	1.163

We used the 36-Item Short Form Health Survey (SF-36) questionnaire, which contains 36 questions regarding the patient's general condition, including physical condition, general health, vitality, social functioning, emotions, mental health, activity, and pain. The number of points recorded in each scale of the questionnaire is transformed into standard values and calibrated on a unique scale with a theoretical minimum of 0 points, indicating poor general health, and a maximum of 100 points, indicating excellent general health. This scale has been used to study the general health status of patients with chronic respiratory diseases, such as COPD, asthma, and bronchiectasis [23].

We also used the Modified Medical Research Council (mMRC) Dyspnea Scale, which is a good indicator of the functional capacity of patients' lungs. Level 0 indicates no dyspnea, Level 1 indicates dyspnea on an incline, Level 2 indicates that the patient walks more slowly than his or her peers, Level 3 indicates that the patient has to stop after walking 100 m, and Level 4 indicates that the patient is unable to leave the house [24].

Finally, we used the HADS, which measures the emotional state of patients and their degree of anxiety and depression. It contains 10 declarations in which the respondent indicates the extent to which they relate to him. Based on the total score, it is determined whether the patient has mild (0–10), moderate (10–25), or severe (25–40) anxiety and depression level [7].

Because certain topics covered in these four administered questionnaires are repeated, a modified survey was developed and adapted to this research. The most important stage in dealing with modified questionnaires (MQs) is calculating the results, or scoring, which is conducted in the following order: (1) entering data, (2) checking the entered data and determining if all questions have been answered, (3) collecting the obtained results, (4) transforming the results into a new score, and (5) checking the previous procedure.

The following parameters of the pulmonary function test were measured: (a) forced expiratory volume in the first second (FEV1) pre- and postadministration of a bronchodilator, (b) forced vital capacity (FVC), and (c) peak expiratory flow (PEF).

TABLE 2: Correlation between the parameters of spirometry, smoking, exacerbations, and the modified questionnaire score.

Female	Smoking	FVC	FEV1	PEF	Exacerbation	MQ score
Smoking	1	0.0895	−0.0958	−0.1988	0.0852	−0.3347
FVC	0.0895	1	0.7983	0.5674	−0.4705	−0.3960
FEV1	−0.0958	0.7983	1	0.8197	−0.4292	−0.2691
PEF	−0.1988	0.5674	0.8197	1	−0.4438	−0.2219
Exacerbation	0.0852	−0.4701	−0.4292	−0.4438	1	0.6015
Score	−0.3347	−0.3960	−0.1691	−0.1219	0.6015	1
Male	Smoking	FVC	FEV1	PEF	Exacerbation	Score
Smoking	1	0.0072	−0.0680	0.0673	0.2357	−0.0009
FVC	0.0072	1	0.8379	0.8556	−0.4899	−0.496
FEV1	−0.0680	0.8379	1	0.8942	−0.3661	−0.4142
PEF	0.0673	0.8558	0.8942	1	−0.3318	−0.4177
Exacerbation	0.2357	−0.4899	−0.3661	−0.3318	1	0.8013
Score	−0.0009	−0.4969	−0.4142	−0.4177	0.8013	1

2.3. Statistical Analysis. The free statistical software Cronbach's alpha (V.1.01) was used to verify the consistency (internal validity) of the modified questionnaire structure. A correlation of ≥0.7 was assumed to indicate that questions within a dimension are likely to measure the same construct.

Data analysis was performed using SPSS version 20.0 (IBM Corp), with a p value < 0.005 indicating statistical significance for correlations (mild, moderate, and highly; $r = \pm 0.26 - \pm 1$) among pulmonary function parameters, smoking habit, and MQ.

Multifactorial nonlinear regression analysis was performed to define the model that would mathematically express the general physical condition, HRQOL, and the emotional state of COPD patients on the basis of pulmonary function parameters, smoking habits, and exacerbation frequency.

3. Results

Of 132 patients examined, 63 female patients had less airway obstruction than men (Table 1) and a similar exacerbation frequency as that of men (mean, 1.956 ± 0.864 versus 2.0 ± 1.163, resp.). Other patient statistics of lung function and exacerbation are shown in Table 1.

Correlations between spirometry, smoking habit, exacerbation frequency, and the MQ score for female and male patients are shown in Table 2.

The MQ score highly correlated with exacerbation frequency in both sexes ($r = 0.60$; $r = 0.80$; $p < 0.005$), moderately correlated with spirometry parameters in males (MQ/FVC, $r = -0.49$; MQ/FEV1, $r = -0.41$; MQ/PEF, $r = -0.41$), and mildly correlated with smoking habits in females (MQ/smoking habits, $r = -0.33$).

Exacerbation frequency mildly correlated with spirometry parameters. The greatest impact was noted in FVC (female, exacerbation/FVC, $r = -0.47$; male, exacerbation/FVC, $r = -0.48$).

The results of verifying the authenticity of customized questionnaires are given in Table 3, which show high reliability. The Cronbach's α was 0.8944, which is approximately the maximum value of 1.

TABLE 3: Cronbach's α coefficient for the five questionnaires conducted.

	Cronbach's α	Std. α	G6 (smc)	Average R
Total	0.8944	1	1	1
MQ	0.95	1	1	1
SGRQ	0.8312	1	1	1
mMRC Dyspnea Scale	0.7674	1	1	1
SF-36 Scale	0.8204	1	1	1
HADS	0.8697	1	1	1

TABLE 4: Multifactorial nonlinear regression analysis values for model development.

Number of observations = 132
Nonlinear iteration limit = 250
Diverging nonlinear iteration limit = 10
Number of nonlinear iterations performed = 5
Residual tolerance = 0.0000000001
Sum of residuals = 2.4163
Average residual = 1.8305
Residual sum of squares (absolute) = 3806.8881
Residual sum of squares (relative) = 3806.8881
Standard error of the estimate = 5.4966
Coefficient of multiple determination (R^2) = 0.6362
Proportion of variance explained = 63.6259%
Adjusted coefficient of multiple determination (R_a^2) = 0.6218251316

Out of all respondents, 25% stated that they had some contact with a psychiatrist, but further analysis of this data was not provided. Indeed, 22% of respondents said they had used psychiatric drugs. Psychiatric heredity was listed as positive in 7.5% of patients, anxiety in 86%, and a depressive syndrome in 63%.

3.1. Development of Mathematical Model. Using the multifactorial nonlinear regression analysis, a statistical model that determined the MQ score using spirometry parameters, exacerbation frequency, and smoking habits was developed. The results of statistical analysis are given in Table 4.

Table 5: Regression variables.

Variable	Value	Standard error	t-ratio	Prob (t)
A	−0.1482	2.7698	−5.351	0.0
B	−5.8662	0.0194	−0.301	0.0341
C	−4.4479	2.6682	−1.666	0.098
D	2.3828	1.1024	2.161	0.032
E	0.1752	1.5025	11.660	0.0
F	3.5046	6.8791	50.945	0.0

A, variable regression for $x1$, smoking habit; B, variable regression for $x2$, value of FVC; C, variable regression for $x3$, value of FEV1; D, variable regression for $x4$, value of PEF; E, variable regression for $x5$, exacerbation frequency; t-ratio, ratio of the estimated parameter and standard deviation of the same; Prob (t), probability that the value of the regression coefficient with the independent variable is 0.

The model used the following definition:

$$Y = \exp(a \times x1 + b \times x2 + c \times x3 + d \times x4 + e \times x5 + f), \quad (1)$$

where Y is the score of the questionnaire; $x1$ is smoking habit; $x2$ is the FVC value; $x3$ is the FEV1 value; $x4$ is the PEF value; $x5$ is exacerbation frequency; and a, b, c, d, e, and f are variable regression values.

A basic assumption made during the process of developing the model is that the dependent variable Y (score) can be determined using independent variables, $x1$–$x5$ (smoking habit, exacerbation frequency, and spirometry parameters).

The adequacy of the selection of independent variables is confirmed by proving the null hypothesis, that is, the regression coefficient of independent variables is equal to 0. This hypothesis is examined using the parameter Prob (t), which is the probability that the value of the regression coefficient with the independent variable is 0. Thus, a Prob (t) value of 0 indicates that the null hypothesis is not true. The fact that the selection of independent parameters of the model was adequate proves that the value of Prob (t), for 50% of coefficients with independent variables, is 0 (Table 5).

Coefficient values for (B), (C), and (D) amount to Prob (t) values of 0.034, 0.098, and 0.032, respectively, and the probability that the values of independent variables (FVC, FEV1, and PEF) will be 0 is 3.84%, 9.8%, and 3.2%, respectively. This result negates the assumption that lung function parameters substantially influence the HRQOL score of patients.

The t-ratio is the ratio of the estimated parameter and standard deviation of the same. The higher the t-ratio value, the more significant is the influence of independent variable on the dependent variable. In our model, the t-ratio for the parameter (E) of 11.660 was the highest, indicating that the influence of the coefficient $x5$, that is, exacerbation frequency, was the highest (Table 5).

The rating of the obtained model is based on the coefficient of determination, R^2 ($0 \leq R^2 \leq 1$; $p = 0.05$). In addition to R^2, an adjusted coefficient of determination, which can be <0, is used because of the introduction of a new factor that has no essential significance for variable-ranking but increases the value of the coefficient of determination. In our model, the resulting value for the coefficient of determination was $R^2 = 0.6362592869$ and the adjusted coefficient of determination was $R^2 = 0.6218251316$. The obtained coefficient of determination values indicate that 63.62% or 62.18% of the variation in the obtained score of the questionnaire can be explained by the developed model.

The model can be considered successful because, in practice, all models with a coefficient of determination $R^2 \geq 0.6$ are accepted.

The final model was as follows:

$$\begin{aligned} \text{SCORE} = \exp(&-0.14 \times \text{smoking habit} - 5.86 \times \text{FVC} \\ &- 4.44 \times \text{FEV1} + 2.38 \times \text{PEF} \\ &+ 0.17 \times \text{exacerbation} + 3.50), \end{aligned} \quad (2)$$

where SCORE is the total results of the MQ, and FVC, FEV1, and PEF are spirometry parameters measured.

4. Discussion

Obstructive lung disease has been the subject of numerous medical and epidemiological studies. Some authors have argued that COPD can be defined as a smoking disease, given that an exposure to smoke is the primary criterion in the definition of the disease. When assessing the risk factors for COPD, spirometry is an important parameter. Thus, it is necessary to carefully evaluate the definition of respiratory obstruction (FEV1/FVC < 0.7) and not to overestimate or underestimate COPD among the elderly and young populations [14].

In several studies, approximately 97.5% of respondents were male; therefore, COPD is considered to be a disease affecting the male population [11]. COPD is highly correlated with smoking behavior, and the ratio of male to female smokers was 10.9 : 1 in Taiwanese adults [17].

In our study, a large number of female smokers (74%) had COPD compared with their total number. The smoking habit negatively correlated with the MQ score in both sexes. Smoking habit noticeably changed the HRQOL in female patients, with a 25% lower HRQOL score than male patients. However, the physiological and neurological factors that contributed to the hypersensitivity of the female body and the bronchial tree, in particular tobacco smoke and harmful substances from cigarettes, are unclear. A biological mechanism that explains the relationship between the smoking index and the HRQOL score in COPD patients has been proposed. A previous study has found that the proinflammatory cytokine IL-6 increased as the COPD stage worsened in smokers [9]. Furthermore, an increase in IL-6 has been found in patients with depression [8], which might lead to poor HRQOL scores in COPD patients. In our study, the lowest FEV1 value for female smokers was 0.6 L and the largest was 3.8 L. In female nonsmokers, the FEV1 values ranged from 1.4 to 4 L. Male smokers with COPD had an FEV1 ranging from 0.7 L (min) to 5 L (max) and nonsmokers had an FEV1 ranging from 1.9 L (min) to 4.2 L (max). In addition, male smokers had a moderate change in the HRQOL scores.

Moreover, our assessment showed a mild correlation between exacerbation frequency and smoking index (Table 2), which confirms the aforementioned research.

An important indicator of COPD severity is the HRQOL assessed using a questionnaire. Pickard et al. have shown that SGRQ scores are associated with a greater statistical power to discriminate among the levels of COPD severity using relative efficiency (RE) ratios rather than generic measures of health. The SGRQ exhibited a strong correlation with clinically measured FEV1 ($r = 0.43$) [15].

In this study, the lung function parameter FEV1 positively correlated with the total MQ score (male MQ/FEV1, $r = 0.41$), which can be used as the relevant indicator of HRQOL. Specifically, in both female and male patients, FVC values moderately correlated with the total MQ score.

The GOLD standard 2016 defines COPD exacerbation as an acute clinical event characterized by the worsening of respiratory symptoms, which is different from usual variation in symptoms. In our research, exacerbation frequency significantly correlated with the MQ score, confirming the previously conducted finding that exacerbations in patients with COPD is related to the HRQOL score [25, 26]. Patients with COPD and comorbid depression have more exacerbations and a reduced HRQOL. Moreover, COPD is a risk factor for the development of depression, particularly in patients with increased disability. Among comorbidities, depression is one of the most frequent because even mild COPD patients have a more than fourfold increase in the prevalence of depression compared with controls [27, 28].

In our study, 22% of COPD patients used psychiatric drugs, anxiety was present in 36%, and a legacy of psychiatric heredity was positive in 7.5%.

In addition, a meta-analysis of the correlation between factors associated with disease-specific HRQOL, as measured by the SGRQ, among COPD patients indicated that dyspnea was a key factor of HRQOL [5].

This study provides a further confirmation of the associations among dyspnea, objective measures lung functioning, and HRQOL. The SGRQ total score declined across GOLD stages 1–4. HRQOL was worse among patients with higher dyspnea (mMRC levels, 2–4) than among those with lower dyspnea (mMRC level, 0-1).

However, the parameters of lung function do not completely measure the mental health, sleep, and fatigue of patients. Therefore, further research is needed on COPD in clinical practice in terms of additional measurements of the health condition of patients [29, 30].

We concluded that smoking, parameters of lung function, and exacerbation frequency can be used to assess HRQOL.

Using multifactorial nonlinear regression analysis, we developed a mathematical model that can precisely determine the HRQOL score. This model enabled us to determine the quality of life of patients in a quick, simple, and efficient way with minimal time and participation. We recommend the use of the model when assessing COPD patients in clinical practice because it precisely confirms the total HRQOL score.

Therefore, we can expect an escalation in the number of female patients with COPD, which was confirmed in our study. According to the World Health Organization, in the last 10 years, the number of female smokers has increased and this trend is ongoing. Montenegro tops the list of European countries with the highest number of women who actively smoke cigarettes.

We hope that our work will promote a wider exploration of the development of the HRQOL model for COPD patients in both clinical practice and research studies. This version of the HRQOL model could enhance the clinical usefulness and acceptability of routine health status assessment by clinicians, thereby saving time and materials.

The limitations of our study are as follows: (1) this study had a relatively small number of patients; (2) although the HADS is commonly used to assess depression and anxiety in other chronic medical disorders [12, 31], it was found to exhibit low diagnostic accuracy for depression in COPD patients [32] and biased when assessing the severity of depression in COPD patients [33]; and (3) this study did not assess passive smoking, which plays a key role in the worsening of respiratory symptoms [31].

5. Conclusion

The HRQOL questionnaire is a good indicator of the health status of COPD patients. Exacerbation frequency and smoking status significantly changed the HRQOL scores. The smoking index reduced the HRQOL by 25% in female patients compared with that in male patients. Using multifactorial nonlinear regression analysis, a mathematical model was developed by which the scoring of the HRQOL questionnaire can be obtained in a simple and easy way using spirometry parameters, smoking habits, and exacerbation frequency during the year. By applying the obtained model, the HRQOL score can be determined and the success of therapy can be predicted. We believe that our work will stimulate the further validation of the model by measuring HRQOL in larger studies as well as use with similar respiratory conditions such as asthma.

Acknowledgments

The authors would like to thank Darinka Kovačić, Department of Pulmonology, Mediterranean Health Center Igalo, for assistance on obtaining data. The authors would like to thank Enago (www.enago.com) for the English language review.

References

[1] A. Buist, M. McBurnie, and W. Vollmer, "International variation in the prevalence of COPD (the BOLD Study): a population-based prevalence study," *The Lancet*, vol. 370, no. 9589, pp. 741–750, 2007.

[2] European Respiratory Society, *The European Lung White Book*, European Respiratory Society Publications Office, Sheffield, UK, 2013.

[3] V. Jørgen, S. H. Suzanne, G. A. Alvar et al., "Global strategy for diagnosis, management, and prevention of COPD: GOLD executive summary," *American Journal of Respiratory and Critical Care Medicine*, vol. 187, no. 4, pp. 347–365, 2013.

[4] Global Initiative for Chronic Obstructive Pulmonary Disease (GOLD), *Global Strategy for the Diagnosis, Management, and Prevention of Chronic Obstructive Pulmonary Disease*, 2016, http://www.goldcopd.org.

[5] M. Miravitlles, J. Molina, J. A. Quintano, A. Campuzano, J. Perez, and C. Roncero, "Factors associated with depression and severe depression in patients with COPD," *Respiratory Medicine*, vol. 108, no. 11, pp. 1615–1625, 2014.

[6] M. W. Zhang, R. C. Ho, M. W. Cheung, E. Fu, and A. Mak, "Prevalence of depressive symptoms in patients with chronic obstructive pulmonary disease: a systematic review, meta-analysis and meta-regression," *General Hospital Psychiatry*, vol. 33, no. 3, pp. 217–223, 2011.

[7] M. Niti, T.-P. Ng, E. H. Kua, R. C. M. Ho, and C. H. Tan, "Depression and chronic medical illnesses in Asian older adults: the role of subjective health and functional status," *International Journal of Geriatric Psychiatry*, vol. 22, no. 11, pp. 1087–1094, 2007.

[8] Y. Liu, R. C. Ho, and A. Mak, "Interleukin (IL)-6, tumour necrosis factor alpha (TNF-α) and soluble interleukin-2 receptors (sIL-2R) are elevated in patients with major depressive disorder: a meta-analysis and meta-regression," *Journal of Affective Disorders*, vol. 139, no. 3, pp. 230–239, 2012.

[9] M. Emami Ardestani and Z. Omid, "Role of serum interleukin 6, albumin and C-reactive protein in COPD patients," *Tanaffos*, vol. 14, no. 2, pp. 134–140, 2015.

[10] Y. Lu, R. Ho, T. K. Lim et al., "Neuropeptide Y may mediate psychological stress and enhance TH2 inflammatory response in asthma," *Journal of Allergy and Clinical Immunology*, vol. 135, no. 4, pp. 1061–1063, 2015.

[11] A. Blakemore, C. Dickens, E. Guthrie et al., "Depression and anxiety predict health-related quality of life in chronic obstructive pulmonary disease: systematic review and meta-analysis," *International Journal of Chronic Obstructive Pulmonary Disease*, vol. 9, pp. 501–512, 2014.

[12] R. C. Ho, K. K. Mak, A. N. Chua, C. S. Ho, and A. Mak, "The effect of severity of depressive disorder on economic burden in a university hospital in Singapore," *Expert Review of Pharmacoeconomics & Outcomes Research*, vol. 13, no. 4, pp. 549–559, 2013.

[13] N. Molinari, P. Chanez, N. Roche, E. Ahmed, I. Vachier, and A. Bourdin, "Rising total costs and mortality rates associated with admissions due to COPD exacerbations," *Respiratory Research*, vol. 17, no. 1, p. 149, 2016.

[14] P. Garrido, J. de Miguel Díez, R. Gutiérrez et al., "Negative impact of chronic obstructive pulmonary disease on the health-related quality of life of patients. Results of the EPIDEPOC study," *Health Qual Life Outcomes*, vol. 4, pp. 31–33, 2006.

[15] A. S. Pickard, Y. Yang, and T. Lee, "Comparison of health-related quality of life measure in chronic obstructive pulmonary disease," *Health and Quality of Life Outcomes*, vol. 9, p. 26, 2011.

[16] C. Santiveri, M. Espinalt, and F. Carrasco, "Evaluation of male COPD patients' health status by proxies," *Respiratory Medicine*, vol. 101, no. 3, p. 43945, 2007.

[17] Y.-T. Chen and Y.-H. Ying, "Study of patients' willingness to pay for a cure of COPD in Taiwan," *International Journal of Environmental Research and Public Health*, vol. 13, no. 3, p. 273, 2016.

[18] P. Jones, *St. George's Respiratory Questionnaire for COPD Patients (SGRQ- C) Manual*, 2008, http://www.healthstatus.sgul.ac.uk.

[19] P. W. Jones, K. I. Adame, G. Nadean, and N. Banik, "Comparisons of health status scores with MRC grades in COPD: implication for COPD GOLD 2011 clasiff," *European Respiratory Journal*, vol. 42, no. 3, pp. 647–654, 2013.

[20] A. C. Akinci, R. Pinar, and T. Damir, "The relation of the subjective dyspnea perception with objective dyspnea, QoL and functional capacity in patients with COPD," *Journal of Clinical Nursing*, vol. 22, no. 7-8, pp. 969–976, 2013.

[21] P. W. Jones, "COPD assessment test–rationale, development, validation and performance," *COPD*, vol. 10, no. 2, pp. 269–271, 2013.

[22] P. W. Jones, F. H. Quirk, C. M. Baveystock, and P. Littlejohns, "A selfcomplete measure of health status for chronic airflow limitation: the St. George's Respiratory Questionnaire," *American Review of Respiratory Disease*, vol. 145, no. 6, pp. 1321–1327, 1992.

[23] J. Ware and C. D. Sherbourne, "The MOS 36-item short-form health survey (SF-36). I. Conceptual framework and item selection," *Medical Care*, vol. 30, no. 6, pp. 473–483, 1992.

[24] J. C. Bestall, E. A. Paul, R. Garrod, R. Garnham, P. W. Jones, and J. A. Wedzicha, "Usefulness of the Medical Research Council (MRC) dyspnoea scale as a measure of disability in patients with chronic obstructive pulmonary disease," *Thorax*, vol. 54, no. 7, pp. 581–586, 1999.

[25] M. Decramer, W. Janssens, and M. Miravitlles, "Chronic obstructive pulmonary disease," *The Lancet*, vol. 379, no. 9823, pp. 1341–1351, 2012.

[26] H. Doll and M. Miravitlles, "Quality of life in acute exacerbations of chronic bronchitis andchronic obstructive pulmonary disease. A review of the literature," *Pharmacoeconomics*, vol. 23, no. 4, pp. 345–363, 2005.

[27] E. Atlantis, P. Fahey, B. Cochrane, and S. Smith, "Bidirectional associations between clinically relevant depression or anxiety and COPD. A systematics review and meta-analysis," *Chest*, vol. 144, no. 3, pp. 766–777, 2013.

[28] A. I. Papaioannou, K. Bartziokas, S. Tsikrika et al., "The impact of depressive symptoms on recovery and outcomes of hospitalised COPD exacerbations," *European Respiratory Journal*, vol. 41, no. 4, pp. 815–823, 2013.

[29] M. B. Parshall, R. M. Schwartzstein, L. Adams et al., "An official American Thoracic Society Statement: update on mechanisms, assessment, and management of dyspnea," *American Journal of Respiratory and Critical Care Medicine*, vol. 185, no. 4, pp. 435–452, 2012.

[30] N. Roche, N. H. Chavannes, and M. Miravitlles, "COPD symptoms in the morning: impact, evaluation and management," *Respiratory Research*, vol. 14, p. 112, 2013.

[31] K. K. Mak, R. C. Ho, and J. R. Day, "The associations of asthma symptoms with active and passive smoking in Hong Kong adolescents," *Respiratory Care*, vol. 57, no. 9, pp. 1398–1404, 2012.

[32] C. Nowak, A. N. Sievi, F. C. Clarenbach et al., "Accuracy of the Hospital Anxiety and Depression Scale for identifying depression in chronic obstructive pulmonary disease patients," *Pulmonary Medicine*, vol. 2014, Article ID 973858, 7 pages, 2014.

[33] W. K. Tang, E. Wong, H. F. Chiu, C. M. Lum, and G. S. Ungvari, "Examining item bias in the anxiety subscale of the Hospital Anxiety and Depression Scale in patients with chronic obstructive pulmonary disease," *International Journal of Methods in Psychiatric Research*, vol. 17, no. 2, pp. 104–110, 2008.

18

Cost Analysis of Noninvasive Helmet Ventilation Compared with Use of Noninvasive Face Mask in ARDS

Kwadwo Kyeremanteng,[1] Louis-Philippe Gagnon,[2] Raphaëlle Robidoux,[3] Kednapa Thavorn,[4,5,6] Dipayan Chaudhuri,[3] Daniel Kobewka,[7] and John P. Kress[8]

[1]*Department of Medicine, Division of Critical Care, University of Ottawa, Ottawa, ON, Canada*
[2]*Department of Critical Care Medicine, Queen's University, Kingston, ON, Canada*
[3]*University of Ottawa, Ottawa, ON, Canada*
[4]*Clinical Epidemiology Program, The Ottawa Hospital Research Institute, The Ottawa Hospital, Ottawa, ON, Canada*
[5]*School of Epidemiology, Public Health and Preventive Medicine, University of Ottawa, Ottawa, ON, Canada*
[6]*Institute of Clinical and Evaluative Sciences (ICES uOttawa), Ottawa, ON, Canada*
[7]*Department of Medicine, Division of General Internal Medicine, University of Ottawa, Ottawa, ON, Canada*
[8]*University of Chicago Medicine, Chicago, IL, USA*

Correspondence should be addressed to Kwadwo Kyeremanteng; kkyeremanteng@toh.ca

Academic Editor: Inmaculada Alfageme

Intensive care unit (ICU) costs have doubled since 2000, totalling 108 billion dollars per year. Acute respiratory distress syndrome (ARDS) has a prevalence of 10.4% and a 28-day mortality of 34.8%. Noninvasive ventilation (NIV) is used in up to 30% of cases. A recent randomized controlled trial by Patel et al. (2016) showed lower intubation rates and 90-day mortality when comparing helmet to face mask NIV in ARDS. The population in the Patel et al. trial was used for cost analysis in this study. Projections of cost savings showed a decrease in ICU costs by $2527 and hospital costs by $3103 per patient, along with a 43.3% absolute reduction in intubation rates. Sensitivity analysis showed consistent cost reductions. Projected annual cost savings, assuming the current prevalence of ARDS, were $237538 in ICU costs and $291682 in hospital costs. At a national level, using yearly incidence of ARDS cases in American ICUs, this represents $449 million in savings. Helmet NIV, compared to face mask NIV, in nonintubated patients with ARDS, reduces ICU and hospital direct-variable costs along with intubation rates, LOS, and mortality. A large-scale cost-effectiveness analysis is needed to validate the findings.

1. Introduction

Our population is aging, hospital admissions are getting more frequent with a longer length of stay (LOS), intensive care and hospital occupancy rates are climbing, and healthcare-associated expenditures are increasing [1, 2]. Intensive care costs alone totalled 108 billion US dollars in 2010, nearly double that of 2000 (56 billion US dollars). ICU costs account for 13.2% of hospital expenditures and 0.72% of the gross domestic product in the United States, a 32% percent rise from 2000 to 2010 [1, 2]. It is estimated that a single day in the intensive care unit (ICU) costs 2500–4300 US dollars per patient, representing a 61.1% increase in costs over the same time period with the use of new medications, technologies, and specialized care [1–4]. Moving forward, finding ways to reduce ICU costs will reduce the financial burden of increasing utilization of ICU care. New practices focusing on cost-effectiveness will be key by evaluating the effectiveness of the practice on patient outcomes as well as the resources required to implement it [5].

Acute respiratory distress syndrome (ARDS) has a worldwide prevalence of 10.4% in ICUs and an overall 28-day mortality of 34.8% [6]. In the absence of a proven mortality benefit, noninvasive ventilation (NIV) is used in up to 30% of patients with ARDS [6–8]. In June 2016, Patel et al. published the first randomized controlled trial comparing helmet and face mask NIV for patients with ARDS [7]. The patients who received helmet NIV had a reduction in intubation rates, ICU LOS, and 90-day mortality, as well as increased ventilator-free days. Intubation rates were 61.5% in the face mask group, as opposed to 18.2% in the helmet group, giving an absolute risk reduction of 43.3% (95% CI 24.3–62.4%, $p < 0.001$). In fact, the trial was stopped early for efficacy at the first interim analysis after one-third of planned patient enrollment.

Increased ventilator days are associated with longer LOS, higher risk of complications of intubation in ARDS such as pneumonia [9], delirium [10], and ICU-acquired weakness [11], and a higher risk of mortality. Reducing intubation rates is therefore expected to reduce the number of complications and have significant cost savings.

Helmet NIV has been shown to provide similar oxygenation when compared to face mask NIV while providing better patient tolerability, less air leaks, and a universal size independent of facial anatomy [12, 13].

This study was conducted to quantify the potential ICU and hospital cost savings of helmet NIV compared to face mask NIV in ARDS.

2. Methods

The population used to calculate ICU and hospital costs consists of patients with ARDS, treated with face mask or helmet NIV, studied in the randomized controlled trial by Patel et al. [7]. The total and individual patient costs of both study groups were calculated based on their reported ICU and hospital LOS. A cost analysis model proposed by Lord et al. [14] based on cost values published by Kahn et al. [15] was used to estimate average daily cost, which was then multiplied by the LOS values. This model calculates daily direct-variable costs in the ICU and on hospital wards. It assumes that ICU days are more expensive than ward days, that all ward days have the same cost, that the first ICU day is the most expensive, and that the ICU cost decreases daily until day 5. All costs were inflated to 2016 US dollars using the overall consumer price index reported by the Bureau of Labor Statistics [16]. We calculated the difference in costs by subtracting the costs of the helmet NIV group from the face mask NIV group. 95% confidence intervals were estimated using bootstrap resampling procedures with 1000 iterations. Potential cost savings were projected by assuming a 10% prevalence of ARDS, 30% use of NIV in ARDS, and identical cost of purchase of helmet and face mask NIV to then multiply average cost savings per patient with the potential number of ARDS patients per year treated with NIV.

3. Results

For the purpose of this paper, the population examined by Patel et al. was used as the study sample (as detailed in [7]). The total number of patients is 83, 39 of which were treated with face mask NIV, and 44 with helmet NIV. Both groups were comparable in terms of age, severity of illness, medical history, reason for acute respiratory failure, $PaO_2 : FiO_2$ ratio, and the amount of respiratory support on NIV. Outcomes are presented in Table 1. There was a statistically significant reduction in endotracheal intubation (−43.3%, $p < 0.001$) and increase in ventilator-free days (8.4, $p < 0.001$) with helmet NIV. There was also a reduction in ICU LOS, hospital LOS, and 90-day mortality with helmet NIV.

Absolute differences in cost are shown in Table 2. With a significant reduction in ICU and hospital LOS in the helmet NIV group, associated ICU and hospital costs were reduced by 2527 US dollars and 3103 US dollars per patient, respectively. The total cost saving in the care of the helmet NIV group was 71842 US dollars.

A sensitivity analysis was conducted to assess potential variations in ICU and hospital costs, according to varying ICU lengths of stay, for either the face mask or the helmet group, or both. As shown in Table 3, even by increasing the helmet group's ICU LOS, helmet NIV consistently represented a cost-saving method to treat patients with ARDS. For example, a one-day increase in ICU LOS for the helmet group and a steady ICU LOS for the face mask group lead to a reduction in ICU and hospital costs of 1712 US dollars and 2288 US dollars per patient, respectively, favoring helmet NIV. To note, these analyses manipulated LOS regardless of outcome, which was expected to remain stable across groups throughout the sensitivity analysis. However, as helmet NIV group patients are expected to show a greater proportion of successful outcomes, the sensitivity analysis may be seen as conservative in the magnitude of the advantage it indicates for helmet use.

4. Discussion

This cost analysis shows a consistent reduction in cost associated with the use of helmet NIV in the ARDS population studied by Patel et al. [7] along with a reduction in intubation rates, LOS, and mortality. Potential savings could be illustrated despite variations in LOS with the sensitivity analysis, and these savings were extrapolated to differing volumes of ARDS. This analysis represents an important step in finding a cost-efficient, well-tolerated, and easily applicable way to deliver care to patients with ARDS who are not intubated at the time of assessment and admission to the ICU. As mentioned, this represents up to 30% of patients with ARDS. Importantly, single interventions with a mortality benefit in the care of ICU patients such as this one are uncommon [17].

The magnitude of potential savings at a national level is immense. 5.7 million patients are admitted to an ICU each year in the United States [18], and 10.4% of them are assumed to have ARDS [6]. This corresponds to 592800 patients who are admitted with ARDS yearly. Assuming that up to 30% of these patients are treated with NIV, which is to say 177840 patients, the use of the helmet interface would lead to potential total savings of 449 million US dollars when compared to the face mask interface.

Limitations to this cost analysis lie in the assumptions of the model. Firstly, calculations were based on a randomized and controlled, but single-center, unblended, and small study population. This center was also accustomed to using

Table 1: Outcomes and adverse events in the Patel et al. [7] study.

	Face mask ($n = 39$)	Helmet ($n = 44$)	Absolute difference (95% CI)	p value
Primary outcomes, n (%)				
Endotracheal intubation	24 (61.5)	8 (18.2)	−43.3 (−62.4 to −24.3)	<0.001
Reason for intubation				
Respiratory failure	20 (83.3)	3 (37.5)	−45.3 (−82.5 to −9.1)	0.01
Circulatory failure	3 (12.5)	0 (0)	−12.5 (−25.7 to 0.7)	0.55
Neurologic failure	1 (4.2)	5 (62.5)	58.3 (24.8 to 92.8)	0.001
Secondary outcomes, median (IQR), days				
Ventilator-free days	12.5 (0.49 to 28)	28 (13.7 to 28)	8.4 (13.4 to 3.4)	<0.001
ICU LOS	7.8 (3.9 to 13.8)	4.7 (2.5 to 8.7)	−2.76 (−6.07 to 0.54)	0.04
Hospital LOS	15.2 (7.8 to 19.7)	10.1 (6.5 to 15.9)	−2.92 (−8.47 to 2.63)	0.16
Mortality, n (%)				
Hospital	19 (48.7)	12 (27.3)	−21.4 (−41.9 to −1.0)	0.04
90 days	22 (56.4)	15 (34.1)	−22.3 (−43.3 to −1.4)	0.02
Adverse events				
Mask deflation	0 (0)	2 (4.5)		
Skin ulceration	3 (7.6)	3 (6.8)		

Table 2: Cost analysis of ARDS population treated with NIV in the Patel et al. [7] study (95% CI) per patient.

	Face mask ($n = 39$)	Helmet ($n = 44$)	Absolute difference (95% CI)
ICU LOS (days)	7.8 (3.9–13.8)	4.7 (2.5–8.7)	—
ICU cost (US dollars)	10773	8246	2527 (2251–2817)
Hospital LOS (days)	15.2 (7.8–19.7)	10.1 (6.5–15.9)	—
Hospital cost (US dollars)	12938	9835	3103 (2829–3392)
Total direct-variable cost for cohort (US dollars)	504582	432740	71842 (69895–73740)

Table 3: Sensitivity analysis assuming variability in ICU LOS in different NIV study groups.

		ICU costs (US dollars)			Hospital costs (US dollars)		
		Face mask	Helmet	Absolute difference	Face mask	Helmet	Absolute difference
Change in ICU LOS (days)	Affected study population						
+1	Face mask	11588	8246	3342	13765	9835	3930
	Helmet	10773	9061	1712	12938	10650	2288
	Face mask and helmet	11588	9061	2527	13765	10650	3115
−1	Face mask	9958	8246	1712	12135	9835	2300
	Helmet	10773	7380	3393	12938	8968	3970
	Face mask and helmet	9958	7380	2578	12135	8968	3167

the helmet NIV interface. In order to avoid unwarranted variability, centers unaccustomed to the use of helmet NIV would need to be included in future studies, to avoid selection bias based on established experience with the interface. Secondly, costs were obtained from a model developed from a separate single-center's financial data. In order to establish that helmet NIV is a truly cost-effective way of treating nonintubated patients with ARDS, a large multicenter health economic evaluation, comparing costs and outcomes of the helmet to the face mask NIV, interfaces would need to be done. Hospitals would track direct costs concurrently and include the cost of the apparatus of NIV (face masks, helmets, etc.) in the analyses, in order to provide exact rather than projected costs. It would not be possible to perform a blinded study as patients and healthcare providers would evidently notice with which group of NIV delivery they were interacting. However, the bias of not being blinded is unlikely to affect results due to the presence of objective indications for intubation and progression of respiratory illness. Also this study's costing methods do not incorporate major cost drivers such as extracorporeal membrane oxygenation (ECMO) or renal replacement therapy, which may be seen in severe cases of ARDS.

It is noteworthy that the majority of costs in the ICU are fixed. An intervention such as the use of helmet NIV in ARDS has the potential to decrease direct-variable ICU costs, which usually account for 20% of yearly ICU expenses. Savings in direct-variable costs would create opportunities to fund other initiatives such as early mobility, which has been shown to increase ventilator-free days and functional outcomes as well as decreasing LOS [19–22].

5. Conclusion

The use of the helmet NIV interface, when compared to the face mask interface in the management of nonintubated patients with ARDS, reduces intubation rates and mortality, as well as ICU and hospital costs. The savings from such an intervention are potentially immense from a national standpoint, and they represent an opportunity to re-distribute direct-variable ICU funds to other evidence-based beneficial therapies, such as early mobility initiatives.

Future studies could conduct a cost-effectiveness analysis comparing cost and health outcomes associated with each NIV interface. Cost-effectiveness analyses are crucial to minimize preventable expenses and ensure sustainability in the health sector, an ever-growing need in today's climate. These analyses could be incorporated in large-scale trials looking at new interventions and clinical guideline development by focusing on cost effectiveness. They could also be integrated in the comparison of two or more therapies with already established benefits for the same disease or syndrome. A relevant example is that of the comparison of outcomes and costs associated with the use of helmet NIV and high-flow nasal oxygen in acute hypoxic respiratory failure. Those potential studies would enrich this domain of research even further and contribute to build a more sustainable healthcare system for aging populations.

Authors' Contributions

Kwadwo Kyeremanteng wrote the article, performed analysis, reviewed the original material, and contributed to manuscript development. Louis-Philippe Gagnon wrote the article and performed analysis. Raphaëlle Robidoux wrote the article and Kednapa Thavorn performed analysis. Dipayan Chaudhuri and Daniel Kobewka contributed in press and manuscript development.

Acknowledgments

The authors acknowledge the work done by Patel, Wolfe, Pohlman, Hall, and Kress in the original study used for analysis of cost benefits.

References

[1] N. A. Halpern, D. A. Goldman, K. S. Tan, and S. M. Pastores, "Trends in critical care beds and use among population groups and medicare and medicaid beneficiaries in the United States: 2000–2010," *Critical Care Medicine*, vol. 44, no. 8, pp. 1490–1499, 2016.

[2] N. A. Halpern and S. M. Pastores, "Critical care medicine in the United States 2000–2005: an analysis of bed numbers, occupancy rates, payer mix, and costs," *Critical Care Medicine*, vol. 38, no. 1, pp. 65–71, 2010.

[3] E. B. Milbrandt, A. Kersten, M. T. Rahim et al., "Growth of intensive care unit resource use and its estimated cost in medicare," *Critical Care Medicine*, vol. 36, no. 9, pp. 2504–2510, 2008.

[4] J. M. Kahn and D. C. Angus, "Reducing the cost of critical care: new challenges, new solutions," *American Journal of Respiratory and Critical Care Medicine*, vol. 174, no. 11, pp. 1167-1168, 2006.

[5] A. S. Detsky and I. G. Naglie, "A clinician's guide to cost-effectiveness analysis," *Annals of Internal Medicine*, vol. 113, no. 2, pp. 147–154, 1990.

[6] G. Bellani, J. G. Laffey, T. Pham et al., "Epidemiology, patterns of care, and mortality for patients with acute respiratory distress syndrome in intensive care units in 50 countries," *JAMA*, vol. 315, no. 8, pp. 788–800, 2016.

[7] B. K. Patel, K. S. Wolfe, A. S. Pohlman, J. B. Hall, and J. P. Kress, "Effect of noninvasive ventilation delivered by helmet vs. face mask on the rate of endotracheal intubation in patients with acute respiratory distress syndrome: a randomized clinical trial," *JAMA*, vol. 315, no. 22, pp. 2435–2441, 2016.

[8] A. W. Thille, D. Contou, C. Fragnoli et al., "Non-invasive ventilation for acute hypoxemic respiratory failure: intubation rate and risk factors," *Critical Care*, vol. 17, no. 6, p. R269, 2013.

[9] American Thoracic Society and Infectious Diseases Society of America, "Management of adults with hospital-acquired and ventilator-associated pneumonia: 2016 Clinical Practice Guidelines by the Infectious Diseases Society of America and the American Thoracic Society," *Clinical Infectious Diseases*, vol. 63, no. 5, pp. e61–e111, 2016.

[10] E. W. Ely, A. Shintani, B. Truman et al., "Delirium as a predictor of mortality in mechanically ventilated patients in the intensive care unit," *JAMA*, vol. 291, no. 14, pp. 1753–1762, 2004.

[11] J. P. Kress and J. B. Hall, "ICU-acquired weakness and recovery from critical illness," *New England Journal of Medicine*, vol. 370, no. 17, pp. 1626–1635, 2014.

[12] T. Principi, S. Pantanetti, F. Catani et al., "Noninvasive continuous positive airway pressure delivered by helmet in hematological malignancy patients with hypoxemic acute respiratory failure," *Intensive Care Medicine*, vol. 30, no. 1, pp. 147–150, 2004.

[13] E. Rodriguez, P. J. Papadakos, M. Carron, R. Cosentini, and D. Chiumello, "Clinical review: helmet and non-invasive mechanical ventilation in critically ill patients," *Critical Care*, vol. 17, no. 2, p. 223, 2013.

[14] R. K. Lord, C. R. Mayhew, R. Korupolu et al., "ICU early physical rehabilitation programs: financial modeling of cost savings," *Critical Care Medicine*, vol. 41, no. 3, pp. 717–724, 2013.

[15] J. M. Kahn, G. D. Rubenfeld, J. Rohrbach, and B. D. Fuchs, "Cost savings attributable to reductions in intensive care unit length of stay for mechanically ventilated patients," *Medical Care*, vol. 46, no. 12, pp. 1226–1233, 2008.

[16] M. Crawford, J. Church, and B. Akin, *Consumer Price Index Detailed Report Data for June 2016*, Bureau of Labor Statistics, Washington, DC, USA, 2016, http://www.bls.gov/cpi/#publications.

[17] G. Landoni, M. Comis, M. Conte et al., "Mortality in multicenter critical care trials: an analysis of interventions with a significant effect," *Critical Care Medicine*, vol. 43, no. 8, pp. 1559–1568, 2015.

[18] M. L. Barrett, M. W. Smith, A. Elixhauser, L. S. Honigman, and J. M. Pines, *Utilization of Intensive Care Services, 2011. Healthcare Cost and Utilization Project*, 2014, http://hcup-us.ahrq.gov/reports/statbriefs/sb185-Hospital-Intensive-Care-Units-2011.jsp.

[19] W. D. Schweickert, M. C. Pohlman, A. S. Pohlman et al., "Early physical and occupational therapy in mechanically ventilated, critically ill patients: a randomised controlled trial," *The Lancet*, vol. 373, no. 9678, pp. 1874–1882, 2009.

[20] Z. Li, X. Peng, B. Zhu, Y. Zhang, and X. Xi, "Active mobilization for mechanically ventilated patients: a systematic review," *Archives of Physical Medicine and Rehabilitation*, vol. 94, no. 3, pp. 551–561, 2013.

[21] J. Adler and D. Malone, "Early mobilization in the intensive care unit: a systematic review," *Cardiopulmonary Physical Therapy Journal*, vol. 23, no. 1, pp. 5–13, 2012.

[22] M. Malkoc, D. Karadibak, and Y. Yildirim, "The effect of physiotherapy on ventilatory dependency and the length of stay in an intensive care unit," *International Journal of Rehabilitation Research*, vol. 32, no. 1, pp. 85–88, 2009.

19

Feasibility and Safety of Pleuroscopic Cryobiopsy of the Pleura: A Prospective Study

Chia-Hung Chen,[1,2,3] Wen-Chien Cheng,[1,4,5] Biing-Ru Wu,[1] Chih-Yu Chen,[1,4,5] Wei-Chun Chen,[1,4,5] Wei-Chih Liao,[1,3,5] and Chih-Yen Tu[1,4,6]

[1]*Division of Pulmonary and Critical Care Medicine, Department of Internal Medicine, China Medical University Hospital, Taichung, Taiwan*
[2]*Department of Respiratory Therapy, China Medical University, Taichung, Taiwan*
[3]*Graduate Institute of Clinical Medical Science, China Medical University, Taichung, Taiwan*
[4]*School of Medicine, China Medical University, Taichung, Taiwan*
[5]*Department of Internal Medicine, Hyperbaric Oxygen Therapy Center, China Medical University, Taichung, Taiwan*
[6]*Department of Life Science, National Chung Hsing University, Taichung, Taiwan*

Correspondence should be addressed to Chih-Yen Tu; chesttu@gmail.com

Academic Editor: Fu-Tsai Chung

Background. The aim of this study was thus to evaluate the feasibility and safety of taking biopsy specimens by cryoprobe from the parietal pleura during semirigid pleuroscope. *Methods.* In a single-center, observational, prospective study, patients with exudative pleural effusion (EPE) were evaluated with a semirigid pleuroscope between January 2015 and July 2017. Each patient underwent pleural biopsy using flexible forceps and flexible cryoprobe through pleuroscope following diagnostic thoracentesis and closed pleural biopsy (CPB). *Results.* A total of 92 patients (median age 64 years) were included in the study, most of whom were men (65.2%). Cytological cell block (CCB) and CPB made definitive diagnoses in 32/92 (34.8%) and 25/92 (27.5%), respectively; flexible forceps biopsy (FFB) and cryoprobe biopsy (CB) established definitive diagnoses in 84/92 (91.3%) and 91/92 (98.9%), respectively. The sample obtained by CB (9.4 ± 4.9 mm) was significantly larger than the other two methods: FFB (4.2 ± 2.3 mm) or CPB (1.9 ± 1.0 mm) ($P < 0.0001$). The immunohistochemical (IHC) staining was more easily performed with CB (98.9%) compared to either FFB (87.0%) or CPB (13.0%). There were no significant complications or procedure-related deaths. *Conclusions.* Based on these results, CB during semirigid pleuroscope has a high diagnostic yield, differentiating EPE of unknown etiology with satisfactory effectiveness and safety.

1. Introduction

Over fifty different pleuropulmonary or systemic disorders can cause pleural effusions. Following diagnostic thoracentesis and closed pleural biopsy (CPB), up to 25 percent of patients remain undiagnosed [1, 2]. Medical thoracoscopy increases the diagnostic yield in these cases because it offers the clinician a "window" for direct visualization and collection of samples from the parietal pleura [3]. Rigid thoracoscopy, with or without video assistance has traditionally been the procedure of choice [4]. A now widely available alternative to the conventional rigid thoracoscope is the semirigid fiber-optic video pleuroscope [5, 6], which has good sensitivity (91%) and specificity (100%) in the diagnosis of exudative pleural effusions (EPEs) and good positive and negative likelihood ratios (4.92 and 0.08, resp.) [7]. A semirigid pleuroscope can also be used therapeutically to aspirate pleural fluid or to separate pleural adhesions [8].

However, the obtained biopsy samples by semirigid pleuroscope are small and insufficient depth due to lack of mechanical power and the small size of the cup of the biopsy forceps [7, 9]. This results in concerns about diagnostic adequacy, especially in patients with significantly thickened pleura, and for this reason, new biopsy instruments are needed. Biopsy via cryoprobe, first used in 1968, has mainly been employed in the management of obstructive endobronchial tumors. Recently, cryotherapy in bronchoscopy has been used for several purposes including management of endobronchial tuberculosis [10], endobronchial tumors [11–13], for diagnosis of interstitial lung disease (ILD) [14–17], and peripheral lung lesion [18]. These studies have demonstrated that the cryoprobe is feasible and a more efficient diagnostic tool with a superior diagnostic rate and ability to obtain a larger specimen with better preserved cellular architecture than forceps biopsy.

There has been an increasing interest in the feasibility and safety of pleural cryobiopsy (CB) during semirigid pleuroscope. Several studies have shown that CB during flexi-rigid pleuroscope is feasible, safe, and effective [19–21]. However, most of these studies were conducted either with small populations or retrospectively. This prospective study thus aimed to evaluate the efficacy and safety of CB during semirigid pleuroscope in diagnosis of EPE. We also assessed the diagnostic yield of CB, quality of biopsy tissue obtained, and feasibility of immunohistochemistry (IHC) staining, in a comparison with conventional methods (CCB, CPB, and FFB).

2. Patients and Methods

The study was performed prospectively between January 2015 and July 2017 at the department of the Division of Pulmonary and Critical Care Medicine in the China Medical University Hospital, which is a 2,146-bed community-based university hospital in Taichung, Taiwan. The study was approved by the China Medical University Hospital Internal Review Board (CMUH103-REC1-112), and written informed consent was obtained from all patients.

2.1. Enrolled Patients. The patients were recruited from inpatient clinics if they met the following criteria: (1) age >18 years, (2) presence of unilateral pleural effusion of unknown origin after less invasive means of diagnosis, and (3) presence of advanced epidermal growth factor receptor (EGFR) mutation positive nonsmall cell lung cancer (NSCLC), (4) clinical resistance to an EGFR tyrosine kinase inhibitor (TKI) (gefitinib, erlotinib, or afatinib), and (5) undergoing a repeat biopsy for tumor genotyping as part of their routine clinical care. Patients with the following criteria were excluded: (1) a tendency for uncontrolled bleeding, (2) unstable cardiovascular status or severe heart failure, unstable hemodynamic status, (3) Eastern Cooperative Oncology Group performance status 4, and (4) persistent hypoxemia.

2.2. Instruments. The instrument that we used was the autoclavable Olympus LTF-240 (Olympus, Tokyo, Japan) semirigid pleuroscope with 2.8 mm inner channel diameter. FFB of the parietal pleural was taken with flexible FB-35C-1 Olympus forceps with cusps being 2.4 mm for the outer diameter and a length of 3.5 mm; the CB sample was obtained using a flexible cryoprobe with a 1.9 mm diameter and a 900 mm length (20416-037, Erbokryo CA, Erbe, Germany) and the CPB sample was sampled via Abram's needle (Figure 1).

2.3. Procedure. We performed diagnostic pleuroscopy in bronchoscopy suite on a spontaneous breathing patient. Bedside thoracic ultrasound was performed prior to the procedure to establish the optimal entry point. The patient was positioned in the lateral decubitus with the involved side upward. Topical anesthesia was achieved by 2% lidocaine mixed with adrenaline, applied subcutaneously and throughout the chest wall to the parietal pleura. Patients received intravenous midazolam for analgesia with sedation. Patients' blood pressure, pulse rate, and saturation were continuously monitored. Supplemental oxygen was given during the procedure. Initially, CPB with Abram's needle was performed before trocar insertion. All pleural fluid was removed after insertion of the semirigid pleuroscope, and the pleural space was thoroughly inspected. Suspected lesions in parietal pleural nodules were taken by flexible forceps biopsy and cryoprobe biopsy. Four sample specimens from CPB, forceps biopsy, and cryoprobe biopsy were taken in each patient. To avoid selection bias, we used forceps biopsy and cryoprobe pleural biopsy in the same parietal pleural nodule. A 14F chest tube was placed at the end of the procedure, and a chest radiograph was obtained afterwards. The drainage amount of pleural effusion and duration of procedures from semirigid pleuroscope insertion to final withdrawal were recorded.

2.4. Tissue Sampling and Complications. CPB was performed prior to the insertion of the semirigid pleuroscope. After giving local anesthesia at a suitable location at the dorsolateral thoracic wall, pleural fluid was sampled via Abram's needle, and four biopsy specimens were taken with an inward motion of the closed biopsy punch.

Conventional FFB was obtained using flexible biopsy forceps that could be accommodated within the working channel of the semirigid pleuroscope. CB was performed following the pleural biopsy using FFB. The cryoprobe tip was applied to the area of parietal pleura to be biopsied, and the cryoprobe was activated for ~3 s by a foot-switch activation mechanism. The probe tip cooled to −89.5°C within seconds after activation. The semirigid pleuroscope and the probe, with the biopsied pleural tissue attached to it, were then withdrawn together. Each biopsy sample was released from the probe by thawing in saline, and then the sample was fixed in formalin. Four biopsy specimens were taken in all procedures.

The biopsy sites were assessed for bleeding each time before further biopsies were performed. The degree of bleeding at the biopsy site was assessed as follows: nil = slight, self-limited; mild bleeding = requiring vasoactive drug (adrenaline) injection; and moderate to severe bleeding = requiring electrocautery or argon plasma coagulation (APC) intervention.

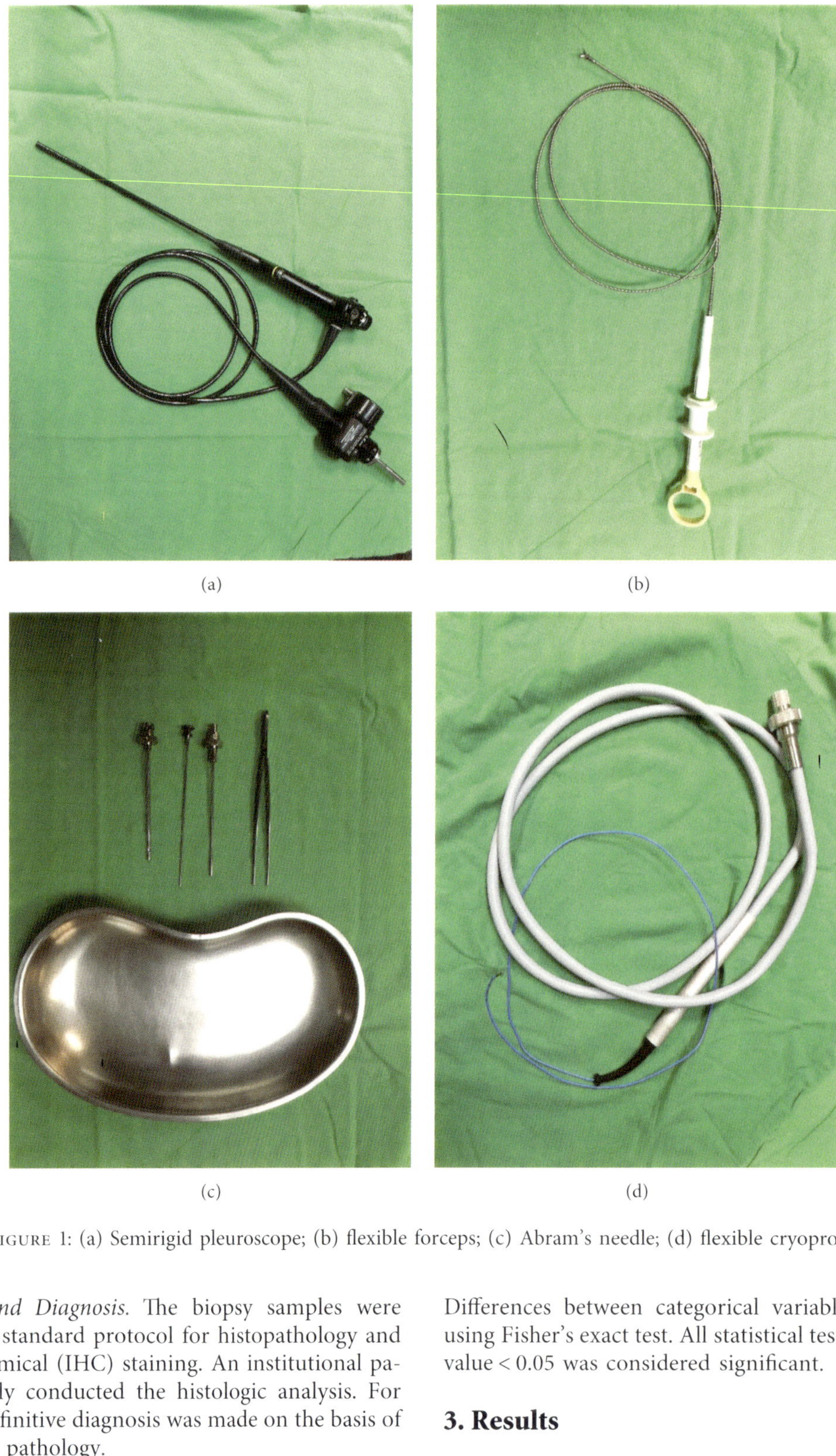

Figure 1: (a) Semirigid pleuroscope; (b) flexible forceps; (c) Abram's needle; (d) flexible cryoprobe.

2.5. Pathology and Diagnosis. The biopsy samples were processed as per standard protocol for histopathology and immunohistochemical (IHC) staining. An institutional pathologist routinely conducted the histologic analysis. For each patient, a definitive diagnosis was made on the basis of the results of the pathology.

2.6. Statistical Analysis. The data were analyzed using SPSS for Windows, version 17.0 (Chicago, IL, USA). Continuous variables were reported as means ± SDs and were compared using 2-tailed Student's t-tests. Categorical variables were reported as the numbers of patients and percentages. Differences between categorical variables were evaluated using Fisher's exact test. All statistical tests were 2 sided; a P value < 0.05 was considered significant.

3. Results

3.1. Characteristics of the Patients and Pleural Effusion. A total 92 patients (32 women, 60 men) with a median age of 64 years (range 22–92) were included in the study (Table 1). Eighty-three patients underwent semirigid pleuroscope for workup of an undiagnosed pleural effusion, and 9 patients with EGFR mutation NSCLC and clinical resistance to an EGFR TKI underwent repeat biopsy for tumor genotyping

TABLE 1: Characteristics of the patients.

Characteristics	Medical pleuroscopy patients ($n = 92$)
Age	64.8 ± 13.9
Sex (n, %)	
Male	60 (65.2)
Female	32 (34.8)
Underlying disease (n, %)	
None	35 (38.0)
Malignancy	26 (28.3)
DM	11 (12.0)
ESRD	5 (5.4)
CHF	5 (5.4)
Reason for medical pleuroscopy (n, %)	
Unknown pleural effusion	83 (90.2)
Rebiopsy	9 (9.8)

by semirigid pleuroscope. The samples were obtained using all techniques (CPB, FFB, and CB). Cytological cell block (CCB) was also analyzed in the diagnosis of pleural effusions. Pleural malignancy (47 lung adenocarcinoma, 1 large cell carcinoma, 2 squamous cell carcinoma, 3 lymphoma, 2 mesothelioma, 2 nasopharyngeal cancer, 2 breast cancer, 2 thyroid cancer, 2 colon cancer, 1 cholangiocarcinoma, 1 angiosarcoma, 1 gastric cancer, 1 cervix cancer, 1 sarcomatoid carcinoma, and 1 urothelial carcinoma) was diagnosed in 69 patients, and benign pleural diseases (8 tuberculosis pleuritic, 2 autoimmune pleuritic, and 13 chronic pleuritic) were diagnosed in 23 patients (Table 2). The average duration of the procedure was 34.2 min (±8.6 min), and the average drainage amount of pleural effusion was 1059 ml (±757 ml). The average duration of chest tube drainage was 2.6 days (±2.4 days), and the average length of stay after procedure was 2.4 days (±2.6 days). There were no deaths within 30 days after the procedure.

TABLE 2: Characteristics of the pleural effusion.

Characteristics	Medical pleuroscopy patients ($n = 92$)
Etiology for pleural effusion	
Malignancy	69 (75)
Lung adenocarcinoma	47 (51.1)
Lung large cell carcinoma	1 (1)
Lung squamous cell carcinoma	2 (2.2)
Lymphoma	3 (3.3)
Mesothelioma	2 (2.2)
Nasopharyngeal cancer	2 (2.2)
Breast cancer	2 (2.2)
Thyroid cancer	2 (2.2)
Colon cancer	2 (2.2)
Sarcomatoid carcinoma	1 (1)
Cholangiocarcinoma	1 (1)
Cervix cancer	1 (1)
Urothelial carcinoma	1 (1)
Gastric cancer	1 (1)
Angiosarcoma	1 (1)
Benign	23 (25)
TB	8 (8.7)
Autoimmune related	2 (2.2)
Chronic pleuritic	13 (14.1)
Drainage amount (ml)	1059 ± 757
Duration of procedure (minutes)	34.2 ± 8.6
Duration of subsequent chest drainage (days)	2.6 ± 2.4
Length of stay after procedure (days)	2.4 ± 2.6
30 days mortality	0

3.2. Diagnostic Yield and Sample Quality. The diagnostic yield was 32/92 (34.8%) in CCB. The CPB yielded a definitive histopathological diagnosis in 25/92 (27.1%) patients. FFB was able to establish a definitive diagnosis in 84/92 (91.3%) patients. A diagnosis from CB was made in 91/92 (98.9%) patients. Evaluation of the 92 patients revealed an advantage for the new technique over conventional technique, with the achieved diagnostic yields of CB being significantly higher than the other three methods of FFB, CPB, and CCB ($P = 0.017$, $P < 0.001$, and $P < 0.001$ resp.). The immunohistochemical (IHC) staining was feasible in CB samples, identifying 91/92 (98.9%) patients with a definite diagnosis, which was significantly higher than that of the other three methods of FFB (80/92, 87.0%, $P = 0.001$), CPB (12/92, 13.0%, $P < 0.0001$), and CCB (12/92, 13.0%, $P < 0.0001$) samples (Table 3). The sizes of specimens obtained by CB (9.4 mm ± 4.9 mm) were significantly bigger than those of the either CPB (1.9 mm ± 1.0 mm) or FFB (4.2 mm ± 2.3 mm) ($P < 0.0001$). Moreover, the CB specimens tended to be artifacts that were less crushed and had better tissue integrity (Figures 2 and 3).

3.3. Complications. The safety data are reported in Table 3. All the procedures were generally well tolerated by the patients. There were no significant complications reported in any patient following the procedures. Mild bleeding, requiring vasoactive drug (adrenaline) injection, was observed in both groups (6/92 patients after FFB and 8/92 patients after CB). No moderate to severe bleeding requiring electrocautery or APC intervention occurred.

4. Discussion

This was a prospective, single-center, controlled study evaluating the novel CB technique in comparison with conventional technique using CCB, CPB, and FB in the diagnosis of EPE during semirigid pleuroscopy. Our study showed that CB during semirigid pleuroscopy was a safe technique with a higher diagnostic yield (98.9%) for the diagnosis of EPE. In addition, IHC staining may be easily

Table 3: The diagnostic yield, size, and quality of samples and complications.

Semirigid pleuroscope patients ($n = 51$)	Close pleural biopsy	Flexible forceps biopsy	Cryoprobe biopsy	Cytology cell block
Diagnostic yield	25 (27.1)	84 (91.3)	91 (98.9)	32 (34.8)
For IHC stain	12 (13.0)	80 (87.0)	91 (98.9)	12 (13.0)
Size, mm	1.9 ± 1.0	4.2 ± 2.3	9.4 ± 4.9	—
Complication				
Bleeding				
Nil	92	86	84	0
Mild	0	6	8	0
Moderate to severe	0	0	0	0

Nil bleeding: slight, self-limited; mild bleeding: needing bosmin injection; moderate to severe: needing coagulation or APC. P value of diagnostic yield: close pleural biopsy versus flexible forceps biopsy: <0.0001; close pleural biopsy versus cryoprobe biopsy: <0.0001; close pleural biopsy versus cytology cell block: 0.929; flexible forceps biopsy versus cryoprobe biopsy: 0.017. P value of IHC stain: close pleural biopsy versus flexible forceps biopsy: <0.0001; close pleural biopsy versus cryoprobe biopsy: <0.0001; close pleural biopsy versus cytology cell block: 0.998; flexible forceps biopsy versus cryoprobe biopsy: 0.001. P value of size: close pleural biopsy versus flexible forceps biopsy: <0.0001; close pleural biopsy versus cryoprobe biopsy: <0.0001; flexible forceps biopsy versus cryoprobe biopsy: <0.0001.

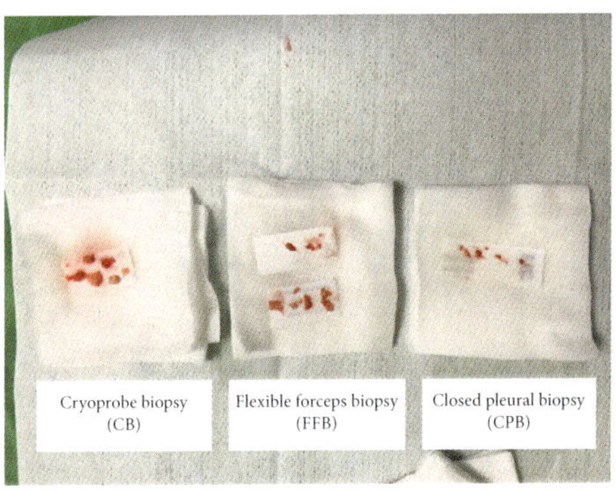

Figure 2: The pleural biopsy obtained by CB had larger tissue size with better tissue integrity compared to the other two methods.

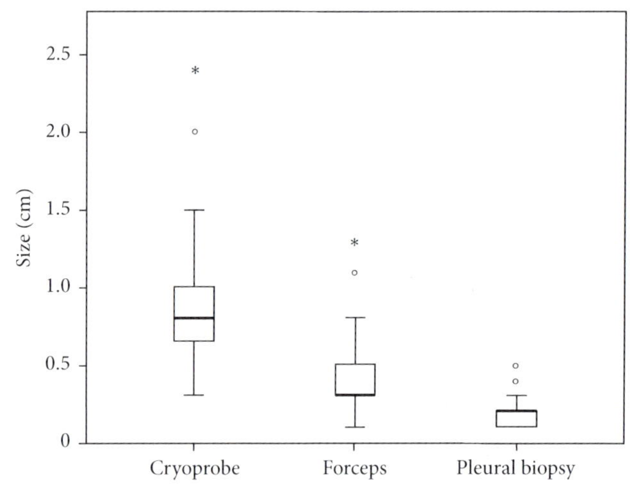

Figure 3: The sample obtained by CB (9.1 ± 4.5 mm) was significantly bigger than the other two methods: FFB (4.0 ± 2.1 mm) or CPB (1.9 ± 1.0 mm) ($P < 0.0001$).

performed in samples obtained by CB (98.9%). Our explanation for this is that CB samples (9.4 mm ± 4.9 mm) are larger and have better tissue integrity than samples from the other techniques. Most importantly, there were no significant complications after CB, with the occurrence of mild bleeding after biopsy being similar in CB and FFB.

Medical thoracoscopy is a useful, effective, and safe method for investigating and managing undiagnosed EPE [22]. It can be performed using either a rigid thoracoscope or a semirigid pleuroscope [3]. Although the samples obtained by semirigid pleuroscope were smaller than those from the rigid thoracoscope, there were no differences in the quality and interpretability of the specimens assessed by the pathologist. In other words, both approaches provide comparable diagnostic yields [9, 23]. However, taking adequate samples from thickened pleura (e.g., in mesothelioma and fibrothorax) remains the most important limitation of the semirigid pleuroscope. This was not only a difficult but also time-consuming task due to the lack of mechanical power and the small size of the cup of the flexible forceps.

In addition, the histological finding of 'nonspecific pleuritis' is common in thoracoscopic forceps biopsies, and their false-negative rate for the detection of pleural malignancy has been determined to be around 5%, with the most frequent false-negative diagnosis being mesothelioma [2, 24, 25]. The mean interval between nondiagnostic thoracoscopy and the final diagnosis was 9.8 (±4.6) months [24], and for mesothelioma, the interval was 8.7 months [26]. To overcome the limitation of small biopsies by semirigid pleuroscope, CB may be another choice. In our study, only one patient (1.1%) without definitive diagnosis which was diagnosed mesothelioma by surgery. As cancer therapy becomes more individualized, larger and better quality tissue obtained at biopsy might facilitate mutational analysis and genetic profiling [27]. Therefore, 9 patients with EGFR mutation lung adenocarcinoma and having clinical resistance to an EGFR TKI underwent repeat biopsy for tumor genotyping by cryoprobe biopsy during semirigid pleuroscopy. CB successfully obtained pleural tissue suitable for histopathological analysis in all 9 patients.

Cryotherapy in bronchoscopy has been used for diagnosis and management of endobronchial lesion [11–14, 28, 29]. Endobronchial CB is safe and increases the diagnostic yield in comparison with conventional FB [11, 30, 31]. The overall superiority of CB is most likely due to the higher quality of the

Table 4: Comparison with similar studies.

Medical pleuroscopy patients ($n = 51$)	Rozman et al. [19]	Thomas et al. [18]	Maturu et al. [20]	Our study
Number of subjects	15	22	6	92
Age	61 (33–83)	72 (47–89)	50 (29–61)	64 (22–92)
Sex (male : female)	12 : 3	21 : 1	4 : 2	2 : 1
Quality of sample				
Size (mm) (CB versus FB)	NA	10 versus 4	9.2 versus 3.7	9.4 versus 4.2
Artifacts on histology				
CB	6/14	2/22	0/6	NA
FB	NA	21/22	3/4	NA
Diagnostic yield				
CB	14/14	20/22	6/6	91/92
FB	15/15	20/22	3/4	84/92
Final diagnosis of mesothelioma	9	11	0	0
Bleeding (CB versus FB)				
Nil	0	17 versus 18	NA	84 versus 86
Mild	14 versus 15	5 versus 4	NA	8 versus 6
Moderate to severe	0	0	0	0

NA: not available.

samples from their significantly larger biopsies regarding size and artifact-free tissue sections, which has been shown in previous studies [14, 28, 31, 32]. The cryotherapy probe also facilitates sampling of target lesions positioned tangentially to the instrument, which are difficult than samples from flexible forceps, especially in narrow airway. The potential advantages of this method are the shortening of the duration of the procedure and avoidance of repeated biopsy-related complications [30].

A number of recent studies have assessed the feasibility and safety of pleural CB during semirigid pleuroscopy. These results are summarized in Table 4. Rozman et al. demonstrated that the samples were of good quality (81% were easily interpretable), with the level of artifacts below 25%. The specimens were adequate for histological diagnosis, IHC staining, and DNA isolation, and a definitive diagnosis was achieved in 20/22 (90%) of the subjects undergoing CB and FFB [20]. Thomas et al. reported that CB (10 mm, 7–15.8) was larger than FFB (4 mm, 3–8) and had better preserved cellular architecture and tissue integrity. Crushed artifacts were less common with CB (2/22) compared with FFB (21/22), and both FFB and CB made definitive diagnoses in 15/15 (100%) and 14/14 (100%) [19]. Maturu et al. also showed that CB was significantly larger ($P = 0.001$) when compared with FFB (9.17 ± 1.84 versus 3.75 ± 0.96 mm), and that crushed artifacts were more frequent with FFB as compared with CB (3/4 versus 0/6). Similarly, the depth of tissue was greater with the cryoprobe. It revealed a higher diagnostic yield for CB (6/6) compared to FFB (3/4) [21]. The present study demonstrated that CB was significantly larger ($P < 0.0001$) when compared with FFB (9.1 ± 4.5 mm versus 4.0 ± 2.1 mm). IHC stains were more easily performed with CB as compared with FFB (91/92 versus 80/91), though not reaching statistical significance. CB has proven to have excellent tissue quality for IHC [28], and we found that the diagnostic yield was higher (but not statistically significant) with CB (50/51) than with FFB (47/51). In the case of the accuracy of diagnosis, it is well known that quality of the specimen is important. Although CB reduces the histological finding of "nonspecific pleuritic," which presents a management dilemma for clinicians, the diagnostic yield of CB was comparable to FFB based on the abovementioned studies. These findings may be explained by the fact that these studies were small and thickened pleura pathologies were lacking in two of the studies.

In spite of the above-favorable evidence, the cryotherapy probe has not been routinely used as a biopsy instrument mainly because of concerns that the immediate pulling of a frozen probe could lead to significant complications, such as bleeding. Rozman et al. reported the assessed degree of bleeding was slight and self-limited, as expected after biopsy and no further interventions were needed [20]. Thomas et al. indicated that mild bleeding was observed in their FFB (4/22) group and CB (5/22) group [19]. Our study also indicated that the incidence of mild bleeding was similar between the CB group (8/92) and FB group (6/92). We did not observe any other complications. These findings also accord with previous studies [19, 20] that found CB during flexi-rigid pleuroscopy was safe.

In spite of our careful study design, we acknowledge a number of limitations in our study. First, only 92 patients were enrolled in our study in a single hospital. Second, the CB was taken after conventional FFB. Bleeding may not be fairly evaluated when samples from the same lesion were taken by CB and FFB. Third, for patients with thickened pleural pathologies where FFB biopsy alone might lead to a false-negative result, no additional diagnostic benefits were found for CB over conventional FFB; one explanation for this is that subjects with mesothelioma or fibrotic pleural pathologies were lacking in our study.

5. Conclusions

The results of the present study may be summarized as CB during semirigid pleuroscope is a safe and feasible technique and it has a diagnostic yield for the diagnosis of undiagnosed EPE that is comparable to conventional pleural biopsy using FFB. CB was also easier to interpret by the pathologist because of the larger tissue samples with better preserved cellular architecture. Larger randomized trials and multicenter studies are required for further evaluation of the routine use of CB during semirigid pleuroscopy.

Abbreviations

EPE: Exudative pleural effusion
CB: Cryoprobe biopsy
CPB: Closed pleural biopsy
CCB: Cytological cell block
FFB: Flexible forceps biopsy
IHC: Immunohistochemical
APC: Argon plasma coagulation
ILD: Interstitial lung disease
NSCLC: Nonsmall cell lung cancer
EGFR: Epidermal growth factor receptor
TKI: Tyrosine kinase inhibitor.

Disclosure

This study was presented as poster in 2017 European Respiratory Society International Congress [33] and in the 40th Annual Meeting of the Japan Society for Respiratory Endoscopy [34].

References

[1] T. R. Collins and S. A. Sahn, "Thoracocentesis: clinical value, complications, technical problems, and patient experience," *Chest*, vol. 91, no. 6, pp. 817–822, 1987.

[2] L. N. Venekamp, B. Velkeniers, and M. Noppen, "Does 'idiopathic pleuritis' exist? Natural history of non-specific pleuritis diagnosed after thoracoscopy," *Respiration*, vol. 72, no. 1, pp. 74–78, 2005.

[3] P. Lee and H. G. Colt, "Rigid and semirigid pleuroscopy: the future is bright," *Respirology*, vol. 10, no. 4, pp. 418–425, 2005.

[4] P. Lee and H. G. Colt, "Pleuroscopy in 2013," *Clinics in Chest Medicine*, vol. 34, no. 1, pp. 81–91, 2013.

[5] B. Thangakunam, DJ. Christopher, P. James, and R. Gupta, "Semi-rigid thoracoscopy: initial experience from a tertiary care hospital," *Indian Journal of Chest Diseases and Allied Sciences*, vol. 52, no. 1, pp. 25–27, 2010.

[6] Z. Wang, Z. H. Tong, H. J. Li et al., "Semi-rigid thoracoscopy for undiagnosed exudative pleural effusions: a comparative study," *Chinese Medical Journal*, vol. 121, no. 15, pp. 1384–1389, 2008.

[7] R. Agarwal, A. N. Aggarwal, and D. Gupta, "Diagnostic accuracy and safety of semirigid thoracoscopy in exudative pleural effusions: a meta-analysis," *Chest*, vol. 144, no. 6, pp. 1857–1867, 2013.

[8] A. N. McLean, S. R. Bicknell, L. G. McAlpine, and A. J. Peacock, "Investigation of pleural effusion: an evaluation of the new Olympus LTF semiflexible thoracofiberscope and comparison with Abram's needle biopsy," *Chest*, vol. 114, no. 1, pp. 150–153, 1998.

[9] A. Rozman, L. Camlek, M. Marc-Malovrh, N. Triller, and I. Kern, "Rigid versus semi-rigid thoracoscopy for the diagnosis of pleural disease: a randomized pilot study," *Respirology*, vol. 18, no. 4, pp. 704–710, 2013.

[10] E. Q. Fu, Y. D. Nan, F. G. Jin, and A. Q. Ma, "Therapeutic effects of sequential therapy by electric coagulation, cryotherapy and balloon dilation with an electronic video bronchoscope," *Experimental and Therapeutic Medicine*, vol. 5, no. 6, pp. 1649–1656, 2013.

[11] Z. Aktas, E. Gunay, N. T. Hoca et al., "Endobronchial cryobiopsy or forceps biopsy for lung cancer diagnosis," *Annals of Thoracic Medicine*, vol. 5, no. 4, pp. 242–246, 2010.

[12] M. Hetzel, J. Hetzel, C. Schumann, N. Marx, and A. Babiak, "Cryorecanalization: a new approach for the immediate management of acute airway obstruction," *Journal of Thoracic and Cardiovascular Surgery*, vol. 127, no. 5, pp. 1427–1431, 2004.

[13] M. O. Maiwand and G. Asimakopoulos, "Cryosurgery for lung cancer: clinical results and technical aspects," *Technology in Cancer Research and Treatment*, vol. 3, no. 2, pp. 143–150, 2004.

[14] A. Babiak, J. Hetzel, G. Krishna et al., "Transbronchial cryobiopsy: a new tool for lung biopsies," *Respiration*, vol. 78, no. 2, pp. 203–208, 2009.

[15] G. L. Casoni, S. Tomassetti, A. Cavazza et al., "Transbronchial lung cryobiopsy in the diagnosis of fibrotic interstitial lung diseases," *PLoS One*, vol. 9, no. 2, article e86716, 2014.

[16] O. Fruchter, L. Fridel, B. A. El Raouf, N. Abdel-Rahman, D. Rosengarten, and M. R. Kramer, "Histological diagnosis of interstitial lung diseases by cryo-transbronchial biopsy," *Respirology*, vol. 19, no. 5, pp. 683–688, 2014.

[17] V. Pajares, C. Puzo, D. Castillo et al., "Diagnostic yield of transbronchial cryobiopsy in interstitial lung disease: a randomized trial," *Respirology*, vol. 19, no. 6, pp. 900–906, 2014.

[18] M. Schuhmann, K. Bostanci, A. Bugalho et al., "Endobronchial ultrasound-guided cryobiopsies in peripheral pulmonary lesions: a feasibility study," *European Respiratory Journal*, vol. 43, no. 1, pp. 233–239, 2014.

[19] R. Thomas, S. Karunarathne, B. Jennings et al., "Pleuroscopic cryoprobe biopsies of the pleura: a feasibility and safety study," *Respirology*, vol. 20, no. 2, pp. 327–332, 2015.

[20] A. Rozman, L. Camlek, M. Marc Malovrh, I. Kern, and N. Schonfeld, "Feasibility and safety of parietal pleural cryobiopsy during semi-rigid thoracoscopy," *Clinical Respiratory Journal*, vol. 10, no. 5, pp. 574–578, 2015.

[21] V. N. Maturu, I. S. Sehgal, S. Dhooria et al., "Pleuroscopic cryobiopsy: case series and systematic review," *Journal of Bronchology and Interventional Pulmonology*, vol. 22, no. 3, pp. e11–e13, 2015.

[22] F. Rodriguez-Panadero, "Medical thoracoscopy," *Respiration*, vol. 76, no. 4, pp. 363–372, 2008.

[23] M. A. Khan, S. Ambalavanan, D. Thomson, J. Miles, and M. Munavvar, "A comparison of the diagnostic yield of rigid and semirigid thoracoscopes," *Journal of Bronchology and Interventional Pulmonology*, vol. 19, no. 2, pp. 98–101, 2012.

[24] H. E. Davies, J. E. Nicholson, N. M. Rahman, E. M. Wilkinson, R. J. Davies, and Y. C. Lee, "Outcome of patients with

nonspecific pleuritis/fibrosis on thoracoscopic pleural biopsies," *European Journal of Cardio-Thoracic Surgery*, vol. 38, no. 4, pp. 472–477, 2010.

[25] J. S. Ferrer, X. G. Munoz, R. M. Orriols, R. W. Light, and F. B. Morell, "Evolution of idiopathic pleural effusion: a prospective, long-term follow-up study," *Chest*, vol. 109, no. 6, pp. 1508–1513, 1996.

[26] J. P. Janssen, S. Ramlal, and M. Mravunac, "The long-term follow up of exudative pleural effusion after nondiagnostic thoracoscopy," *Journal of Bronchology*, vol. 11, no. 3, pp. 169–174, 2004.

[27] M. Tiseo, G. Rossi, M. Capelletti et al., "Predictors of gefitinib outcomes in advanced non-small cell lung cancer (NSCLC): study of a comprehensive panel of molecular markers," *Lung Cancer*, vol. 67, no. 3, pp. 355–360, 2010.

[28] J. Hetzel, M. Hetzel, C. Hasel, P. Moeller, and A. Babiak, "Old meets modern: the use of traditional cryoprobes in the age of molecular biology," *Respiration*, vol. 76, no. 2, pp. 193–197, 2008.

[29] L. Yarmus, J. Akulian, C. Gilbert et al., "Cryoprobe transbronchial lung biopsy in patients after lung transplantation: a pilot safety study," *Chest*, vol. 143, no. 3, pp. 621–626, 2013.

[30] J. Hetzel, R. Eberhardt, F. J. Herth et al., "Cryobiopsy increases the diagnostic yield of endobronchial biopsy: a multicentre trial," *European Respiratory Journal*, vol. 39, no. 3, pp. 685–690, 2012.

[31] C. Schumann, J. Hetzel, A. J. Babiak et al., "Cryoprobe biopsy increases the diagnostic yield in endobronchial tumor lesions," *Journal of Thoracic and Cardiovascular Surgery*, vol. 140, no. 2, pp. 417–421, 2010.

[32] K. J. Franke, M. Szyrach, G. Nilius et al., "Experimental study on biopsy sampling using new flexible cryoprobes: influence of activation time, probe size, tissue consistency, and contact pressure of the probe on the size of the biopsy specimen," *Lung*, vol. 187, no. 4, pp. 253–259, 2009.

[33] C. H. Chen, W. H. Cheng, B. R. Wu et al., "Feasibility and safety of pleuroscopic cryobiopsy of the pleura: a prospective study," in *Proceedings of the 2017 European Respiratory Society International Congress*, Milan, Italy, September 2017.

[34] C. H. Chen, W. H. Cheng, B. R. Wu et al., "Feasibility and safety of pleuroscopic cryobiopsy of the pleura: a prospective study," in *Proceedings of the 40th Annual Meeting of the Japan Society for Respiratory Endoscopy*, Nagasaki, Japan, June 2017.

20

Daytime Sleepiness in Patients Diagnosed with Sarcoidosis Compared with the General Population

Andreas Hinz[1] **Kristina Geue,**[1] **Markus Zenger,**[2,3] **Hubert Wirtz,**[4] **and Andrea Bosse-Henck**[4]

[1]*Department of Medical Psychology and Medical Sociology, University of Leipzig, Leipzig, Germany*
[2]*Faculty of Applied Human Studies, University of Applied Sciences Magdeburg and Stendal, Stendal, Germany*
[3]*Integrated Research and Treatment Center (IFB) Adiposity Diseases-Behavioral Medicine, Medical Psychology and Medical Sociology, University of Leipzig, Leipzig, Germany*
[4]*Department of Respiratory Medicine, University of Leipzig, Leipzig, Germany*

Correspondence should be addressed to Andreas Hinz; andreas.hinz@medizin.uni-leipzig.de

Academic Editor: Pierachille Santus

Background. The aim of this study was to analyze daytime sleepiness in a sample of patients diagnosed with sarcoidosis. *Methods.* A sample of 1197 German sarcoidosis patients was examined with the Epworth Sleepiness Scale (ESS), the Fatigue Assessment Scale, the Hospital Anxiety and Depression Scale, the Pittsburgh Sleep Quality Index, and the Short-Form Health Survey (SF-8). The patients' ESS mean scores were compared with those obtained from a large general population sample. *Results.* Exactly 50% of the patients reached the criterion (ESS > 10) for excessive daytime sleepiness, compared with only 22.1% in the general population. The effect size for the mean score difference between both samples was $d = 0.62$. The number of affected organs and the number of concomitant diseases proved to be significant independent predictors of daytime sleepiness. Sleepiness was associated with fatigue ($r = 0.45$), anxiety ($r = 0.23$), depression ($r = 0.28$), sleep problems ($r = 0.23$), and detriments in physical ($r = -0.29$) and mental ($r = -0.28$) quality of life. *Conclusions.* The issue of excessive daytime sleepiness should be considered in the management of sarcoidosis.

1. Introduction

Sarcoidosis is a multisystem inflammatory disease, characterized by epitheloid granulomas [1]. Almost all organs of the body can be involved, but the lungs are the most frequently affected organ. Sarcoidosis patients suffer from a broad spectrum of symptoms such as muscle pain, weight loss, fever, night sweats, cough, breathlessness, and reduced exercise capacity, which results in reduced quality of life (QoL) [2, 3]. Fatigue is a symptom that is particularly prevalent in these patients [4]. This symptom is associated with poor sleep quality and excessive daytime sleepiness (EDS), which is defined as difficulty in maintaining an alert awake state in everyday situations [5]. EDS is associated with insomnia [6], obstructive sleep apnea [7], cognitive impairment [8, 9], cardiovascular diseases [10, 11], psychiatric disorders [12, 13], and low socioeconomic status [14]. The relationship between daytime sleepiness and QoL is less clear. A general population study [15] found small but consistent associations between daytime sleepiness and both physical and mental components of QoL, while among patients suffering from obstructive sleep apnea [16] daytime sleepiness was associated with physical but not mental QoL. Several studies have been performed to analyze fatigue [17, 18] and poor sleep quality [19] in patients suffering from sarcoidosis, but the role daytime sleepiness plays in sarcoidosis patients is largely unknown.

The instrument most often used for measuring daytime sleepiness is the Epworth Sleepiness Scale (ESS) [20]. Convergent, discriminant [21], and ecological validity [22] of the scale have been proved. The items of the ESS were included in the item banks of the Patient-Reported Outcomes Measurement

Information System (PROMIS) "sleep disturbance and sleep-related" [23]. Using the ESS, a British study [24] compared sarcoidosis patients with healthy controls and found markedly elevated levels of daytime sleepiness among the sarcoidosis patients ($M = 8.0$ versus $M = 4.7$ in the ESS); however, the sample sizes were low (73 sarcoidosis patients and 82 controls), and the controls were not representative of the general population.

The aims of this study were (a) to determine the degree of EDS in sarcoidosis patients in comparison with the general population and to test psychometric properties of the ESS in a large sample of sarcoidosis patients, (b) to analyze the impact of affected organs and concomitant diseases on EDS, and (c) to investigate associations between daytime sleepiness and QoL.

2. Methods

2.1. Study Participants. All members of the German Sarcoidosis Society ($n = 4100$) were invited to take part in the study and received a booklet with several questionnaires, along with the regular newsletter. Among other scales, the booklet included the ESS. The study was approved by the Ethics Committee of the Medical Faculty of the University of Leipzig. All participating individuals gave informed consent. The inclusion criteria were a diagnosis of sarcoidosis, age 18 years and above, and the willingness to take part in the study.

The scores of the general population were taken from a recent large normative study ($n = 9711$) also performed in Germany [25]. We had access to the original data and selected a random subsample ($n = 7990$) so that the gender distribution (65.5% women) and the mean age ($M = 54.2$ years) were nearly identical with the sample of the sarcoidosis patients.

2.2. Instruments. The ESS [20, 26] was designed to quantify a person's likelihood of falling asleep in several everyday situations and the degree to which sleepiness interferes with their daytime functioning. Eight items have to be answered on a four-point scale. The ESS total score is the sum of the ratings of the items, and it can range from 0 to 24. Scores of 11 and above are frequently considered indicative of EDS [27]. German normative values of the ESS are available [25].

In addition to the ESS, several other questionnaires were used in this study: the Pittsburgh Sleep Quality Index (PSQI) [28], the Fatigue Assessment Scale (FAS) [29], the Hospital Anxiety and Depression Scale (HADS) [30], and the quality of life instrument Short Form Health Survey (SF-8) [31]. Furthermore, self-reported clinical variables (affected organs, concomitant diseases, time since diagnosis, and therapy) were obtained.

2.3. Statistical Techniques. Because the proportion of females in the patients' sample was higher than in the normative study, we calculated weighted means for items and sum scores of the general population with the weights corresponding to the gender distribution of the patients' sample to enable unbiased comparisons. The resulting general population means are therefore slightly different from those reported for the total general population study. Group differences in ESS mean scores were statistically tested with t-tests. Effect sizes d were used to express the mean score difference, related to the pooled standard deviation [32]. A multiple regression analysis (method = enter) was performed to test the combined influence of several predictors of EDS. All calculations were performed with SPSS version 20.

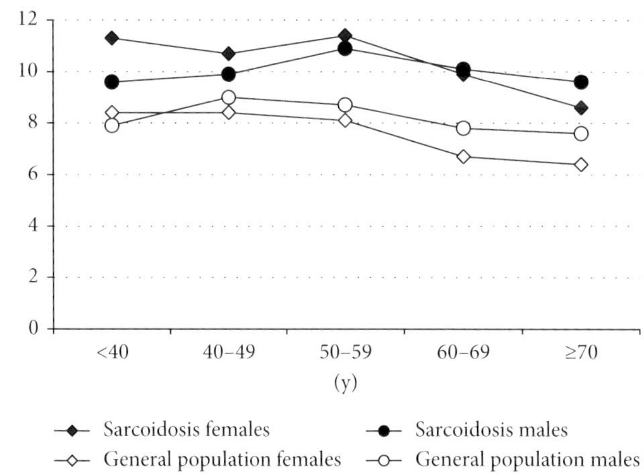

FIGURE 1: ESS mean scores for sarcoidosis patients and the general population, broken down by gender and age groups.

3. Results

3.1. Sample Characteristics. Of the 4100 patients invited to participate, 1270 (31%) returned the questionnaire. 73 of these questionnaires could not be used because of missing data. In total, data from 1197 participants were ultimately included in the analysis. The sample consisted of 783 females (65.4%) and 414 males with an overall mean age of 54.3 ± 11.6 years. The mean time since first diagnosis was 12.8 years (range, 0–64 years). 542 patients (45.3%) were receiving steroid therapy at the time of the survey. The most often affected organs were lungs (89.2%), followed by skin (24.5%) and lymphatic nodes (20.8%). In 39.7% of the patients, only one organ was affected, 28.2% had two affected organs, and 32.1% reported at least three affected organs.

3.2. EDS Mean Scores Compared with the General Population. Figure 1 shows ESS mean scores of the patients and the general population [25]. There was no consistent gender difference between the male and the female patients. In the first three age decades, female patients reported more EDS than male patients, while the trend was opposite for the age groups 60–69 years and ≥70 years.

Every age group of sarcoidosis patients reported higher levels of EDS compared with the general population (Figure 1). The mean of the male patients was 10.18 ± 4.77, while the corresponding mean of the female patients was somewhat higher (10.56 ± 4.91), resulting in a total mean score of 10.43 ± 4.87 of the patients. The corresponding mean scores of the general population were 8.26 ± 3.53 (males) and 7.55 ± 3.77 (females). This results in effect sizes of $d = 0.45$ (males) and

Table 1: ESS items and global mean scores.

	Patients		General population		d	p	r_{it}	Alpha del.
	M	(SD)	M	(SD)				
1 Sitting/reading	1.43	(1.01)	1.09	(0.89)	0.36	<0.001	0.63	0.78
2 Watching TV	1.97	(0.99)	1.77	(0.93)	0.21	<0.001	0.49	0.81
3 Public place	1.21	(0.97)	0.92	(0.82)	0.32	<0.001	0.66	0.78
4 Car passenger	1.21	(1.05)	0.81	(0.92)	0.41	<0.001	0.56	0.80
5 Afternoon	2.41	(0.85)	2.06	(0.91)	0.40	<0.001	0.36	0.82
6 Sitting/talking to someone	0.39	(0.60)	0.13	(0.40)	0.52	<0.001	0.58	0.80
7 After lunch	1.45	(1.02)	1.01	(0.87)	0.47	<0.001	0.61	0.79
8 Traffic	0.32	(0.62)	0.14	(0.41)	0.35	<0.001	0.48	0.81
ESS total score	10.43	(4.87)	7.95	(3.73)	0.58	<0.001	–	0.82

Note. M: mean; SD: standard deviation; d: effect size; *p*: significance; r_{it}: part-whole-corrected test-item correlation; alpha del.: Cronbach's alpha if item is deleted.

$d = 0.71$ (females) for the comparison between sarcoidosis patients and the general population; the effect size of the total sample was $d = 0.62$.

Expressed in terms of patients with scores above the cutoff point for excessive daytime sleepiness (ESS > 10), the percentages were 48.1% for the male patients and 51.0% for the female patients. The corresponding percentages from the general population were 25.0% (males) and 20.6% (females) [25]. In the total sample of the sarcoidosis patients, 598 (50.0%) of the 1197 patients had scores above the cutoff point, while the corresponding percentage in the general population was 22.1%.

3.3. Item Analyses. Item mean scores are presented in Table 1. As in the general population, the afternoon is the situation with the highest chance to fall asleep. In all eight items, the patients reported more sleepiness than the general population. All items positively contributed to the ESS total score. The reliability (Cronbach's alpha) of the ESS was 0.82.

3.4. Effect of Clinical Variables on ESS. Table 2 shows the impact of the affected organs on EDS, expressed in univariate analyses. The sequence of the organs is arranged according to the frequency with which they were affected by the disease. Muscles and bones are the organs with the highest effect sizes. Among the concomitant diseases, sleep apnea was most strongly associated with EDS ($d = 0.61$). There was no statistical significant association between time since diagnosis and daytime sleepiness. Participants receiving steroid therapy were significantly more affected by daytime sleepiness than participants without that therapy.

The results of the multivariate analysis are presented in Table 3. The number of affected organs as well as the number of concomitant diseases proved to be independent factors for predicting EDS. The multiple r of this analysis was 0.21.

3.5. Associations between Daytime Sleepiness and Other Scales. The correlations between the ESS and other scales are given in Table 4. The strongest association was found for fatigue ($r = 0.44$). All the coefficients were statistically significant with $p < 0.001$.

4. Discussion

Excessive daytime sleepiness is common among patients suffering from sarcoidosis. Exactly 50% of the sarcoidosis patients fulfilled the criterion of EDS, while only 22.1% of the adult general population reported experiencing EDS. The effect size of the mean score difference was $d = 0.62$. Half a standard deviation ($d = 0.50$) is a frequently used criterion for clinical relevance [33]. The burden of EDS is prevalent in all age groups to a similar degree. Female patients were slightly more affected by EDS than males, though most normative studies [25,34–36] found higher degrees of sleepiness among males.

The ESS proved to be a reliable instrument for measuring EDS in sarcoidosis patients, and the alpha coefficient (0.82) was even higher than the coefficients obtained in other studies [37, 38]. All items contributed positively to the total score, and all items showed a statistically significant difference between the patients and the general population.

If the burden of patients is to be assessed in relation to the burden perceived by healthy controls, it is possible to examine a specifically selected sample of healthy controls or to refer to normative values. We used the second approach, which is more convenient and which provides more profound comparisons. The study with sarcoidosis and idiopathic pulmonary fibrosis patients [24], for example, included a control group of 82 persons with an ESS mean score of 4.7 and a HADS depression mean score of 2.1 which are markedly below the normative scores obtained in larger general population studies. Using such healthy controls can lead to an overestimation of the differences to the patient groups and to an imprecise estimation of the disease burden.

Among the affected organs, muscles and bones were seen to have the highest impact on EDS. A compromised musculoskeletal system may lead to physical inactivity and lack of exercise [39], and a low degree of physical fitness may be associated with EDS. Sarcoidosis patients experience improvements in fatigue levels when they participate in physical exercise programs [40], and they should be encouraged to be

Table 2: The association between clinical variables and daytime sleepiness.

Organs/comorbidity		N	M ± SD	d	t	p
Organs						
Lungs	Yes	1086	10.5 ± 4.8	0.12	1.08	0.279
	No	111	9.9 ± 5.0			
Skin	Yes	293	10.9 ± 4.9	0.13	1.85	0.065
	No	904	10.3 ± 4.8			
Lymphatic nodes	Yes	249	11.0 ± 4.9	0.14	2.06	0.040
	No	948	10.3 ± 4.9			
Eyes	Yes	191	10.4 ± 5.0	0.00	0.25	0.804
	No	1006	10.4 ± 4.8			
Liver	Yes	141	11.1 ± 5.0	0.16	1.87	0.062
	No	1056	10.3 ± 4.8			
Muscles	Yes	113	12.1 ± 5.1	0.37	3.87	<0.001
	No	1084	10.3 ± 4.8			
Nerves	Yes	108	11.0 ± 5.3	0.12	1.29	0.196
	No	1089	10.4 ± 4.8			
Bones	Yes	105	12.0 ± 5.2	0.34	3.39	0.001
	No	1092	10.3 ± 4.8			
Heart	Yes	95	10.9 ± 4.8	0.10	1.08	0.281
	No	1102	10.4 ± 4.9			
Kidneys	Yes	60	10.7 ± 5.2	0.06	0.49	0.622
	No	1037	10.4 ± 4.8			
Number of organs	<3	813	10.1 ± 4.8	0.23	3.81	<0.001
	≥3	384	11.2 ± 4.9			
Comorbidity						
Arterial hypertension[a]	Yes	452	10.6 ± 5.0	0.06	1.02	0.306
	No	738	10.3 ± 4.8			
Disease of thyroid gland[a]	Yes	320	10.6 ± 5.0	0.06	0.99	0.323
	No	869	10.3 ± 4.8			
Obesity (BMI ≥30)[a]	Yes	320	11.3 ± 5.0	0.24	3.87	<0.001
	No	875	10.1 ± 4.8			
Restless legs syndrome[a]	Yes	186	11.4 ± 5.2	0.24	3.00	0.003
	No	998	10.2 ± 4.8			
Diabetes mellitus[a]	Yes	134	10.9 ± 5.2	0.10	1.26	0.209
	No	1060	10.4 ± 4.8			
Sleep apnea[a]	Yes	104	13.1 ± 5.0	0.61	5.95	<0.001
	No	1084	10.1 ± 4.8			
Pulmonary hypertension[a]	Yes	38	10.9 ± 5.5	0.10	0.67	0.503
	No	1138	10.4 ± 4.8			
Number of concomitant diseases	<3	1002	10.1 ± 4.8	0.40	4.30	<0.001
	≥3	195	12.1 ± 5.1			
Time since diagnosis and therapy						
Time since diagnosis[a]	≤10 y	625	10.7 ± 4.8	0.10	1.72	0.086
	>10 y	566	10.2 ± 5.0			
Steroid therapy	Yes	542	10.8 ± 4.9	0.14	2.62	0.009
	No	655	10.1 ± 4.8			

Note. d: effect size; t: t value of the t-test; p: significance; [a]case numbers not added to 1197 due to missing values.

physically active even when they are bothered by EDS. However, it should be taken into account that patients whose muscles or bones are affected often have other affected organs too, and that the mean number of concomitant diseases is higher in these patient subgroups.

Concomitant diseases have an impact on EDS, in particular sleep apnea (effect size $d = 0.61$). This corresponds to the findings of other studies [41–43]. Sleep apnea is an interruption of sleep due to the collapse of upper airways, and it can lead to hypoxic episodes. This reduced sleep quality is also associated with daytime sleepiness. The number of affected organs as well as the number of comorbidities proved to be independent prognostic factors for EDS in the multiple regression analysis. This indicates that there are additive effects of the affected organs and concomitant diseases which should be taken into account when treating this patient population. The frequency of several concomitant diseases in the patients' sample was

Table 3: Demographic and medical factors as predictors of EDS.

	B	SE (B)	Beta	T	*p*
Affected organs (sum)	0.399	0.102	0.116	3.933	<0.001
Comorbidity (sum)	0.545	0.117	0.141	4.652	<0.001
Age	−0.054	0.012	−0.128	4.294	<0.001
Sex (female)	0.030	0.296	0.003	0.101	0.920

Table 4: Correlations between the ESS and other scales.

Scale	*r*
PSQI	
Sleep problems	0.23
FAS	
Fatigue	0.44
HADS	
Anxiety	0.23
Depression	0.28
SF-8	
Physical functioning	−0.28
Role-physical	−0.32
Bodily pain	−0.25
General health	−0.25
Vitality	−0.27
Social functioning	−0.30
Role-emotional	−0.32
Mental health	−0.26
Physical component score	−0.29
Mental component score	−0.28

higher than in the general population. Therefore, it is difficult to clarify which proportion of the heightened EDS level is due to sarcoidosis itself and which proportion can be attributed to comorbidity. However, even if the causal relationship between sarcoidosis and comorbidity is unclear, clinicians should know that patients with sarcoidosis experience heightened levels of daytime sleepiness. The clinicians should advise their patients to maintain correct sleep hygiene.

Patients receiving steroid therapy were more strongly affected by EDS than patients without that therapy (Table 2). However, even the patients not receiving steroid therapy had markedly higher daytime sleepiness scores ($M = 10.1$) than people from the general population ($M = 7.95$). This means that sarcoidosis itself (and not the therapy) is the main reason for the heightened levels of sleepiness.

All correlations between the ESS scores and the QoL and mental health scales were statistically significant and clinically meaningful. The strongest association was found with fatigue ($r = 0.45$) which underlines the impact of EDS on symptoms such as fatigue. Consistent with the Chinese [15] and the German [25] general population study, daytime sleepiness was associated with both physical and mental components of QoL, and the correlations with the physical component score ($r = -0.28$) and the mental component score ($r = -0.29$) were nearly identical. This might help explain the strong association with fatigue, a concept which also consists of both physical and mental components. This cross-sectional study does not allow for drawing conclusions about causality. EDS might cause fatigue and vice versa.

Some *limitations* of the study should be noted. The presence of sarcoidosis in the sample was not determined by clinical diagnosis, and all clinical data were self-reported. The representativeness of the patients' sample is difficult to assess, thus possibly introducing a selection bias. The univariate analyses presented in Table 2 do not take into account the combined effects of affected organs and concomitant diseases.

In summary, EDS is a problem for one out of every two sarcoidosis patients. Not only sleep quality and depression but also daytime sleepiness should be considered when treating patients suffering from sarcoidosis.

Acknowledgments

The authors thank the German Sarcoidosis Association for its support to the study.

References

[1] D. Valeyre, A. Prasse, H. Nunes et al., "Sarcoidosis," *The Lancet*, vol. 383, no. 9923, pp. 1155–1167, 2014.

[2] J. de Vries and M. Drent, "Quality of life and health status in sarcoidosis: a review of the literature," *Clinics in Chest Medicine*, vol. 29, no. 3, pp. 525–532, 2008.

[3] M. A. Judson, "Quality of life in sarcoidosis," *Seminars in Respiratory and Critical Care Medicine*, vol. 38, no. 4, pp. 546–558, 2017.

[4] W. P. E. de Kleijn, J. de Vries, E. E. Lower et al., "Fatigue in sarcoidosis: a systematic review," *Current Opinion in Pulmonary Medicine*, vol. 15, no. 5, pp. 499–506, 2009.

[5] American Academy of Sleep Medicine, *International Classification of Sleep Disorders*, American Academy of Sleep Medicine, Darien, IL, USA, 3rd edition, 2005.

[6] C. L. Drake, I. Vargas, T. Roth et al., "Quantitative measures of nocturnal insomnia symptoms predict greater deficits across multiple daytime impairment domains," *Behavioral Sleep Medicine*, vol. 13, no. 1, pp. 73–87, 2015.

[7] J. A. Cvengros, V. M. Rodríguez, S. Snyder et al., "An adaptive treatment to improve positive airway pressure (PAP) adherence in patients with obstructive sleep apnea: a proof of concept trial," *Behavioral Sleep Medicine*, vol. 15, no. 5, pp. 345–360, 2017.

[8] I. Jaussent, J. Bouyer, M. L. Ancelin et al., "Excessive sleepiness is predictive of cognitive decline in the elderly," *Sleep*, vol. 35, no. 9, pp. 1201–1207, 2012.

[9] E. Byun, J. Kim, and B. Riegel, "Associations of subjective sleep quality and daytime sleepiness with cognitive impairment in adults and elders with heart failure," *Behavioral Sleep Medicine*, vol. 15, no. 4, pp. 302–317, 2017.

[10] A. B. Newman, C. F. Spiekerman, P. Enright et al., "Daytime sleepiness predicts mortality and cardiovascular disease in older adults: the Cardiovascular Health Study Research Group,"

Journal of the American Geriatrics Society, vol. 48, no. 2, pp. 115–123, 2000.

[11] I. Jaussent, J. P. Empana, M. L. Ancelin et al., "Insomnia, daytime sleepiness and cardio-cerebrovascular diseases in the elderly: a 6-year prospective study," *PLoS One*, vol. 8, no. 2, Article ID e56048, 2013.

[12] I. Jaussent, J. Bouyer, M. L. Ancelin et al., "Insomnia and daytime sleepiness are risk factors for depressive symptoms in the elderly," *Sleep*, vol. 34, no. 8, pp. 1103–1110, 2011.

[13] T. H. Ng, K.-F. Chung, C.-T. Lee et al., "Eveningness and its associated impairments in remitted bipolar disorder," *Behavioral Sleep Medicine*, vol. 14, no. 6, pp. 650–664, 2016.

[14] D. C. Jarrin, J. J. McGrath, J. E. Silverstein et al., "Objective and subjective socioeconomic gradients exist for sleep quality, sleep latency, sleep duration, weekend oversleep, and daytime sleepiness in adults," *Behavioral Sleep Medicine*, vol. 11, no. 2, pp. 144–158, 2013.

[15] S. Wu, R. Wang, X. Ma et al., "Excessive daytime sleepiness assessed by the Epworth Sleepiness Scale and its association with health related quality of life: a population-based study in China," *BMC Public Health*, vol. 12, no. 1, p. 849, 2012.

[16] W. Lee, S.-A. Lee, H. U. Ryu et al., "Quality of life in patients with obstructive sleep apnea: relationship with daytime sleepiness, sleep quality, depression, and apnea severity," *Chronic Respiratory Disease*, vol. 13, no. 1, pp. 33–39, 2016.

[17] M. Drent, E. E. Lower, and J. D. Vries, "Sarcoidosis-associated fatigue," *European Respiratory Journal*, vol. 40, no. 1, pp. 255–263, 2012.

[18] B. Strookappe, J. de Vries, M. Elfferich et al., "Predictors of fatigue in sarcoidosis: the value of exercise testing," *Respiratory Medicine*, vol. 116, pp. 49–54, 2016.

[19] A. Bosse-Henck, H. Wirtz, and A. Hinz, "Subjective sleep quality in sarcoidosis," *Sleep Medicine*, vol. 16, no. 5, pp. 570–576, 2015.

[20] M. W. Johns, "A new method for measuring daytime sleepiness–the Epworth Sleepiness Scale," *Sleep*, vol. 14, no. 6, pp. 540–545, 1991.

[21] B. Kaambwa, C. Mpundu-Kaambwa, R. Adams et al., "Suitability of the Epworth Sleepiness Scale (ESS) for economic evaluation: an assessment of its convergent and discriminant validity," *Behavioral Sleep Medicine*, 2016, In press.

[22] J. E. Broderick, D. U. Junghaenel, S. Schneider et al., "Pittsburgh and Epworth sleep scale items: accuracy of ratings across different reporting periods," *Behavioral Sleep Medicine*, vol. 11, no. 3, pp. 173–188, 2013.

[23] L. Yu, D. J. Buysse, A. Germain et al., "Development of short forms from the PROMIS™ sleep disturbance and Sleep-Related Impairment item banks," *Behavioral Sleep Medicine*, vol. 10, no. 1, pp. 6–24, 2011.

[24] C. P. Atkins, D. Gilbert, C. Brockwell et al., "Fatigue in sarcoidosis and idiopathic pulmonary fibrosis: differences in character and severity between diseases," *Sarcoidosis Vasculitis and Diffuse Lung Diseases*, vol. 33, pp. 130–138, 2016.

[25] C. Sander, U. Hegerl, K. Wirkner et al., "Normative values of the Epworth Sleepiness Scale (ESS), derived from a large German sample," *Sleep and Breathing*, vol. 20, no. 4, pp. 1337–1345, 2016.

[26] K. E. Bloch, O. D. Schoch, J. N. N. Zhang et al., "German version of the Epworth Sleepiness Scale," *Respiration*, vol. 66, no. 5, pp. 440–447, 1999.

[27] M. Johns and B. Hocking, "Daytime sleepiness and sleep habits of Australian workers," *Sleep*, vol. 20, no. 10, pp. 844–847, 1997.

[28] D. J. Buysse, C. F. Reynolds, T. H. Monk et al., "Quantification of subjective sleep quality in healthy elderly men and women using the Pittsburgh Sleep Quality Index (PSQI)," *Sleep*, vol. 14, no. 4, pp. 331–338, 1991.

[29] J. D. Vries, H. Michielsen, G. L. van Heck et al., "Measuring fatigue in sarcoidosis: the Fatigue Assessment Scale (FAS)," *British Journal of Health Psychology*, vol. 9, no. 3, pp. 279–291, 2004.

[30] A. S. Zigmond and R. P. Snaith, "The hospital anxiety and depression scale," *Acta Psychiatrica Scandinavica*, vol. 67, no. 6, pp. 361–370, 1983.

[31] J. E. Ware, M. Kosinski, J. E. Dewey et al., *How to Score and Interpret Single-Item Health Status Measures: A Manual For Users of The SF-8™ Health Survey*, QualityMetric Incorporated, Lincoln, RI, USA, 2001.

[32] J. Cohen, *Statistical Power Analysis for the Behavioral Sciences*, Erlbaum, Hillsdale, NJ, USA, 1988.

[33] G. R. Norman, J. A. Sloan, and K. W. Wyrwich, "Interpretation of changes in health-related quality of life—the remarkable universality of half a standard deviation," *Medical Care*, vol. 41, no. 5, pp. 582–592, 2003.

[34] S. Pallesen, I. H. Nordhus, S. Omvik et al., "Prevalence and risk factors of subjective sleepiness in the general adult population," *Sleep*, vol. 30, no. 5, pp. 619–624, 2007.

[35] N. Tsuno, I. Jaussent, Y. Dauvilliers et al., "Determinants of excessive daytime sleepiness in a French community-dwelling elderly population," *Journal of Sleep Research*, vol. 16, no. 4, pp. 364–371, 2007.

[36] P. H. Gander, N. S. Marshall, R. Harris et al., "The Epworth Sleepiness Scale: Influence of age, ethnicity, and socioeconomic deprivation. Epworth sleepiness scores of adults in New Zealand," *Sleep*, vol. 28, no. 2, pp. 249–253, 2005.

[37] N. H. Chen, M. W. Johns, H. Y. Li et al., "Validation of a Chinese version of the Epworth sleepiness scale," *Quality of Life Research*, vol. 11, no. 8, pp. 817–821, 2002.

[38] S. A. Beaudreau, A. P. Spira, A. Stewart et al., "Validation of the Pittsburgh Sleep Quality Index and the Epworth Sleepiness Scale in older black and white women," *Sleep Medicine*, vol. 13, no. 1, pp. 36–42, 2012.

[39] M. A. Spruit, M. J. Thomeer, R. Gosselink et al., "Skeletal muscle weakness in patients with sarcoidosis and its relationship with exercise intolerance and reduced health status," *Thorax*, vol. 60, no. 1, pp. 32–38, 2005.

[40] R. Marcellis, M. van der Veeke, I. Mesters et al., "Does physical training reduce fatigue in sarcoidosis?," *Sarcoidosis Vasculitis and Diffuse Lung Diseases*, vol. 32, no. 1, pp. 53–62, 2015.

[41] K. C. Patterson, F. Huang, J. M. Oldham et al., "Excessive daytime sleepiness and obstructive sleep apnea in patients with sarcoidosis," *Chest*, vol. 143, no. 6, pp. 1562–1568, 2013.

[42] A. P. Spira, S. A. Beaudreau, K. L. Stone et al., "Reliability and validity of the Pittsburgh Sleep Quality Index and the Epworth Sleepiness Scale in older men," *Journals of Gerontology Series A—Biological Sciences and Medical Sciences*, vol. 67, no. 4, pp. 433–439, 2012.

[43] C. Sauter, S. Asenbaum, R. Popovic et al., "Excessive daytime sleepiness in patients suffering from different levels of obstructive sleep apnoea syndrome," *Journal of Sleep Research*, vol. 9, no. 3, pp. 293–301, 2000.

21

Preliminary Results of the Adoption and Application of the Integrated Comprehensive Care Bundle Care Program When Treating Patients with Chronic Obstructive Pulmonary Disease

Jason R. Guertin,[1,2,3,4] James M. Bowen,[1,2,5] Carolyn Gosse,[5] Gord Blackhouse,[1,2] Daria J. O'Reilly,[1,2,5] Emanuel Baltaga,[5] Gerard Cox,[5,6] Donna Johnson,[5] Brandi Le Blanc,[5] Jane Loncke,[5] Stewart Pugsley,[5,6] Ravi Sivakumaran,[5] Laura Wheatley,[5] Kevin Smith,[5,6] and Jean-Eric Tarride[1,2,5,7]

[1] *Programs for Assessment of Technology in Health, The Research Institute of St. Joe's Hamilton, St. Joseph's Healthcare Hamilton, Hamilton, ON, Canada*
[2] *Department of Health Research Methods, Evidence, and Impact, Faculty of Health Sciences, McMaster University, Hamilton, ON, Canada*
[3] *Department of Social and Preventive Medicine, Université Laval, Quebec City, QC, Canada*
[4] *Centre de Recherche du CHU de Québec, Université Laval, Axe Santé des Populations et Pratiques Optimales en Santé, Hôpital du St-Sacrement, Quebec City, QC, Canada*
[5] *St. Joseph's Healthcare Hamilton, Hamilton, ON, Canada*
[6] *Department of Medicine, DeGroote School of Medicine, McMaster University, Hamilton, ON, Canada*
[7] *Center for Health Economics and Policy Analysis, McMaster University, Hamilton, ON, Canada*

Correspondence should be addressed to Jean-Eric Tarride; tarride@mcmaster.ca

Academic Editor: Alice M. Turner

Background. St. Joseph's Health System has implemented an integrated comprehensive care bundle care (ICC) program with the hopes that it would improve patients' care while reducing overall costs. The aim of this analysis was to evaluate the performance of the ICC program within patients admitted with chronic pulmonary obstructive disease (COPD). *Methods.* We conducted a retrospective observational cohort study comparing ICC patients to non-ICC patients admitted to St. Joseph's Healthcare Hamilton for COPD being discharged with support services between June 2012 and March 2015, using administrative data. Confounding adjustment was achieved through the use of propensity score matching. Medical resource utilizations during the initial hospitalization and within the 60 days following discharge were compared using regression models. *Results.* All 76 patients who entered the ICC program (100.0%) were matched 1 : 1 to 76 eligible non-ICC patients (28.4%). Length of stay (6.47 [7.29] versus 9.55 [10.21] days) and resource intensity weights (1.16 [0.80] versus 1.64 [1.69]) were lower in the ICC group within the initial hospitalization but, while favoring the ICC program, healthcare resource use tended not to differ statistically following discharge. *Interpretation.* The ICC program was able to reduce initial medical resource utilization without increasing subsequent medical resource use.

1. Introduction

Healthcare demand and costs are rising in Canada and abroad with the fear that this continuous rise could affect the sustainability of the healthcare systems. Many attempts have been made to curb this increase through the use of multiple hospital/physician/healthcare provider organizations funding models with various degrees of success [1–7]. Most successful attempts tended to encourage coordination of care by multiple healthcare providers which included retroaction to the clinical team in hopes of improving care, aligned incentives for care integration across multiple providers, and

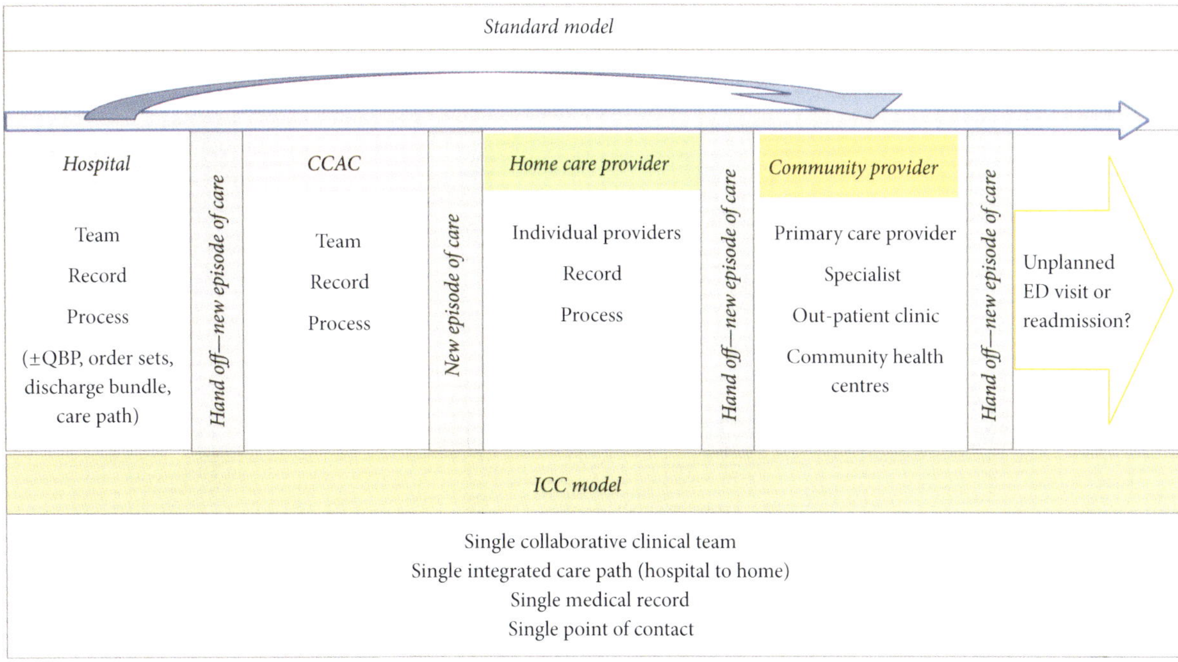

FIGURE 1: Standard model and ICC model of patient care. CCAC: Community Care Access Centre; ED: emergency department; ICC: integrated comprehensive care; QBP: quality-based procedures.

optimized resource utilization by the medical teams. In April 2012, St. Joseph's Health System (SJHS) set up a novel patient-centered integrated funding model pilot within the Hamilton (Ontario) region, hereby referred to as the integrated comprehensive care bundle care (ICC) program, designed with these criteria in mind. A detailed description of the ICC program can be found elsewhere [8]. Briefly, the ICC program was designed to integrate care across the hospital and home care continuum, with a single team and care management model that provided homecare support for patients' admitted at St. Joseph's Healthcare Hamilton (SJHH) in collaboration with a lead home care provider, St. Joseph's Home Care (SJHC). Its creation was designed with seven elements in mind: (1) client centered care to empower clients with knowledge, participation, and self-care; (2) integrated care coordinators who would follow clients across the continuum of care; (3) integrated interdisciplinary teams standardizing care pathways spanning hospital and community; (4) use of shared electronic health record which would also serve as a hub for communication; (5) use of simple and available technology to provide flexibility in communication; (6) community-based 24 hours a day, seven days a week access to healthcare; and (7) flexibility in the delivery of care in hopes of continually improving the processes of care. This contrasts with the standard model in which patients' care is in silos and involves multiple additional independent actors including Community Care Access Centres (CCAC) and home care and community providers (Figure 1).

The current ICC model in place at the SJHH is composed of three registered health care professionals who act as the ICC coordinators for all of the clinical streams and are supported by an administrative/research support position. Patients followed within the ICC program have access to the ICC team 24 hours a day, seven days a week through a toll free telephone number. In addition to the ICC personnel, the ICC program leverages an independent version of the SJHC Information System (Procura® ContinuLink® [Victoria, British Columbia]) to provide real-time remote access to client files. Remote access to these files is accomplished by using tablets, laptops, or desktop computers to securely access the information and clinical documentation remotely and provide the option to take digital pictures when required (e.g., wounds).

The ICC program is currently offered to patients in four clinical streams (i.e., thoracic surgery, total joint replacement, congestive heart failure, and chronic obstructive pulmonary disease [COPD]). It was hypothesized that the ICC program could potentially (1) reduce inpatient length of stay (LOS) of the index admission by favoring earlier evaluation for homecare intervention, (2) provide added benefits following discharge, and (3) improve patient and provider experience.

A previous evaluation of the ICC program within the thoracic surgery clinical stream at SJHH showed that, despite having minimal impact within the initial hospitalization, the ICC program was associated with lower proportions of emergency department visits and hospitalization in the post-discharge phase and with a tendency to reduce overall costs [9]. However, it is unknown if these results apply to different populations.

The current manuscript provides the results of our initial evaluation of the performance of the pilot ICC program within the COPD clinical stream for patients admitted to SJHH.

2. Methods

2.1. Design and Setting. We conducted a comparative retrospective cohort study using data from the Canadian Institute for Health Information (CIHI) Discharge Abstract Database (DAD) linked to the SJHC dataset maintained in Procura ContinuLink.

2.2. Study Population. We used CIHI Case Mix Group (CMG) classifications to identify all patients admitted at SJHH for COPD between June 1, 2012, and March 31, 2015. All eligible patients (i.e., community dwelling patients with a hospital admission driven by COPD, requiring home care supports to transition from hospital to home that were not currently receiving care by CCAC, not on a wait list for long-term care or a day program) were approached by the ICC coordinator on the first day of their admission (or on the day of COPD diagnosis for incident COPD cases) for enrollment into the ICC program. Patients in this group who accepted enrollment and were subsequently discharged home formed the ICC group.

Concurrent comparator patients who were admitted to SJHH for COPD and discharged with standard support services during the study follow-up period were eligible to act as comparator patients (hereby defined as the non-ICC group) (Figure 2). In the event that a patient in the non-ICC group had multiple eligible admissions during the examined time-frame, this patient's index admission was randomly selected among all eligible admissions.

2.3. Outcomes. The primary outcome of this study was the in-hospital LOS for the index admission. Secondary outcomes included other in-hospital medical resource utilization rates and included the resource intensity weights (RIW) (i.e., a standard index used by CIHI to reflect intensity of care associated with each hospital admission) [10] of the index admission, the proportion of atypical admissions (defined as admissions in which a patient either has died, was transferred in or out of the hospital, or experienced a long LOS) [11] during the index admission, the number of hospital readmissions, and the total number of days admitted up to 60 days following discharge from index admission. Although 60-day follow-up was considered to be a relevant time-horizon for this study, it could potentially downsize the total number of days patients were admitted during follow-up. As such, this outcome was evaluated using two approaches: (1) a truncated approach where patients' LOS was truncated at the end of the examined time-window and (2) a nontruncated approach where if a patient remained admitted beyond the examined time-window (i.e., 30 or 60 days), the full LOS would be counted (e.g., if a patient was admitted for 5 days on the 29th day of 30-day follow-up, this patient would be assigned a 1-day LOS in the truncated approach and a 5-day LOS in the nontruncated approach).

2.4. Statistical Analyses. Discrete data are presented in absolute (number) and relative (percentage) values and continuous data are presented as mean (standard deviation [SD]) or as average rate of event (95% confidence intervals [CI]) per 100 persons; rates were defined per 100 persons per month or per two months in function of the examined follow-up period (i.e., 30 or 60 days). Baseline sociodemographics of all patients included within the ICC and non-ICC group were assessed on the index admission's admission date as well as the numbers of time they were admitted in the 60 days prior to their index admission.

We used propensity score (PS) matching to control for measured baseline confounding between the two groups [12]. Patients' PS were estimated using a multivariate logistic regression PS model which included the following covariates: age, sex, fiscal quarter at the time of patients' discharge from the index admission (fiscal years in Canada go from April 1 to March 31, as such fiscal quarter 1: April to June; fiscal quarter 2: July to September; fiscal quarter 3: October to December; fiscal quarter 4: January to March), and the number of admissions (0, 1 or ≥ 2) in the 60 days prior to the index admission. Following the selection of the PS model, PS were assessed for all patients included within the ICC and non-ICC groups and matching was conducted using a greedy nearest neighbor 1 : 1 matching algorithm. Matching occurred if the difference in the logit of the PS between nearest neighbors was within 0.2 times the SD of the cohort's PS [13]. Patients selected by the matching algorithm formed the matched population.

Between group balance in terms of the baseline characteristics within the unmatched and matched populations was assessed using absolute standardized differences (ASDD); ASDD > 0.10 were assumed to indicate lack of balance between groups [14, 15]. Proportion of atypical index admission and proportion of patients readmitted within 60 days following discharge of the index admission between the ICC and non-ICC groups were compared using chi-square or Fisher's exact test, when appropriate. Between group differences in terms of LOS for the index admission were compared using negative binomial regressions [16–18] whereas between group differences in the index admission's RIW were compared using generalized linear model with log link and gamma family function [17, 19]. Differences in the rate of hospital readmissions and of in-hospital LOS during follow-up between the ICC and non-ICC patients were compared using zero-inflated negative binomial (ZINB) regressions [17, 19]. These types of model are used when there are a large proportion of 0s in the data (e.g., 135 [88.8%] of 152 matched patients were not hospitalized at 30 days). Rather than using a single distribution to model the count data (e.g., negative binomial distribution), ZINB models use two distributions to account for the excess zeros by implicitly modeling two populations. The first part of the model assumes that some individuals will never be hospitalized using a binary link function (e.g., logit function) while the second part of the model assumes that other individuals can or cannot be hospitalized following a negative binomial distribution. Due to its two-part structure, the ZINB models generate two sets of parameters, one for each part of the model (i.e., zero-inflated part and negative binomial part). All analyses were conducted using the SAS 9.3 Program (Cary, North Carolina). We interpreted 2-tailed P values < 0.05 as significant.

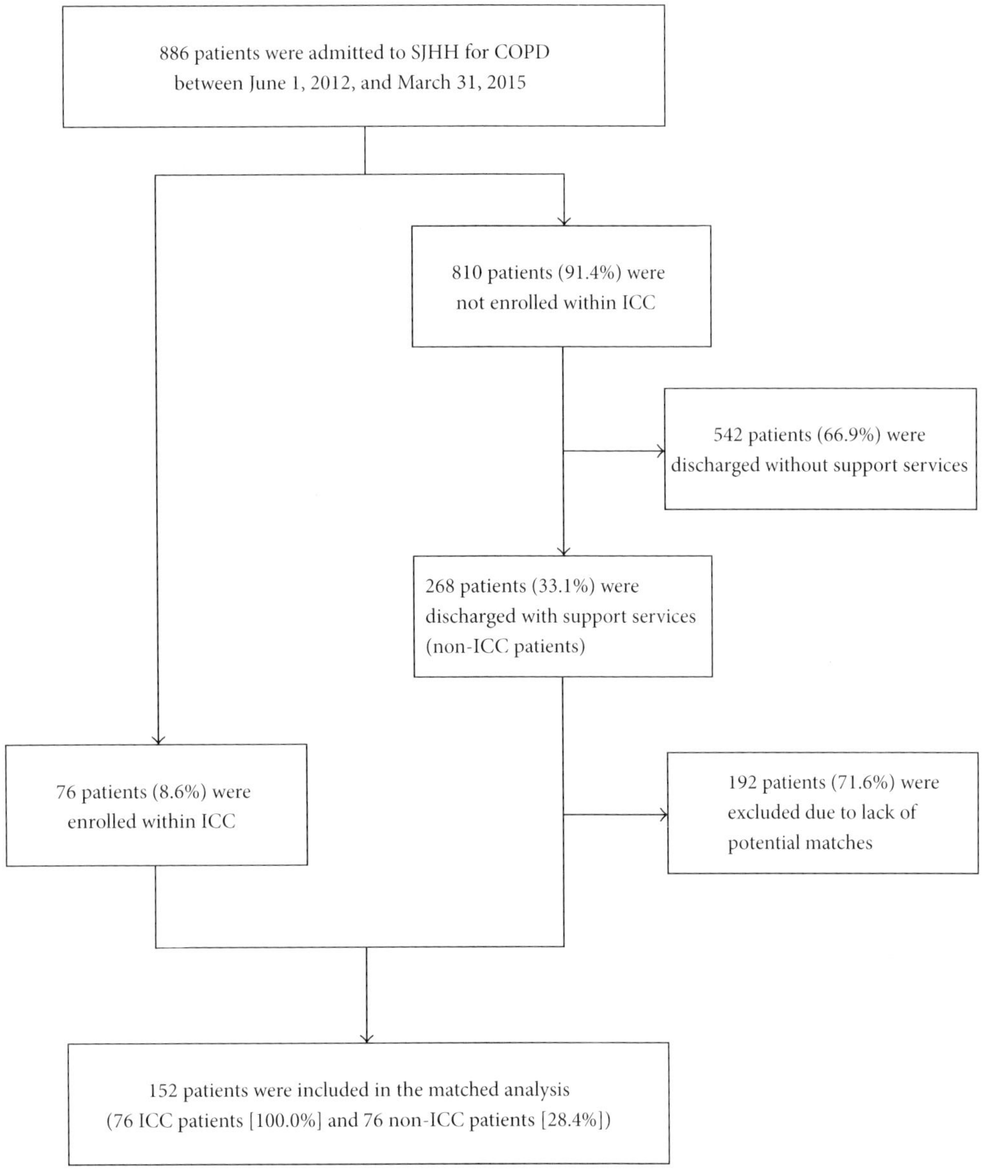

FIGURE 2: Patient flow-chart of patients admitted for chronic obstructive pulmonary disease at St. Joseph's Healthcare Hamilton. COPD: chronic obstructive pulmonary disease; ICC: integrated comprehensive care; SJHH: St. Joseph's Healthcare Hamilton.

3. Results

3.1. Study Population. A patient flow-chart is shown in Figure 2. Seventy-six patients admitted to SJHH for COPD and discharged home between June 10, 2012, and February 16, 2015, were enrolled within the ICC COPD clinical stream. Aside from these 76 patients, a total of 810 patients have been admitted to SJHH for COPD between June 1, 2012, and March 31, 2015. Of these 810 patients, a total 268 patients (33.1%) admitted to SJHH for COPD and discharged with support services between June 1, 2012, and March 31, 2015, composed the non-ICC group.

3.2. Unmatched Analyses. Baseline comparison of the ICC and non-ICC group is shown in Table 1. Although patients in the ICC and non-ICC groups tended to be similar regarding most of the examined baseline characteristics, patients included within ICC group tended to have been admitted to a hospital more frequently in the 60 days prior to the index admission than patients within the non-ICC group (an average of 0.49 [0.72] versus 0.35 [0.66] admission per patient [ASDD = 0.20]), thus justifying the need to adjust for these differences.

3.3. Propensity Score Adjusted Analyses. Matched non-ICC comparators were found for all 76 patients in the ICC group. PS matching attained balance on all examined baseline characteristics (Table 2). Outcomes within the ICC group and their matched non-ICC comparators are provided within Table 3 (beta-estimates of the regression models are provided

TABLE 1: Baseline characteristics within the unmatched ICC and eligible COPD patients.

	ICC group	Non-ICC comparator group*	Absolute standardized differences†
Number of patients	$N = 76$	$N = 268$	
Male sex, *n* (%)	38 (50.00)	130 (48.51)	0.03
Age, mean (SD)	73.62 (9.18)	73.66 (10.75)	0.00
N per quarter (proxy for seasonality), *n* (%)			
FYQ1	18 (23.68)	57 (21.27)	0.06
FYQ2	17 (22.37)	48 (17.91)	0.11
FYQ3	17 (22.37)	79 (29.48)	0.16
FYQ4	24 (31.58)	84 (31.34)	0.01
Prior admission in the 60 days prior to baseline			
No admission, *n* (%)	47 (61.84)	198 (73.88)	0.26
1 prior admission, *n* (%)	23 (30.26)	51 (19.03)	0.26
2 or more prior admissions, *n* (%)	6 (7.89)	19 (7.09)	0.03
N of admissions in the 60 days prior to baseline admission, mean (SD)	0.49 (0.72)	0.35 (0.66)	0.20

FYQ, fiscal year quarter; *N*, number; SD, standard deviation. *The comparator group within this table was composed of all patients who did not enter within the ICC group and who were admitted for COPD to St. Joseph's Healthcare Hamilton and discharged between June 1, 2012, and March 31, 2015. †Absolute standardized differences > 0.10 are generally assumed to indicate lack of balance between groups.

TABLE 2: Baseline characteristics within the matched population.

	ICC group	Matched non-ICC group*	Absolute standardized differences†
Number of patients	$N = 76$	$N = 76$	
Male sex, *n* (%)	38 (50.00)	38 (50.00)	0.00
Age, mean (SD)	73.62 (9.18)	74.49 (9.90)	0.09
N per quarter (proxy for seasonality), *n* (%)			
FYQ1	18 (23.68)	15 (19.74)	0.10
FYQ2	17 (22.37)	18 (23.68)	0.03
FYQ3	17 (22.37)	17 (22.37)	0.00
FYQ4	24 (31.58)	26 (34.21)	0.06
Prior admission in the 60 days prior to baseline			
No admission, *n* (%)	47 (61.84)	47 (61.84)	0.00
1 prior admission, *n* (%)	23 (30.26)	22 (28.95)	0.03
2 or more prior admissions, *n* (%)	6 (7.89)	7 (9.21)	0.05
N of admission in the 60 days prior to baseline admission, mean (SD)	0.49 (0.72)	0.49 (0.70)	0.00

FYQ, fiscal year quarter; *N*, number; SD, standard deviation. *The comparator group within this table was composed of eligible non-ICC patients that were propensity score-matched to an ICC patient. Patients were matched on patients' gender, age, the fiscal quarter in which they were discharged from the hospital for a COPD admission, and number of prior admissions in the last 60 days. †Absolute standardized differences > 0.10 are generally assumed to indicate lack of balance between groups.

in Table 4). Results indicated that patients within the ICC group had shorter index LOS (6.47 [7.29] versus 9.55 [10.21] days) and used less RIW (1.16 [0.80] versus 1.64 [1.69]) than their matched comparators. In the follow-up period, results failed to indicate any statistically significant difference in terms of readmission rates after discharge at 30-day follow-up (11.84 [4.41; 19.27] versus 13.16 [3.76; 22.56] readmissions per 100 persons) or at 60-day follow-up (23.68 [11.96; 35.41] versus 25.00 [12.55; 37.45] readmissions per 100 persons). Despite this lack of difference in terms of readmission rates, results did indicate that the ICC group had less in-hospital LOS at 30 days after discharge when

Table 3: Medical resource utilization within the index admission and up to 60-day follow-up within the matched population.

	ICC group	Matched non-ICC comparator group*	P value	
Number of patients	$N = 76$	$N = 76$		
Length of stay during initial hospitalization (days) (mean (SD); min–max)	6.47 (7.29) [1; 42]	9.55 (10.21) [1; 57]	<0.01	
Resource intensity weight (RIW) during initial hospitalization (mean (SD); min–max)	1.16 (0.80) [0.17; 5.53]	1.64 (1.69) [0.73; 11.63]	<0.01	
Proportion of atypical index admission, n (%)	4 (5.26)	4 (5.26)	1.00	
Proportion of patients with at least 1 readmission, n (%)				
At 30 days	9 (11.84)	8 (10.53)	0.80	
At 60 days	15 (19.74)	15 (19.74)	1.00	
Average readmission rates per 100 persons (95% CI)				
At 30 days	11.84 (4.41; 19.27)	13.16 (3.76; 22.56)	0.07‡	0.99§
At 60 days	23.68 (11.96; 35.41)	25.00 (12.55; 37.45)	0.72‡	0.76§
Average LOS per 100 persons (95% CI)				
Truncated at 30 days	94.74 (27.58; 161.89)	136.84 (27.36; 246.33)	0.11‡	0.78§
Truncated at 60 days	236.84 (103.71; 369.97)	285.53 (73.10; 497.95)	0.43‡	0.80§
Average LOS (nontruncated) per 100 persons (95% CI)†				
At 30 days	122.37 (31.68; 213.05)	536.84 (0.00; 1189.14)	<0.01‡	0.56§
At 60 days	260.53 (110.56; 410.49)	609.21 (0.00; 1261.88)	0.07‡	0.76§

LOS, length of stay; N, number; SD, standard deviation. No adjustment beyond the propensity score matching was conducted. Beta-estimates (95% CI) for each statistical comparison are provided within Table 4. *The comparator group within this table was composed of eligible non-ICC patients that were propensity score-matched to an ICC patient. Patients were matched on patients' gender, age, the fiscal quarter in which they were discharged from the hospital for a COPD admission, and number of prior admissions in the last 60 days. †For patients still admitted at the end of the examined time-horizon, the complete LOS was included in the analysis even if it extended beyond the examined time-horizon. ‡P value within the negative binomial part of the ZINB regression. §P value within the zero-inflated part of the ZINB regression.

analyzed under the nontruncated approach (122.37 [31.68; 213.05] versus 536.84 [0.00; 1,189.14] days per 100 patients).

4. Interpretation

4.1. Main Findings. Evaluation of the ICC program is fundamental to adequately assess its value to patients and the healthcare system [20]. Our study represents the first evaluation of the application of the ICC program to a chronic disease population. Our results indicate that the LOS and RIW within the index admission were lower within the ICC group than within the non-ICC group (Table 3). Such results could raise concerns of the presence of selection bias (i.e., that the ICC coordinators favored less severe cases). However, seeing as the baseline comparisons within the unmatched population indicated that ICC patient utilized more resources prior to baseline (Table 1), such concerns seem unwarranted. With respect to follow-up outcomes, numerical differences in favor of ICC were observed for the 30- and 60-day readmission rates and LOS per 100 persons although most of these results did not attain statistical significance (Table 3). This could be partially explained by the relatively small sample size available for analyses.

4.2. Relationship to Other Studies. This is the second pilot evaluation of the performance of the ICC program within SJHH. Though none of the results regarding the ICC program in either stream would indicate worse outcomes with the ICC program, added benefits provided by the ICC program seem to differ between streams. For example, within the COPD stream, benefits with the ICC program were generally observed within the index hospitalization (Table 3), whereas benefits provided within the thoracic surgery stream tended to be in the postdischarge phase [9]. Continued assessment of the performance of the ICC program within these two streams is required to better comprehend if these results reflect true differences regarding the performance of the ICC program at SJHH (i.e., that ICC program provides benefits solely within the index hospitalization within the COPD stream and only within the postdischarge phase within the thoracic surgery stream) or if both studies lacked statistical power to detect a statistically significant result in both phases. Regardless of the case, seeing as the results may differ between

Table 4: Results of the statistical comparisons of the outcomes within the matched population.

	Beta-estimates (95% CI)			P value
Length of stay during initial hospitalization	−0.39 (−0.67−−0.11)			<0.01
Resource intensity weight (RIW) during initial hospitalization	−0.34 (−0.53−−0.16)			<0.01
Proportion of atypical index admission*	—			1.00
Proportion of patients with at least 1 readmission*				
At 30 days	—			0.80
At 60 days	—			1.00
	Negative binomial part Beta-estimates (95% CI)	P value	Zero-inflated part Beta-estimates (95% CI)	P value
Average readmission rates per 100 persons				
At 30 days	−1.37 (−2.86−0.12)	0.07	−14.52 (−2324.47−2295.43)	0.99
At 60 days	−0.27 (−1.72−1.18)	0.72	−0.50 (−3.74−2.74)	0.76
Average LOS per 100 persons				
At 30 days	−0.50 (−1.11−0.11)	0.11	−0.15 (−1.16−0.87)	0.78
At 60 days	−0.27 (−0.94−0.40)	0.43	−0.10 (−0.92−0.72)	0.80
Average LOS (nontruncated) per 100 persons				
At 30 days	−1.75 (−3.01−−0.49)	<0.01	−0.31 (−1.38−0.75)	0.56
At 60 days	−0.95 (−1.99−0.08)	0.07	−0.14 (−1.02−0.74)	0.76

* P values estimated by chi-square or Fischer's exact test. The comparator group used for these analyses was composed of eligible non-ICC patients that were propensity score-matched to an ICC patient. Patients were matched on patients' gender, age, the fiscal quarter in which they were discharged from the hospital for a COPD admission, and number of prior admissions in the last 60 days.

the two previously examined streams, evaluation of the two streams which have yet to be evaluated (i.e., total joint replacement and congestive heart failure) is warranted as the performance of the ICC program within these two streams may also differ.

4.3. Implications for Practice. Despite these positive results, concerns regarding the fact that both currently available evaluations of the ICC program have been conducted within a research university hospital center and that the results we show may not be reproducible within community hospitals could be raised. It is important to note that the ICC program was later expanded in September 2013 to another SJHS hospital, St. Mary's General Hospital, a community hospital center in Kitchener-Waterloo, Ontario [21]. Although preliminary, initial positive results observed within the SJHS also seem to be observed within this nontertiary setting (full evaluation of this second program is currently underway). These positive and promising results partly support the recent decision of the Ministry of Health and Long-Term Care of Ontario to expand the ICC (for both COPD and CHF patients) program across the Hamilton Niagara Haldimand Brant Local Health Integration Network [22, 23].

4.4. Limitations. Our study has several limitations. First, we had access to limited patients' baseline characteristics as well as a limited sample size. Although we used PS matching to further select balanced comparator groups, we may not exclude the risk that we did not fully adjust for measured confounding (e.g., adjusting for seasonality of the index admission would not be able to adjust for acute temporal variability in service-related confounding) nor can we fully exclude the risk of confounding due to unmeasured confounders (e.g., patients' smoking status which was not available within the in-hospital database) [12, 24]. Second, we only had access to the CIHI DAD to conduct this evaluation. Future work evaluating the ICC program will require access to additional CIHI databases, such as the National Ambulatory Care Reporting System, Ontario Case Costing Initiative databases as well as the Client Health Related Information System, and the Registered Persons database, and to be able to link patients' data across these databases to fully examine the ICC program's impact on patients' morbidity and mortality as well as its short- and long-term economic implications. Fourth, our results also highlight the fact that only a limited subset of patients admitted to SJHH for COPD during the study's follow-up period entered within the ICC program (76 [22.1%] out of 344 patients). This observation may reflect issues with the ICC program's capacity which we were unable to evaluate within the current study. Future work will be required to identify the optimal number of ICC coordinators which will be required to fully manage all potential patients. Finally, we recognize that our analyses could have lacked power to detect a significant difference between groups. However, as this evaluation was conducted in a pilot setting where the primary objective was to assess the feasibility of the ICC program not its performance, we did not conduct a power calculation or a sample size estimation prior to conducting

TABLE 5: Baseline characteristics within the unselected population.

	ICC group	Unselected COPD comparison group*	Absolute standardized differences†
Number of patients	$N = 76$	$N = 810$	
Male sex, n (%)	38 (50.00)	406 (50.12)	0.00
Age, mean (SD)	73.62 (9.18)	72.17 (11.42)	0.14
N per quarter (proxy for seasonality), n (%)			
FYQ1	18 (23.68)	161 (19.88)	0.09
FYQ2	17 (22.37)	155 (19.14)	0.08
FYQ3	17 (22.37)	231 (28.52)	0.14
FYQ4	24 (31.58)	263 (32.47)	0.02
Prior admission in the 60 days prior to baseline, n (%)			
No admission	47 (61.84)	645 (79.63)	0.40
1 prior admission	23 (30.26)	126 (15.56)	0.36
2 or more prior admissions	6 (7.89)	39 (4.81)	0.13
N of admissions in the 60 days prior to baseline admission, mean (SD)	0.49 (0.72)	0.27 (0.60)	0.33

FYQ, fiscal year quarter; N, number; SD, standard deviation. *The comparison group within this table is composed of all 810 patients admitted to St. Joseph's Healthcare Hamilton for COPD between June 1, 2012, and March 31, 2015, who did not enter within the ICC group. †Absolute standardized differences > 0.10 are generally assumed to indicate lack of balance between groups.

the study and did not expect to detect a significant difference in any of the examined outcomes. Despite these limitations, our results regarding the value of the ICC program remain strong (Table 3).

4.5. Recommendations for Future Evaluations. From a broader perspective, this evaluation also depicts issues associated with evaluating an intervention which is offered in a nonrandomized manner. Unlike results observed within a randomized controlled study, any differences, or lack of differences, observed within a nonrandomized study may be due to confounding. To address this potential issue, we had determined a priori that confounding adjustment would be conducted in a stepwise approach. First, the ICC program's performance would be evaluated only in patients who could be eligible for inclusion within the ICC program (i.e., those discharged alive with support services following an admission for COPD) and second, subsequent differences in measured baseline characteristics would be further adjusted thanks to a PS matching approach [25]. Had we not selected an appropriate comparator group (baseline comparison of the 76 ICC patients and of the 810 patients admitted to SJHH for COPD is shown in Table 5), we would not have been able to identify that the ICC program could reduce the initial LOS (6.47 [7.29] days in the ICC versus 7.78 [13.92] days in the non-ICC group) (Table 6).

We recommend that any research team planning to conduct a similar analysis reflect on the following points. Firstly, identification and selection of an optimal comparator group are pivotal for the appropriate evaluation of the program. Secondly, all nonrandomized studies are subject to confounding bias; following the selection of the comparator group, researchers must thoroughly examine all available characteristics to identify the level of balance between both groups. Thirdly, following identification of unbalanced characteristics, comparisons must be conducted using optimal adjustment methods (e.g., PS matching). Finally, as shown within our example, full access to all relevant databases and the ability to link data between these databases must be obtained in order to extensively evaluate all short- and long-term implications of such programs across both inpatient and outpatient healthcare services. In addition, the evaluation of these complex healthcare interventions must move beyond the traditional first-level indicators (e.g., readmission [yes versus no]) to better appreciate their impact across the whole spectrum of care.

4.6. Conclusion. In conclusion, based on our preliminary results, implementation of the ICC program to the COPD clinical stream within the SJHH statistically reduced patients' index LOS which should reduce in-hospital costs and showed a potential for a reduction in the number of days patients were hospitalized in the 30 and 60 days after discharge. Additional analyses focusing on patients' outcome following discharge, their perception regarding outpatient care, and a full economic evaluation of the ICC program must be conducted prior to concluding on its full value.

TABLE 6: Example of the unadjusted analyses using the inappropriate COPD comparator group.

	ICC group	Unselected COPD comparison group*		P value
Number of patients	$N = 76$	$N = 810$		
Length of stay during initial hospitalization (days) (mean (SD); min–max)	6.47 (7.29) [1; 42]	7.78 (13.92) [1; 226]		0.13
Resource intensity weight (RIW) during initial hospitalization (mean (SD); min–max)	1.16 (0.80) [0.17; 5.53]	1.56 (2.09) [0.18; 27.32]		<0.01
Proportion of atypical index admission, n (%)	4 (5.26)	71 (8.77)		0.39
Proportion of patients with at least 1 readmission, n (%)				
At 30 days	9 (11.84)	73 (9.01)		0.42
At 60 days	15 (19.74)	128 (15.80)		0.37
Average readmission rates per 100 persons (95% CI)				
At 30 days	11.84 (4.41; 19.27)	9.63 (7.45; 11.81)	0.82‡	1.00§
At 60 days	23.68 (11.96; 35.41)	18.64 (15.44; 21.85)	0.87‡	0.82§
Average LOS per 100 persons (95% CI)				
At 30 days	94.74 (27.58; 161.89)	64.81 (44.98; 84.65)	0.80‡	0.39§
At 60 days	236.84 (103.71; 369.97)	148.89 (110.59; 187.19)	0.43‡	0.36§
Average LOS (nontruncated) per 100 persons (95% CI)†				
At 30 days	122.37 (31.68; 213.05)	149.14 (70.07; 228.20)	0.34‡	0.31§
At 60 days	260.53 (110.56; 410.49)	212.59 (130.95; 294.23)	0.96‡	0.39§

LOS, length of stay; N, number; SD, standard deviation. Beta-estimates (95% CI) for each statistical comparison are provided in Table 7. *The comparison group within this table is composed of all 810 patients admitted to St. Joseph's Healthcare Hamilton for COPD between June 1, 2012, and March 31, 2015, who did not enter within the ICC group. †For patients still admitted at the end of the examined time-horizon, the complete LOS was included in the analysis even if it extended beyond the examined time-horizon. ‡P value within the negative binomial part of the ZINB regression. §P value within the zero-inflated part of the ZINB regression.

TABLE 7: Results of the statistical comparisons of the outcomes within the inappropriate COPD comparator group.

	Beta-estimates (95% CI)			P value
Length of stay during initial hospitalization	−0.18 (−0.42–0.05)			0.13
Resource intensity weight (RIW) during initial hospitalization	−0.29 (−0.46–−0.13)			<0.01
Proportion of atypical index admission*	—			0.39
Proportion of patients with at least 1 readmission*				
At 30 days	—			0.42
At 60 days	—			0.37
	Negative binomial part		Zero-inflated part	
	Beta-estimates (95% CI)	P value	Beta-estimates (95% CI)	P value
Average readmission rates per 100 persons				
At 30 days	−0.12 (−1.21–0.96)	0.82	−14.57 (−6017.00–5987.87)	1.00
At 60 days	0.10 (−1.07–1.27)	0.87	−0.34 (−3.19–2.52)	0.82
Average LOS per 100 persons				
At 30 days	0.09 (−0.61–0.78)	0.80	−0.33 (−1.08–0.43)	0.39
At 60 days	0.23 (−0.34–0.81)	0.43	−0.29 (−0.90–0.33)	0.36
Average LOS (nontruncated) per 100 persons				
At 30 days	−0.57 (−1.74–0.60)	0.34	−0.46 (−1.34–0.42)	0.31
At 60 days	−0.02 (−0.81–0.77)	0.96	−0.30 (−0.97–0.37)	0.39

*P values estimated by chi-square or Fischer's exact test. The comparison group used in these analyses is composed of all 810 patients admitted to St. Joseph's Healthcare Hamilton for COPD between June 1, 2012, and March 31, 2015, who did not enter within the ICC group.

Disclosure

Portions of this work have been presented in abstract form at the 2016 Annual CAPT Conference and at the 2017 CADTH Symposium.

Acknowledgments

The integrated comprehensive care bundle care program was funded by the Ontario Ministry of Health and Long-Term Care.

References

[1] G. Browky, *HSOs, HMOs, and CHOs: the continuing history of capitation-funded healthcare. can fam physician*, vol. 36, 1990.

[2] F. Beland, H. Bergman, P. Lebel et al., "A system of integrated care for older persons with disabilities in canada: results from a randomized controlled trial," *The Journals of Gerontology Series A: Biological Sciences and Medical Sciences*, vol. 61, no. 4, pp. 367–373, 2006.

[3] J. C. Robinson, "The dynamics and limits of corporate growth in health care," *Health Affairs*, vol. 15, no. 2, pp. 155–169, 1996.

[4] P. P. Budetti, S. M. Shortell, T. M. Waters et al., "Physician and health system integration," *Health Affairs*, vol. 21, no. 1, pp. 203–210, 2002.

[5] K. M. Duvalko, M. Sherar, and C. Sawka, "Creating a system for performance improvement in cancer care: cancer care Ontario's clinical governance framework," *Journal of The Moffitt Cancer Center*, vol. 16, no. 4, pp. 293–302, 2009.

[6] G. R. Baker and A. MacIntosh-Murray, "Governance for quality and patient safety: the impact of the Ontario excellent care for all act, 2010," *Healthcare quarterly*, vol. 15, pp. 44–50, 2012.

[7] J. L. Kwan, M. W. Morgan, T. E. Stewart, and C. M. Bell, "Impact of an innovative inpatient patient navigator program on length of stay and 30-day readmission," *Journal of Hospital Medicine*, vol. 10, no. 12, pp. 799–803, 2015.

[8] L. Wheatley, W. Doyle, C. Evans, C. Gosse, and K. Smith, "Integrated comprehensive care a case study in nursing leadership and system transformation," *Nursing Leadership*, vol. 30, pp. 33–42, 2017.

[9] Y. Shargall, W. C. Hanna, L. Schneider et al., "The integrated comprehensive care program: a novel home care initiative after major thoracic surgery," *Seminars in Thoracic and Cardiovascular Surgery*, vol. 28, no. 2, pp. 574–582, 2016.

[10] Canadian Institute for Health Information, Canadian MIS Database—Hospital Financial Performance Indicators, 1999–2000 to 2009–2010, Methodological Notes.

[11] Canadian Institute for Health Information, "Patient cost estimator: methodological notes and glossary".

[12] P. R. Rosenbaum and D. B. Rubin, "The central role of the propensity score in observational studies for causal effects," *Biometrika*, vol. 70, no. 1, pp. 41–55, 1983.

[13] P. C. Austin, "Optimal caliper widths for propensity-score matching when estimating differences in means and differences in proportions in observational studies," *Pharmaceutical Statistics*, vol. 10, no. 2, pp. 150–161, 2011.

[14] P. C. Austin, "Balance diagnostics for comparing the distribution of baseline covariates between treatment groups in propensity-score matched samples," *Statistics in Medicine*, vol. 28, no. 25, pp. 3083–3107, 2009.

[15] M. Mamdani, K. Sykora, P. Li et al., "Reader's guide to critical appraisal of cohort studies: 2. assessing potential for confounding," *British Medical Journal*, vol. 330, no. 7497, pp. 960–962, 2005.

[16] J. L. Moran and P. J. Solomon, "A review of statistical estimators for risk-adjusted length of stay: analysis of the Australian and new Zealand intensive care adult patient data-base, 2008-2009," *BMC Medical Research Methodology*, vol. 12, Article ID 68, 2012.

[17] A. C. Cameron and P. K. Trivedi, *Regression Analysis of Count Data*, 2nd edition, 2013.

[18] R. Winkelmann, *Econometric Analysis of Count Data*, Springer-Verlag, Heidelberg, Germany, 5th edition, 2008.

[19] W. H. Greene, *Econometric Analysis*, Wiley, Hoboken, NJ, USA, 4th edition, 2000.

[20] S. Rosenbaum and T. Burke, "Accountable Care Organizations," *Public Health Reports*, vol. 126, no. 6, pp. 875–878, 2011.

[21] "St. Mary's General Hospital. Successful model for complex care patients expands to St. Mary's," http://www.smgh.ca/successful-model-for-complex-care-patients-expands-to-st-marys/.

[22] "Ontario ministry of health and long-term care. bundled care (integrated funding models): queen's printer for Ontario," http://www.health.gov.on.ca/en/pro/programs/ecfa/funding/ifm/.

[23] R. Collier, "10 health stories that mattered this week," http://www.cmaj.ca/site/earlyreleases/4september15_10_health_stories_that_mattered_this_week.xhtml.

[24] J. M. Brooks and R. L. Ohsfeldt, "Squeezing the balloon: propensity scores and unmeasured covariate balance," *Health Services Research*, vol. 48, no. 4, pp. 1487–1507, 2012.

[25] J. M. Wooldridge, *Econometric Analysis of Cross section and Panel Data*, MIT Press, Mass, USA, 2nd edition, 2001.

Risk of Cardiovascular Events Associated with Inhaled Corticosteroid Treatment in Patients with Chronic Obstructive Pulmonary Disease

Xia Jing,[1] Yufeng Li,[2] and Jianying Xu[1]

[1]*Department of Respiratory Diseases, Shanxi Dayi Hospital Affiliated to Shanxi Medical University, Taiyuan, Shanxi, China*
[2]*Department of Neurology, Shanxi Dayi Hospital Affiliated to Shanxi Medical University, Taiyuan, Shanxi, China*

Correspondence should be addressed to Jianying Xu; 18734583616@163.com

Academic Editor: Alice M. Turner

Background. The cardiovascular (CV) safety of inhaled corticosteroids (ICSs) in chronic obstructive pulmonary disease (COPD) is controversial because different studies have suggested that ICSs either increase or reduce the risk of CV events in COPD patients. In this meta-analysis, we assess the CV safety of ICS therapy in COPD. *Methods.* A meta-analysis of randomized, double-blind, parallel-group, placebo-controlled trials of ICS treatment for COPD that include at least 4 weeks of follow-up was performed. A random-effects model was used to evaluate the effects of ICS treatment on CV events. CV events were documented in each trial, and the relative risk (RR) and 95% confidence intervals (CIs) for ICSs were estimated. *Results.* Thirty-one trials were included in this meta-analysis. The risk of CV events was not different between ICS-treated and control groups (RR: 0.99; 95% CI: 0.93 to 1.06; $P = 0.801$). In a subgroup analysis, there were no significant differences in CV events between an ICS combined with long-acting β_2 agonist (LABA) (ICS + LABA) group and an LABA-only group (RR: 1.00; 95% CI: 0.90 to 1.10; $P = 0.930$), as well as between a combination group (ICS + LABA) and a long-acting muscarinic antagonist (LAMA) combined with LABA (LAMA + LABA) group (RR: 0.78; 95% CI: 0.39 to 1.55; $P = 0.473$). In addition, there was no difference in the risk of CV events between ICS treatment and control groups (RR: 0.99; 95% CI: 0.90 to 1.09; $P = 0.872$). *Conclusions.* These results demonstrate that ICSs do not increase the risk of CV events in COPD patients.

1. Introduction

Chronic obstructive pulmonary disease (COPD) is currently the fourth leading cause of death in the world [1] and is projected to be the third leading cause of death worldwide by 2020 [2]. Inflammatory changes in the airway and lung parenchyma are responsible for pulmonary function decline [3]. Inhaled corticosteroids (ICSs) are effective in reducing airway inflammation, nonspecific airway hyperresponsiveness, and airway obstruction in patients with COPD [4]. An ICS combined with a long-acting β_2 agonist (LABA) is more effective than monotherapy in improving lung function, reducing symptoms, increasing exercise tolerance, decreasing the frequency of exacerbation and hospitalization, and improving patient health [5]. According to the current Global Initiative for Chronic Obstructive Lung Disease (GOLD) guidelines, ICSs in combination with LABAs are suggested for patients with moderate-to-very severe COPD [6]. ICSs, such as fluticasone and budesonide, are widely used in COPD treatment, and other formulations of ICSs approved for use in COPD are fluticasone with salmeterol and budesonide with formoterol [7].

COPD is significantly associated with subclinical atherosclerosis [8], a recognized marker of cardiovascular (CV) disease. CV disease, which is a frequent and important comorbidity in COPD, is a fatal cause of morbidity and mortality among COPD patients during exacerbations [9]. ICSs may potentially reduce CV events by reducing exacerbations, alleviating hypoxia, and relieving the systemic inflammatory reaction to atherogenesis in patients with COPD [10]. Nevertheless, after prolonged treatment, the potential benefits of an ICS may be offset by its adverse systemic effects, such as increased extracellular volume, hypertension, glucose intolerance, and dyslipidemia, which are well-recognized risk factors for CV disease [11, 12]. Several studies have shown that ICS treatment can alleviate CV symptoms in COPD patients [3, 13–15], while other studies have suggested that ICSs lead to an increased risk of CV events [16, 17]. Critical evaluation is required to assess whether ICS treatment can reduce or increase the risk of CV events in COPD patients. Therefore, we conducted this meta-analysis to evaluate the effect of ICS treatment on CV events in COPD patients compared with controls.

2. Materials and Methods

2.1. Register and Search Strategy. This systematic review and meta-analysis were reported in accordance with the Preferred Reporting Items for Systematic Reviews and Meta-Analyses (PRISMA) Statement and registered at the International Prospective Register of Systematic Reviews (number CRD42017066017).

We searched PubMed, Embase, the Cochrane Library, Web of Knowledge, the United States Food and Drug Administration (US FDA) website, the http://ClinicalTrials.gov database, and the GSK (GlaxoSmithKline) Clinical Study Register for eligible trials. The search strategy used for PubMed was "inhaled corticosteroids" OR "ICS" OR "budesonide" OR "fluticasone" OR "flunisolide" OR "beclomethasone" OR "beclometasone" OR "triamcinolone" AND "COPD" OR "chronic obstructive pulmonary disease" OR "chronic obstructive lung disease" OR "COAD" OR "chronic obstructive airway disease" OR "pulmonary disease, chronic obstructive" OR "airflow obstruction, chronic" OR "chronic airflow obstruction" AND "mortality" OR "death" OR "myocardial" OR "cardiovascular" AND "clinical trial," based on previously published meta-analyses [18, 19]. We also conducted a manual search using the reference lists of key articles published in English. We considered all potentially eligible studies for review, irrespective of the primary outcome or language. Those searches aimed at identifying studies which were published between January 1, 1980, and January 24, 2018.

2.2. Eligibility Criteria. The inclusion criteria for our trials were as follows: (1) studies that were randomized controlled trials (RCTs) with a double-blind, parallel-group, placebo-controlled design and more than 4 weeks of follow-up and the title or abstract including any ICS (flunisolide, fluticasone, beclomethasone, budesonide, or triamcinolone); (2) studies that used standardized diagnostic criteria for COPD (spirometry is required for diagnosis in this clinical context, and the presence of a postbronchodilator FEV1/FVC (forced expiratory volume in the first second/forced vital capacity) ratio <0.70 confirms the presence of a persistent airflow limitation, and thus the presence of COPD, in patients with appropriate symptoms and significant exposures to noxious stimuli [20]); (3) studies that included any subtype of COPD, severity of disease, and sex or race of study participant subjects; (4) studies that used an ICS as the intervention drug versus a control treatment, which consisted of an ICS versus placebo, an ICS in combination with an LABA versus an LABA alone, or the combination of an ICS and an LABA versus the combination of a long-acting muscarinic antagonist (LAMA) and an LABA; (5) trials that provided the details of CV events (coronary artery disorders, cardiac arrhythmias, heart failures, cardiac disorder signs and symptoms, myocardial disorders, cardiac valve disorders, pericardial disorders, central nervous system vascular disorders, arteriosclerosis, stenosis, vascular insufficiencies and necrosis, aneurysms and artery dissections, embolisms, thrombosis, and hypertension) and explicitly reported data (including zero events) for at least one such event, but the outcome does not include stroke or peripheral arterial disease. New onset cases of cardiac disorders and cardiovascular death were included; and (6) studies whose full text can be found on a search site.

2.3. Exclusion Criteria. Our exclusion criteria were as follows: (1) studies that were less than 4 weeks in duration, as we were interested in long-term CV event risks; (2) studies that mixed groups of participants with asthma; (3) trials that did not compare an ICS with another treatment; and (4) studies that provided no raw data regarding the number of CV events in ICS-treated patients with COPD.

2.4. Outcome Measures and Data Extraction. The initial outcomes were CV adverse events. The CV events were defined as coronary artery disorders, cardiac arrhythmias, heart failures, cardiac disorder signs and symptoms, myocardial disorders, cardiac valve disorders, pericardial disorders, central nervous system vascular disorders, hypertension, arteriosclerosis, stenosis, vascular insufficiencies and necrosis, aneurysms and artery dissections, embolisms, and thrombosis. Two reviewers (XJ and YFL) independently and individually extracted the outcome data with an agreement value (κ) of 94.5%, and a third reviewer (JYX) provided additional insight when a discrepancy occurred. If the primary outcomes were not available in the original article, we searched for details using http://ClinicalTrials.gov, the US FDA website, and the manufacturer's clinical trial registry website. We used the Jadad scoring system to evaluate all trials [21], and a score >2 was required for a trial to be kept in our analysis.

2.5. Statistical Analysis. We pooled trial data using Stata Version 12.0 and calculated the relative risk (RR) and 95% confidence intervals (CIs) for the primary outcomes. A two-sided α value of 0.05 was defined as statistically significant. The magnitude of heterogeneity was estimated by the I^2 statistic and Cochran's Q test, and an I^2 value greater than 50% was indicative of moderate-to-high heterogeneity. If substantial statistical heterogeneity was found, we explored the sources of heterogeneity and the effect of individual study characteristics and subgroups on the risk estimates. The funnel plots and Begg's and Egger's tests were used to assess the publication bias.

Subgroup analyses were conducted with the data separated by three different groups (ICS versus placebo, ICS + LABA versus LABA, and ICS + LABA versus LAMA + LABA).

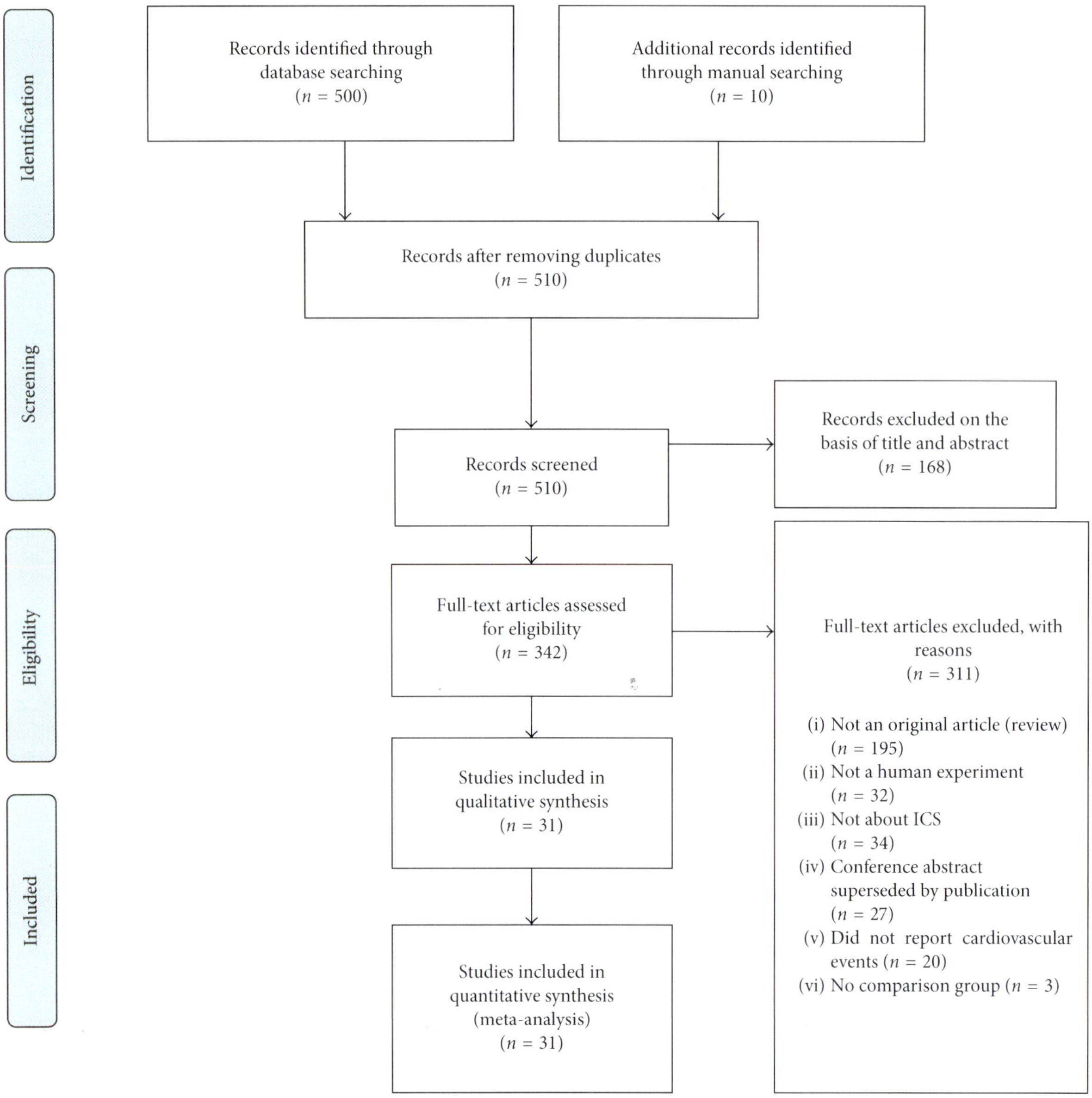

FIGURE 1: Study selection process.

An influence analysis was performed to evaluate the influence of individual studies on the summary effect. Because the effect of ICS on CV disease is a long-term effect, we conducted a sensitive analysis including studies with longer-term follow-up (>2 years).

3. Results

3.1. Characteristics of the Identified Studies. A total of 31 trials including 57031 patients fulfilled the inclusion criteria and were selected for analysis. The details of the study selection strategy are shown in Figure 1, and the main characteristics of the included trials are shown in Table 1. All trials were of high quality (Jadad score >2). These trials enrolled a total of 29171 participants who received an ICS and 27860 participants who received control therapies. Among the 31 studies, the main outcome of 13 studies was cardiovascular events, but there was no exact definition of cardiovascular events in these studies. In 31 studies, 5 studies resulted in cardiac arrhythmias, 2 in atrial fibrillation, 3 in cardiac failure, 3 in cardiac ischemia, 1 in acute myocardial infarction, 1 in angina pectoris, 1 in coronary artery stenosis, 1 in acute coronary syndrome, 2 in hypertension, and 15 in cardiovascular death. Inhaled fluticasone was evaluated in 26 trials [3, 16, 17, 22–44], inhaled budesonide in 4 trials [15, 45–47], and inhaled beclomethasone in only 1 trial [48]. The range of mean age in patients was from 52.4 to 67.6. The majority of the participants were male, with the proportion of current smokers ranging from 24% [22] to 83% [31]. The duration of the trials ranged from 4 to 156 weeks, with 18 trials being longer than 52 weeks in duration [3, 15, 22–26, 28, 30, 32, 33, 35, 39, 42, 44, 45, 47]. Most trials enrolled participants with severe COPD, as the mean predicted FEV1 of the participants was >50% in 7 trials [15, 23, 29, 33, 37, 38, 47] compared to ≤50% in 17 trials [3, 16, 17, 22, 24, 28,

Table 1: Characteristics of included studies.

Author	Year	J	Drug	Male (%)	Mean age (years)	FEV1 (% predicted)	Current smokers (%)	Treatment duration (weeks)
Aaron et al. [22]	2007	7	SFC versus SAL	57.9	67.5 ± 8.9	39.4 ± 11.9	32.4	52
				57.4	67.6 ± 8.2	38.0 ± 13.1	24.3	
Burge et al. [23]	2000	5	FP versus placebo	75	63.7 ± 7.1	50.3 ± 14.9	36.4	156
				74.2	63.8 ± 7.1	50.0 ± 14.9	39.2	
Calverley et al. [24]	2003	5	SFC versus SAL; FP versus placebo	75	62.7 ± 8.7	44.8 ± 14.7	52	52
				70	63.2 ± 8.6	44.3 ± 13.8	51	
				70	63.5 ± 8.5	45 ± 13.6	53	
				75	63.4 ± 8.6	44.2 ± 13.7	47	
Calverley et al. [25]	2007	6	SFC versus SAL; FP versus placebo	75	65 ± 8.3	44.3 ± 12.3	43	156
				76	65.1 ± 8.2	43.6 ± 12.6	43	
				75	65 ± 8.4	44.1 ± 12.3	43	
				76	65 ± 8.2	44.1 ± 12.3	43	
Ferguson et al. [26]	2008	7	SFC versus SAL	58.3	64.9 ± 9.0	39.8 ± 13.9	40	52
				52.0	65.0 ± 9.1	50.6 ± 15.4	38	
FLTA3025 [41]	2000	5	FP versus placebo	66	63.3 ± 10	NA	NA	24
				72	65.2 ± 8.7			
Hanania et al. [27]	2003	7	SFC versus SAL	61	63 ± NA	41 ± 11	43	24
				58	64 ± NA	42 ± 12	51	
Kardos et al. [28]	2007	4	SFC versus SAL	74	63.8 ± 8.3	40.4 ± 8.9	49.7	52
				77.6	64 ± 8.2	40.3 ± 8.5	49.9	
Lofdahl et al. [15]	2007	5	Budesonide versus placebo	73.5	52.5 ± 7.5	76.8 ± 12.4	39.4	156
				72.2	52.4 ± 7.7	76.9 ± 13.2	39.2	
Paggiaro et al. [29]	1998	5	FP versus placebo	99	62 ± NA	59 ± 18	49	24
				78	64 ± NA	55 ± 17	49	
Rennard et al. [45]	2009	6	Budesonide/FOR versus placebo	62.5	63.2 ± 8.9	33.8 ± 11.4	34.8	52
				65.3	62.9 ± 9.1	35.5 ± 11.9	39.5	
SCO100250 [40]	2007	6	SFC versus SAL	51	65.4 ± NA	NA	NA	52
				57	65.3 ± NA			
SCO100470 [42]	2005	6	SFC versus SAL	78.3	63.5 ± 9.3	NA	42	24
				77.2	63.7 ± 9.0		44	
SCO40041 [43]	2007	5	SFC versus SAL	59.7	65.4 ± 8.4	NA	NA	156
				62.7	65.9 ± 9.5			
SFCT01/SCO30002 [44]	2005	5	FP versus placebo	83.9	64.6 ± 8.7	NA	NA	52
				80	65.7 ± 9.0			
Tashkin et al. [46]	2008	4	Budesonide/FOR versus FOR	67.9	63 ± NA	33.7 ± 11.8	40.8	26
				65.5	64 ± NA	33.6 ± 11.3	38.4	
			Budesonide versus placebo	67.6	63 ± NA	33.5 ± 10.8	40.0	
				69.0	63 ± NA	34.6 ± 10.5	36.0	
Vestbo et al. [47]	1999	5	Budesonide versus placebo	58.6	59.0 ± 8.3	86.2 ± 20.6	75.9	156
				62.1	59.1 ± 9.7	86.9 ± 21.1	77.2	
Wouters et al. [30]	2005	4	SFC versus SAL	73	63 ± 7.9	47.4 ± 13.9	39	52
				75	64 ± 7.7	48.2 ± 12.9	35	
Boscia et al. [31]	2012	4	FF/VI versus placebo	46	57.9 ± 9.2	49.8 ± 10.6	83	4
Vestbo et al. [32]	2009	4	FP versus placebo	75	64.8 ± NA	44.7 ± NA	43	144
				77	64.9 ± NA	44.4 ± NA	42	
			SFC versus SAL	75	64.9 ± NA	44.8 ± NA	43	
				77	64.8 ± NA	44.1 ± NA	43	
Vestbo et al. [39]	2016	6	FF versus placebo	74	65 ± 8	59.6 ± 6.1	47	152
				75	65 ± 8	59.7 ± 6.1	47	
			FF/VI versus VI	76	65 ± 8	59.7 ± 6.1	45	
				75	65 ± 8	59.7 ± 6.1	47	
Kerwin et al. [34]	2013	4	FF versus placebo	64	62.7 ± 9.5	41.5 ± 13.13	54	24
				68	62.1 ± 8.8	42.4 ± 12.80	54	
			FF/VI versus VI	67	62.3 ± 8.5	42.3 ± 12.74	54	
				68	63.4 ± 9.6	44.5 ± 12.78	54	
Dransfield et al. [3]	2013	6	FF/VI versus VI	57.3	63.6 ± 9.1	45.7 ± 12.9	NA	52
				58.4	63.6 ± 9.4	44.3 ± 13.2		

Table 1: Continued.

Author	Year	J	Drug	Male (%)	Mean age (years)	FEV1 (% predicted)	Current smokers (%)	Treatment duration (weeks)
Calverley et al. [35]	2010	7	SFC versus SAL	75	65.0 ± 8.3	NA	43	144
				76	65.2 ± 8.2		43	
			FP versus placebo	75	65.1 ± 8.4		43	
				76	65.1 ± 8.1		43	
Martinez et al. [16]	2013	5	FF/VI versus VI	71	61.9 ± 8.8	48.1 ± 12.85	53	24
				74	61.2 ± 8.6	48.5 ± 12.89	55	
			FF versus placebo	74	61.8 ± 8.3	48.4 ± 12.17	56	
				74	61.9 ± 8.1	48.3 ± 12.71	53	
Donohue et al. [36]	2015	5	FSC versus UMEC/VI	69	63.0 ± 8.91	48.3 ± 10.82	41	12
				72	62.5 ± 9.05	48.6 ± 10.71	45	
Singh et al. [37]	2015	4	FSC versus UMEC/VI	71	61.4 ± 8.06	51.1 ± 10.50	61	12
				73	61.8 ± 7.94	50.2 ± 10.85	57	
Zheng et al. [17]	2015	5	FF/VI versus placebo	93	65.1 ± 9.19	49.6 ± 13.19	52	24
				90	64.7 ± 8.78	48.6 ± 13.39	56	
Wedzicha et al. [48]	2014	5	BDP/FOR versus FOR	69	64.6 ± 8.6	41.9 ± 6.0	39	48
				69	63.9 ± 8.6	41.6 ± 6.0	40	
Vogelmeier et al. [38]	2013	7	SFC versus QVA149	71.6	63.4 ± 7.7	60.0 ± 10.7	48.1	48
				70.2	63.2 ± 8.2	60.5 ± 10.5	47.7	
Vestbo et al. [33]	2016	7	FF/VI versus placebo	50	67 ± 10	NA	45	144
				48	67 ± 10		47	

The quality (Q) of each study was based on the Jadad scoring system. J: Jadad score; FP: fluticasone propionate; SAL: salmeterol xinafoate; SFC: combination of salmeterol xinafoate and fluticasone propionate; BDP: beclomethasone dipropionate; FOR: formoterol; TIO: tiotropium; UMEC: umeclidinium; QVA149: combination of indacaterol (a long-acting β_2 agonist) with glycopyrronium (a long-acting muscarinic antagonist) as a dual bronchodilator; FF: fluticasone furoate; VI: vilanterol; NA: not applicable.

30–32, 34, 36, 45, 46, 48], whereas 7 trials did not report the details of FEV1.

The modified Jadad scale is used to assess the methodological quality of a clinical trial judging the effectiveness of blinding. The score range is from zero (very poor) to seven (rigorous).

3.2. Main Findings. In total, all 31 studies reported at least one CV event. The ICS treatment did not increase the risk of CV events in COPD patients compared with the controls (RR: 0.99; 95% CI: 0.93 to 1.06; $P = 0.801$; Figure 2), and there was no evidence of statistical heterogeneity ($I^2 = 0\%$, $P = 0.846$).

3.3. Subgroup Analyses. ICS use was not associated with a significant effect on the risk of CV events when used in the combination of ICS + LABA compared to LABA alone (RR: 1.00; 95% CI: 0.90 to 1.10; $P = 0.930$ (Figure 2); $I^2 = 0\%$, $P = 0.643$). In addition, there was no significant difference between the ICS + LABA combination and the LAMA + LABA combination in the number of CV events (RR: 0.78; 95% CI: 0.39 to 1.55; $P = 0.473$ (Figure 2); $I^2 = 0\%$, $P = 0.238$). ICS treatment did not increase the risk of CV events compared with placebo (RR: 0.99; 95% CI: 0.90 to 1.09; $P = 0.872$ (Figure 2); $I^2 = 0\%$, $P = 0.816$).

3.4. Sensitivity Analysis. We implemented a sensitivity analysis by using influence analysis to verify whether an individual study influenced the results, and no combined outcomes were changed by any given study. In analysis including studies with a longer-term period (>2 years), the pooled RR and 95% CI were 0.99 (0.92–1.06), and there was no evidence of statistical heterogeneity either ($I^2 = 0\%$, $P = 0.787$).

3.5. Publication Bias. Moreover, the funnel plot that was used to assess publication bias appeared to be symmetrical and showed no publication bias (Figure 3). Meanwhile, there was no publication bias shown using Egger's test ($P = 0.733$). In sensitivity analysis, there was no publication bias shown using Egger's test either ($P = 0.735$).

4. Discussion

Our meta-analysis did not show any consistent association between ICS therapy and CV events in COPD patients, either as monotherapy or in combination with LABAs, when compared to placebo, LABA, and LABA/LAMA controls.

COPD is not simply a pulmonary disease [49]; it is associated with increased extrapulmonary complications. COPD often coexists with other chronic diseases that can influence patients' physical status and prognosis [50]. Patients with COPD are at higher risk of CV events than age-matched and sex-matched individuals without COPD [9, 51]. Meanwhile, more patients with COPD die from CV events than from the respiratory consequences of airflow limitation [52] because the hypoxemia, respiratory alkalosis caused by hyperventilation, and inflammation in people with lung function decline could result in higher CV morbidity and mortality [53]. In contrast, prevention and

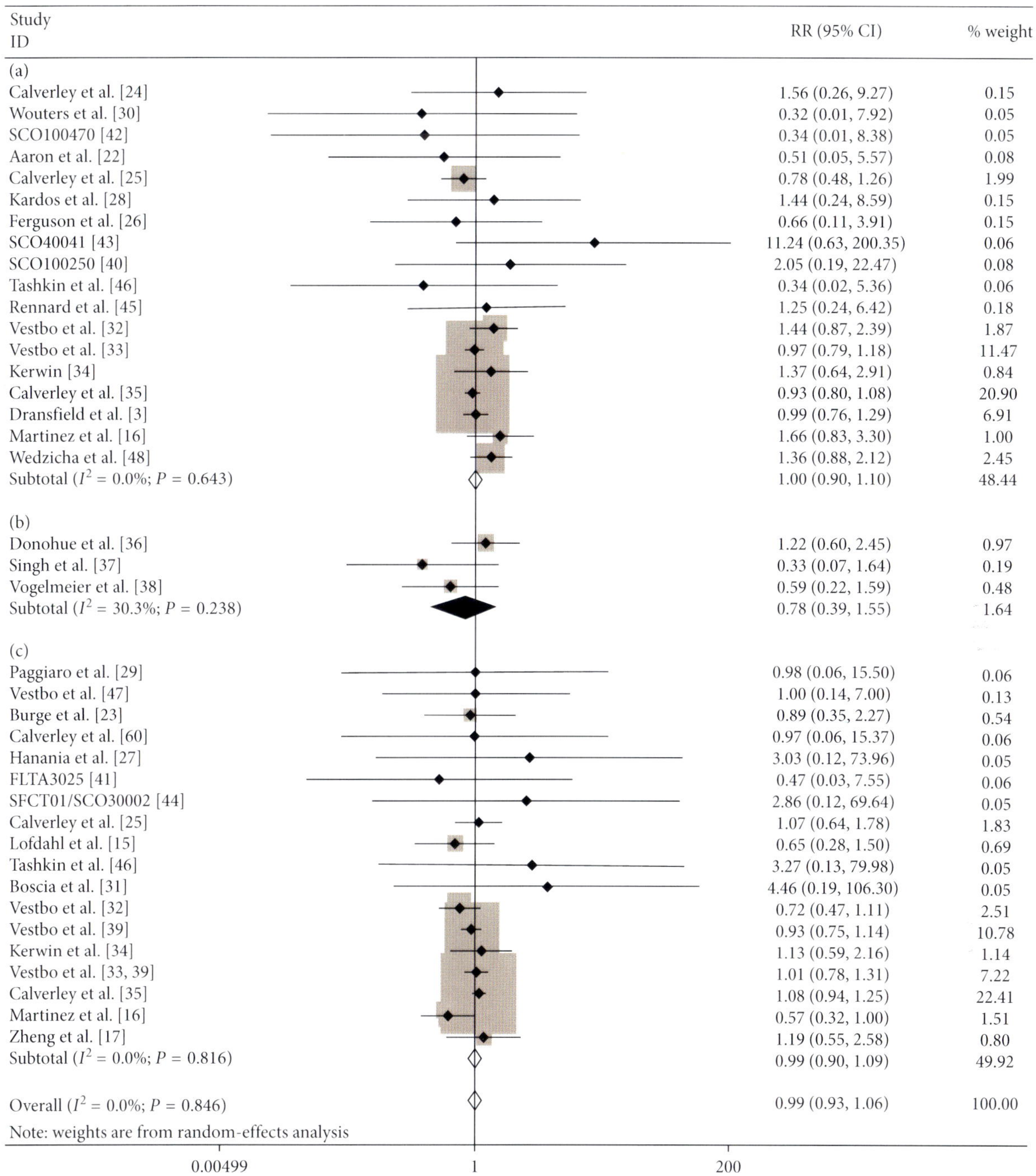

FIGURE 2: Meta-analysis of RCTs of ICSs versus controls for risk of CV events. (a) ICS + LABA versus LABA; (b) ICS + LABA versus LAMA + LABA; (c) ICS versus placebo. LABA: long-acting β_2 agonist; LAMA: long-acting muscarinic agonist.

treatment of exacerbations have been identified by GOLD as a priority since they are associated with impaired pulmonary function. Consequently, treatments that increase lung function and reduce exacerbations [54] would be expected to reduce both respiratory and adverse CV events. The recommendation of ICS therapy combined with an LABA in patients with moderate-to-very severe airflow limitations is based on evidence for reduced exacerbations. The pathophysiology of COPD includes systemic inflammation disorder and/or alterations in repair mechanisms. There are potential mechanisms linking COPD with an increased risk of CV events, including common risk factors (e.g., smoking), systemic inflammation [55], and vascular dysfunction [56]. The overexpression of inflammatory mediators into the circulatory system of COPD patients is relevant to the progression of CV events [57]. A mechanism for the reduction in CV-related deaths associated with ICS therapy is not clear. Potential explanations include a reduction in COPD exacerbations, which lead to hypoxia and instability that may predispose patients to CV events, a reduction in systemic inflammatory reactions to atherosclerosis [58], or a reduction in adaptive immune responses. Nevertheless,

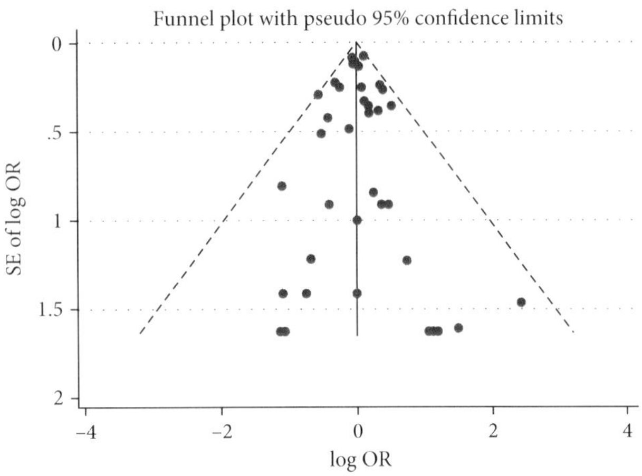

FIGURE 3: Funnel plots of RCTs of ICSs versus controls for risk of CV events.

ICS therapy may have limited CV benefits because ICS treatment does not reduce the inflammatory marker levels in systemic circulation (serum levels of C-reactive protein or interleukin 6), and ICS therapy also has little impact on neutrophil inflammatory responses or extracellular matrix remodeling linked to CV disease in COPD [57, 59].

The results of our analysis are consistent with other published studies showing that ICSs have no increased risks of CV events in COPD patients. Calverley et al. [60] reported that most of the deaths were events related to COPD, and only a few were related to CV events in COPD patients treated with budesonide. Furthermore, Calverley et al. [35] observed that the probability of COPD patients having an adverse CV event within 3 years of treatment was 24.3% for fluticasone propionate (FP) and 24.2% for placebo. Moreover, Dransfield et al. [3] reported that different doses of fluticasone furoate/vilanterol (FF/VI) combinations did not increase the risk of CV events compared with the risk associated with vilanterol (VI) alone. In addition, Loke et al. [61] concluded that ICS use was not associated with a significant risk of myocardial infarction when combined ICS + LABA therapy was compared to LABA treatment alone (RR: 0.92; 95% CI: 0.63 to 1.35; $P = 0.67$) or when ICS treatment was compared to placebo (RR: 0.97; 95% CI: 0.67 to 1.40; $P = 0.87$). They also found that ICS use was not associated with a significant risk of CV-related death when combined ICS + LABA therapy was compared to LABA treatment alone (RR: 1.12; 95% CI: 0.79 to 1.58; $P = 0.53$) or when ICS was evaluated against placebo (RR: 0.95; 95% CI: 0.71 to 1.27; $P = 0.74$). According to a recent study, the CV endpoint in the fluticasone furoate (FF) (hazard ratio (HR): 0.90; 95% CI: 0.73 to 1.1) groups did not differ from that in the placebo group [33]. Meanwhile, FF/VI had no effect on composite CV events (HR: 0.93; 95% CI: 0.75 to 1.14) with similar findings for VI (HR: 0.99; 95% CI: 0.80 to 1.22) [33].

There are certain discrepancies between the results of our meta-analysis and the outcomes of previous studies. A number of studies have suggested that ICSs may potentially confer CV benefits. Two observational studies [13, 14] reported a significant association between ICS exposure and a reduction in CV-related deaths but did not specify details on the causes of death. Macie et al. [14] concluded that an ICS-induced reduction in mortality was particularly notable for CV-associated deaths but not for COPD. Lee et al. [13] found that ICS exposure was associated with a 20% decrease in the odds of a CV-related death (odds ratio (OR): 0.80; 95% CI: 0.72 to 0.88). A pooled analysis of these two studies showed a significant reduction in CV-associated deaths (RR: 0.79; 95% CI: 0.72 to 0.86; $P < 0.0001$) [61]. Similar beneficial effects were also verified in RCTs. Lofdahl et al. [15] found that patients treated with inhaled budesonide had a significantly lower incidence of ischemic cardiac events (RR: 0.58; 95% CI: 0.35 to 0.98; $P = 0.043$) than those receiving placebo. Additionally, in a previous study [3], the risk of CV events decreased with increasing doses of FF; specifically, there was a CV benefit of FF/VI therapy compared with VI therapy alone with respect to patient-reported outcomes. Nevertheless, ICSs were not associated with a significantly reduced risk of myocardial infarction (RR: 0.83; 95% CI: 0.63 to 1.08) in an observational study [62]. Furthermore, another analysis conducted by Calverley et al. [25] showed that there was no significant reduction in cardiac disorders among patients treated with fluticasone (reported as CV event rates per study year: 0.113 in the placebo group, 0.102 in the fluticasone group, 0.114 in the salmeterol group, and 0.087 in the combination therapy group). Conversely, another study [16] suggested that FF/VI treatment resulted in increased CV effects compared with VI treatment alone. Similarly, in a study of Asian patients treated with FF/VI, high-dose FF was associated with increased CV events compared to those with low-dose FF [17].

There are several limitations to our research that make it difficult to reach a definitive conclusion. First, the RCTs did not use specific definitions of a CV event, and inconsistent adverse event reporting may result in some missing outcome data. Second, most of the included trials were not specifically designed to monitor the risk of CV events, which might have resulted in incomplete reporting of CV events. Third, the data used in this analysis were based on the judgment of the investigators, which might result in discrepancies between studies. Despite these limitations, we believe that our analysis adds more positive evidence for CV safety of ICS therapies in COPD patients. We will investigate the intraclass differences in the risk of CV events between different ICS therapies in our future meta-analysis. Our follow-up reanalysis of patient-level data (gender, age, smoking history, pulmonary function, and preexisting ICS use) may clarify the optimal role of ICS use in COPD.

5. Conclusions

In summary, despite certain limitations, our findings still have potential implications. We performed a meta-analysis of 31 RCTs, and the outcome indicates that ICSs do not increase the risk of CV events in COPD patients. This analysis also provides further evidence of safety for this important treatment option. Further studies are needed to validate our results in independent cohorts of patients with larger sample sizes and a wider range of clinical courses.

Acknowledgments

The authors thank Miaomiao Hou for her help with data abstraction and Jie Niu for his help with picture processing. This research was supported by a grant from the Natural Science Foundation of China (no. 81470240).

References

[1] Collaborators GBDCRD, "Global, regional, and national deaths, prevalence, disability-adjusted life years, and years lived with disability for chronic obstructive pulmonary disease and asthma, 1990-2015: a systematic analysis for the Global Burden of Disease Study 2015," *The Lancet Respiratory Medicine*, vol. 5, pp. 691–706, 2017.

[2] B. N. Mccullagh, A. P. Comellas, Z. K. Ballas, J. J. Newell, M. B. Zimmerman, and A. E. Azar, "Antibody deficiency in patients with frequent exacerbations of chronic obstructive pulmonary disease (COPD)," *PLoS One*, vol. 12, no. 2, Article ID e0172437, 2017.

[3] M. T. Dransfield, J. Bourbeau, P. W. Jones et al., "Once-daily inhaled fluticasone furoate and vilanterol versus vilanterol only for prevention of exacerbations of COPD: two replicate double-blind, parallel-group, randomised controlled trials," *The Lancet Respiratory Medicine*, vol. 1, no. 3, pp. 210–223, 2013.

[4] M. Bonay, C. Bancal, and B. Crestani, "Benefits and risks of inhaled corticosteroids in chronic obstructive pulmonary disease," *Drog Safety*, vol. 25, no. 1, pp. 57–71, 2002.

[5] D. Stolz, H. H. Hirsch, D. Schilter et al., "Intensified therapy with inhaled corticosteroids and LABA at the onset of URTI to prevent COPD exacerbations-a multicentre, randomised, double-blind, placebo-controlled trial," *American Journal of Respiratory and Critical Care Medicine*, vol. 197, no. 9, pp. 1136–1146, 2017.

[6] C. F. Vogelmeier, G. J. Criner, F. J. Martinez et al., "Global strategy for the diagnosis, management, and prevention of chronic obstructive lung disease 2017 report. GOLD executive summary," *Archivos de Bronconeumología*, vol. 53, no. 3, pp. 128–149, 2017.

[7] A. V. Gonzalez, J. Coulombe, P. Ernst, and S. Suissa, "Long-term use of inhaled corticosteroids in COPD and the risk of fracture," *Chest*, vol. 153, no. 2, pp. 321–328, 2017.

[8] P. Ambrosino, R. Lupoli, G. Cafaro et al., "Subclinical carotid atherosclerosis in patients with chronic obstructive pulmonary disease: a meta-analysis of literature studies," *Annals of Medicine*, vol. 49, no. 6, pp. 513–524, 2017.

[9] S. M. Curkendall, C. DeLuise, J. K. Jones et al., "Cardiovascular disease in patients with chronic obstructive pulmonary disease, Saskatchewan Canada cardiovascular disease in COPD patients," *Annals of Epidemiology*, vol. 16, no. 1, pp. 63–70, 2006.

[10] D. D. Sin and S. F. Paul Man, "Cooling the fire within: inhaled corticosteroids and cardiovascular mortality in COPD," *Chest*, vol. 130, no. 3, pp. 629–631, 2006.

[11] D. Pandya, A. Puttanna, and V. Balagopal, "Systemic effects of inhaled corticosteroids: an overview," *Open Respiratory Medicine Journal*, vol. 8, no. 1, pp. 59–65, 2014.

[12] S. Battaglia, I. Cardillo, F. Lavorini, M. Spatafora, and N. Scichilone, "Safety considerations of inhaled corticosteroids in the elderly," *Drugs and Aging*, vol. 31, no. 11, pp. 787–796, 2014.

[13] T. A. Lee, A. S. Pickard, D. H. Au, B. Bartle, and K. B. Weiss, "Risk of death associated with medications for recently diagnosed chronic obstructive pulmonary disease," *Annals of Internal Medicine*, vol. 149, no. 6, pp. 380–390, 2008.

[14] C. Macie, K. Wooldrage, J. Manfreda, and N. R. Anthonisen, "Inhaled corticosteroids and mortality in COPD," *Chest*, vol. 130, no. 3, pp. 640–646, 2006.

[15] C. G. Lofdahl, D. S. Postma, N. B. Pride, J. Boe, and N. A. Thoren, "Possible protection by inhaled budesonide against ischaemic cardiac events in mild COPD," *European Respiratory Journal*, vol. 29, no. 6, pp. 1115–1119, 2007.

[16] F. J. Martinez, J. Boscia, G. Feldman et al., "Fluticasone furoate/vilanterol (100/25; 200/25 μg) improves lung function in COPD: a randomised trial," *Respiratory Medicine*, vol. 107, no. 4, pp. 550–559, 2013.

[17] J. Zheng, T. de Guia, J. Wang-Jairaj et al., "Efficacy and safety of fluticasone furoate/vilanterol (50/25 mcg; 100/25 mcg; 200/25 mcg) in Asian patients with chronic obstructive pulmonary disease: a randomized placebo-controlled trial," *Current Medical Research and Opinion*, vol. 31, no. 6, pp. 1191–1200, 2015.

[18] M. T. Halpern, J. K. Schmier, M. D. Van Kerkhove, M. Watkins, and C. J. Kalberg, "Impact of long-term inhaled corticosteroid therapy on bone mineral density: results of a meta-analysis," *Annals of Allergy, Asthma and Immunology*, vol. 92, no. 2, pp. 201–207, 2004.

[19] N. Xia, H. Wang, and X. Nie, "Inhaled long-acting β2-agonists do not increase fatal cardiovascular adverse events in COPD: a meta-analysis," *PLoS One*, vol. 10, no. 9, Article ID e0137904, 2015.

[20] C. F. Vogelmeier, G. J. Criner, F. J. Martinez et al., "Global strategy for the diagnosis, management and prevention of chronic obstructive lung disease 2017 report: GOLD executive summary," *Respirology*, vol. 22, no. 3, pp. 575–601, 2017.

[21] A. R. Jadad, R. Andrew Moore, D. Carroll et al., "Assessing the quality of reports of randomized clinical trials: is blinding necessary?," *Controlled Clinical Trials*, vol. 17, no. 1, pp. 1–12, 1996.

[22] S. D. Aaron, K. L. Vandemheen, D. Fergusson et al., "Tiotropium in combination with placebo, salmeterol, or fluticasone-salmeterol for treatment of chronic obstructive pulmonary disease: a randomized trial," *Annals of Internal Medicine*, vol. 146, no. 8, pp. 545–555, 2007.

[23] P. S. Burge, P. M. Calverley, P. W. Jones, S. Spencer, J. A. Anderson, and T. K. Maslen, "Randomised, double blind, placebo controlled study of fluticasone propionate in patients with moderate to severe chronic obstructive pulmonary disease: the ISOLDE trial," *BMJ*, vol. 320, no. 7245, pp. 1297–1303, 2000.

[24] P. Calverley, R. Pauwels, J. Vestbo et al., "Combined salmeterol and fluticasone in the treatment of chronic obstructive pulmonary disease: a randomised controlled trial," *The Lancet*, vol. 361, no. 9356, pp. 449–456, 2003.

[25] P. M. Calverley, J. A. Anderson, B. Celli et al., "Salmeterol and fluticasone propionate and survival in chronic obstructive pulmonary disease," *New England Journal of Medicine*, vol. 356, no. 8, pp. 775–789, 2007.

[26] G. T. Ferguson, A. Anzueto, R. Fei, A. Emmett, K. Knobil, and C. Kalberg, "Effect of fluticasone propionate/salmeterol (250/50 μg) or salmeterol (50 μg) on COPD exacerbations," *Respiratory Medicine*, vol. 102, no. 8, pp. 1099–1108, 2008.

[27] N. A. Hanania, P. Darken, D. Horstman et al., "The efficacy and safety of fluticasone propionate (250 μg)/salmeterol

(50 μg) combined in the Diskus inhaler for the treatment of COPD," *Chest*, vol. 124, no. 3, pp. 834–843, 2003.
[28] P. Kardos, M. Wehcker, T. Glaab, and C. Vogelmeier, "Impact of salmeterol/fluticasone propionate versus salmeterol on exacerbations in severe chronic obstructive pulmonary disease," *American Journal of Respiratory and Critical Care Medicine*, vol. 175, no. 2, pp. 144–149, 2007.
[29] P. L. Paggiaro, R. Dahle, I. Bakran, L. Frith, K. Hollingworth, and J. Efthimiou, "Multicentre randomised placebo-controlled trial of inhaled fluticasone propionate in patients with chronic obstructive pulmonary disease," *The Lancet*, vol. 351, no. 9105, pp. 773–780, 1998.
[30] E. F. Wouters, D. S. Postma, B. Fokkens et al., "Withdrawal of fluticasone propionate from combined salmeterol/fluticasone treatment in patients with COPD causes immediate and sustained disease deterioration: a randomised controlled trial," *Thorax*, vol. 60, no. 6, pp. 480–487, 2005.
[31] J. A. Boscia, K. K. Pudi, M. T. Zvarich, L. Sanford, S. K. Siederer, and C. Crim, "Effect of once-daily fluticasone furoate/vilanterol on 24-hour pulmonary function in patients with chronic obstructive pulmonary disease: a randomized, three-way, incomplete block, crossover study," *Clinical Therapeutics*, vol. 34, no. 8, pp. 1655.e5–1666.e5, 2012.
[32] J. Vestbo, J. A. Anderson, P. M. Calverley et al., "Adherence to inhaled therapy, mortality and hospital admission in COPD," *Thorax*, vol. 64, no. 11, pp. 939–943, 2009.
[33] J. Vestbo, J. A. Anderson, R. D. Brook et al., "Fluticasone furoate and vilanterol and survival in chronic obstructive pulmonary disease with heightened cardiovascular risk (SUMMIT): a double-blind randomised controlled trial," *The Lancet*, vol. 387, no. 10030, pp. 1817–1826, 2016.
[34] E. M. Kerwin, C. Scott-Wilson, L. Sanford et al., "A randomised trial of fluticasone furoate/vilanterol (50/25 μg; 100/25 μg) on lung function in COPD," *Respiratory Medicine*, vol. 107, no. 4, pp. 560–569, 2013.
[35] P. M. Calverley, J. A. Anderson, B. Celli et al., "Cardiovascular events in patients with COPD: TORCH study results," *Thorax*, vol. 65, no. 8, pp. 719–725, 2010.
[36] J. F. Donohue, S. Worsley, C. Q. Zhu, L. Hardaker, and A. Church, "Improvements in lung function with umeclidinium/vilanterol versus fluticasone propionate/salmeterol in patients with moderate-to-severe COPD and infrequent exacerbations," *Respiratory Medicine*, vol. 109, no. 7, pp. 870–881, 2015.
[37] D. Singh, S. Worsley, C. Q. Zhu, L. Hardaker, and A. Church, "Umeclidinium/vilanterol versus fluticasone propionate/salmeterol in COPD: a randomised trial," *BMC Pulmonary Medicine*, vol. 15, p. 91, 2015.
[38] C. F. Vogelmeier, E. D. Bateman, J. Pallante et al., "Efficacy and safety of once-daily QVA149 compared with twice-daily salmeterol–fluticasone in patients with chronic obstructive pulmonary disease (ILLUMINATE): a randomised, double-blind, parallel group study," *The Lancet Respiratory Medicine*, vol. 1, no. 1, pp. 51–60, 2013.
[39] J. Vestbo, D. Leather, N. D. Bakerly et al., "Effectiveness of fluticasone furoate-vilanterol for COPD in clinical practice," *New England Journal of Medicine*, vol. 375, no. 13, pp. 1253–1260, 2016.
[40] GlaxoSmithKline. Study No. SCO100250.
[41] GlaxoSmithKline. Study No. FLTA3025.
[42] GlaxoSmithKline. Study No. SCO100470.
[43] GlaxoSmithKline. Study No. SCO40041.
[44] GlaxoSmithKline. Study No. SFCT01/SCO30002.
[45] S. I. Rennard, D. P. Tashkin, J. McElhattan et al., "Efficacy and tolerability of budesonide/formoterol in one hydrofluoroalkane pressurized metered-dose inhaler in patients with chronic obstructive pulmonary disease: results from a 1-year randomized controlled clinical trial," *Drugs*, vol. 69, no. 5, pp. 549–565, 2009.
[46] D. P. Tashkin, S. I. Rennard, P. Martin et al., "Efficacy and safety of budesonide and formoterol in one pressurized metered-dose inhaler in patients with moderate to very severe chronic obstructive pulmonary disease: results of a 6-month randomized clinical trial," *Drugs*, vol. 68, no. 14, pp. 1975–2000, 2008.
[47] J. Vestbo, T. Søorensen, P. Lange, A. Brix, P. Torre, and K. Viskum, "Long-term effect of inhaled budesonide in mild and moderate chronic obstructive pulmonary disease: a randomised controlled trial," *The Lancet*, vol. 353, no. 9167, pp. 1819–1823, 1999.
[48] J. A. Wedzicha, D. Singh, J. Vestbo et al., "Extrafine beclomethasone/formoterol in severe COPD patients with history of exacerbations," *Respiratory Medicine*, vol. 108, no. 8, pp. 1153–1162, 2014.
[49] L. M. Fabbri and K. F. Rabe, "From COPD to chronic systemic inflammatory syndrome?," *The Lancet*, vol. 370, no. 9589, pp. 797–799, 2007.
[50] J. Vestbo, S. S. Hurd, A. G. Agusti et al., "Global strategy for the diagnosis, management, and prevention of chronic obstructive pulmonary disease: GOLD executive summary," *American Journal of Respiratory and Critical Care Medicine*, vol. 187, no. 4, pp. 347–365, 2013.
[51] D. M. Mannino, D. Thorn, A. Swensen, and F. Holguin, "Prevalence and outcomes of diabetes, hypertension and cardiovascular disease in COPD," *European Respiratory Journal*, vol. 32, no. 4, pp. 962–969, 2008.
[52] N. R. Anthonisen, M. A. Skeans, R. A. Wise et al., "The effects of a smoking cessation intervention on 14.5-year mortality: a randomized clinical trial," *Annals of Internal Medicine*, vol. 142, no. 4, pp. 233–239, 2005.
[53] S. Sidney, M. Sorel, C. P. Quesenberry, C. DeLuise, S. Lanes, and M. D. Eisner, "COPD and incident cardiovascular disease hospitalizations and mortality: Kaiser Permanente Medical Care Program," *Chest*, vol. 128, no. 4, pp. 2068–2075, 2005.
[54] J. A. Wedzicha, T. A. Seemungal, P. K. MacCallum et al., "Acute exacerbations of chronic obstructive pulmonary disease are accompanied by elevations of plasma fibrinogen and serum IL-6 levels," *Thrombosis and Haemostasis*, vol. 84, no. 2, pp. 210–215, 2000.
[55] D. D. Sin and S. F. Man, "Why are patients with chronic obstructive pulmonary disease at increased risk of cardiovascular diseases? The potential role of systemic inflammation in chronic obstructive pulmonary disease," *Circulation*, vol. 107, no. 11, pp. 1514–1519, 2003.
[56] J. D. Maclay, D. A. McAllister, N. L. Mills et al., "Vascular dysfunction in chronic obstructive pulmonary disease," *American journal of Respiratory and Critical Care Medicine*, vol. 180, no. 6, pp. 513–520, 2009.
[57] P. J. Barnes and B. R. Celli, "Systemic manifestations and comorbidities of COPD," *European Respiratory Journal*, vol. 33, no. 5, pp. 1165–1185, 2009.
[58] D. E. Sholter and P. W. Armstrong, "Adverse effects of corticosteroids on the cardiovascular system," *Canadian Journal of Cardiology*, vol. 16, no. 4, pp. 505–511, 2000.
[59] D. D. Sin, S. F. Man, D. D. Marciniuk et al., "The effects of fluticasone with or without salmeterol on systemic biomarkers of inflammation in chronic obstructive pulmonary disease," *American Journal of Respiratory and Critical Care Medicine*, vol. 177, no. 11, pp. 1207–1214, 2008.

Verification of a Motion Sensor for Evaluating Physical Activity in COPD Patients

Seiko Miyamoto, Yoshiaki Minakata, Yuichiro Azuma, Kazumi Kawabe, Hideya Ono, Ryuta Yanagimoto, and Tadatoshi Suruda

Department of Clinical Laboratory, National Hospital Organization Wakayama Hospital, 1138 Wada Mihama-cho, Hidaka-gun, Wakayama 644-0044, Japan

Correspondence should be addressed to Yoshiaki Minakata; minakaty@wakayama2.hosp.go.jp

Academic Editor: Leonida Compostella

Background. Objective evaluation of the physical activity (PA) in patients with chronic obstructive pulmonary disease (COPD) is important. We validated a triaxial accelerometer, Active Style Pro HJA-750C® (HJA), and evaluated the necessary conditions for obtaining reproducible data. *Methods.* The PA measured by HJA was compared with that measured by two already validated accelerometers in 11 patients with COPD (age: 76.6 ± 6.9, FEV1% predicted: 57.6 ± 18.6). Then, the influence of weather and holidays on the PA and the required number of days to obtain repeatability were examined in 21 patients with COPD (age: 73.0 ± 8.0, FEV1% predicted: 58.7 ± 19.0). *Results.* The PA values measured by HJA and those by DynaPort Move Monitor® (DMM) or Actimarker® (AM) were significantly correlated at all intensities ($p = 0.024$ at ≥4.0 METs by DMM and $p < 0.0001$ at the rest) except at ≥4.0 METs by AM, though the values measured by HJA were higher than those by AM which was reported to underestimate PA. The durations of PA on rainy days were significantly shorter than those on nonrainy days, but those on holidays were not different from those on weekdays. The values of ICC for 3, 4, or 5 days were higher than 0.8 at all intensities. The PA measured by HJA was correlated with the dyspnea scale FVC and age and tended to correlate with FEV1. *Conclusions.* The HJA was validated for evaluating the PA in patients with COPD. This trial is registered with UMIN000016363.

1. Introduction

Physical activity (PA) in patients with chronic obstructive pulmonary disease (COPD) is an important issue because it is related to the decline of lung function [1], hospitalizations [2], and mortality [3]. Furthermore, the PA level evaluated by an accelerometer is the strongest predictor of all-cause mortality in COPD [4].

The reports of PA in patients with COPD measured by accelerometers have rapidly increased [5–7]. Recently, the associations between the intensity of PA in COPD and several factors including dyspnea [8], limitation of tidal volume expansion [9], and leg muscle oxygen availability [10] have been reported. DynaPort Activity Monitor® (McRoberts BV, The Hague, Netherlands), its upgraded version, DynaPort Move Monitor (DMM; McRoberts BV, The Hague, Netherlands) [11–14], and SenseWear Armband® (BodyMedia, Pittsburgh, USA) [15–17] are frequently used in Western countries, but are not available in Japan. A compact-sized triaxial accelerometer, the Actimarker (AM; Panasonic, Osaka, Japan), had been available [8, 18–21], but production of the AM ended several years ago. An Activity Monitoring and Evaluation System (Solid Brains Inc., Kumamoto, Japan) is used for COPD [22, 23], but 2 accelerometers are required, and it is rather heavy and relatively complex to use for physicians. Recently, a new compact triaxial accelerometer, Active Style Pro HJA-750C (HJA; Omron Healthcare Co., Ltd, Kyoto, Japan), became available in Japan. Its metabolic equivalent (MET) value is calculated from three different linear regression formulas (sedentary, household, and locomotion) [24, 25]. However, the validity of HJA for patients with COPD has not been evaluated. Furthermore, when the PA is evaluated by HJA, the reproducibility of the data is very important, especially for evaluating the effects of medical intervention on PA.

The main hypothesis in this study was that the HJA is valid for evaluating the PA in patients with COPD. To prove this hypothesis, we tested the reproducibility of HJA compared to that of DMM or AM, which had been validated for patients with COPD. Then, in order to obtain repeatable data, we investigated the influence of weather or holidays on the duration of PA and also the minimal number of days required for analysis. Furthermore, we evaluated the relationships between PA and several demographic factors.

2. Materials and Methods

2.1. Subjects. For study 1, patients with stable COPD aged 40 or older were recruited from the National Hospital Organization Wakayama Hospital from April to September 2015. For studies 2 and 3, outpatients with stable COPD without any other diseases that might obviously interfere with walking were recruited from the same institute from May 2015 to January 2016 and from November 2016 to October 2017. COPD was defined as postbronchodilator forced expiratory volume in one second (FEV1)/forced vital capacity (FVC) < 0.7. The participants had not been diagnosed with asthma or bronchiectasis [26]. This study was conducted in accordance with the Declaration of Helsinki and was approved by the local ethics committee (IRB Committee of National Hospital Organization Wakayama Hospital; approval number: 1 and 8; approval date: October 31, 2014, and March 20, 2015, resp.).Written informed consent was obtained from all participants.

2.2. Design

2.2.1. Study 1. In order to evaluate the validity of the device, HJA compared to DMM or AM, patients attached three devices at the same time in the daytime except while bathing for 7 days (Supplementary S1). When the total measurement duration was less than 8 hours, the data were considered invalid [27, 28]. The data from the first and last days were excluded because the patients went to the hospital for the setup or removal of the devices and were recorded only part of the day [19, 29]. The data from the first 3 valid days include holidays per each patient employed for analysis because the minimal required number of days for evaluated PA in COPD was reported to be 2 to 7 [11, 18, 28, 30–32], and the data from at least 3 days could be obtained from all participants when the invalid days were excluded from measured 7 days (Supplementary S2). Then, the durations of PA according to the intensity (≥2.0 METs, ≥3.0 METs, and ≥4.0 METs) were compared. For DMM, the duration of locomotion (walking + cycling) was employed as an index of the PA.

2.2.2. Study 2. To investigate the influence of the weather or holiday on the duration of PA and determine the minimal required number of days for analysis, the HJA was attached throughout the day except while bathing for 2 weeks. The description of a diary in relation to weather and the kinds of activities was required during the measurement of PA. During the 2 weeks, the data of the first and last days were excluded [19, 29]. When the total measurement duration was less than 8 hours [27, 28] or when unusual activities (e.g., traveling, etc.) were performed, the data were excluded as invalid. The durations of PA on rainy days were compared with those on nonrainy days, and those on holidays (Saturday, Sunday, and legal holidays) were compared with those on weekdays. To determine how many days of measurement are necessary to ensure the repeatability of the measurements, the intraclass correlation coefficient (ICC) values of the duration of PA from the first 2, 3, 4, and 5 days among all evaluable days were evaluated (Supplementary S3).

2.2.3. Study 3. To evaluate the influenced factor for PA, the values of pulmonary function tests and other demographic factors were compared with the values of PA among the patients of study 2. The values of PA were calculated as mean values from the data of the first three nonrainy days except the first and last days (Supplementary S3).

2.3. Measurement of PA. HJA, AM, and DMM are all triaxial accelerometers that are compact and worn only at the waist. HJA and AM can record the duration of PA according to the intensity, and DMM can record the time spent in inactive (lying and sitting), static (standing and shuffling), moving (walking, stair walking, and cycling), and not worn.

HJA is a small (40 mm × 52 mm × 12 mm) and lightweight (23.0 g) accelerometer that can continuously monitor the PA for 45 days. The HJA collects the data of triaxial acceleration at a rate of 32 Hz to 12-bit accuracy. The range of the acceleration data of each axis is ±6 G, resulting in a resolution of 3 mG. The acceleration signals, calculated as the average of the absolute values of the accelerometer output of each axis from 10-second epochs at the middle of each activity, were processed for various acceleration output variables. The MET value is calculated from three different linear regression formulas (sedentary, household, and locomotion) produced by the relationship between the value of acceleration and the MET value measured by indirect calorimetry [24, 25].

3. Statistical Analysis

Statistical analysis was performed using GraphPad Prism 5 (GraphPad Software, San Diego, CA) and IBM SPSS Statistics (IBM Japan, Tokyo, Japan). The relationships between the PA evaluated by HJA and DMM or AM were assessed by Spearman's rank correlation, and those between HJA and AM were assessed by Bland–Altman plots. The influences of rainy days and holidays were assessed by the Wilcoxon signed-rank test. The repeatability of the data among measured days was assessed by ICC, in which ICC ≥ 0.8 is a generally accepted value for multiple ICCs in accelerometer studies [31–34]. The relationships between the PA and demographic factors were assessed by Spearman's rank

Table 1: Characteristics.

	Study 1	Study 2
Age (years)	76.6 ± 6.9	73.0 ± 8.0
Gender (M/F) (n)	11/1	20/1
Smoking history		
Pack-years	96.1 ± 47.5	56.7 ± 36.7
Curr/ex/non (n)	4/7/1	7/13/1
Body mass index	19.9 ± 2.5	20.4 ± 4.0
GOLD stage (I/II/III/IV) (n)	1/5/6/0	3/10/7/1
mMRC scale (0/1/2/3/4) (n)	1/4/1/6/0	6/9/3/3/0
Pulmonary function		
FVC (L)	2.78 ± 0.60	2.92 ± 0.64
FEV1 (L)	1.43 ± 0.37	1.57 ± 0.52
FEV1/FVC (%)	51.7 ± 9.2	53.1 ± 8.6
FEV1% predicted (%)	57.6 ± 18.6	58.7 ± 19.0
Occupation (yes/no)	8/4	15*/6

*Farmer: 7; forestry: 2; fisherman: 1; driver: 1; carpenter: 1; concrete work: 1; iron industry: 1; clerical: 1; M: male; F: female; curr: current smoker; ex: ex-smoker; non: nonsmoker; GOLD: Global Initiative for Chronic Obstructive Lung Disease; mMRC: modified Medical Research Council; FVC: forced vital capacity; FEV1: forced expiratory volume in one second. Data are presented as means ± SD.

correlation and the Kruskal–Wallis test. The significance was considered as less than 0.05.

4. Results

4.1. Study 1. Eleven outpatients with COPD aged 76.6 ± 6.9 were recruited (Table 1). Correlations between the PA measured by HJA and DMM were statistically significant for all indices of PA including duration at ≥2.0 METs and duration of locomotion (r = 0.808, $p < 0.0001$), ≥3.0 METs and locomotion (r = 0.801, $p < 0.0001$), and ≥4.0 METs and locomotion (r = 0.376, p = 0.024) (Figure 1(a)). Correlations between the PA measured by HJA and AM were also statistically significant for the duration at ≥2.0 METs (r = 0.832, $p < 0.0001$) and ≥3.0 METs (r = 0.718, $p < 0.0001$) but not at ≥4.0 METs (r = −0.045, p = 0.795) (Figure 1(b)). The durations at ≥4.0 METs measured by HJA were 0 min in 10 of 36 cases, but those measured by AM were 28 of 36 cases. There were fixed biases between the values of PA measured by HJA and those by AM at all intensities, when a Bland–Altman plot was applied (at ≥2.0 METs: average 95% confidence interval (95% CI) 29.1, 17.1 and limit of agreement (LOA) −11.5, 57.7; at ≥3.0 METs: 95% CI 14.7, 4.8 and LOA −8.61, 28.17; at ≥4.0 METs: 95% CI 2.07, 0.81 and LOA −2.23, 5.12). Most of the values of PA by HJA were higher than those by AM.

4.2. Study 2. Twenty-one outpatients with COPD aged 73.0 ± 8.0 were recruited (Table 1). In one patient, there was no rainy weather during the measurement period, so the effect of rainy days on PA was evaluated with the data of 20 patients. The number of rainy days was 2.6 ± 1.3, nonrainy days 10.0 ± 1.8, holidays 4.0 ± 0.9, and weekdays 8.3 ± 1.2. The durations of PA on rainy days were significantly shorter than those on nonrainy days at ≥2.0 METs ($p < 0.001$) and ≥3.0 METs ($p < 0.01$) but not at ≥4.0 METs (P = 0.062) (Figure 2). The durations of PA on holidays were not significantly different from those on weekdays (≥2.0 METs, p = 0.165; ≥3.0 METs, p = 0.121; and ≥4.0 METs, p = 0.096) (Figure 3). The values of ICC for 2 days were less than 0.8 at ≥4.0 METs, but those for 3, 4, or 5 days were more than 0.8 at all intensities (Figure 4).

4.3. Study 3. The durations of PA were positively correlated with FVC% predicted and negatively with modified Medical Research Council (mMRC) dyspnea scale score and age and tended to be positively correlated with FEV1% predicted (Table 2).

5. Discussion

5.1. Overviews. The correlations of PA at ≥2.0, ≥3.0, and ≥4.0 METs measured by HJA were confirmed with those measured by DMM or AM except at ≥4.0 METs by AM. However, most of the values of the duration of PA by HJA were higher than those measured by AM. When the PA of COPD was evaluated by HJA, the duration of PA was significantly shorter on rainy days than that on nonrainy days at ≥2.0 and ≥3.0 METs. In order to obtain reproducibility in the duration of PA measured by HJA, the data of at least 3 nonrainy days were necessary at all intensities. An available new triaxial accelerometer, the HJA, was validated, and the method for selecting the repeatable data was demonstrated in the current study. These results could provide Japanese physicians with the available method for evaluating the PA in patients with COPD.

5.2. Validation of HJA with AM and DMM (Study 1). HJA is a more compact triaxial accelerometer than AM, and the two accelerometers can evaluate the same parameters. DMM is distributed widely mainly in Europe [14] and is one of the recommended devices for evaluating PA in patients with COPD [30]. DMM can evaluate the duration of PA according to the kinds of activities, which are not entirely the same parameters as those for HJA. Both DMM and AM have been used for the measurement of PA in patients with COPD

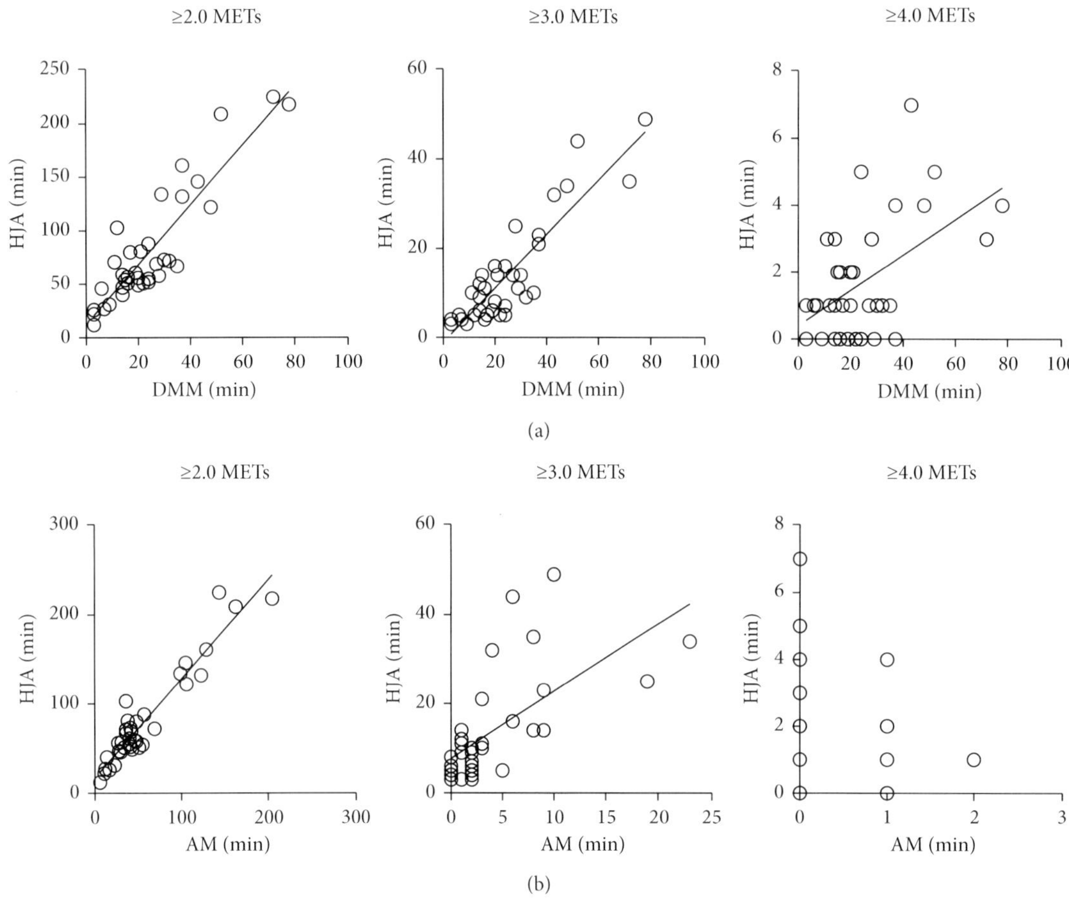

Figure 1: Correlations between the durations of PA measured by HJA and those by DMM and AM. (a) Comparison between HJA and DMM; (b) comparison between HJA and AM. The variables measured by HJA and AM were the duration of PA at ≥2.0 METs, ≥3.0 METs, or ≥4.0 METs. The variables measured by DMM were the duration of locomotion. METs: metabolic equivalents; HJA: Active Style Pro HJA-750C; AM: Actimarker; DMM: DynaPort Move Monitor.

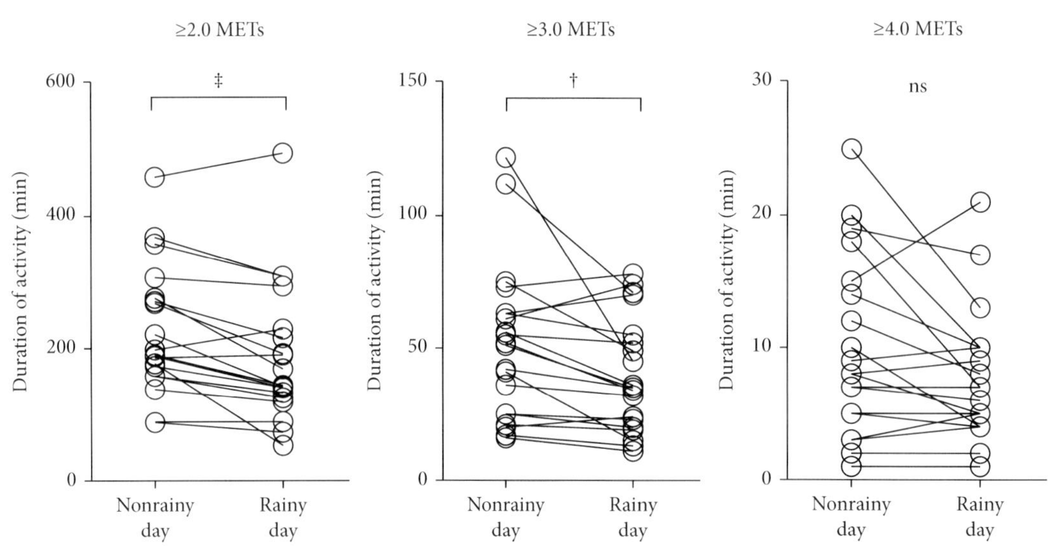

Figure 2: Effect of rainy days on the duration of PA. METs: metabolic equivalents; PA: physical activity; ‡: $p < 0.001$; †: $p < 0.01$.

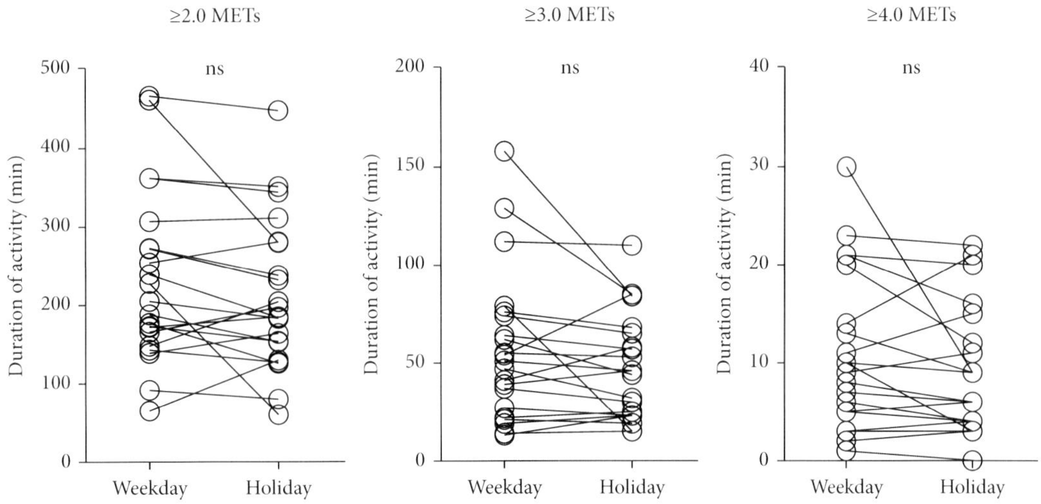

Figure 3: Effect of holidays on the duration of PA. METs: metabolic equivalents; PA: physical activity.

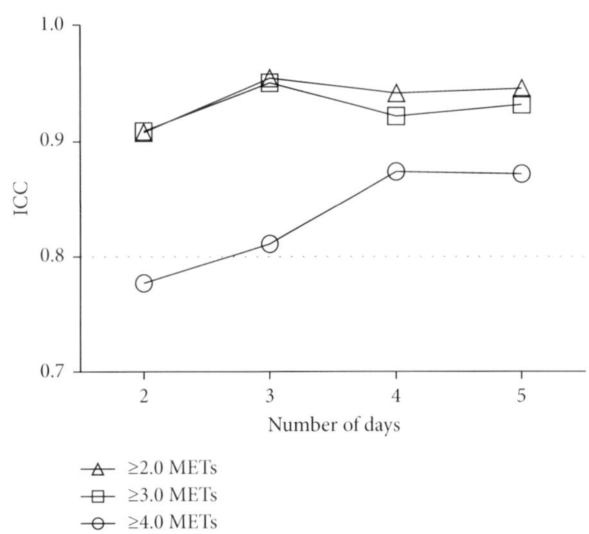

Figure 4: Repeatability of the measurement. Triangle indicates the duration at ≥2.0 METs; square indicates the duration at ≥3.0 METs; circle indicates the duration at ≥4.0 METs. METs: metabolic equivalents; ICC: intraclass correlation coefficient.

Table 2: Correlations between physical activity and demographic factors.

	≥2.0 METs		≥3.0 METs		≥4.0 METs	
	r value	p value	r value	p value	r value	p value
Age	0.061	0.792	−0.293	0.197	−0.437	0.048
BMI	0.024	0.918	0.031	0.895	0.240	0.296
Smoking (pack-year)	−0.170	0.462	0.194	0.399	0.331	0.143
mMRC score	—	0.024	—	0.004	—	0.038
Goddard score	−0.405	0.068	−0.289	0.204	−0.197	0.392
FVC% predicted	0.403	0.070	0.487	0.025	0.448	0.041
FEV1/FVC	0.244	0.286	0.341	0.130	0.349	0.121
FEV1% predicted	0.409	0.066	0.424	0.056	0.381	0.088
IC	−0.335	0.138	−0.055	0.806	0.068	0.769

BMI: body mass index; mMRC: modified Medical Research Council; FVC: forced vital capacity; FEV1: forced expiratory volume in one second; IC: inspiratory capacity.

[14, 18]. In the current study, significant correlations were confirmed between HJA and DMM or AM at all intensities except ≥4.0 METs by AM, though the durations of PA at ≥2.0, ≥3.0, and ≥4.0 METs by HJA were compared to the duration of locomotion by DMM.

For the PA at ≥4.0 METs, AM could detect only 28% of cases (10 out of 36), but HJA could detect 74% of cases (28 out of 36). This might be the reason why no correlation was observed between AM and HJA. Furthermore, most of the values of PA measured by AM were also lower than those by HJA at ≥2.0 and ≥3.0 METs, and fixed biases between HJA and AM were observed with Bland–Altman plots. The AM underestimated METs for all nonlocomotive activities except for hanging clothes and for all locomotive activities except for climbing down the stairs compared to the energy expenditure evaluated by the expired gas using the Douglas bag method [35]. The HJA might detect the PA more precisely than AM. On the other hand, the PA measured by DMM can well reflect the activity-related energy expenditure measured by the doubly labelled water indirect-calorimetry method [14].

5.3. Conditions for Measurement of PA (Study 2). As the composition of day-to-day variations in PA is important for evaluating the PA, factors that could affect the values of PA should be minimized. First, inclement weather might be one of the factors that could suppress PA. The PA on rainy days was significantly lower than that on nonrainy days at all intensities. These results were compatible with those of previous reports [18, 36]. Second, holidays might be another factor. The PA in COPD on holidays was not different from that on weekdays at all intensities. Steele et al. showed that the amount of physical activity performed during weekdays or weekend days is similar in retired persons [5], which is compatible with our results. However, Pitta et al. reported that the data of weekend days and holidays should be excluded [11]. Tudor-Locke et al. also reported that Sunday should be the last day to enter the analysis [34]. These differences might be affected by whether the subject is employed or not. In the current study, 6 patients had no occupation and 10 out of 15 patients who had occupations worked on both weekdays and holidays (farmer, forestry, and fisherman). This might be the reason why the PA was not different between holidays and weekdays in this study.

In order to obtain repeatability for the PA results at all intensities (ICC ≥ 0.8), the data of 3 days were required. In most of the previous reports that evaluated the PA in COPD with an accelerometer, the data of 3 to 5 days were required [5, 18, 31]. These reports are compatible with our results. Pitta et al. reported that 2 days were enough, but they evaluated the repeatability with ICC ≥ 0.7, which was less reliable than that of the current report (ICC ≥ 0.8) [11]. These results suggest that, for the purpose of obtaining reproducible data, it would be better to analyze the data from 3 nonrainy days.

5.4. Influenced Factor for PA (Study 3). The durations of PA were negatively correlated with the mMRC grade. PA in COPD was reported to be correlated with mMRC [8, 12, 37], and the cutoff value was mMRC 2 [8]. These findings are compatible with our results. Dyspnea might be a key element in modulating the PA in COPD. The durations of PA were correlated with FVC% predicted and tended to correlate with FEV1% predicted. It was reported that a correlation between pulmonary function and PA was observed but it was weak [7, 12, 38], which was also compatible with our results. The durations of PA at ≥4.0 METs were negatively correlated with age. Older people were more likely to be inactive than younger people [39]. In recommendation from the American College of Sports Medicine and the American Heart Association, the recommended level of PA is lower in older people than that in younger ones [39, 40]. Recently, the associations between the intensity of PA in COPD and limitation of tidal volume expansion [9] or leg muscle oxygen availability [10] have also been reported.

5.5. Limitations. There are several limitations that need to be addressed: first, the numbers of recruited subjects in both studies were small. The small number might have influence on the effects of holidays in study 2 and on the correlation with pulmonary function especially FEV1 in study 3. Second, though the effects of weather and holidays were evaluated, seasonal effects were not evaluated. Since the weather or temperature might influence the PA in COPD [36, 41], further study is required to determine such possible effects. Third, comorbidities and psychological conditions were not evaluated in this study. Many factors might have influence on the PA, especially on the results of study 3. Effects of these factors should be evaluated in other studies.

6. Conclusions

A new triaxial accelerometer, the HJA, was validated by comparing it with DMM and AM, which had already been validated for measuring the PA in patients with COPD. When the PA in COPD was measured with HJA, the data of 3 nonrainy days were necessary for obtaining reproducible data. The PA was associated with the dyspnea grade and pulmonary function.

Abbreviations

PA: Physical activity

COPD: Chronic obstructive pulmonary disease

DMM: DynaPort Move Monitor

AM: Actimarker

HJA: Active Style Pro HJA-750C

ICC: Intraclass correlation coefficient

METs: Metabolic equivalents.

Authors' Contributions

Seiko Miyamoto and Yoshiaki Minakata created the conception and design and analyzed the data. Yoshiaki Minakata, Yuichiro Azuma, Kazumi Kawabe, Hideya Ono, Ryuta Yanagimoto, and Tadatoshi Suruda acquired the data. All authors interpreted the data, drafted the manuscript, approved the version to be published, and agreed to be accountable for all aspects of the work. Seiko Miyamoto and Yoshiaki Minakata equally contributed to this manuscript.

Acknowledgments

The authors thank Mr. Brent Bell for reading the manuscript. This study was supported by JSPS KAKENHI Grant no. 15KO9187.

Supplementary Materials

Supplementary 1. Figure S1: setup of 3 triaxial accelerometers. HJA: Active Style Pro HJA-750C; AM: Actimarker; DMM: DynaPort Move Monitor.
Supplementary 2. Figure S2: numbers of patients and measurement days of study 1. HJA: Active Style Pro HJA-750C; AM: Actimarker; DMM: DynaPort Move Monitor.
Supplementary 3. Figure S3: numbers of patients and measurement days of studies 2 and 3. HJA: Active Style Pro HJA-750C.

References

[1] J. Garcia-Aymerich, P. Lange, M. Benet, P. Schnohr, and J. M. Anto, "Regular physical activity modifies smoking-related lung function decline and reduces risk of chronic obstructive pulmonary disease: a population-based cohort study," *American Journal of Respiratory and Critical Care Medicine*, vol. 175, no. 5, pp. 458–463, 2007.

[2] F. Pitta, T. Troosters, V. S. Probst, M. A. Spruit, M. Decramer, and R. Gosselink, "Physical activity and hospitalization for exacerbation of COPD," *Chest*, vol. 129, no. 3, pp. 536–544, 2006.

[3] J. Myers, M. Prakash, V. Froelicher, D. Do, S. Partington, and J. E. Atwood, "Exercise capacity and mortality among men referred for exercise testing," *New England Journal of Medicine*, vol. 346, no. 11, pp. 793–801, 2002.

[4] B. Waschki, A. Kirsten, O. Holz et al., "Physical activity is the strongest predictor of all-cause mortality in patients with COPD: a prospective cohort study," *Chest*, vol. 140, no. 2, pp. 331–342, 2011.

[5] B. G. Steele, L. Holt, B. Belza, S. Ferris, S. Lakshminaryan, and D. M. Buchner, "Quantitating physical activity in COPD using a triaxial accelerometer," *Chest*, vol. 117, no. 5, pp. 1359–1367, 2000.

[6] H. Watz, B. Waschki, C. Boehme, M. Claussen, T. Meyer, and H. Magnussen, "Extrapulmonary effects of chronic obstructive pulmonary disease on physical activity: a cross-sectional study," *American Journal of Respiratory and Critical Care Medicine*, vol. 177, no. 7, pp. 743–751, 2008.

[7] F. Pitta, M. Y. Takaki, N. H. Oliveira et al., "Relationship between pulmonary function and physical activity in daily life in patients with COPD," *Respiratory Medicine*, vol. 102, no. 8, pp. 1203–1207, 2008.

[8] A. Hayata, Y. Minakata, K. Matsunaga, M. Nakanishi, and N. Yamamoto, "Differences in physical activity according to mMRC grade in patients with COPD," *International Journal of Chronic Obstructive Pulmonary Disease*, vol. 11, pp. 2203–2208, 2016.

[9] E. A. Kortianou, A. Aliverti, Z. Louvaris et al., "Limitation in tidal volume expansion partially determines the intensity of physical activity in COPD," *Journal of Applied Physiology*, vol. 118, no. 1, pp. 107–114, 2015.

[10] Z. Louvaris, E. A. Kortianou, S. Spetsioti et al., "Intensity of daily physical activity is associated with central hemodynamic and leg muscle oxygen availability in COPD," *Journal of Applied Physiology*, vol. 115, no. 6, pp. 794–802, 2013.

[11] F. Pitta, T. Troosters, M. A. Spruit, V. S. Probst, M. Decramer, and R. Gosselink, "Characteristics of physical activities in daily life in chronic obstructive pulmonary disease," *American Journal of Respiratory and Critical Care Medicine*, vol. 171, no. 9, pp. 972–977, 2005.

[12] F. Pitta, T. Troosters, V. S. Probst, S. Lucas, M. Decramer, and R. Gosselink, "Potential consequences for stable chronic obstructive pulmonary disease patients who do not get the recommended minimum daily amount of physical activity," *Jornal Brasileiro de Pneumologia*, vol. 32, no. 4, pp. 301–308, 2006.

[13] V. T. Van Hees, S. M. Slootmaker, G. De Groot, W. Van Mechelen, and R. C. Van Lummel, "Reproducibility of a triaxial seismic accelerometer (DynaPort)," *Medicine & Science in Sports & Exercise*, vol. 41, no. 4, pp. 810–817, 2009.

[14] R. A. Rabinovich, Z. Louvaris, Y. Raste et al., "Validity of physical activity monitors during daily life in patients with COPD," *European Respiratory Journal*, vol. 42, no. 5, pp. 1205–1215, 2013.

[15] K. Hill, T. E. Dolmage, L. Woon, R. Goldstein, and D. Brooks, "Measurement properties of the SenseWear armband in adults with chronic obstructive pulmonary disease," *Thorax*, vol. 65, no. 6, pp. 486–491, 2010.

[16] D. Donaire-Gonzalez, E. Gimeno-Santos, E. Balcells et al., "Physical activity in COPD patients: patterns and bouts," *European Respiratory Journal*, vol. 42, no. 4, pp. 993–1002, 2013.

[17] K. M. Beeh, H. Watz, L. Puente-Maestu et al., "Aclidinium improves exercise endurance, dyspnea, lung hyperinflation, and physical activity in patients with COPD: a randomized, placebo-controlled, crossover trial," *BMC Pulmonary Medicine*, vol. 14, no. 1, p. 209, 2014.

[18] A. Sugino, Y. Minakata, M. Kanda et al., "Validation of a compact motion sensor for the measurement of physical activity in patients with chronic obstructive pulmonary disease," *Respiration*, vol. 83, no. 4, pp. 300–307, 2012.

[19] Y. Minakata, A. Sugino, M. Kanda et al., "Reduced level of physical activity in Japanese patients with chronic obstructive pulmonary disease," *Respiratory Investigation*, vol. 52, no. 1, pp. 41–48, 2014.

[20] Y. Minakata, Y. Morishita, M. Hiramatsu et al., "Effect of transdermal tulobuterol patch on the physical activity in eight male subjects with chronic obstructive pulmonary disease," *Clinical Research in Pulmonology*, vol. 2, no. 1, p. 1010, 2014.

[21] Y. Minakata, Y. Morishita, T. Ichikawa et al., "Effects of pharmacologic treatment based on airflow limitation and breathlessness on daily physical activity in patients with chronic obstructive pulmonary disease," *International Journal of Chronic Obstructive Pulmonary Disease*, vol. 10, pp. 1275–1282, 2015.

[22] A. Kawagoshi, N. Kiyokawa, K. Sugawara et al., "Quantitative assessment of walking time and postural change in patients with COPD using a new triaxial accelerometer system," *International Journal of Chronic Obstructive Pulmonary Disease*, vol. 8, pp. 397–404, 2013.

[23] A. Kawagoshi, N. Kiyokawa, K. Sugawara et al., "Effects of low-intensity exercise and home-based pulmonary rehabilitation with pedometer feedback on physical activity in elderly patients with chronic obstructive pulmonary disease," *Respiratory Medicine*, vol. 109, no. 3, pp. 364–371, 2015.

[24] K. Ohkawara, Y. Oshima, Y. Hikihara, K. Ishikawa-Takata, I. Tabata, and S. Tanaka, "Real-time estimation of daily physical activity intensity by a triaxial accelerometer and a gravity-removal classification algorithm," *British Journal of Nutrition*, vol. 105, no. 11, pp. 1681–1691, 2011.

[25] Y. Oshima, K. Kawaguchi, S. Tanaka et al., "Classifying household and locomotive activities using a triaxial accelerometer," *Gait & Posture*, vol. 31, no. 3, pp. 370–374, 2010.

[26] Global Initiative for Chronic Obstructive Lung Disease, *Global Strategy for the Diagnosis, Management, and Prevention of Chronic Obstructive Pulmonary Disease*, 2017, http://www.goldcopd.org/.

[27] H. Watz, T. Troosters, K. M. Beeh et al., "ACTIVATE: the effect of aclidinium/formoterol on hyperinflation, exercise capacity, and physical activity in patients with COPD," *International Journal of Chronic Obstructive Pulmonary Disease*, vol. 12, pp. 2545–2558, 2017.

[28] B. Byrom and D. A. Rowe, "Measuring free-living physical activity in COPD patients: deriving methodology standards for clinical trials through a review of research studies," *Contemporary Clinical Trials*, vol. 47, pp. 172–184, 2016.

[29] M. J. Mador, A. N. Patel, and J. Nadler, "Effects of pulmonary rehabilitation on activity levels in patients with chronic obstructive pulmonary disease," *Journal of Cardiopulmonary Rehabilitation and Prevention*, vol. 31, no. 1, pp. 52–59, 2011.

[30] H. Watz, F. Pitta, C. L. Rochester et al., "An official European Respiratory Society statement on physical activity in COPD," *European Respiratory Journal*, vol. 44, no. 6, pp. 1521–1537, 2014.

[31] H. Watz, B. Waschki, T. Meyer, and H. Magnussen, "Physical activity in patients with COPD," *European Respiratory Journal*, vol. 33, no. 2, pp. 262–272, 2009.

[32] C. E. Matthews, B. E. Ainsworth, R. W. Thompson, and D. R. Bassett Jr., "Sources of variance in daily physical activity levels as measured by an accelerometer," *Medicine & Science in Sports & Exercise*, vol. 34, no. 8, pp. 1376–1381, 2002.

[33] T. Baranowski and C. de Moor, "How many days was that? Intra-individual variability and physical activity assessment," *Research Quarterly for Exercise and Sport*, vol. 71, no. 2, pp. S74–S78, 2000.

[34] C. Tudor-Locke, L. Burkett, J. P. Reis, B. E. Ainsworth, C. A. Macera, and D. K. Wilson, "How many days of pedometer monitoring predict weekly physical activity in adults?," *Preventive Medicine*, vol. 40, no. 3, pp. 293–298, 2005.

[35] Y. Hikihara, S. Tanaka, K. Ohkawara, K. Ishikawa-Takata, and I. Tabata, "Validation and comparison of 3 accelerometers for measuring physical activity intensity during nonlocomotive activities and locomotive movements," *Journal of Physical Activity and Health*, vol. 9, no. 7, pp. 935–943, 2012.

[36] A. D. Alahmari, A. J. Mackay, A. R. Patel et al., "Influence of weather and atmospheric pollution on physical activity in patients with COPD," *Respiratory Research*, vol. 16, no. 1, p. 71, 2015.

[37] H. Demeyer, E. Gimeno-Santos, R. A. Rabinovich et al., "Physical activity characteristics across GOLD quadrants depend on the questionnaire used," *PLoS One*, vol.11, no.3, article e0151255, 2016.

[38] S. Singh and M. D. Morgan, "Activity monitors can detect brisk walking in patients with chronic obstructive pulmonary disease," *Journal of Cardiopulmonary Rehabilitation*, vol. 21, no. 3, pp. 143–148, 2001.

[39] W. L. Haskell, I. M. Lee, R. R. Pate et al., "Physical activity and public health: updated recommendation for adults from the American College of Sports Medicine and the American Heart Association," *Medicine & Science in Sports & Exercise*, vol. 39, no. 8, pp. 1423–1434, 2007.

[40] M. E. Nelson, W. J. Rejeski, S. N. Blair et al., "Physical activity and public health in older adults: recommendation from the American College of Sports Medicine and the American Heart Association," *Medicine & Science in Sports & Exercise*, vol. 39, no. 8, pp. 1435–1445, 2007.

[41] L. Sewell, S. J. Singh, J. E. Williams, and M. D. Morgan, "Seasonal variations affect physical activity and pulmonary rehabilitation outcomes," *Journal of Cardiopulmonary Rehabilitation and Prevention*, vol. 30, no. 5, pp. 329–333, 2010.

24

The Effect of Mechanical Ventilation on TASK-1 Expression in the Brain in a Rat Model

Buqi Na,[1] Hong Zhang,[2] Guangfa Wang,[2] Li Dai,[1] and Guoguang Xia[1]

[1]*Department of Respiratory and Critical Care Medicine, Beijing Jishuitan Hospital, Beijing 100035, China*
[2]*Department of Respiratory and Critical Care Medicine, Peking University First Hospital, Beijing 100034, China*

Correspondence should be addressed to Hong Zhang; 13520222956@163.com

Academic Editor: Emmanuel Charbonney

Background and Objective. TWIK-related acid-sensitive potassium channel 1 (TASK-1) is closely related to respiratory central control and neuronal injury. We investigated the effect of MV on TASK-1's functions and explored the mechanism using a rat model. *Methods.* Male Sprague-Dawley rats were randomized to three groups: (1) high tidal volume (HVt): MV for four hours with Vt at 10 mL/kg; (2) low Vt (LVt): MV for four hours with Vt at 5 mL/kg; (3) basal (BAS): anesthetized and unventilated animals. We measured lung histology and plasma and brain levels of proteins (IL-6, TNF-α, and S-100B) and determined TASK-1 levels in rat brainstems as a marker of respiratory centre activity. *Results.* The LISs (lung injury scores) were significantly higher in the HVt group. Brain inflammatory cytokines levels were different to those in serum. TASK-1 levels were significantly lower in the MV groups ($P = 0.002$) and the HVt group tended to have a lower level of TASK-1 than the LVt group. *Conclusion.* MV causes not only lung injury, but also brain injury. MV affects the regulation of the respiratory centre, perhaps causing damage to it. Inflammation is probably not the main mechanism of ventilator-related brain injury.

1. Introduction

Although mechanical ventilation (MV) is often a lifesaving method in critically ill patients, it is associated with many potential complications. MV causes not only ventilation-induced lung injury, but also distal organ dysfunction [1, 2], including the brain. Acute respiratory distress syndrome (ARDS) patients may develop non-muscle related ventilator-dependence, which is probably induced by ventilation. Long-term survivors of acute lung injury (ALI)/ARDS often have significant neurocognitive and emotional morbidity, while brain injury patients are more prone to lung complications [3–5]. Thus, the brain and lung have an integrity of function. It is important to explore the interaction between the lung and the brain in patients undergoing MV; however, studies on the impact of MV on the brain are limited and mainly focused on neonates [6, 7], and how MV influenced respiratory centre activity remains poorly understood.

K^+ currents have a key role in setting, maintaining, and regulating membrane potential and cellular activity and K_{2P} channels are major contributors to those background currents [8]. TWIK-related acid-sensitive potassium channel 1 (TASK-1) is in this family, which produces instantaneous open-rectifier (i.e., "leak") K^+ currents, and plays key role in the regulation of cell membrane potential [9, 10]. It has TASK-1~5 subtypes; among them, the pK of TASK-1 is ~ 7.4, which is very close to the normal acid and alkaline environment of the human body [11]. They are widely expressed in the central nervous system (CNS), especially in brainstem respiratory neurons and motor neuron [9, 12], including the pre-Bötzinger complex of the medulla oblongata, which is the generator of basic respiratory rhythm [9, 11–13]. Thus, TASK-1 plays a role in respiratory rhythm generation [10, 12–14]. Inhibition of the TASK-1 leads to an increased excitability of brainstem respiratory neurons, through further depolarization of cell membrane [11], thus enhancing the respiratory drive [13, 14]. Accompanied by its unique pharmacological profile, TASK-1 plays an extensive role in various physiological regulation activities including stress and inflammation and neuroimmune responses and is implicated in processes such as neuronal apoptosis [15].

We investigated the effect of MV on the brain in a rat model using TASK-1 functions as indicators. We compared TASK-1 expression in rats ventilated with two different ventilator strategies, a high tidal volume (Vt) group and a low Vt group, and compared with basal level rats.

2. Methods

2.1. Animal Preparation. This study was approved by the Animal Ethics Committee of Peking University First Hospital. We used 24 adult male Sprague-Dawley rats weighing 350 to 400 grams, which were assigned randomly to one of three experimental groups ($n = 8$ in each group): (i) the high Vt group (HVt), ventilated with 10 mL/kg and a positive end-expiratory pressure (PEEP) of 0 cm H_2O (ZEEP) for four hours; (ii) the low Vt group (LVt), ventilated with 5 mL/kg and ZEEP for four hours; and (iii) the basal group (BAS), unventilated animals, which were immediately exsanguinated after induction of anaesthesia. Anaesthesia was performed by intraperitoneal urethane (1.2 g/kg) and paralysis was achieved using intravenous rocuronium (1 mL/kg/h). Additional anaesthesia was given when necessary. An endotracheal tube (2.5 mm inner diameter) was inserted and tightly tied to avoid air leaks. MV group animals were connected to an HX-300 ventilator (Thai Union Technology, Chengdu, China) and ventilated for four hours. Volume-controlled ventilation was used with a respiratory rate of 60 to 70 breaths/min to yield a partial pressure of carbon dioxide in arterial blood ($PaCO_2$) of 35 to 40 mm Hg at baseline. A positive end-expiratory pressure of 0 mm Hg and an inspiration : expiration ratio of 1 : 1.25 were applied. The inspiratory oxygen fraction was kept at 0.3 throughout the experiment. The left carotid artery was cannulated and connected to a pressure transducer to monitor mean arterial pressure (MAP) and heart rate (HR). The right jugular vein was cannulated for fluid infusion. Fluid replacement was provided by administration of Ringer's lactate solution 10 $mL{\cdot}kg^{-1}{\cdot}h^{-1}$ (or in accordance with the hemodynamics).

2.2. Experimental Protocol. The MAP and HR values were measured at baseline and hourly thereafter; arterial blood gases were measured at baseline, 2 h, and 4 h. Fluid management was identical in both groups. Rats were euthanized by exsanguination at the end of the four-hour period, and 8 mL of blood was collected through the arterial catheter. We stored the plasma at −80°C for protein determinations. Rat brainstems were removed and immediately frozen and stored at −80°C. Hearts and lungs were removed en bloc, and the left lung was frozen for additional pathological examination.

2.3. Measurements

2.3.1. Histological Analysis. Left lower lobes were fixed by instillation of formalin into the airway at a pressure of 5 cm H_2O and immersed in the same fixative. A senior pathologist, who was blinded to experimental groups, calculated the histological scores after haematoxylin-eosin (HE) staining at a magnification of ×400. Lung damage was determined using a lung injury score (LIS), based on the evaluation of alveolar oedema, haemorrhage, leukocyte infiltration, alveolar septal thickening, and alveolar inflation in each animal. Each parameter was scored from 0 to 4. Subsequently, the total LIS was calculated by adding the individual scores for each parameter, up to a maximum score of 16.

2.3.2. Plasma and Brain Protein Immunoassays. Commercially available enzyme-linked immunosorbent assay (ELISA) kits (Biosource, Camarillo, CA, USA) were used to determine the levels of the following proteins in plasma/brain homogenates: tumour necrosis factor-alpha (TNF-α), interleukin-6 (IL-6), and S-100B. Analyses of all samples, standards, and controls were run in duplicate, following the manufacturer's recommendations.

2.3.3. Western Blotting for TASK-1. Rats lower brainstems were homogenized using lysis buffer containing 30 ml tris(hydroxymethyl) aminomethane hydrochloride (pH 7.5), 250 mL sucrose, 150 mL sodium chloride, 1.0 mL dichlorodiphenyltrichloroethane, and a protease inhibitor cocktail (Sigma; St. Louis, MO, USA), buffer containing another protease inhibitor mixture and phosphatase inhibitor mixture (both from Roche Applied Science, Indianapolis, IN, USA). Supernatants were collected after centrifugation at 11,180g at 4°C for 10 min. The protein concentration of each sample was measured using a bicinchoninic acid assay kit (KeyGEN BioTECH, Jiangsu, China) using bovine serum albumin (BSA) as a standard. An equal amount of protein extract from each sample (50 mg) was loaded and separated on a 10% Tris-glycine SDS polyacrylamide gel and transferred electrophoretically onto a nitrocellulose membrane (Pujinkangli, Beijing, China). The membrane was blocked with 5% nonfat dry milk in Tris-buffered saline containing 0.1% Tween 20 for 1 h at 25°C and then incubated for 24 h with anti-TASK-1 antibodies (1 : 200 dilution) (Alomone Labs, Jerusalem, JRS, Israel) at 4°C. The blots were then washed and incubated with goat-anti-rabbit secondary antibodies (1 : 5,000 dilution) (Zhongshanjinqiao, Beijing, China). Visualization was performed using enhanced chemiluminescence (Visual Protein Biotechnology, Taipei, Taiwan). Protein bands were quantified (the integrated optical density value of each band was calculated and corrected to that of GAPDH) using the AlphaEaseFC image analysis software package (version 3.5, Eastman Kodak, Rochester, NY, USA).

2.4. Statistical Analysis. All values are expressed as the mean ± SD. Mann–Whitney nonparametric U tests were used to analyse differences between groups, under the supervision of an expert statistician, in the SPSS 17.0 software (Chicago, IL, USA). A P value < 0.013 was considered statistically significant after Bonferroni correction.

3. Results

3.1. Physiological Variables. MAP remained stable and within the normal range throughout the four-hour period of MV in all groups (Figure 1). Oxygen saturation was relatively low at baseline, increased after two hours, and remained stable throughout the rest of the experiment. $PaCO_2$ returned to a

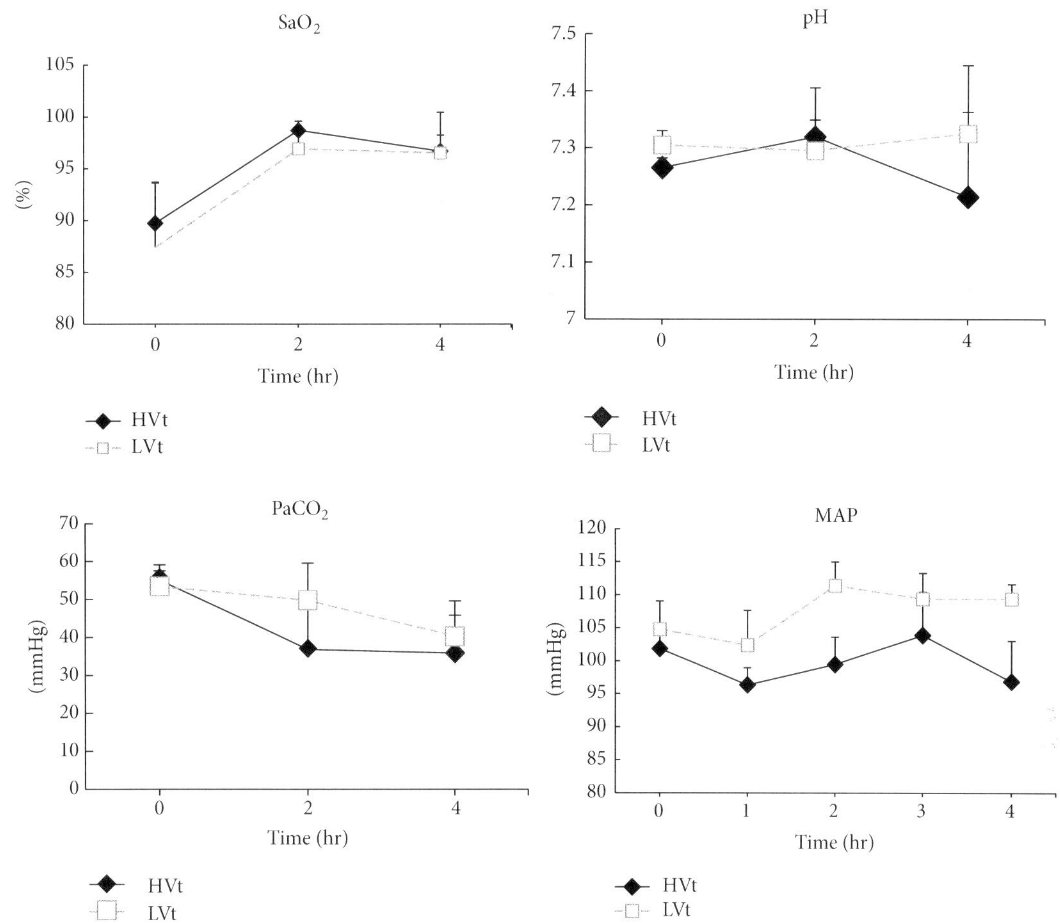

FIGURE 1: *Hemodynamic and respiratory characteristics of rats during the four-hour period of ventilation.* No differences between groups were observed at baseline. MAP remained stable in both groups. There were no differences between the LVt and HVt for arterial oxygen saturation (SaO_2). $PaCO_2$ in LVt animals was higher than in HVt animals. The pH decreased slightly in the HVt animals at four hours. But neither $PaCO_2$ nor pH had significant difference between two ventilatory groups during 4-hour period. Data are presented as the mean ± SD. $N = 8$ animals per group. MAP, mean arterial pressure; BAS, basal; LVt, low tidal volume; HVt, high tidal volume; SaO_2, arterial oxygen saturation; $PaCO_2$, partial pressure of carbon dioxide in arterial blood.

normal range at two hours in the HVt group and remained relatively high in the LVt animals; however, no significant difference was found between the MV groups. There was a decline in the pH value in the HVt group at four hours, although it was not significant compared with that of the LVt group.

3.2. Histology. Figure 2 shows representative images of the lungs in rats from each experimental group. Lung tissues of the MV groups showed obvious damage. The LISs were significantly higher in the MV rats compared with that in the unventilated rats ($P = 0.001$), and the LIS of the HVt group was significantly higher than that of the LVt group ($P = 0.001$).

3.3. Plasma and Brain Protein Levels. Figure 3 shows the plasma and brain levels of proinflammatory mediators. MV increased the plasma levels of IL-6 ($P = 0.001$) and TNF-α (HVt versus BAS $P = 0.01$, LVt versus BAS $P = 0.001$) significantly. In the brain, the HVt group showed reduced levels of IL-6 ($P = 0.001$) and TNF-α ($P = 0.05$) compared with the baseline level. IL-6 and TNF-α levels were similar in the LVt and basal groups. In the plasma, S-100B increased significantly in the HVt group ($P = 0.001$). In brain, S-100B decreased in HVt and increased in LVt group. Taken together, the inflammatory response was different in brain compared with the peripheral blood. In serum, there was higher inflammatory response in the MV groups. In the brain, LVt group showed a similar inflammatory response to the basal animals. By contrast, the HVt group exhibited a much lower inflammatory response. As for S100B, in serum, significant increase was seen in HVt group. In brain, LVt group had a higher S100B level compared to baseline, whereas there was a decrease in S100B level in HVt group.

3.4. TASK-1 Expression in Brainstem. Figure 4 shows the TASK-1 levels in the rat brains. Differences in TASK-1 channel levels in the three groups of rats were observed. Compared with basal rats, TASK-1 channel levels were significantly lower in the HVt and LVt groups (both $P = 0.002$). In ventilated

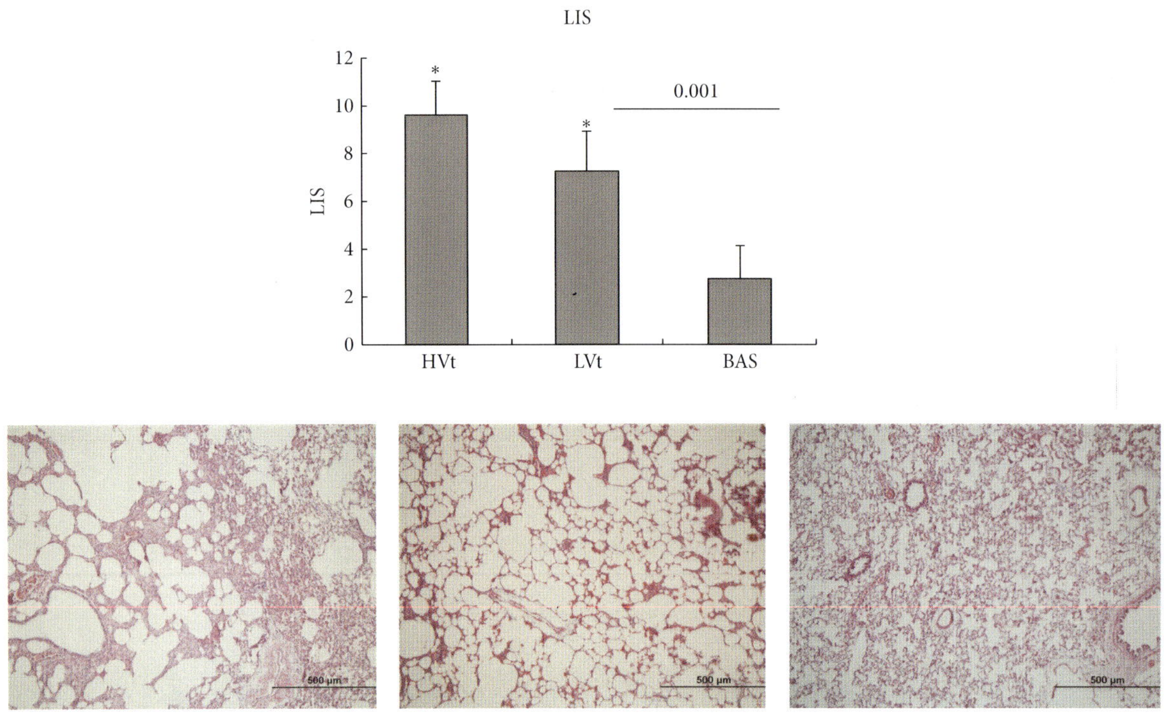

FIGURE 2: *Representative images of lungs in each group after haematoxylin and eosin staining and associated LISs.* Lung tissue of the MV group showed obvious damage, including significant alveolar oedema, haemorrhage, inflammatory cell infiltration, alveolar septal thickening, and alveolar overexpansion or atelectasis. LIS increased with MV and was significantly higher in the HVt group compared with that in the LVt group. Results are represented as the mean ± SD. $^*P < 0.013$ versus the basal group. $N = 8$ animals per group. MV, mechanical ventilation; BAS, basal; LVt, low tidal volume; HVt, high tidal volume; LIS, lung injury score.

rats, the HVt group had lower levels of TASK-1 compared with that in the LVt group; however, the difference did not reach statistical significance.

4. Discussion

4.1. Ventilation-Induced Lung Injury and Systemic Inflammation. Ventilator-associated lung injury (VILI) includes barotrauma, volutrauma, atelectrauma, and biotrauma, among which volutrauma, the overexpansion produced by high tidal volume, is the major cause of VILI [1, 16, 17]. Using histopathological analysis, we found that ventilated rats had lung injuries, with a significantly higher LIS than basal rats. Moreover, the LIS was significantly higher in the HVt group compared with that in the LVt group, indicating that MV induced lung injury, and the extent of damage increased with increasing tidal volume size, which was consistent with previous studies.

Some scholars use the concept of "organ crosstalk" to describe the effects of mechanical ventilation on multiple organs and the interactions between them [4]. However, how the lung-brain crosstalk occurs is unclear. Studies have shown that the ventilation-induced inflammatory response not only aggravates lung injury, but also leads to distal organ damage through circulation [18–21], which is the "biotrauma" mentioned above. Some researchers have suggested that inflammatory mediators in the blood can be sensed by the brain; thus, altering the permeability of the blood-brain barrier might be one possible mechanism of ventilation-related brain injury [22, 23]. However, previous studies focused on the lung and peripheral inflammation, and few addressed the inflammation status of the CNS [18, 19]. We measured IL-6 and TNF-α in the serum and brain and found that MV increased the blood IL-6 and TNF-α significantly, irrespective of the tidal volume level, whereas in the brain, a significant decrease in IL-6 was observed in the HVt group compared with that in the basal group. MV induced lung injury and the release of inflammatory cytokines into the circulation, but this systemic inflammation did not affect the brain, indicating that inflammation is not the only cause of ventilator-related brain injury.

4.2. Effect of MV on the Brain and TASK-1 Expression. Previous studies showed MV might promote brain activation [18] and influence cerebral tissue oxygenation and metabolism [20] and even brain tissue damage and disintegration of the blood-brain barrier [24–26]. TASK-1, is a two-pore (2P) domain potassium channel, which plays key role in the regulation of cell membrane potential [9, 10]. It is expressed widely in the CNS, especially in brainstem respiratory neurons and motor neurons [9, 27], including the pre-Bötzinger complex of the medulla oblongata, which is the generator of the basic respiratory rhythm [9, 11–13]. Therefore, TASK-1 plays a role in respiratory rhythm generation [10, 12, 14].

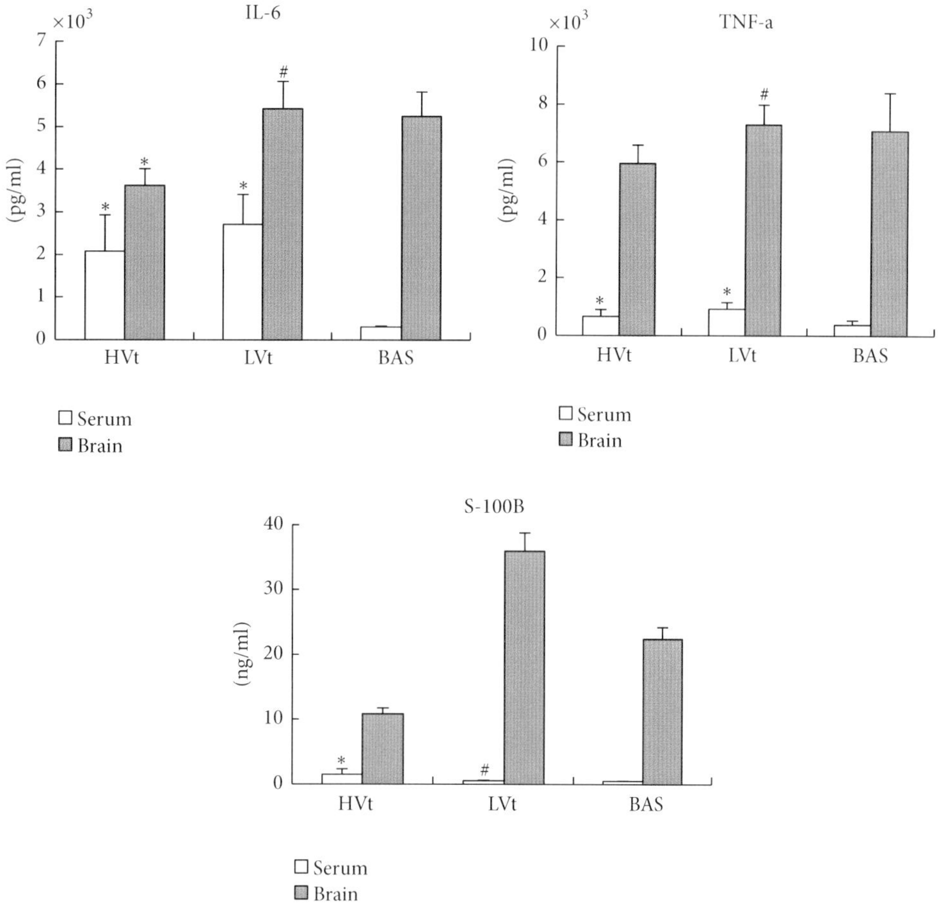

Figure 3: *Cytokine concentrations in plasma and brain homogenates.* MV increased plasma IL-6 and TNF-α significantly, irrespective of the Vt level (LVt or HVt) ($P < 0.013$). In the brain, IL-6 and TNF-α decreased in the HVt group. There was no difference in IL-6 and TNF-α levels between the LVt and basal groups. In the plasma, S-100B increased significantly in the HVt group. In brain, no correlation between S100B levels and tidal volume levels was seen. Results are presented as the mean ± SD. $^*P < 0.013$ versus the basal group and $^\#P < 0.013$ versus the HVt group. $N = 8$ animals per group. MV, mechanical ventilation; BAS, basal; LVt, low tidal volume; HVt, high tidal volume.

Inhibition of TASK-1 leads to an increased excitability of brainstem respiratory neurons, through depolarization of the cell membrane [11], thus enhancing the respiratory drive [13, 14]. Our results showed a significant decrease in TASK-1 channel levels in both the HVt and LVt groups, and there was a trend for the HVt group to have a lower level of TASK-1 compared with that in the LVt group. This suggested that MV might have an effect on respiratory centre function via changing the excitability of respiratory neurons, and this effect might correlate with the tidal volume level.

S100B is a calcium binding protein physiologically produced and released predominantly by astrocytes, because their levels may increase in CSF and blood in several brain pathologies including cell death [24–26]; it is considered to be a marker of neuronal damage. Bickenbach et al. [20] investigated the effects of different tidal volume ventilation on cerebral tissue oxygenation and metabolism in pig and found that low tidal volume (6 ml/kg) group significantly improved brain tissue oxygenation and micrometabolism compared to high tidal volume (12 ml/kg) group. In addition, serum S100B protein levels significantly increased in high tidal volume group compared to baseline level, indicating neuronal damage. In pig model of hypoxemia, Fries et al. [28] found increase of S100B in ALI pig serum, while visible damage was observed in hippocampal neurons under microscope. Also, studies showed that S100B over a certain threshold (ng/ml as a unit of measurement) [29, 30] are indicators of prior brain damage and bear clinical significance as predictors of poor outcome. As neurologic injury markers in blood are hampered by many confounding factors, some scholars proposed that biochemical markers in brain might be more accurate reflectors of cerebral pathological changes [24, 30]. But there are few studies comparing the prognostic value of S100B in serum and brain (CSF or brain homogenates) and the result differs [31, 32]. We for the first time measured S100B in both serum and brain during mechanical ventilation and observed that, in serum, S100B increased significantly in HVt group, which suggested neuronal damage in this group. In brain, LVt group had a higher S100B level than basal group, whereas there was a decrease in S100B level in HVt group.

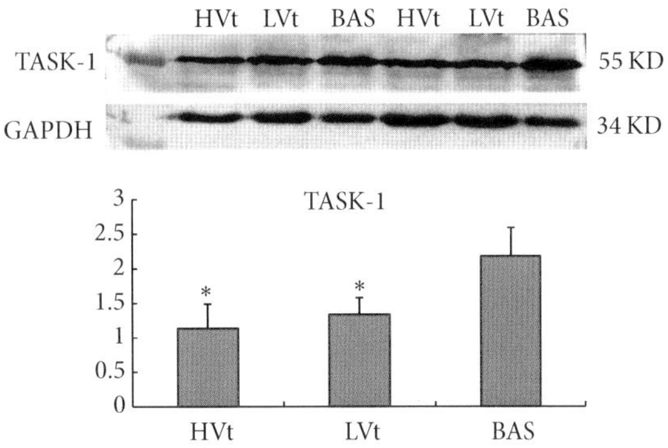

Figure 4: *Western blotting analysis of TASK-1 levels in each group.* Significant decreases in the TASK-1 channel levels in the HVt and LVt groups were observed. The HVt group tended to have a lower level of TASK-1 than the LVt group. Results are presented as mean ± SD. $^*P < 0.013$ versus the basal group (HVt versus BAS $P = 0.002$, $U = 3$) (LVt versus BAS $P = 0.002, U = 2$). $N = 8$ animals per group. BAS, basal; LVt, low tidal volume; HVt, high tidal volume.

MV can induce apoptosis in distant organs (including the kidney, intestine, heart, and liver) through different pathways [22]. Although many studies have speculated that potassium channels induce neuronal apoptosis [33, 34] or immune inflammatory injury [35], increasing evidence suggests that an important emerging therapeutic mechanism underlying neuroprotection is the activation/opening K_{2P} channels. Inflammatory plaques of human multiple sclerosis patients displayed profoundly lowered expression of TASK isoforms [15]. Rao et al. found that traumatic brain injury led to a downregulation of potassium channels (RK5, TWIK, and X62859) in the injured cortex, leading to decreased posttraumatic axonal conductance and epilepsy [36]. Liu et al. determined that K_{2P} channels (TASK-1, 2, 3) protected cells effectively from cytotoxic stress by preventing activation of apoptotic pathways [37]. Increased membrane excitability by TASK channel inhibition could contribute to increased electrical activity and subsequent neuronal degeneration caused by intracellular sodium and calcium accumulation, which is known as "excitotoxicity," the most common pathological mechanism leading to neuronal death. Meuth et al. [15] observed hypoxia depolarized central neurons after specific inhibition of TASK-1; they proposed that upregulation of functional TASK channel expression might exert a neuroprotective effect by dampening neuronal excitability. Neurons expressing nitric oxide (NO) synthase (NOS-I), which is upregulated in many human chronic neurodegenerative diseases, are highly susceptible to neurodegeneration. González-Forero et al. [38] showed that the autocrine activation of the neuronal NO/cGMP pathway induced by XIIth nerve injury enhanced excitability of the motor neuron pool and fully suppressed TASK currents via a protein kinase G-(PKG-) dependent mechanism. Finally, they proposed a hypothesis whereby TASK channel inhibition via persistent autocrine activation of the NO/cGMP/PKG cascade could sensitize NOS-expressing neurons to excitotoxic damage in brain neurodegenerative processes via a sustained increase in their excitability. Moreover, Mazzone and Nistri [39] used a validated in vitro model of spinal cord injury induced by kainate-mediated excitotoxicity to explore relation of S100B levels and damage severity and found that S100B represents a useful biomarker of lesion progression as its level is related to the occurrence and severity of neuronal loss due to excitotoxicity. Therefore, MV might cause neuronal damage directly in the brain or cause apoptosis by reducing the protective factor-TASK-1 channel expression. TASK channel inhibition-mediated sensitization of neurons to excitotoxic damage might be the mechanism of the latter [36].

Our study had certain limitations: (1) as anaesthetized animals soon develop respiratory failure, a group of spontaneously breathing rats was not set in this study; thus the results did not allow us to discriminate the role played by surgical procedures. (2) We hypothesized that mechanical ventilation affects TASK-1, thereby affecting the respiratory centre activity, based on the fact that TASK1 is closely related to respiratory neuron excitability. Functional change in neuron physiology was not determined in our study. As leak conductance of TASK-1 channel under different ventilatory settings can not be measured in vivo via patch clamp techniques, a better experimental design is needed in future research to determine functional status of TASK-1 channel during MV. (3) We measured S100B as a biomarker of neuronal damage and found the change of serum S100B was consistent with literature, indicating neuronal damage in HVt, but in brain, we did not observe correlation between S100B levels and tidal volume levels. Ahmed et al. [40] had found the CSF levels of biomarkers including S100B had time-dependent changes, with first peak appearing at 6 h after the injury and second peak at 24 h or 72 h, indicating that determining S100B continuously at different time intervals might reflect neuronal injury of brain more accurately. Moreover, in subsequent studies we should detect the neuronal apoptosis by TUNEL method in frozen slices of brainstem from different groups to reflect neuronal apoptosis directly and verify the significance of serum or brain S100B in predicting neuronal damage during mechanical ventilation. (4) To explore the mechanism through which MV influenced the brain, we measured IL-6 and TNF-a in serum and brain, respectively, to reflect the difference of inflammatory response in peripheral and central nervous system and obtained some different result from previous studies [22, 23]. Taking the fact that proinflammatory cytokines IL-6 and TNF-a could be influenced by many confounding factors and blood-brain barrier as well, we would like to assess immune cells in both serum and brain during MV in subsequent studies to further reflect peripheral and central inflammatory status. Moreover, we would like to differentiate and quantify immune cells in bronchoalveolar lavage fluid of different groups in supplementary experiment to explore the effect of MV on the immunoinflammatory status of lung, peripheral blood, and CNS, respectively.

5. Conclusion

In conclusion, MV downregulated the TASK-1 channel level in the rat brainstem, and the effect seemed to correlate positively with the tidal volume level, indicating that MV has an effect on the respiratory centre, possibly causing damage to it by increasing neuronal excitability. We also explored the mechanism through which MV influences the brain and found that (1) MV induced lung injury, which correlated with tidal volume size; (2) MV triggered proinflammatory responses in the circulation, but this systemic inflammation did not influence the brain, which was not consistent with the broadly accepted inflammatory mechanism hypothesis.

Abbreviations

TASK-1:	TWIK-related acid-sensitive potassium channel 1
MV:	Mechanical ventilation
HVt:	High tidal volume
LVt:	Low tidal volume
BAS:	Basal
MAP:	Mean arterial pressure
$PaCO_2$:	Partial pressure of carbon dioxide in arterial blood
LISs:	Lung injury scores
ARDS:	Acute respiratory distress syndrome
ALI:	Acute lung injury
CNS:	Central nervous system
PEEP:	Positive end-expiratory pressure
HR:	Heart rate
HE:	Haematoxylin-eosin
TNF-α:	Tumour necrosis factor-alpha
IL-6:	Interleukin-6
VILI:	Ventilator-associated lung injury
NOS-I:	Nitric oxide synthase
PKG:	Protein kinase G.

Acknowledgments

The authors thank Hongjun Hao, Cheng Zhang, Hui Dong, LiSu, and Peng Jia for technical assistance. This study was funded by the Beijing Natural Science Foundation of China Grant no. 7132187, 2013.

References

[1] N. de Prost, J. Ricard, G. Saumon, and D. Dreyfuss, "Ventilator-induced lung injury: historical perspectives and clinical implications," *Annals of Intensive Care*, vol. 1, no. 1, p. 28, 2011.

[2] E. K. Wolthuis, A. P. J. Vlaar, G. Choi, J. J. T. H. Roelofs, N. P. Juffermans, and M. J. Schultz, "Mechanical ventilation using non-injurious ventilation settings causes lung injury in the absence of pre-existing lung injury in healthy mice.," *Critical care (London, England)*, vol. 13, no. 1, p. R1, 2009.

[3] V. M. Ranieri, P. M. Suter, C. Tortorella et al., "Effect of mechanical ventilation on inflammatory mediators in patients with acute respiratory distress syndrome: a randomized controlled trial," *Journal of the American Medical Association*, vol. 282, no. 1, pp. 54–61, 1999.

[4] M. E. Quílez, J. López-Aguilar, and L. Blanch, "Organ crosstalk during acute lung injury, acute respiratory distress syndrome, and mechanical ventilation," *Current Opinion in Critical Care*, vol. 18, no. 1, pp. 23–28, 2012.

[5] J. Bickenbach, I. Biener, M. Czaplik et al., "Neurological outcome after experimental lung injury," *Respiratory Physiology and Neurobiology*, vol. 179, no. 2-3, pp. 174–180, 2011.

[6] G. R. Polglase, S. L. Miller, S. K. Barton et al., "Initiation of resuscitation with high tidal volumes causes cerebral hemodynamic disturbance, brain inflammation and injury in preterm lambs," *PLoS ONE*, vol. 7, no. 6, Article ID e39535, 2012.

[7] B. Skiöld, Q. Wu, S. B. Hooper et al., "Early detection of ventilation-induced brain injury using magnetic resonance spectroscopy and diffusion tensor imaging: An in vivo study in preterm lambs," *PLoS ONE*, vol. 9, no. 4, Article ID e95804, 2014.

[8] S. A. N. Goldstein, D. Bockenhauer, I. O'Kelly, and N. Zilberberg, "Potassium leak channels and the KCNK family of two-P-domain subunits," *Nature Reviews Neuroscience*, vol. 2, no. 3, pp. 175–184, 2001.

[9] E. M. Talley, Q. Lei, J. E. Sirois, and D. A. Bayliss, "TASK-1, a two-pore domain K^+ channel, is modulated by multiple neurotransmitters in motoneurons," *Neuron*, vol. 25, no. 2, pp. 399–410, 2000.

[10] C. P. Washburn, J. E. Sirois, E. M. Talley, P. G. Guyenet, and D. A. Bayliss, "Serotonergic raphe neurons express TASK channel transcripts and a TASK-like pH- and halothane-sensitive K+ conductance," *Journal of Neuroscience*, vol. 22, no. 4, pp. 1256–1265, 2002.

[11] F. Duprat, I. Lauritzen, A. Patel, and E. Honoré, "The TASK background K2P channels: chemo- and nutrient sensors," *Trends in Neurosciences*, vol. 30, no. 11, pp. 573–580, 2007.

[12] S. Trapp, M. I. Aller, W. Wisden, and A. V. Gourine, "A role for TASK-1 (KCNK3) channels in the chemosensory control of breathing," *Journal of Neuroscience*, vol. 28, no. 35, pp. 8844–8850, 2008.

[13] H. Koizumi, S. E. Smerin, T. Yamanishi, B. R. Moorjani, R. Zhang, and J. C. Smith, "TASK channels contribute to the K+-dominated leak current regulating respiratory rhythm generation in vitro," *Journal of Neuroscience*, vol. 30, no. 12, pp. 4273–4284, 2010.

[14] D. A. Bayliss, E. M. Talley, J. E. Sirois, and Q. Lei, "TASK-1 is a highly modulated pH-sensitive leak K+ channel expressed in brainstem respiratory neurons," *Respiration Physiology*, vol. 129, no. 1-2, pp. 159–174, 2001.

[15] S. G. Meuth, T. Kanyshkova, N. Melzer et al., "Altered neuronal expression of TASK1 and TASK3 potassium channels in rodent and human autoimmune CNS inflammation," *Neuroscience Letters*, vol. 446, no. 2-3, pp. 133–138, 2008.

[16] Y. Sutherasan, M. Vargas, and P. Pelosi, "Protective mechanical ventilation in the non-injured lung: review and meta-analysis," *Critical Care*, vol. 18, no. 2, article no. 211, 2014.

[17] J. W. Kuiper, F. B. Plötz, A. J. Groeneveld et al., "High tidal volume mechanical ventilation-induced lung injury in rats is greater after acid instillation than after sepsis-induced acute lung injury, but does not increase systemic inflammation: An experimental study," *BMC Anesthesiology*, vol. 11, article no. 26, 2011.

[18] M. Quilez, G. Fuster, J. Villar et al., "Injurious mechanical ventilation affects neuronal activation in ventilated rats," *Critical Care*, vol. 15, no. 3, p. R124, 2011.

[19] M. A. Hegeman, M. P. Hennus, C. J. Heijnen et al., "Ventilator-induced endothelial activation and inflammation in the lung and distal organs," *Critical Care*, vol. 13, no. 6, p. R182, 2009.

[20] J. Bickenbach, N. Zoremba, M. Fries et al., "Low tidal volume ventilation in a porcine model of acute lung injury improves cerebral tissue oxygenation," *Anesthesia and Analgesia*, vol. 109, no. 3, pp. 847–855, 2009.

[21] S. P. Yu, C.-H. Yeh, S. L. Sensi et al., "Mediation of neuronal apoptosis by enhancement of outward potassium current," *Science*, vol. 278, no. 5335, pp. 114–117, 1997.

[22] Y. Imai, J. Parodo, O. Kajikawa et al., "Injurious mechanical ventilation and end-organ epithelial cell apoptosis and organ dysfunction in an experimental model of acute respiratory distress syndrome," *Journal of the American Medical Association*, vol. 289, no. 16, pp. 2104–2112, 2003.

[23] R. Gonzalvo, O. Martí-Sistac, L. Blanch, and J. López-Aguilar, "Bench-to-bedside review: Brain-lung interaction in the critically ill - A pending issue revisited," *Critical Care*, vol. 11, no. 3, article no. 216, 2007.

[24] R. Brouns, B. de Vil, P. Cras, D. de Surgeloose, P. Mariën, and P. P. de Deyn, "Neurobiochemical markers of brain damage in cerebrospinal fluid of acute ischemic stroke patients," *Clinical Chemistry*, vol. 56, no. 3, pp. 451–458, 2010.

[25] M. L. Chaves, A. L. Camozzato, E. D. Ferreira et al., "Serum levels of S100B and NSE proteins in Alzheimer's disease patients," *Journal of Neuroinflammation*, vol. 7, article 6, 2010.

[26] J. Steiner, H. Bielau, H.-G. Bernstein, B. Bogerts, and M. T. Wunderlich, "Increased cerebrospinal fluid and serum levels of S100B in first-onset schizophrenia are not related to a degenerative release of glial fibrillar acidic protein, myelin basic protein and neurone-specific enolase from glia or neurones," *Journal of Neurology, Neurosurgery and Psychiatry*, vol. 77, no. 11, pp. 1284–1287, 2006.

[27] C. P. Washburn, D. A. Bayliss, and P. G. Guyenet, "Cardiorespiratory neurons of the rat ventrolateral medulla contain TASK-1 and TASK-3 channel mRNA," *Respiratory Physiology Neurobiology*, vol. 138, no. 1, p. pp, 2003.

[28] M. Fries, J. Bickenbach, D. Henzler et al., "S-100 protein and neurohistopathologic changes in a porcine model of acute lung injury," *Anesthesiology*, vol. 102, no. 4, pp. 761–767, 2005.

[29] N. Marchi, R. P. Fau, M. Kapural et al., *Janigro D Peripheral Markers of Brain Damage And Blood-Brain Barrier Dysfunction*, 2003.

[30] I. Kellermann, A. Kleindienst, N. Hore, M. Buchfelder, and S. Brandner, "Early CSF and serum S100B concentrations for outcome prediction in traumatic brain injury and subarachnoid hemorrhage," *Clinical Neurology and Neurosurgery*, vol. 145, pp. 79–83, 2016.

[31] A. Petzold, P. Michel, M. Stock, and M. Schluep, "Glial and axonal body fluid biomarkers are related to infarct volume, severity, and outcome," *Journal of Stroke and Cerebrovascular Diseases*, vol. 17, no. 4, pp. 196–203, 2008.

[32] A. Kleindienst and M. R. Bullock, "A critical analysis of the role of the neurotrophic protein S100B in acute brain injury," *Journal of Neurotrauma*, vol. 23, no. 8, pp. 1185–1200, 2006.

[33] C. D. Bortner, F. M. Hughes Jr., and J. A. Cidlowski, "A primary role for K+ and Na+ efflux in the activation of apoptosis," *Journal of Biological Chemistry*, vol. 272, no. 51, pp. 32436–32442, 1997.

[34] I. Lauritzen, M. Zanzouri, E. Honoré et al., "K+-dependent cerebellar granule neuron apoptosis. Role of TASK leak K+ channels," *Journal of Biological Chemistry*, vol. 278, no. 34, pp. 32068–32076, 2003.

[35] S. Bittner, S. G. Meuth, K. Göbel et al., "TASK1 modulates inflammation and neurodegeneration in autoimmune inflammation of the central nervous system," *Brain*, vol. 132, no. 9, pp. 2501–2516, 2009.

[36] V. L. R. Rao, V. K. Dhodda, G. Song, K. K. Bowen, and R. J. Dempsey, "Traumatic brain injury-induced acute gene expression changes in rat cerebral cortex identified by GeneChip analysis," *Journal of Neuroscience Research*, vol. 71, no. 2, pp. 208–219, 2003.

[37] C. Liu, J. F. Cotton, J. A. Schuyler et al., "Protective effects of TASK-3 (KCNK9) and related 2P K channels during cellular stress," *Brain Research*, vol. 1031, no. 2, pp. 164–173, 2005.

[38] D. González-Forero, F. Portillo, L. Gómez, F. Montero, S. Kasparov, and B. Moreno-López, "Inhibition of resting potassium conductances by long-term activation of the NO/cGMP/protein kinase G pathway: A new mechanism regulating neuronal excitability," *Journal of Neuroscience*, vol. 27, no. 23, pp. 6302–6312, 2007.

[39] G. L. Mazzone and A. Nistri, "S100β as an early biomarker of excitotoxic damage in spinal cord organotypic cultures," *Journal of Neurochemistry*, vol. 130, no. 4, pp. 598–604, 2014.

[40] F. Ahmed, A. Gyorgy, A. Kamnaksh et al., "Time-dependent changes of protein biomarker levels in the cerebrospinal fluid after blast traumatic brain injury," *Electrophoresis*, vol. 33, no. 24, pp. 3705–3711, 2012.

25

Chest Ultrasonography in Modern Day Extreme Settings: From Military Setting and Natural Disasters to Space Flights and Extreme Sports

Francesco Feletti,[1,2] Viviana Mucci,[3] and Andrea Aliverti[2]

[1]*Department of Diagnostic Imaging, AUSL Romagna, S. Maria delle Croci Hospital, Ravenna, Italy*
[2]*Dipartmento di Elettronica, Informazione e Bioingegneria (DEIB), Politecnico di Milano, Milan, Italy*
[3]*Antwerpen University Research Centre for Equilibrium and Aerospace (AUREA), Antwerp, Belgium*

Correspondence should be addressed to Francesco Feletti; feletti@extremesportmed.org

Academic Editor: Christophe Leroyer

Chest ultrasonography (CU) is a noninvasive imaging technique able to provide an immediate diagnosis of the underlying aetiology of acute respiratory failure and traumatic chest injuries. Given the great technologies, it is now possible to perform accurate CU in remote and adverse environments including the combat field, extreme sport settings, and environmental disasters, as well as during space missions. Today, the usage of CU in the extreme emergency setting is more likely to occur, as this technique proved to be a fast diagnostic tool to assist resuscitation manoeuvres and interventional procedures in many cases. A scientific literature review is presented here. This was based on a systematic search of published literature, on the following online databases: PubMed and Scopus. The following words were used: "chest sonography," " thoracic ultrasound," and "lung sonography," in different combinations with "extreme sport," "extreme environment," "wilderness," "catastrophe," and "extreme conditions." This manuscript reports the most relevant usages of CU in the extreme setting as well as technological improvements and current limitations. CU application in the extreme setting is further encouraged here.

1. Introduction

In the past two decades, the prehospital treatment in extreme settings has greatly advanced [1, 2]. Extreme settings are known for posing additional challenges to medical operations. Extreme settings are described as situations characterized by austere nature and specific inherent threats encountered (e.g., avalanches). These can vary from war scenarios to natural disasters, high-altitude missions, and extreme sport scenarios (e.g., deserted areas, savage seas, and high mountains) [3]. Medical operations in extreme settings usually require the need for integration of medical and rescue skills, as well as the demand for prehospital medicine and expanded care protocols [3, 4].

The military field has implemented over the year specific extreme condition infield trauma management techniques [5]. In addition to this, they have developed specific protocols and procedures including logistical plans for medical evacuation of casualties and for climatic control for medical devices [6, 7].

Extreme environments are also considered remote and adverse locations where most extreme sports are practiced. Extreme sports have exponentially grown in popularity for the past 40 years [8]; these activities are often performed in austere environments (tumbling rivers, canyons, and glaciers) far away from medical assistance [9] and difficult to be reached.

Similarly, complex medical assistance is also present when considering space missions. Commercial orbital and suborbital space flights are becoming a solid reality, since Red Bull Stratos and StratEx Space Dive have opened a new era in the last year [10, 11]. In addition to these, other extreme medical settings are going to be present in the next decades due to climate change. With regard to this topic, climate change is leading to a change in distribution of infectious diseases and an increased risk for unexpected weather events capable of destroying infrastructures and creating a wilderness, isolated environment in a previously urban context [3, 12].

An efficient tool to improve medical management in the above described extreme setting is ultrasound. Clinicians in the extreme setting are challenged by the uncomfortable, often unsafe, and dangerous locations, with limited supplied and appropriate equipment.

Chest ultrasonography (CU) is a versatile, accurate diagnostic, low-cost, nonionising tool. It is based on noninvasive techniques [13] that can be easily performed in the field, through its portable device version. CU can be used as the tool for quick and accurate diagnosis prior to reaching organized medical facilities or during transportation [14–17]. Moreover, CU can also assist in resource allocation, decisions, screening for conditions, and patient management [18].

Given the multifunction of CU, this manuscript focuses on the usage of CU when dealing with respiratory failure as well as traumatic thoracic injuries in extreme settings. Thoracic injuries and respiratory failure are possible life-threatening conditions when considering extreme settings Chest injuries are representing about a quarter of the causes of death related to traumas, and they are commonly reported in extreme settings [1, 19]. Chest imaging is essential when dealing with critically ill patients, and CU has been used as a role in the prevention, assessment, and treatment of many traumatic and nontraumatic emergencies [20, 21]. Indeed, CU is a type of examination that offers more details and more sensible data compared to the traditional radiological exam for the diagnosis of many conditions, including pneumothorax, pleural effusion, and lung contusion [22–24]. In addition, CU is able to guide the decision-making process and to assist interventional procedures [21, 25].

This paper aims to review the scientific literature about the usages of CU in extreme settings, in order to elucidate the applications of this imaging method in extreme emerging situations. Secondly, we performed an overview on the current limitations of commercially available CU devices, and we proposed new technological solutions to address them. Lastly, operator-training models and trainings for advancing the use of CU in all extreme conditions are discussed here. Based on the current review, we hypothesized that, in the future, the use of CU in extreme settings will increase.

2. Methods

This review was performed using the following database: PubMed and Scopus. We used the following search term categories in combination: "chest sonography," " thoracic ultrasound," and "lung sonography," in different combinations with "extreme sport," "extreme environment," "wilderness," "catastrophe," and "extreme conditions."

Papers were also included using the ancestry approach in order to include anecdotal but relevant reports.

3. Results

The scientific literature related to the use of CU in extreme settings is still sparse Table 1, it is possible to observe the principle applications of CU and its usages reported in the literature.

In Table 2, conditions for which assessment and treatment CU have been proposed in the wilderness setting are given.

4. Discussion

4.1. CU for Traumas. In trauma, CU provides immediate yes/no diagnostic answers to the operators during emergency treatment. Consequently, CU is usually integrated in the focused assessment sonography for trauma (FAST) protocol with the name of extended FAST protocol (e-FAST) or chest abdominal FAST (CA-FAST).

The latter in addition to the upper right and left abdomen, cardiac and pelvic views of the FAST examination, includes also pleura, lung, and pericardium assessment [24]. Repeatability is of particular relevance when considering a trauma. For example, the repeated assessment of pericardial effusion allows a prompt diagnosis of tamponade, a life-threatening condition, also reported in the extreme sport scenario [42].

In addition, many wilderness casualties can be assessed without the help of X-ray examination, but just by using CU. More in detail, CU allows to easily diagnosing chest wall injuries, including muscular lesions and hematomas and bony cage fractures and their complications [17, 18, 43–45].

4.2. CU in Nontraumatic Conditions. In addition to the assessment of traumatic injuries, CU has been shown to be of great advantage during the assessment of pulmonary edema (PE) in high-altitude missions as well as after apnea diving (Table 1).

Pratali et al. reported that, among climbers with the usage of CU, an inverse correlation between O_2 saturation and the progressive increase of B-lines during ascent sports [35] was detected. On the other hand, in a study by Frassi et al. on breath-hold deep divers assessed by means of CU, an increase of B-lines within 10 minutes after immersion in 45% of the participants was documented. The change, only in 28% of the cases, was associated with clinical symptoms [32]. Given those observations, the usages of CU reported here clearly show that this technology allows detecting even subclinical episodes of lung fluid accumulation, as the one reported in extreme sport participants. CU also proved high diagnostic accuracy for the diagnosis of pneumonia and chest wall infections in extreme low-resource settings [17, 18, 44, 46]. The usage of CU allowed to identify and to promptly treat vulnerable subjects on the spot [47].

4.3. CU Assistance in Resuscitation Manoeuvres and Interventional Procedures. In extreme settings, CU may additionally assist interventional procedures as part of resuscitation manoeuvres and patient stabilization, including positioning of

Table 1: Applications of CU in extreme settings according to the literature.

Authors	Kind of study	Number of subjects	Setting	Condition assessed
Farrow [26]	*Pilot study*	19	UNMIL Hospital in Dili, East Timor, or with 3rd Health Support Battalion (3H SB)	Hemothorax and hemopericardium
Cremona et al. [27]	*Prospective study*	262	Monte Rosa mountain (4559 m)	PE
Strode et al. [28]	*Original research*	5	U.S. Army Combat Support Hospital, remotely placed in the field 20 miles from tertiary care	Pericardial effusion
Foale et al. [29]	*Original research*	1	International Space Station (ISS)	Normal anatomy
Fagenholz et al. [30]	*Original research*	11	Himalayan Rescue Association Clinic, Pheriche, Nepal (4240 m)	PE
Dean et al. [31]	*Original research*	3	Aftermath of Hurricane Stan (out of total 139 US examinations in 9 days)	Pleura and lung injuries
Frassi et al. [32]	*Prospective study*	31	International Apnea Diving Championship, Sharm El Sheikh, Egypt	PE
Otto et al. [33]	*Brief report*	2	Advanced Base Camp on Mount Everest (6400 m)	PE
Madill [34]	*Case report*	1	Forward operating base in combat scenario, Afghanistan	Pneumothorax
Pratali et al. [35]	*Observational study*	18	Trekking Gokyo and Khumbu Valley, Kathmandu (1350 m), Namche Bazaar (3440 m), Gokyo (4790 m), and Gorak Shep (5130 m), Nepal	PE
Pingitore et al. [36]	*Original research*	31	Ironman Triathlon (3.8 km swimming + 180 km cycling + 42 km running); Pisa, Italy (30 m above the sea level)	PE
Boussuges et al. [37]	*Original research*	30	Apnea diving competition in the Mediterrenean Sea (autumn and winter)	PE
Shorter and Macias [38]	*Retrospective observational*	6	7-Richter magnitude earthquake	Hemodynamic monitoring, PE, consolidation, atelectasis, and lung recruitment
Yin et al. [39]	*Retrospective analysis*	97	Lushan earthquake	Hemodynamic monitoring, PE, consolidation, atelectasis, and lung recruitment

PE = pulmonary edema.

catheters and tubes, pericardiocentesis, needle thoracostomy, and cricothyroidotomy [21, 25, 48]. In particular, CU has been shown to accurately and quickly evaluate the position of the endotracheal tube and its malpositioning in wilderness settings, including during air medical transports, where capnography is not available and auscultation is impossible due to noise [48].

During the resuscitation evaluation process, the CU usage is able to provide insights about hemodynamic monitoring, drug administration, and potential building up of fluids and blood products [21], since it is also used to estimate the intravascular volume status and to determine the opportunity of CPR continuation [25, 49].

Assessing intravascular volume status by measuring the IVC diameter has been previously shown to be particularly important during resuscitation evaluation. Some examples of the implementation of this technique have been described with young healthy military members, as well as extreme sport participants, since they generally have a large cardiovascular reserve and may be more severely volume depleted than their initial vital signs may suggest [44].

4.4. CU in the War Setting. The US military has pointed out that many clinicians are forced to "do more with less" in austere and deployment environments [6].

Iraq and Afghanistan wars were the most recent wars that required trained physicians and emergency medical crew. While during the First Gulf War, a mature multiservice medical system was never established during the latest events; hence, such a team was implemented [44]. Today, the emergency team plays a key role in the combat environment, due to their unique trainings for critically ill and traumatically injured patients [50].

Emergency ultrasonography usage for treating trauma was quickly embraced by the military, after 1997, when such devices became smaller and portable. Indeed, a small handheld ultrasound device that was light, portable, durable, and battery powered was needed only in such

Table 2: Conditions for which the use of CU has been proposed in the scientific literature.

Interesting contribution to diagnosis	Ultrasonographic method	Signs	Treatment
Pericardial effusion [28]	*Direct visualization*	Hypoanechoic layer posterior to the heart	Monitoring
Pericardial tamponade [17]	*Repeated assessment of pericardial effusion*	50% IVC change in diameter during inspiration (sensitive/nonspecific)/RA collapse that exceeds one-third of cardiac cycle is nearly 100% sensitive and specific/RV diastolic collapse (nonsensitive)/inspiratory septal shift is not specific	Ultrasound-guided long-needle periocardiocentesis
Intravascular volume depletion estimation [40]	*Measurement of the diameter of the IVC just below the diaphragm*	cIVC (IVCmax – IVCmin)/IVCmax >42%	Follow-up after fluid administration
PE [36, 41]	*Assessment of lung sonographic artifacts*	Presence of B-line artifacts: absence of A-line artifacts	Monitoring
Pneumothorax [34]	*Lung sliding detection*	Absence of lung sliding and lung points	To guide decompression of the correct pleural space
Pleural effusion [25]	*Direct visualization*	Hypoanechoic layer of polygonal area under the pleural line	Chest tube placement and verification
Pulmonary contusion [25]	*Direct visualization*	Lung hepatization: B-lines and shred sign	Monitoring
Soft tissue infection of the chest wall [18]	*Direct visualization*	Cellulitis has cobblestone appearance/abscesses are complex structures	Guide planning for the best location for incision and drainage
Bony thoracic cage fractures	*Direct visualization of the fracture and evaluation of complications* (e.g., *pneumothorax, pleural effusion, lung contusion, and hematoma of the chest wall)*	Chimney phenomenon, interruption of cortical bone, and soft tissue hematoma	

IVC: inferior vena cava; RV: right ventricle; RA: right atrium; cIVC: inferior vena cava collapsibility index; IVCmax: inferior vena cava maximum diameter; IVCmin: inferior vena cava minimum diameter; PE: pulmonary edema.

a way CU could be used on the battlefield. Nowadays, with the new technological advancement, such a technology exists [44, 50].

Throughout the years, the military emergency teams gained more experience with emergency ultrasonography, creating what is now named a tactical use of the ultrasound technology. Tactical ultrasound is the use of emergency ultrasound to guide decision-making in the diagnosis, treatment, and disposition of patients when resources are scarce and testing is severely limited [44]. CU is included in tactical ultrasound in the form of e-FAST protocol [44].

4.5. Chest Ultrasonography in Weather Disasters. CU has been shown to be a useful diagnostic tool to be implemented outside the hospital setting such as for mass casualties after natural disasters, including earthquakes, tropical storms, hurricanes, tornadoes, volcanoes, avalanches, mudslides, and floods [51].

Extreme weather conditions are likely to become more and more common due to global warming in the next decades [52].

CU has already been successfully implemented during the Armenian earthquake in 1988 and the Wenchuan earthquake in 2008. During the Armenian disaster, three major cities were affected, and more than 100 villages were destroyed [50]. Out of the 400 patients who were screened sonographically, 304 demonstrated no clinically significant pathology. In almost 25% of the cases (96 patients), a pathological condition was diagnosed by the use of ultrasound [2]. In their prospective observational study about the use of a portable ultrasound in the Amazon Jungle, Blaivas et al. [20] suggest the use of CU in either blunt or penetrating thoracic trauma in remote settings. It is mainly used to diagnose or rule out hemothorax, pericardial effusion, fractures, diaphragmatic rupture, and pneumothorax, as well as a guide to obtaining vascular access.

4.6. Chest Ultrasound in Space. Space is another extreme setting where CU has been shown to increase medical performances [53]. Today, ultrasound is the only imaging tool available in space on board of the International Space Station [53]. At this stage, CU is mostly used for monitoring the drastic physiological changes occurring in microgravity, as well as used a primary diagnostic tool [53].

The first ultrasound system in space was flown on Salyut 6 and 7 to study cardiovascular changes, such as heart chamber sizes and left ventricular systolic functions [53]. The use of ultrasound has enabled to increase the knowledge on fluid shifting occurring during space adaptations.

Back pain, contusion, and strain are common complains among astronauts [53]. Ultrasound technology was able to detect that, during microgravity exposure, the space between the vertebrae increases [53], possibly explaining why complains of back pain are common after space flights.

Ultrasound in space can be used for many purposes including the assessment of tendon, ligament, and bursa diseases, as well as during traumas. The risk of catastrophic and trauma events is generally low in space due to microgravity (Figure 1); however, penetrating traumas can occur, especially during extra vehicular activities (EVAs). As a result, models on Earth using parabolic flights have assessed the potential use of FAST examinations for space missions. Some common thoracic conditions may be considered as particularly severe in space; for example, pneumothorax, in which treatment will require a chest tube placement. This is considered as a mission-terminating event [54]. Therefore, the use of CU in such an event will be crucial for the decision-making process.

One study carried out in ISS analyzed the ability of nonphysician crewmembers to obtain ultrasound images [2]. In this study, crewmembers underwent limited ultrasound training before their mission. The ultrasound examination was conducted onboard of the ISS and transmitted via satellite to a radiologist at NASA Mission Control Centre. The radiologist viewed the images and instructed the crewmember on how to adjust the machine, its settings, and the probe placement. This assessment concluded that crewmembers could successfully perform ultrasound and provide via telemedicine relevant data to the flight surgeon [2]. Ultrasound training programs performed for astronauts and cosmonauts allowed the usage of CU as an easy tool to assess injuries in real time with remote assistance (Figure 2).

For these reasons, CU will continue to play a crucial role as a diagnostic method and treatment tool for medical contingencies in space (Figures 3 and 4) [53].

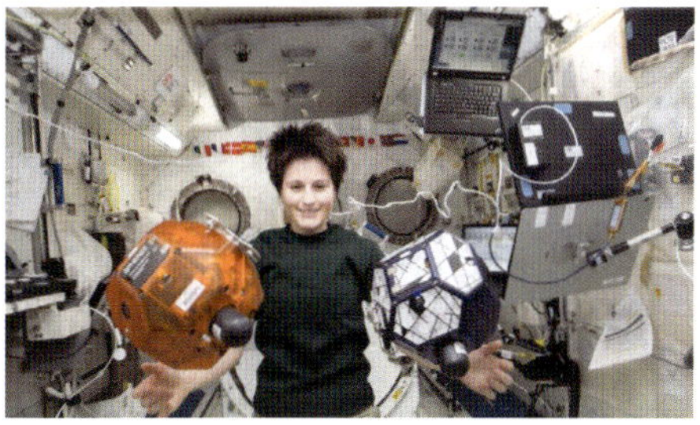

Figure 1: ESA astronaut S. Cristoforetti in microgravity onboard of the International Space Station.

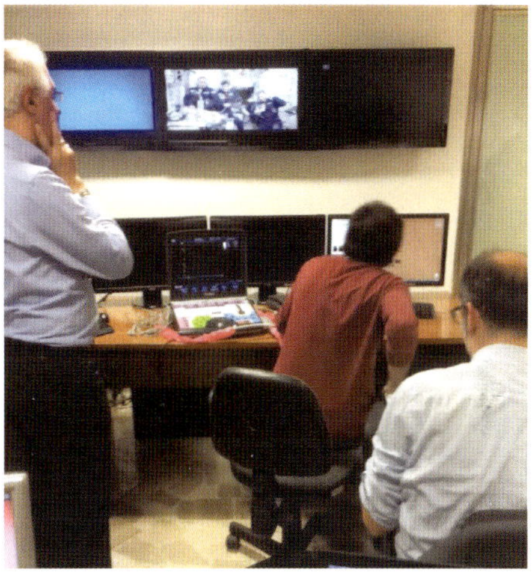

Figure 2: Mission control guiding the astronaut Cristoforetti and the other crewmembers to use the Vivid q CU device during the space mission Futura onboard of the International Space Station.

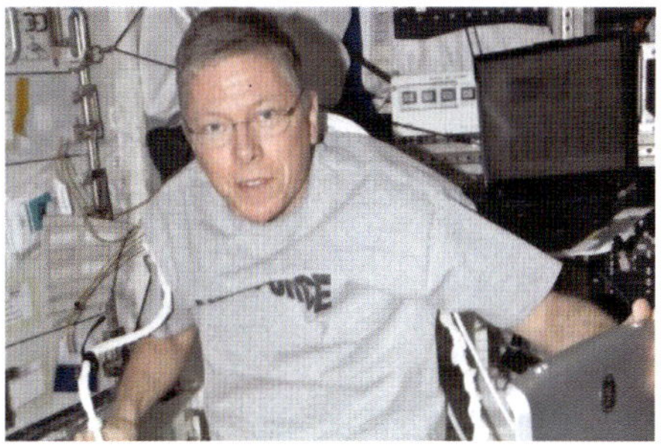

Figure 3: American astronaut Michael E. Fossum working with CU onboard of the International Space Station.

4.7. Chest Ultrasonography in Extreme Sports. The so-called extreme sports are a group of sporting activities where a likely outcome of a mistake or an accident is death due to the practice in adverse environments or to extreme psychophysical performance required [8, 9, 55]. At the moment, the literature describing or reporting CU in extreme sports is scarce. Nevertheless, the usefulness of this imaging technique in specific extreme sports, namely, skateboarding, skiing, apnea diving, climbing, mountaineering, and Ironman races, has already been established [32, 33, 35–37, 45]. Extreme sports are often practiced in remote locations, and evacuation of participants after trauma may require complicated terrestrial rescue operations or the use of helicopters or specific watercrafts. Potentially life-threatening conditions may be quickly assessed with CU directly on the scene without any delay in the evacuation [42]. Even if CU usage in extreme sports compared to other wilderness extreme fields seems limited, the use of CU for chest trauma in extreme sports is one of the most promising areas for future applied studies [45]. In extreme sports, CU may be used to assess the increase in lung fluid content [36]. PE can affect participants of particular extreme sports, such as the one that are exposed to hypo- and/or hyperbaric condition, such as climbers exposed to high altitude (above 4000 m), and divers exposed to a depth of −100 m under the sea level [47]. In these settings, PE may occur as a result of a

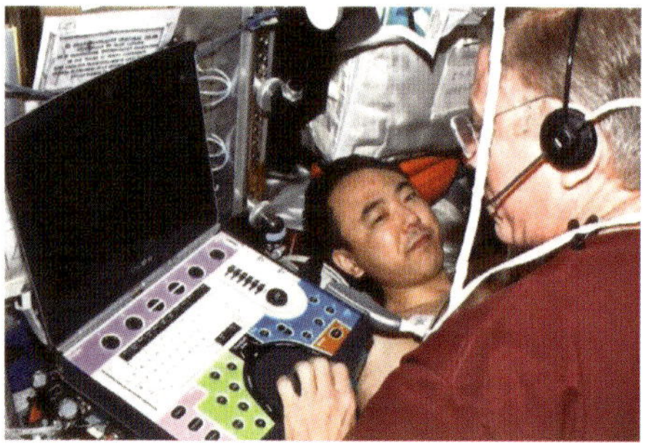

FIGURE 4: American astronaut Michael E. Fossum assessing the Japanese astronaut with CU device onboard of the International Space Station.

combination of hemodynamic, mechanical, hypoxemic, and biochemical mechanisms [47]. However, also in the normal environment, ultraendurance extreme sports may cause lung tissue and microvascular endothelial damage, as a consequence of thermal, hormonal, and metabolic stress [36].

After Ironman race (which consists of swimming required for a distance equal to 3.86 km, riding a bike for a distance equal to 180 km, and running a marathon), CU detected a significant increase of B-lines. This was associated with a decrease in spirometric indices as well as in ventilatory performance [36]. In some cases, the transient subclinical increase in lung fluid content may represent a paraphysiological adaptation, but in others, it may represent an important marker of individual vulnerability to potentially life-threatening PE [47].

4.8. Devices and Future Advancements. Recently, the development of portable ultrasound for commercial use has delivered two main types of products [18]. The first one is represented by the portable devices, which also include power supply and case. These devices are easy to be transported and relatively small. They usually fit in a backpack such as the Vscan (GE, Chicago, IL), Lumify (Philips, Andover, MA), and iViz (SonoSite, Bothell, WA).

These systems are also able to transfer images wireless or via text messages or e-mail. Secondly, the other types of devices are the total wireless ultrasound technologies, which are receiving the images directly on the connected smartphone. Some examples are Clarius (Burnaby, Canada) and Signostics (Bothell, WA) [18].

Despite having new accurate devices able to be used in multiple ways, which are light and easy to be moved, yet there is no CU specifically designed for the extreme setting, currently commercially available. CU designed for the extreme setting should be waterproof, given the wide range of water sports. They should be resistant to cold conditions, in order to be used, for example, in sports performed on snow, as well as to strong vibrations and bright lights. Today, a totally waterproof ultrasound device is still lacking. Water can easily damage the electronic components of the device and the batteries [18]. In sea environments, the saltiness of the water can also be a crucial damaging component. Therefore, it would be worth to develop water-resistant ultrasounds for the future. The new extreme setting CU device should also be designed "bulletproof" for sands and dust, elements often present in extreme settings (e.g., deserts). At high altitude, with low atmospheric pressure and cold, the ultrasound devices can report issues at spinning hard drives. Consequently, it is best to use a system with a solid memory system and without moving components. It has been described before that the immersion of a transduction in warm water was a successful countermeasure for maintaining the functioning of the system [56]. In cold environments, the battery duration can be diminished; as a result, a new way to recharge the device should be developed. On the other hand, when the devices are exposed to heat, a special cooling system should be implemented.

As stated in previous studies, looking at a monitor full sole can be extremely difficult and disturbing for the clinicians [18]. This can be even worse when the screen is reflecting the sun or the snow in extreme settings. For this reason, it may be worth considering the screen-covering tools. The covering tools could range from a solid screen cover to small curtains to cover the operator and the screen. However, which material to use and how to build it, in order also not to overheat the physician and the devices, still remain to be explored. Watercrafts, helicopters, and other vehicles used to rescue the patients are often releasing high vibrations [18]. Reducing or diminishing the movements from the ultrasound scan is crucial to obtain good quality images. However, this can be very challenging in rescue vehicles normally used for remote areas. The development of specific vibration insulated litters could solve this problem. Ergonomics should also be considered.

4.9. Training/Guidelines and Future Perspectives. Aside from the technological advancements, it is essential that every team member, for example, of rescue teams adopting CU, is receiving the adequate CU trainings. The evidence-based application for using CU as a standard of care has greatly increased and with it now the efforts to integrate focused CU training into medical school curricula [57].

Multiple studies have shown that it is possible to learn the basic components of the CU with training programs lasting between two hours and four months to a number of supervised scans between 20 and 80 [58, 59]. For example, when considering medical students, a course, requiring generally 5 to 30 hours in total commitment over several weeks, was able to provide the key components of CU such as terminology, knobology, and image acquisition [57]. Given the technological advancement also in the trainings, CU education should become a routine for physicians of all kinds. Indeed, presently, CU can also be touched through the use of virtual reality. Heer [60] has previously demonstrated that virtual reality can easily facilitate students to learn how to perform CU and to read the images. For example, virtual reality programs are able to enhance the use of a simulator when teaching intraoperative transesophageal echocardiography (TEE). In such studies, it was indicated that the use of virtual reality and simulators led to a superior teaching method [61].

The time required to achieve basic competency in TEE was shortened than that with a curriculum that relies solely on experience with actual patients. Given that such technologies can easily be integrated during the courses, teaching ultrasound should no longer start from exclusive theoretical basis. In addition to this, the use of virtual reality could standardize the learning curriculum of CU, also across multiple countries [61, 62]. Virtual reality for teaching CU can enhance performances by providing repetitive training on selected cases of increasing difficulties, as well as including controlled exposure to rare cases as previously described [60–62]. Nevertheless, yet the integration of such courses is still in its primary phases. On the other hand, CU for extreme settings should also be touched to nonmedically trained team members. Specific studies about the exact time needed to train and different levels of training for the normal population are still missing. It is still unclear how much time is required to be able to perform the best possible imaging recording with basic medical knowledge. What is known is that CU teaching should incorporate different levels of training [29]. If these trainings were well developed and available to all, the usage of CU in extreme settings may increase.

Healthcare professionals could also follow up the patient with the use of telemedicine. A study presented by Strode [28] has demonstrated that, with telemedicine, it is possible to place critical patient information one step closer to a team of expert, from a remote setting, such as during combat triage or in extreme remote areas to a hospital. With these regards, the telemedicine examples provided by the past space missions [53] could represent the first step to create new telemedicine programs on Earth for CU in extreme settings.

Specific guidelines for CU should be implemented for extreme settings and with regard to specific conditions. The power of such a tool relies within the precision of the operators; as a result, the examinations must be performed accurately.

5. Conclusions

This review presented different usages of CU in multiple extreme environments and settings. Despite the usage of CU is well known for certain extreme environments such as for the military, it is still in a developmental phase for others such as in extreme sports. This review showed the versatility of CU and how it has been successfully implemented for treating multiple respiratory and chest conditions. Despite the technological improvements presented, it is clear that a specific CU device for the extreme setting is still missing. Suggestions on new potential aspects to consider in the design and development of specific CU for extreme conditions were also reported. Lastly, the usages of CU can only improve and increase with a parallel rise in its training. For this reason, an overview on trainings for clinicians and nonclinicians was also debated. With these examples, the usage of CU is encouraged for the near future for all extreme settings.

Acknowledgments

The authors wish to acknowledge GE Healthcare and Dr. Cristina Gabardi for the images.

References

[1] L. F. Littlejohn, "Treatment of thoracic trauma: lessons from the battlefield adapted to all austere environments," *Wilderness & Environmental Medicine*, vol. 28, no. 2, pp. 69–73, 2017.

[2] O. J. Ma, J. G. Norvell, and S. Subramanian, "Ultrasound applications in mass casualties and extreme environments," *Critical Care Medicine*, vol. 35, no. 5, pp. 275–279, 2007.

[3] J. M. Sholl and E. P. Curcio, "An introduction to wilderness medicine," *Emergency Medicine Clinics of North America*, vol. 22, no. 2, pp. 265–279, 2004.

[4] D. G. Sward and B. L. Bennett, "Wilderness medicine," *World Journal of Emergency Medicine*, vol. 5, no. 1, pp. 5–15, 2014.

[5] S. M. Galvagno, R. L. Mabry, J. Maddry et al., "Measuring US Army medical evacuation: metrics for performance improvement," *Journal of Trauma and Acute Care Surgery*, vol. 84, no. 1, pp. 150–156, 2018.

[6] R. Richards, J. M. Awrey, S. E. Medeiros, and J. P. McGahan, "Color and power Doppler sonography for pneumothorax detection," *Journal of Ultrasound in Medicine*, vol. 36, no. 10, pp. 2143–2147, 2017.

[7] E. M. Hindle and J. D. Henning, "Critical care at extremes of temperature: effects on patients, staff and equipment," *Journal of the Royal Army Medical Corps*, vol. 160, no. 4, pp. 279–285, 2014.

[8] F. Feletti, A. Aliverti, M. Henjum, M. Tarabini, and E. Brymer, "Incidents and injuries in foot-launched flying extreme sports," *Aerospace Medicine and Human Performance*, vol. 88, no. 11, pp. 1016–1023, 2017.

[9] F. Feletti, "Preface," in *Extreme Sports Medicine*, pp. 7-8, Springer, Berlin, Germany, 2017.

[10] RedBull.com Team, *Final findings of the Red Bull Stratos Scientific Summit*, California Science Center, Los Angeles, CA, USA, 2013, https://issuu.com/redbullstratos/docs/red_bull_stratos_summit_report_final_050213.

[11] Strat Ex, *Alan Eustace and the Paragon StratEx Team Make Stratospheric Exploration History at over 135,000 Feet*, Paragon Space Development Corporation, 2015, http://www.paragonsdc.com/stratex/#one.

[12] A. Rossati, "Global warming and its health impact," *International Journal of Occupational and Environmental Medicine*, vol. 8, no. 1, pp. 7–20, 2017.

[13] S. Wongwaisayawan, R. Suwannanon, S. Sawatmongkorngul, and R. Kaewlai, "Emergency thoracic US: the essentials," *Radiographics*, vol. 36, no. 3, pp. 640–659, 2016.

[14] F. Corcoran, A. Bystrzycki, S. Masud, S. M. Mazur, D. Wise, and T. Harris, "Ultrasound in pre-hospital trauma care," *Trauma*, vol. 18, no. 2, pp. 101–110, 2015.

[15] D. A. Lichtenstein, "BLUE-protocol and FALLS-protocol: two applications of lung ultrasound in the critically ill," *Chest*, vol. 147, no. 6, pp. 1659–1670, 2015.

[16] E. R. Melnick, "Ultrasound in emergency medicine portable ultrasound for remote environments, part I," *Feasibility of Field Deployment*, vol. 40, no. 2, pp. 190–197, 2011.

[17] C. T. C. Russell and P. F. Crawford, "Ultrasound in the austere environment: a review of the history, indications, and specifications," *Military Medicine*, vol. 178, no. 1, pp. 21–28, 2013.

[18] L. Gharahbaghian, K. L. Anderson, V. Lobo, R. W. Huang, C. M. Poffenberger, and P. D. Nguyen, "Point-of-care

ultrasound in austere environments: a complete review of its utilization, pitfalls, and technique for common applications in austere settings," *Emergency Medicine Clinics of North America*, vol. 35, no. 2, pp. 409–441, 2017.

[19] D. H. Livingston and C. J. Hauser, "Trauma to the chest wall and lung," in *Trauma*, E. E. Moore, D. V. Feliciano, and K. I. Mattox, Eds., pp. 507–537, McGraw-Hill Medical, NewYork, NY, USA, 5th edition, 2003.

[20] M. Blaivas, W. Kuhn, B. Reynolds et al., "Change in differential diagnosis and patient management with the use of portable ultrasound in a remote setting," *Wilderness & Environmental Medicine*, vol. 16, no. 1, pp. 38–41, 2005.

[21] G. Gardelli, F. Feletti, A. Nanni, M. Mughetti, A. Piraccini, and M. Zompatori, "Chest ultrasonography in the ICU," *Respiratory Care*, vol. 57, no. 5, pp. 773–781, 2012.

[22] M. Yousefifard, M. Baikpour, P. Ghelichkhani et al., "Screening performance characteristic of ultrasonography and radiography in detection of pleural effusion; a meta-analysis," *Emergency*, vol. 4, no. 1, pp. 1–10, 2016.

[23] W. Kirkpatrick, M. Sirois, K. B. Lupland et al., "Hand-held thoracic sonography for detecting post-traumatic pneumothoraces: the Extended Focused Assessment with Sonography for Trauma (EFAST)," *Journal of Trauma: Injury, Infection, and Critical Care*, vol. 57, no. 2, pp. 288–295, 2004.

[24] M. Zanobetti, A. Coppa, P. Nazerian et al., "Chest abdominal-focused assessment sonography for trauma during the primary survey in the emergency department: the CA-FAST protocol," *European Journal of Trauma and Emergency Surgery*, pp. 1–6, 2015.

[25] L. A. Galdamez, J. B. Clark, and E. L. Antonsen, "Point-of-care ultrasound utility and potential for high altitude crew recovery missions," *Aerospace Medicine and Human Performance*, vol. 88, no. 2, pp. 128–136, 2017.

[26] G. B. Farrow, "Portable ultrasound on deployment: a pilot study," *ADF Health*, vol. 2, pp. 55–58, 2001.

[27] G. Cremona, R. Asnaghi, P. Baderna et al., "Pulmonary extravascular fluid accumulation in recreational climbers: a prospective study," *The Lancet*, vol. 359, no. 9303, pp. 303–309, 2002.

[28] C. A. Strode, B. J. Rubal, R. T. Gerhardt et al., "Satellite and mobile wireless transmission of focused assessment with sonography in trauma," *Academic Emergency Medicine*, vol. 10, no. 12, pp. 1411–1414, 2003.

[29] C. M. Foale, A. Y. Kaleri, A. E. Sargsyan et al., "Diagnostic instrumentation aboard ISS: just-in-time training for non-physician crewmembers," *Aviation, Space, and Environmental Medicine*, vol. 76, no. 6, pp. 594–598, 2005.

[30] P. J. Fagenholz, J. A. Gutman, A. F. Murray, and N. S. Harris, "Treatment of high altitude pulmonary edema at 4240 m in Nepal," *High Altitude Medicine & Biology*, vol. 8, no. 2, pp. 139–146, 2007.

[31] A. J. Dean, B. S. Ku, and E. M. Zeserson, "The utility of handheld ultrasound in an austere medical setting in Guatemala after a natural disaster," *American Journal of Disaster Medicine*, vol. 2, no. 5, pp. 249–256, 2007.

[32] F. Frassi, A. Pingitore, D. Cialoni, and E. Picano, "Chest sonography detects lung water accumulation in healthy elite apnea divers," *Journal of the American Society of Echocardiography*, vol. 21, no. 10, pp. 1150–1155, 2008.

[33] C. Otto, D. R. Hamilton, B. D. Levine et al., "Into thin air: extreme ultrasound on Mt Everest," *Wilderness & Environmental Medicine*, vol. 20, no. 3, pp. 283–289, 2009.

[34] J. J. Madill, "In-flight thoracic ultrasound detection of pneumothorax in combat," *Journal of Emergency Medicine*, vol. 39, no. 2, pp. 194–197, 2010.

[35] L. Pratali, M. Cavana, R. Sicari, and E. Picano, "Frequent subclinical high-altitude pulmonary edema detected by chest sonography as ultrasound lung comets in recreational climbers," *Critical Care Medicine*, vol. 38, no. 9, pp. 1818–1823, 2010.

[36] A. Pingitore, E. Garbella, P. Piaggi et al., "Early subclinical increase in pulmonary water content in athletes performing sustained heavy exercise at sea level: ultrasound lung comet-tail evidence," *American Journal of Physiology-Heart and Circulatory Physiology*, vol. 301, no. 5, pp. 2161–2167, 2011.

[37] A. Boussuges, M. Coulange, J. Bessereau et al., "Ultrasound lung comets induced by repeated breath-hold diving, a study in underwater fishermen," *Scandinavian Journal of Medicine & Science in Sports*, vol. 21, no. 6, pp. 384–392, 2011.

[38] M. Shorter and D. J. Macias, "Portable handheld ultrasound in austere environments: use in the Haiti disaster," *Prehospital and Disaster Medicine*, vol. 27, no. 2, pp. 172–177, 2012.

[39] W. Yin, R. Zhou, H. Wu et al., "Value of focused critical ultrasound in the treatment of critical patients in Lushan earthquake," *Zhonghua Yi Xue Za Zhi*, vol. 94, no. 15, pp. 1135–1138, 2014.

[40] N. Airapetian, J. Maizel, O. Alyamani et al., "Does inferior vena cava respiratory variability predict fluid responsiveness in spontaneously breathing patients?," *Critical Care*, vol. 19, p. 400, 2015.

[41] Y. Wimalasena, J. Windsor, and M. Edsell, "Using ultrasound lung comets in the diagnosis of high altitude pulmonary edema: fact or fiction?," *Wilderness & Environmental Medicine*, vol. 24, no. 2, pp. 159–164, 2013.

[42] F. Yamaji, H. Okada, Y. Nakajima et al., "Blunt cardiac injury due to trauma associated with snowboarding: a case report," *Journal of Medical Case Reports*, vol. 11, no. 1, p. 80, 2017.

[43] R. K. Lee, J. F. Griffith, A. W. Ng, and J. C. Sitt, "Sonography of the chest wall: a pictorial essay," *Journal of Clinical Ultrasound*, vol. 43, no. 9, pp. 525–537, 2015.

[44] R. M. Ferre, J. Johnson, B. Hall et al., *Military and Tactical Ultrasound*, 2017, https://www.acep.org/WorkArea/linkit.aspx?ItemID=86787.

[45] C. S. Evans and N. S. Harris, "Ultrasound and ski resort clinics: mapping out the potential benefits," *Wilderness & Environmental Medicine*, vol. 23, no. 3, pp. 239–247, 2012.

[46] L. E. Ellington, R. H. Gilman, M. A. Chavez et al., "Lung ultrasound as a diagnostic tool for radiographically-confirmed pneumonia in low resource settings," *Respiratory Medicine*, vol. 128, pp. 57–64, 2017.

[47] E. Garbella, G. Catapano, L. Pratali, and A. Pingitore, "Pulmonary edema in healthy subjects in extreme conditions," *Pulmonary Medicine*, vol. 2011, Article ID 275857, 9 pages, 2011.

[48] R. Chun, A. W. Kirkpatrick, M. Sirois et al., "Where's the tube? Evaluation of hand-held ultrasound in confirming endotracheal tube placement," *Prehospital and Disaster Medicine*, vol. 19, no. 4, pp. 366–369, 2004.

[49] J. R. Richards and J. P. McGahan, "Focused Assessment with Sonography in Trauma (FAST) in 2017: what radiologists can learn," *Radiology*, vol. 283, no. 1, pp. 30–48, 2017.

[50] J. A. Nations and R. F. Browning, "Battlefield applications for handheld ultrasound," *Ultrasound Quarterly*, vol. 27, no. 3, pp. 171–176, 2011.

[51] S. P. Stawicki, J. M. Howard, J. P. Pryor, D. P. Bahner, M. L. Whitmill, and A. J. Dean, "Portable ultrasonography in mass casualty incidents: the CAVEAT examination," *World Journal of Orthopedics*, vol. 1, no. 1, pp. 10–19, 2010.

[52] D. G. Huber and J. Gulledge, *Extreme Weather and Climate Change: Understanding the Link and Managing the Risk*, Science

and Impacts Program, Center for Climate and Energy Solutions, Arlington, VA, USA, 2011, http://www.c2es.org/publications/extreme-weather-and-climate-change.

[53] J. Law and P. B. Macbeth, "Ultrasound: from earth to space," *McGill Journal of Medicine*, vol. 13, no. 2, pp. 2–5, 2011.

[54] D. Hamilton, K. Smart, S. Melton, J. D. Polk, and K. Johnson-Throop, "Autonomous medical care for exploration class space," *Journal of Trauma: Injury, Infection, and Critical Care*, vol. 64, no. 4, pp. 354–363, 2008.

[55] T. Immonen, E. Brymer, D. Orth et al., "Understanding action and adventure sports participation-an ecological dynamics perspective," *Sports Medicine-Open*, vol. 3, no. 1, p. 18, 2017.

[56] P. J. Fagenholz, A. F. Murray, V. E. Noble et al., "Ultrasound for high altitude research," *Ultrasound in Medicine & Biology*, vol. 38, no. 1, pp. 1–12, 2012.

[57] D. P. Bahner and N. A. Royall, "Advanced ultrasound training for fourth-year medical students: a novel training program at The Ohio State University College of Medicine," *Academic Medicine*, vol. 88, no. 2, pp. 206–213, 2013.

[58] G. Bedetti, L. Gargani, A. Corbisiero et al., "Evaluation of ultrasound lung comets by hand-held echocardiography," *Cardiovascular Ultrasound*, vol. 4, no. 34, 2006.

[59] U. A. P. Flato, H. P. Guimaraes, G. Petisco et al., "Use of lung ultrasonography in the detection of pneumothorax among medical students and emergency physicians," *Critical Care*, vol. 15, no. 2, p. 1, 2015.

[60] I. M. Heer, K. Middendorf, S. Müller-Egloff, M. Dugas, and A. Strauss, "Ultrasound training: the virtual patient," *Ultrasound in Obstetrics and Gynecology*, vol. 24, no. 4, pp. 440–444, 2004.

[61] A. Jelacic, K. Bowdle, K. Togashi, and P. Vonhomeyer, "The use of TEE simulation in teaching basic echocardiography skills to senior anesthesiology residents," *Journal of Cardiothoracic and Vascular Anesthesia*, vol. 27, no. 4, pp. 670–675, 2013.

[62] L. Konge, E. Albrecht-Beste, and M. B. Nielsen, "Virtual-reality simulation-based training in ultrasound," *Ultraschall in der Medizin-European Journal of Ultrasound*, vol. 35, no. 2, pp. 95–97, 2014.

Effects of Habenular Stimulation Frequencies on Obstructive Sleep Apnea Induced by Stimulation of Insular Cortex

Jing Kang[1,2] and Ming-Xian Li[1]

[1]*The First Affiliated Hospital of Jilin University, Changchun 130021, China*
[2]*Jilin Medical University, Jilin 132013, China*

Correspondence should be addressed to Ming-Xian Li; limingxian_118@163.com

Academic Editor: Emmanuel Charbonney

Objective. To investigate the effects of high-frequency stimulation of the habenula (Hb) on obstructive sleep apnea (OSA) induced by stimulation of the insular cortex *Method*. After OSA was induced by stimulating the insular cortex (Ic) with concentric stimulating electrodes at 100 Hz in rats, the Hb was stimulated at different frequencies (50 Hz, 120 Hz, 130 Hz, and 280 Hz). The changes of apnea events and electromyography (EMG) of the genioglossus were compared before and after stimulation of the Hb. *Results*. With stimulation of the Ic at 100 Hz, apnea events were successfully induced with disappearance of EMG of the genioglossus. After stimulation of the Hb at 130 Hz, apnea events disappeared with significantly increased genioglossal EMG. However, such a change failed to be found at the stimulation frequencies of 50 Hz, 120 Hz, and 280 Hz. *Conclusion*. Stimulation of the Hb at the frequency of 130 Hz could effectively inhibit OSA events induced by stimulation of the Ic.

1. Introduction

Abnormal sleep position, alcohol consumption, drug intake, and obesity can induce obstructive sleep apnea (OSA) [1–3]. Such a complex and highly individualized disease has been associated with multiple cardiovascular diseases. OSA induces chronic hypoxia and hypoventilation that may cause pulmonary hypertension and pulmonary heart disease [4–7]. The predominant pathological causes of OSA include contractility of upper airway muscles, abnormal airway anatomical features, loop gain, and arousal threshold [8]. Since the genioglossus tongue muscle contraction stabilizes and enlarges the portion of the upper airway which is vulnerable to collapse, relaxation of the genioglossus has been implicated in OSA.

According to electroencephalography patterns, which can be used to confirm different stages of sleep, there is a higher likelihood for muscles around the upper airway to relax during deep sleep, thus increasing the possibility of OSA to occur [9]. Previous studies also demonstrated that the electromyography (EMG) activity of the genioglossus is reduced during deep sleep [9]. Subsequently, systolic function decreases with muscle relaxation, which might cause the pharyngeal wall to collapse [10]. Hence, stenosis or closure of the upper airway is usually associated with reduced ventilation or OSA [11–13]. Although recent advancement in neurophysiology has been made in understanding the role of neuronal activity in respiratory movement regulation [13], the pathways regulating the motor control of respiration is not fully explored, especially those regulating the genioglossus contraction, and could be involved in OSA pathogenesis.

Respiratory movement originates from the brainstem and could be regulated by chemoreceptors and mechanoreceptors [12]. In addition, the respiratory movement can also be influenced by signals from the upper portion of the pons and the cerebral cortex [6]. Functional magnetic resonance imaging (fMRI) and animal studies have implicated that the insula cortex plays a major role in the provoking of OSA [7, 8]. In addition, the insular cortex could cause cardiovascular system dysfunction, which is consistent in OSA patients [9]. On the other hand, previous studies have shown that the Hb can mediate the neuronal signaling from the insula cortex. Inhibition of the Hb was able to abrogate

OSA induced by electrical stimulation of the insula cortex [10]. However, it is unclear whether the amplitude of the frequency used to stimulate the Hb is critical to achieve the maximum response in OSA. In this study, we investigated the effect of different Hb stimulation frequencies on obstructive sleep apnea. The breathing pattern as well as the EMG activities of the genioglossus was recorded before and after OSA was induced.

2. Materials and Methods

2.1. Animal Preparation. This study was carried out in accordance with the Guide for the Care and Use of Laboratory Animals of the National Institutes of Health. The protocol was approved by the Animal Care and Use Committee of the Jilin University (Permit number: SCXK, Kyrgyzstan, 2007-0003, and SYXK, Kyrgyzstan, 2007-0011). Wistar rats (200–280 g, 6–8 weeks old, $N = 92$) were obtained from the Jilin University Norman Bethune Medical Department Laboratory Animal Center. The animals were housed under a 12/12-hour light/dark cycle in a temperature-controlled room (maintained at $22 \pm 2^{\circ}$C) with ad libitum access to food and water [11]. All surgical and animal handling procedures were performed in accordance with Guidance Suggestions for the Care and Use of Laboratory Animals issued by the Ministry of Science and Technology of the People's Republic of China. The animals were randomly divided into three groups, the OSA group ($n = 24$), Hb group ($n = 48$), and control group ($n = 20$), using SPSS software. For the OSA group, the insula cortex was stimulated to induce OSA. For the Hb group, the insula cortex and Hb were stimulated with four different frequencies ($n = 12$ for each frequency). For the control group, the surrounding tissue of either the insula cortex ($n = 10$) or the Hb ($n = 10$) was stimulated. The breathing pattern and the EMG activities of the genioglossus and diaphragm were recorded before and after stimulation.

All experimental procedures were performed under anesthesia via intraperitoneal injection of 20% urethane (6 mL/kg), and all efforts were made to minimize suffering. During the surgery, the animals were breathing steadily and maintained in a state of light anesthesia (sensitive corneal reflex and forceps pinch produced withdrawal but no sustained response and no voluntary activities) [14] throughout the experimental procedure. Anesthesia was supplemented if needed during the experiment. The animals were maintained at 36°C rectal temperature with a heating pad. During the experiment, the animals were fixed under the stereotaxic instruments (Takahashi Company, Japan) with blunt ear bars, and a small craniotomy was performed. For the OSA group, an electrode was implanted into the insula cortex (anterior/posterior: 1.0 mm; medial/lateral: 5.4-5.5 mm; and dorsal/ventral: 4.2–4.4 mm), according to the rat brain atlas [15]. Whereas in the Hb group, electrodes were implanted into the insula cortex (Ic) and Hb (anterior/posterior: −3.2 mm; medial/lateral: 0.3–0.6 mm; and dorsal/ventral: 3.8–4.2 mm). The control group received electrical stimulation with the same parameters, but the electrode locations were at four points (top, bottom, left, and right) within a 1 mm^2 range around the Ic. The rats were fixed in a ventral decubitus position and breathed spontaneously during the experiments.

2.2. Electrical Stimulation and Recording Protocols. Electrical stimulation device (Nihon Kohden, Japan) and concentric stimulating electrodes (Nihon Kohden, Japan; outer diameter of 2.0 mm and impedance of 10–15 MΩ; Figure 1) were used for stimulation. OSA was induced by stimulating the Ic at 100 Hz, 0.4 mA, and 1 ms interval for 9 s [16]. Signs of apnea and respiratory distresses were used as indicators of successful induction during the experiment. Histology analysis of induction site was also performed. No signs of apnea and respiratory distress were observed in the control group. In the Hb group, the Hb was stimulated continuously for at least 30 min at 50 Hz, 120 Hz, 130 Hz, or 280 Hz before and after the insula cortex was stimulated.

The breathing pattern and EMG were recorded using a data logger (BL-420S, Chengdu Taimeng Technology Co., Ltd.). A respiratory flow transducer and a tension transducer were utilized to monitor the respiratory flow via endotracheal intubation and respiratory rates, respectively. The lead electrode was inserted to the genioglossus and diaphragm to record the EMG signals in the genioglossus and diaphragm, respectively.

2.3. Data Analysis. The electromyography (EMG) of the genioglossus and diaphragm, as well as the respiratory amplitude and respiratory rate, was compared before and after the stimulation of the Hb. SPSS 19.0 was used for all statistical analysis. Data were presented as mean ± standard deviation ($X \pm S$). $P < 0.05$ was considered as statistically significant.

3. Results

Concentric stimulation of the Ic was performed in 12 OSA rats. During stimulation, weakened genioglossus contraction, apnea, interruption of airflow, and reduction of the respiratory rate were observed in OSA rats. Whereas, after stimulation, signs including intermittent apnea, a significant reduction of airflow (from 89.08 ± 4.21 breaths/min to 12.19 ± 8.49 breaths/min), transbreathing, reduction in the respiratory rate, deep breathing after stimulation, airflow return to baseline in few seconds, and significant reduction of genioglossus discharge were observed (Figure 2). Subsequently, the Hb was stimulated continuously for 30 min at 50 Hz, 120 Hz, 130 Hz, and 280 Hz in the same rat. Simultaneous concentric stimulation of the Ic was performed using the same parameters, and the breath and EMG activities of the genioglossus were monitored. As shown in Figure 3, the respiration rate and amplitude as well as EMG patterns of the genioglossus were returned within normal ranges after 130 Hz stimulation. Notably, the respiration rate changes at different stimulation frequencies of the Hb in OSA-induced animal models (Figure 4).

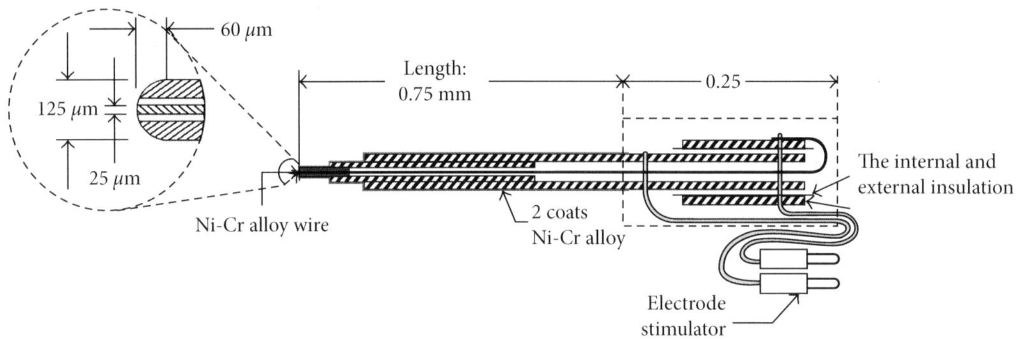

FIGURE 1: Schematic of stimulation electrode. The experimental stimulation electrode is a Ni-Cr alloy wire concentric exciter electrode of Japanese Narishige Company.

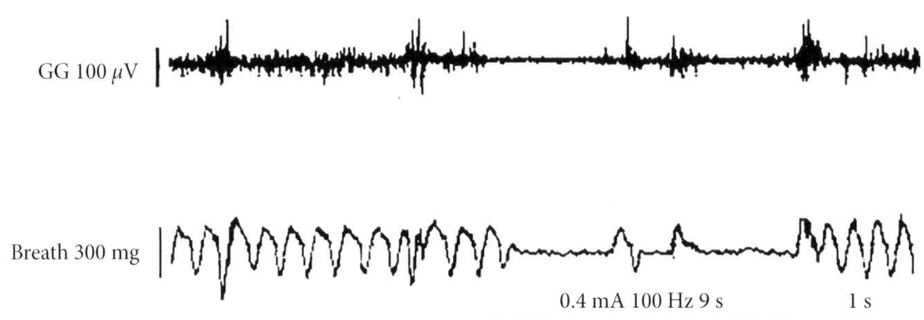

FIGURE 2: Typical changes in respiration and genioglossus EMG patterns before, during, and after stimulation in the IC with 100 Hz.

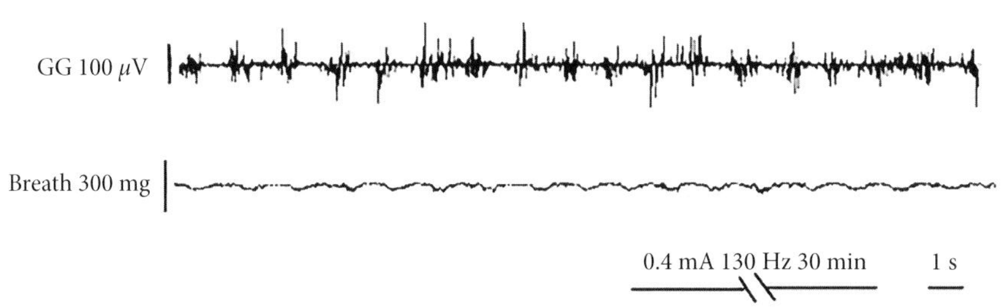

FIGURE 3: Typical respiration and genioglossus EMG patterns after 130 Hz stimulation of the Hb in the OSA-induced animal.

4. Discussion

The genioglossus has been commonly considered as the pathophysiology of OSA. Horner et al. reported that the genioglossus contractile function was significantly decreased during sleep [17]. Our results showed a reduction in genioglossus contraction in OSA rats, which is consistent with a previous study showing that genioglossus activity significantly reduced during sleep in OSA patients with subsequent weakening in contraction resulting in muscle relaxation in the pharyngeal wall [18]. As a consequence, a reduction in the respiratory rate was observed (Figure 2), which may be attributed to the subsequent collapse of the upper airway, thus reducing ventilation [18]. It should be noted that, despite the application of excitatory neurotransmitter serotonin (5-hydroxytryptamine, 5-HT), sleep could not prevent genioglossus diastole [19]. Thus, the main reason for the occurrence of OSA is associated with respiratory disorders, suggesting that the genioglossus could play an important role in OSA. The genioglossus electrical activity weakens during sleep, causing the muscles to relax and a reduction in ventilation. Consequently, chronic intermittent hypoxia or hypercapnia (chronic intermittent hypopnea or hypercapnia, CIHH) occurs, or even acidosis.

Our results showed that 100 Hz concentric stimulation of the Ic could induce OSA in rats. The Ic, a region of the limbic system, can change the genioglossus tension, as well as the breathing depth and rate. Many neurotransmitters regulating the limbic system are associated with many diseases [20–23]. Signals propagating from the Ic to the Hb could reduce the release of 5-HT in the raphe nuclei. Subsequently, the activity of hypoglossal nucleus would decrease, resulting in the reduction of genioglossus contractile function. Consequently, genioglossus relaxation occurs, which can cause airway to collapse, and thus OSA. It should be mentioned that the Ic is involved in regulating OSA and has been related to respiratory motion adjustments [11]. The activities in the Ic increased during OSA, and inhibition could occur in the raphe nucleus that reduces the release of 5-HT. Subsequently, the activity of the hypoglossal

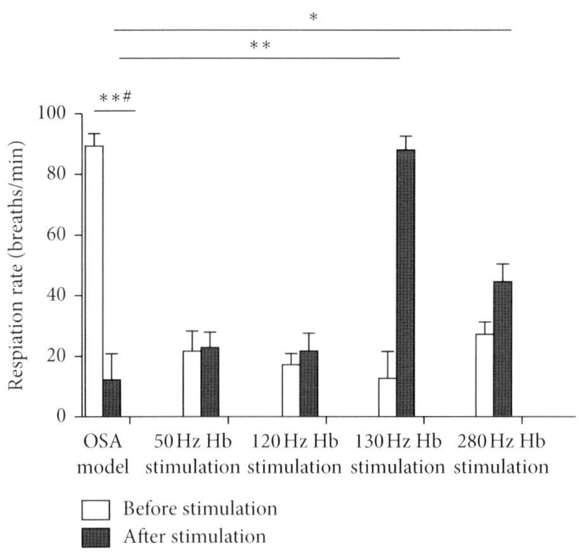

Figure 4: Respiration rate changes at different stimulation frequencies of the Hb in OSA-induced animal models. **# denotes $P < 0.001$ before and after stimulation in the insula cortex, while ** and * denote $P < 0.001$ and $P < 0.05$, respectively, between the OSA model and different stimulation frequencies in the habenula.

nucleus and the hypoglossal nerve excitability are reduced. Thus, the genioglossus contraction is weakened, and the upper airway will be more vulnerable to collapse causing OSA.

When the Hb was stimulated continuously for 30 min at 130 Hz, the EMG patterns of the genioglossus returned within normal ranges. These results indicate that such a stimulation can be used to treat OSA. The Hb plays an important role in OSA, since the Hb mediates signals from the Ic to the downstream. Consequently, 130 Hz stimulation may block the Hb, resulting in genioglossus contraction, and thus, the upper airway may open and ultimately improve ventilation. These results indicate that inhibition of the Hb can block downstream signal propagation from the Ic, thereby avoiding the formation of OSA. Our results reveal the relationship between Hb, OSA, and Ic and may also provide a new therapeutic strategy in OSA.

5. Conclusion

Electrical stimulation of 130 Hz could inhibit Hb, which reduces downstream signal propagation initiated by the Ic. This, in turn, will cause the genioglossus contractile function to recover, avoiding the formation of obstructive sleep apnea.

Acknowledgments

The authors thank Professor Shao Wang for assistance with the experiments, who passed away 2 years ago; he provided constructive advice to conceive the study. The authors are grateful to all the participators of the Department of Physiology Lab and the Center of Medical Laboratory of Jilin Medical University. The study was supported by the National Natural Science Foundation of China (81670080) and the National College Students Innovation and Entrepreneurship Training Program (201613706024). The sponsor had no role in the design or conduct of this research. The authors thank Sleep Medicine for presenting this work as an abstract in December 2017.

References

[1] F. G. Issa and C. E. Sullivan, "Alcohol, snoring and sleep apnea," *Journal of Neurology, Neurosurgery, and Psychiatry*, vol. 45, no. 4, pp. 353–359, 1982.

[2] W. Richard, D. Kox, C. den Herder, M. Laman, H. van Tinteren, and N. de Vries, "The role of sleep position in obstructive sleep apnea syndrome," *European Archives of Oto-Rhino-Laryngology*, vol. 263, no. 10, pp. 946–950, 2006.

[3] A. Romero-Corral, S. M. Caples, F. Lopez-Jimenez, and V. K. Somers, "Interactions between obesity and obstructive sleep apnea: implications for treatment," *Chest*, vol. 137, no. 3, pp. 711–719, 2010.

[4] N. A. Dewan, F. J. Nieto, and V. K. Somers, "Intermittent hypoxemia and OSA: implications for comorbidities," *Chest*, vol. 147, no. 1, pp. 266–274, 2015.

[5] S. Q. Yang, L. L. Han, X. L. Dong et al., "Mal-effects of obstructive sleep apnea on the heart," *Sleep and Breathing*, vol. 16, no. 3, pp. 717–722, 2012.

[6] M. Kohler and J. R. Stradling, "OSA and hypertension: do we know all the answers?," *Chest*, vol. 144, no. 5, pp. 1433–1435, 2013.

[7] M. X. Li, J. H. Wang, M. Huang et al., "Blockage of the habenular nucleus can eliminate dyspnea induced by electrostimulation of the insular cortex," *Neural Regeneration Research*, vol. 5, no. 13, pp. 1025–1029, 2010.

[8] J. P. Saboisky, N. L. Chamberlin, and A. Malhotra, "Potential therapeutic targets in obstructive sleep apnoea," *Expert Opinion on Therapeutic Targets*, vol. 13, no. 7, pp. 795–809, 2009.

[9] A. Vakulin, A. D'Rozario, J. W. Kim et al., "Quantitative sleep EEG and polysomnographic predictors of driving simulator performance in obstructive sleep apnea," *Clinical Neurophysiology*, vol. 127, no. 2, pp. 1428–1435, 2016.

[10] L. K. Huon, S. Y. Liu, T. T. Shih, Y. J. Chen, M. T. Lo, and P. C. Wang, "Dynamic upper airway collapse observed from sleep MRI: BMI-matched severe and mild OSA patients," *European Archives of Oto-Rhino-Laryngology*, vol. 273, no. 11, pp. 4021–4026, 2016.

[11] L. Cui, J. H. Wang, M. Wang et al., "Injection of L-glutamate into the insular cortex produces sleep apnea and serotonin reduction in rats," *Sleep and Breathing*, vol. 16, no. 3, pp. 845–853, 2012.

[12] J. Li, M. X. Li, S. N. Liu et al., "Is brain damage really involved in the pathogenesis of obstructive sleep apnea?," *Neuroreport*, vol. 25, no. 8, pp. 593–595, 2014.

[13] M. X. Li, C. Y. Yan, and S. Wang, "New insights on the role of the insular cortex and habenula in OSA," *Sleep and Breathing*, vol. 19, no. 4, pp. 1347–1353, 2015.

[14] H. L. Fields, J. Bry, I. Hentall, and G. Zorman, "The activity of neurons in the rostral medulla of the rat during withdrawal from noxious heat," *Journal of Neuroscience*, vol. 3, no. 12, pp. 2545–2552, 1983.

[15] P. George and W. Charles, *The Rat Brain in Stereotaxic Coordinates*, Academic Press, Cambridge, MA, USA, 6th edition, 2006.

[16] S. Wang, Q. Fu, and J. Fu, "Modulation of preoptic area on discharges of parafasc insular pain neurons," *Ke Xue Tong Bao*, vol. 28, pp. 401–405, 1983.

[17] R. L. Horner, X. Liu, H. Gill, P. Nolan, H. Liu, and S. Sood, "Effects of sleep-wake state on the genioglossus vs. diaphragm muscle response to CO(2) in rats," *Journal of Applied Physiology*, vol. 92, no. 2, pp. 878–887, 2002.

[18] S. A. Shea, J. K. Edwards, and D. P. White, "Effect of wake-sleep transitions and rapid eye movement sleep on pharyngeal muscle response to negative pressure in humans," *Journal of Physiology*, vol. 520, no. 3, pp. 897–908, 1999.

[19] K. A. Sillay, D. Rusy, L. Buyan-Dent, N. L. Ninman, and K. K. Vigen, "Wide-bore 1.5 T MRI-guided deep brain stimulation surgery: initial experience and technique comparison," *Clinical Neurology and Neurosurgery*, vol. 127, pp. 79–85, 2014.

[20] S. Vallabhajosula, I. U. Haq, N. Hwynn et al., "Low-frequency versus high-frequency subthalamic nucleus deep brain stimulation on postural control and gait in Parkinson's disease: a quantitative study," *Brain Stimulation*, vol. 8, no. 1, pp. 64–75, 2015.

[21] A. M. Lozano, L. Fosdick, M. M. Chakravarty et al., "A phase II study of fornix deep brain stimulation in mild Alzheimer's disease," *Journal of Alzheimer's Disease*, vol. 54, no. 2, pp. 777–787, 2016.

[22] J. A. Espinoza Martinez, G. J. Arango, E. T. Fonoff et al., "Deep brain stimulation of the globus pallidus internus or ventralis intermedius nucleus of thalamus for Holmes tremor," *Neurosurgical Review*, vol. 38, no. 4, pp. 753–763, 2015.

[23] S. K. Yadav, R. Kumar, P. M. Macey, M. A. Woo, F. L. Yan-Go, and R. M. Harper, "Insular cortex metabolite changes in obstructive sleep apnea," *Sleep*, vol. 37, pp. 951–958, 2014.

27

EZH2 Inhibition Ameliorates Transverse Aortic Constriction-Induced Pulmonary Arterial Hypertension in Mice

Zhan-Li Shi, Kun Fang, Zhi-Hui Li, Dan-Hong Ren, Jia-Ying Zhang, and Jing Sun

Department of Intensive Care Unit, Hangzhou Red Cross Hospital/Zhejiang Chinese Medicine, Western Medicine Integrated Hospital, Hangzhou 310003, China

Correspondence should be addressed to Jing Sun; sunjing_hz@aliyun.com

Academic Editor: Du Lei

Background. EPZ005687 is a selective inhibiter of methyltransferase EZH2. In this article, we investigated the protective role and mechanism of EPZ005687 in transverse aortic constriction-induced pulmonary arterial hypertension in mice. *Methods.* We assigned 15 (6–8 weeks old) male balb/c mice to 3 groups randomly: Sham control + DMSO group, TAC + DMSO group, and TAC + EPZ005687 group (10 mg kg^{-1}, once a week for 4 weeks). On day 28 following TAC operation, the right ventricular systolic blood pressure (RVSBP) was measured, and lung tissues were collected for laboratory examinations (DHE, Western blot, real-time PCR, and ChIP). *Results.* Murine PAH model was successfully created by TAC operation as evidenced by increased RVSBP and hypertrophic right ventricle. Compared with the sham control, TAC-induced PAH markedly upregulated the expression of EZH2 and ROS deposition in lungs in PAH mice. The inhibiter of methyltransferase EZH2, EPZ005687 significantly inhibits the development of TAC-induced PAH in an EZH2-SOD1-ROS dependent manner. *Conclusion.* Our data identified that EZH2 serves a fundamental role in TAC-induced PAH, and administration of EPZ005687 might represent a novel therapeutic target for the treatment of TAC-induced PAH.

1. Introduction

There is a growing body of literature that recognizes the end stage of left ventricle heart failure often leading to pulmonary artery hypertension (PAH) and right ventricle heart failure [1–3]. Abundant evidences have investigated the mechanism and therapeutic strategy of heart failure (HF) [4–6]. Yet, there is poorly published data concerning the PAH induced by HF. Recent evidences suggest that the accumulation of reactive oxygen species (ROS) may contribute to the pathogenesis and development of PAH [7, 8]. Furthermore, antioxidant treatments delay the development of PAH, intimating that pulmonary oxidative stress mediates the development of PAH [1, 8].

Epigenetic gene regulations are vital to cardiovascular diseases (CVDs) [9, 10]. Various histone modifications on the promoter involved in genetic expression pattern, activation, or repression; histone H3 lysine 27 trimethylation (H3K27me3) exerts a key role in gene repression [11]. Evidences suggest that H3K27me3 is an important factor for cardiac hypertrophy [12] and generation of ROS [13, 14]. Suppressor of enhancer of zeste homolog 2 (EZH2) is a methyltransferase responsible for laying down the H3K27me3 mark on the chromatin [15, 16]. EZH2 was initially discovered as crucial regulator centrally involved in the regional organization of homeotic gene expression implicated in the assembly of chromatin domains and the regulation of chromatin of repressive protein complexes in chromatin [17]. Although EZH2 was reported to inhibit cardiac hypertrophy by recruiting H3K27me3 on prohypertrophic genes like ANP, BNP [18], and CaMKII [19], it remains obscure how EZH2 may contribute to the pathogenesis of TAC-induced PAH.

The aim of this essay is to discuss the relationship between H3K27me3 modification statuses in TAC-induced PAH. EPZ005687 is a selective inhibitor of the lysine-specific histone methyltransferase EZH2 [20]. Therefore, another objective of this study was to determine whether the administration of EPZ005687 attenuated the progression of PAH induced by TAC. Here, we report that upregulation of EZH2 accompanies SOD1 downregulation in the lung during TAC-induced PAH. Pharmaceutical inhibition of EZH2 delays progression of TAC-induced PAH in mice through inhibiting oxidative stress in lung.

2. Methods

2.1. Animal Preparation. This study was approved by the Animal Ethics Committee of Zhejiang Chinese Medicine and Western Medicine Integrated Hospital. Balb/c mice (Shanghai Biomodel Organism Science & Technology Development Co., Ltd.) were used for the described experiment. Balb/c mice (6–8 weeks) were assigned randomly to three experimental groups: (a) sham control group, injected peritoneally with DMSO for 4 weeks once a week; (b) TAC group, injected peritoneally with DMSO for 4 weeks once a week; and (c) TAC group, injected peritoneally with EPZ005687 (10 mg kg^{-1}) for 4 weeks once a week. The injection was performed at 1, 8, 15, and 22 days post-TAC or sham operation.

2.2. Transverse Aortic Constriction (TAC) Procedure. In brief, 6–8 weeks old male mice (body weight ranging from 22 to 25 g) were operated on using a TAC operation. Before the operation, the mice were anaesthetized with a mixture of ketamine (120 mg kg^{-1}) and xylazine (6 mg kg^{-1}) (i.p.). A horizontal incision 5 mm in length is made at the level of the suprasternal notch to allow direct access to the transverse aorta without damaging the pleural space. Aortic constriction is performed by ligating the aorta between the right innominate artery and the left carotid artery over a 27-gauge needle using 6-0 silk sutures for approximately 70% aortic constriction. After aorta ligation, the needle is then quickly removed; leave the constriction in place and then the thoracic cavity was closed. Successful constriction of the aorta was identified and confirmed by Doppler echocardiogram. Sham-operated animals underwent the same surgical procedure without partial aorta ligation [4].

2.3. RV Pressure Measurements. At the end of the study protocol, open-chest RV catheterization was performed to detect RV Pressure under general anesthesia in all animals (isoflurane 2.0%) as described. The right ventricle was approached via a lateral right thoracotomy through the fifth intercostal space. RV pressures were recorded by the use of a 1.2-F pressure catheter (Scisense Inc., Ontario, Canada) [21].

2.4. Histological Analysis. Heart weight (HW), lung weight (LW), and body weight (BW) were measured. For ROS detection, frozen lung sections (5 μm) were stained with DHE (2 μmol/l Selleck) in a light-protected humidified chamber at 37°C for 30 min. The slides were visualized by confocal fluorescence microscopy (Zeiss).

2.5. Western Blot. Whole lysates were obtained with RIPA buffer (50 mM Tris pH 7.4, 150 mM NaCl, 1% Triton X-100) with freshly added protease inhibitor cocktail tablet (Roche); the protein concentrations were measured by using the Pierce® BCA Protein Assay Kit (23225, Thermo Fisher Scientific, Waltham, MA, USA). The nitrocellulose membranes (1620112, Bio-Rad) were subsequently blocked in TBST containing 5% skimmed milk powder for 90 minutes at room temperature and incubated with anti-EZH2 (Peninsula Laboratories Inc.), anti-SOD1 (Santa Cruz Biotechnology), anti–nitrotyrosine (Santa Cruz Biotechnology), and anti-β-actin (Sigma) overnight at 4°C. On following day, the membranes were incubated with secondary antibodies, respectively, and the signals were visualized with a SignalFire(tm) ECL Reagent (6883S, Cell Signaling Technology, USA).

2.6. RNA Extraction and Quantitative Real-Time PCR. Total RNA was isolated using TRIzol (Invitrogen) according to the manufacturer's instructions. cDNA was synthesized from 1 μg of RNA with the One Step RT-PCR Kit (Takara). Quantitative PCR was processed as described before [22]. Primer pairs used for real-time PCR are as follows: SOD1, forward 5′-ACTGGTGGTCCATGAAAAAGC-3′ and reverse 5′-AACGACTTCCAGCGTTTCCT-3′; [23] EZH2, forward 5′-TGGACCACAGTGTTACCAGCA-3′ [24] and reverse 5′-TGGGCGTTTAGGTGGTGTCT-3′; GAPDH, forward 5′-TGGTTCACACCCATCACAAACA-3′ and reverse 5′-GGTGAAGGTCGGTGTGAACGG-3′. The relative amount of each gene in each sample was estimated by the ΔΔCT method. Results were normalized to Gapdh RNA level.

2.7. Chromatin Immunoprecipitation, ChIP. ChIP assays were performed as previously described [25]. In brief, Chromatin was cross-linked with 1% formaldehyde. Cells were incubated in lysis buffer (150 mM NaCl, 25 mM Tris pH 7.5, 1% Triton X-100, 0.1% SDS, 0.5% deoxycholate) supplemented with protease inhibitor tablet. DNA was fragmented into ~500 bp pieces using a Branson 250 sonicator. Aliquots of lysates containing 100 μg of protein were used for each immunoprecipitation reaction with anti-LSD1 (Abcam) and anti-trimethylated H3K27 (Abcam). Precipitated genomic DNA was amplified by real-time PCR with the following primers: Gapdh promoter region, 5′-ATCACTGCCACCCAGAAGACTGTGGA-3′, and 5′-CTCATACCAGGAAATGAGCTTGACAAA-3′; Sod1 promoter region, 5′-AATAGCGACTTTCCCAGCTC-3′, and 5′-AAACGAAGGTGCAAAACGAG-3′.

2.7. Statistical Analysis. All data are presented as the mean ± standard error. Data of two groups were compared with unpaired *t*-test. One-way analysis of variance with post hoc Scheffe analyses was performed using an SPSS package. Grouping was performed in a randomized manner.

3. Results

3.1. Pulmonary Arterial Hypertension Induced by TAC Simulates EZH2 Expression. First of all, whether the PAH murine model was successfully induced by TAC surgery

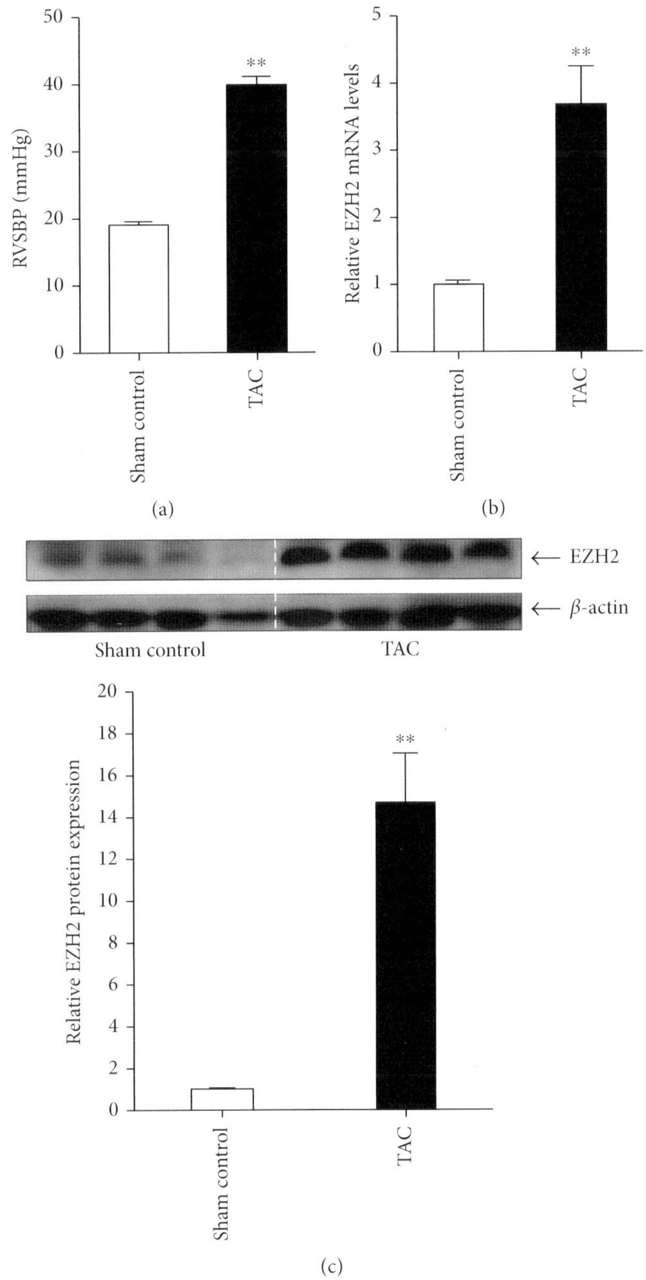

Figure 1: Expression of EZH2 is upregulated in lungs in TAC-induced PAH mice. (a) Right ventricular systolic blood pressure (RVSBP) at day 28 after TAC procedure ($n = 4$ for each group, $^{**}P < 0.001$ versus sham control). Relative mRNA (b) and protein (c) levels of EZH2 in lungs in sham control mice or TAC mice on day 28 following TAC procedure ($n = 4$ for each group, $^{**}P < 0.001$ versus sham control).

should be verified. Additional 8 balb/c mice were used for sham control and TAC procedure without any treatment. As was shown Figure 1(a), on day 28, TAC group mice developed PAH as evidenced by the increase in right ventricular systolic pressure (RVSBP), an index of pulmonary arterial systolic blood pressure (PABP). To investigate the role of EZH2 in the progression of PAH induced by TAC, we measured the EZH2 levels in lung tissues in mice. Western blot analysis and quantitative real-time PCR demonstrated that TAC-induced PAH resulted in a significant induction of EZH2 in PAH lungs as compared with sham control lungs (Figures 1(b) and 1(c)). These results suggest that PAH is successfully induced by TAC, and expression of EZH2 in lungs is notably activated by TAC-induced PAH, which indicates that EZH2 may be involved in TAC-induced PAH.

3.2. EZH2 Inhibition Protects against TAC-Induced PAH In Vivo. To assess the biological impact of EZH2 on the development of pulmonary hypertension, we first measured the RVSP as an indicator of pulmonary artery pressure in spontaneously breathing mice, following sham control and TAC operation, EPZ005687 or DMSO was injected peritoneally as described in methods. On day 28 after TAC, the

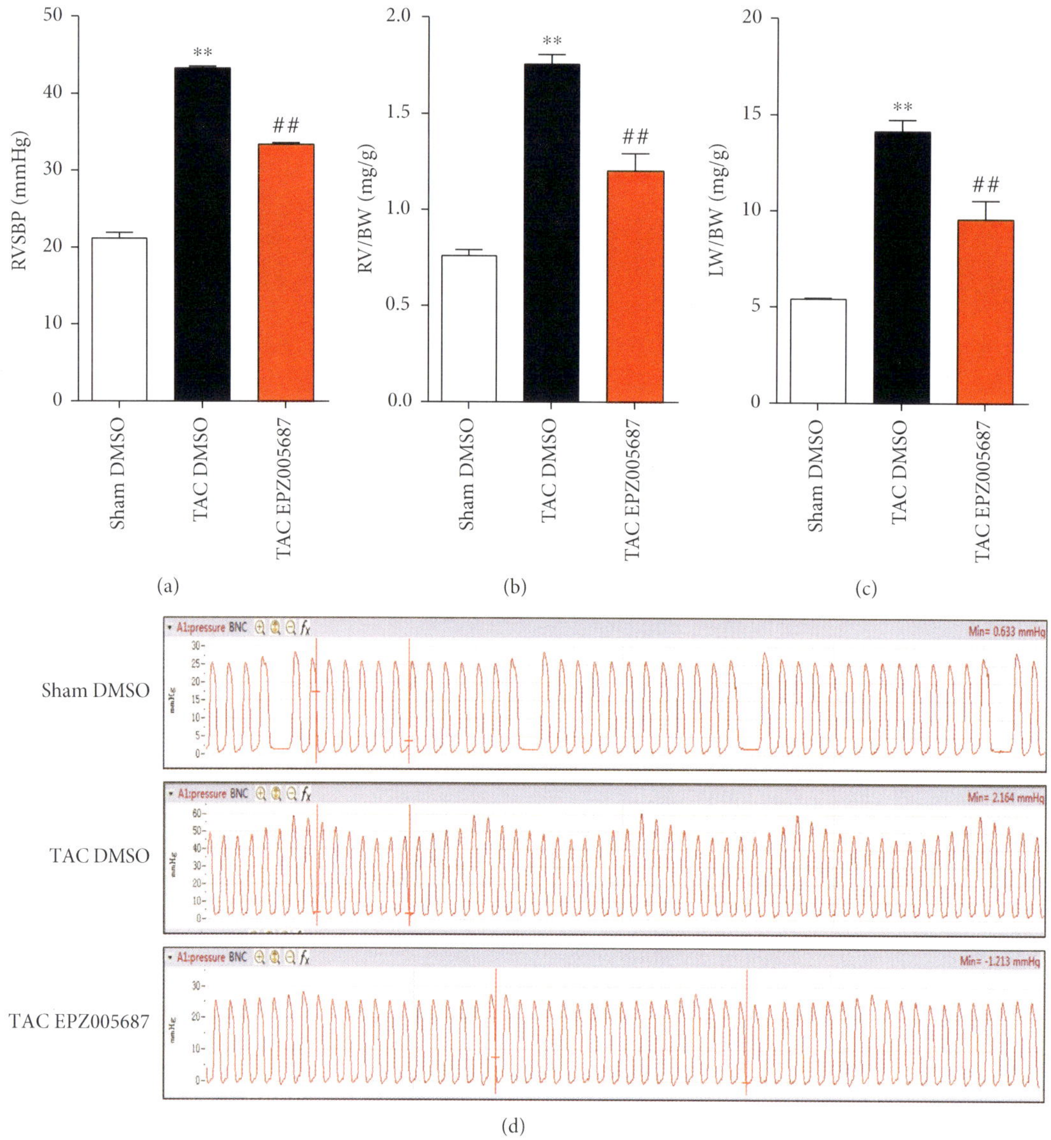

FIGURE 2: Inhibition of EZH2 with EPZ005687 attenuates TAC-induced PAH. (a) Right ventricular systolic blood pressure (RVSBP) at day 28 after TAC procedure. (b) Ratios of LV weight to body weight. (c) Ratios of lung weight to body weight ($n = 5$ for each group, $^{**}P < 0.001$ versus sham control, $^{\#\#}P < 0.001$ versus TAC DMSO). (d) RVSBP and the effect of EPZ005687 on pulmonary vessel tension.

RVSBP was markedly higher in the TAC group than in the sham control group (Figures 2(a) and 2(d)). Besides, as shown in Figures 2(b) and 2(c), ratios of RV and lung weight to body weight were significantly increased 2.1-fold and 2.6-fold in TAC mice compared to sham control mice, respectively. EPZ005687 treatment significantly alleviated the further increase of RVSBP, ratios of LV and lung weight to body weight, respectively. These findings suggest that EPZ005687 treatment might have a prominent role in protecting against TAC-induced PAH and RV hypertrophy in vivo.

3.3. EZH2 Inhibition Regulates Oxidative Reactions in Lungs. ROS are important parts of physiological and pathological processes. Recently, ROS are thought to be signaling molecules to mediate specific cellular responses in the vasculature [26]. Moreover, evidence shows that the accumulation of ROS contributes to the development of PAH [7, 8]. To investigate the role of ROS in our TAC-induced PAH model, DHE fluorescence probe was utilized to detect ROS production in murine frozen lung sections. Figure 3(a) showed that EZH2 silencing prevented the induction of ROS production by TAC-induced PAH from 18.3 fold to 4.8 fold compared with sham control. As anticipated, the increase of lung nitrotyrosine caused by TAC-induced PAH was significant inhibited by EPZ005687 treatment (Figure 3(b)). These findings suggest that inhibition of EZH2 reduces oxidative reaction in lungs caused by TAC-induced PAH.

3.4. EZH2 Suppresses SOD1 Transexpression in Lung in TAC-Induced PAH Mice. SOD1 is responsible for destroying free superoxide radicals in the body. In accordance with the

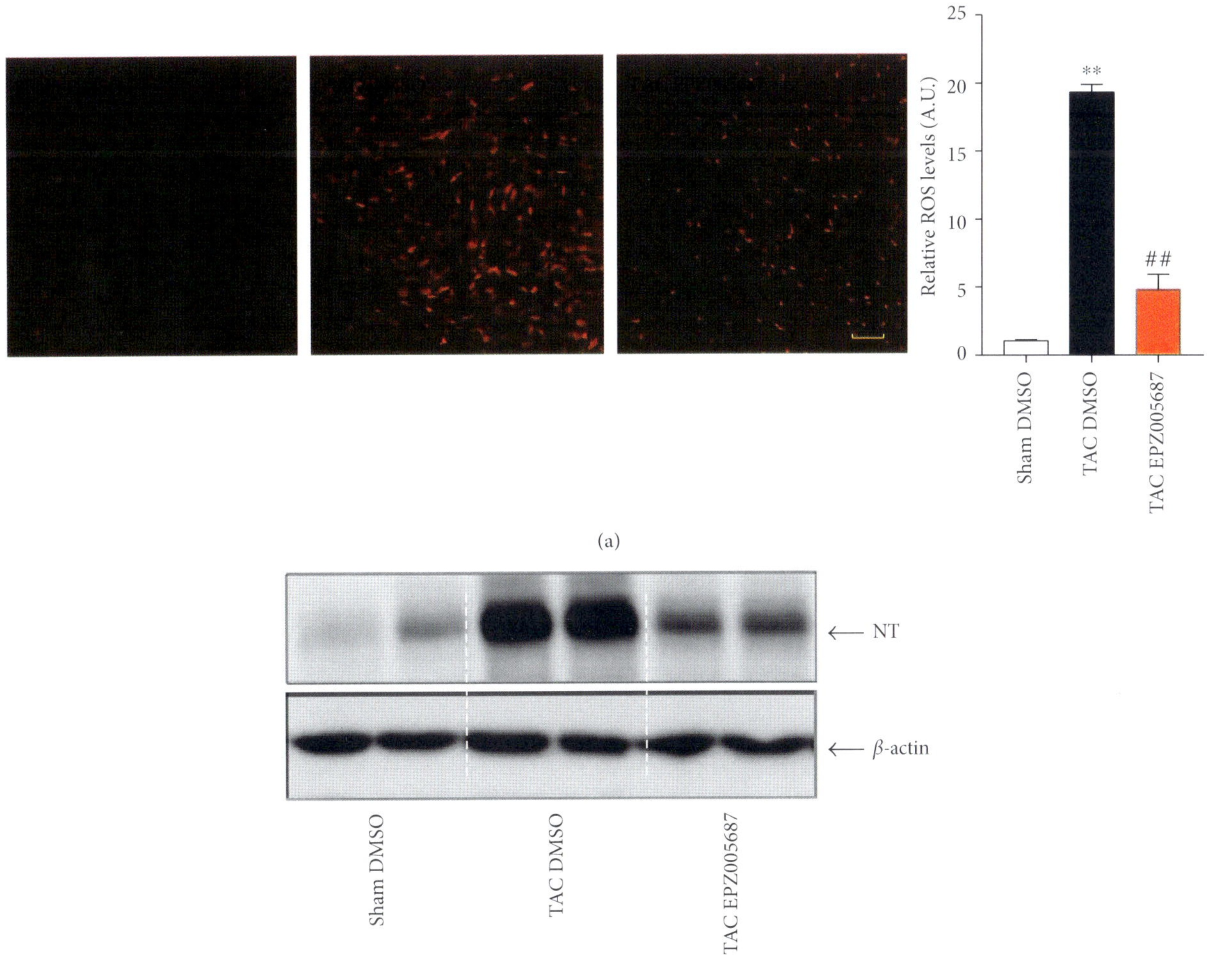

Figure 3: EPZ005687 treatment inhibits oxidative reactions in lungs in TAC-induced PAH mice. (a) Lung tissues ROS levels were evaluated by DHE staining (scale bar, 50 μm, $n = 5$ for each group, $^{**}P < 0.001$ versus sham control, $^{\#\#}P < 0.001$ versus TAC DMSO). (b) The expression of nitrotyrosine in lung lysate was detected by western blot.

oxidative reaction in lungs, the expression of SOD1 was significantly downregulated and the expression of EZH2 was upregulated in TAC + DMSO group as compared with sham control, respectively (Figures 4(a) and 4(b)). Due to the negative correlation between EZH2 and SOD1 expression, and next, we tackled the relationship between EZH2 and SOD1. Interestingly, we observed EPZ005687 treatment could inhibit the expression of EZH2 and reverse the decreased expression of SOD1 (Figures 4(a) and 4(b)). Thus, we hypothesized that EZH2 might promote TAC-induced PAH by targeting SOD1. Chromatin immunoprecipitation (ChIP) assay showed that EZH2 and trimethylated histone H3K27 (H3K27Me3) accumulated on the SOD1 promoter but not the Gapdh promoter in TAC + DMSO group. EPZ005687 treatment was used to validate the role of EZH2 in SOD1 transrepression. Indeed, EPZ005687 treatment could reverse the increased accumulation of EZH2 and H3K27Me3 on SOD1 promoter (Figure 4(c)) and increase SOD1 expression in lung in TAC-induced PAH mice (Figures 4(a) and 4(b)). Combined, these data suggest that EZH2 regulates intracellular ROS levels in response to TAC-induced PAH stimulation through repressing SOD1 transcription.

4. Discussion

In this study, we investigated epigenetic treatment impact of EPZ005687 on TAC-induced PAH. At the end stage, left ventricle heart failure always leads to right ventricle heart failure, pulmonary remodeling, and pulmonary artery hypertension, which cause heavy economic and healthy burdens worldwide [1]. In this essay, we identified that the specific EZH2 inhibitor EPZ005687 attenuates TAC-induced PAH in an ROS-dependent manner through influencing histone H3K27 trimethylation on the SOD1 promoter.

There are abundant and consistent data for increased levels of ROS in patients and animal models of PAH [27, 28]. Notwithstanding, there is much diversity of research about the mechanisms that are responsible for the increased ROS, very few studies have investigated the influence of histone methylation modifications on ROS generation in PAH.

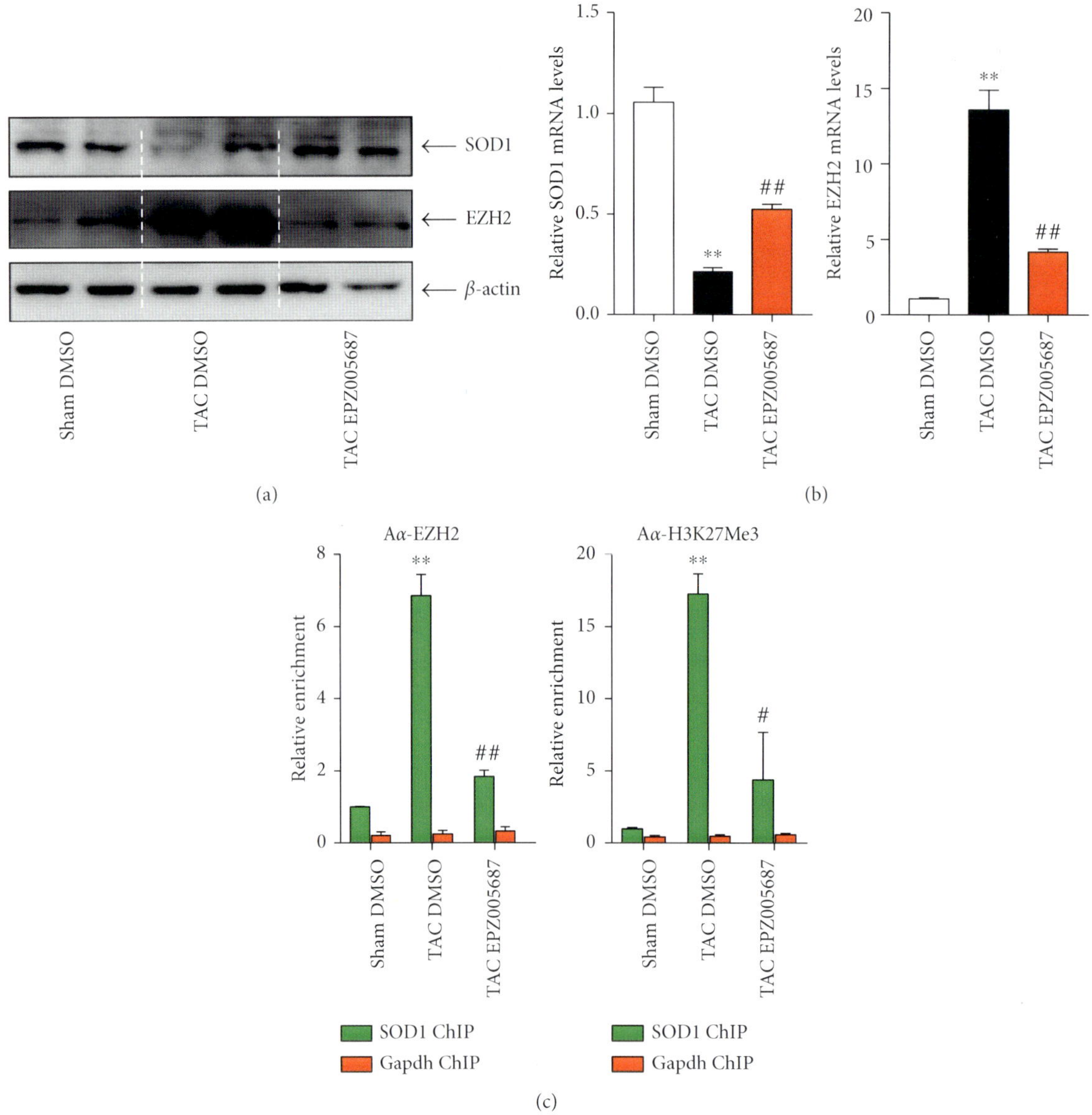

Figure 4: EZH2 regulates TAC-induced PAH by targeting SOD1. Expression levels of SOD1 and EZH2 were measured by (a) Western blot and (b) qPCR ($n = 5$ for each group, $^{**}P < 0.001$ versus sham control, $^{##}P < 0.001$ versus TAC DMSO). (c) ChIP assays were performed with anti-EZH2 and anti-H3K27Me3 using lung tissues in indicated mice ($n = 5$ for each group, $^{**}P < 0.001$ versus sham control, $^{##}P < 0.001$, $^{#}p < 0.01$ versus TAC DMSO).

Histone methylation modifications play vital roles in gene expression.

Different histone methyltransferases are specific for the lysine residue they modify. On histone H3, for example, SET1, Ash2, WDR5, catalyze methylation of H3K4 in mammalian cells [5, 10, 22, 25], H3K4, H3K36, and H3K79 methylation generally represent gene activation. SUV39-h1 and SUV39-h2 histone methyltransferases that catalyze methylation of H3K9 [9], G9a [29], and EZH2 [30] are responsible for methylation of H3K27, whereas methylation on histones H3K9 and H3K27 is usually associated with gene repression.

Polycomb repressive complex 2 (PRC2) catalyze methylation of H3K27 and EZH2 is the catalytic subunit of the PRC2 complex [31]. EZH2-mediated methylation of lysine 27 on histone on target gene promoter suppresses target gene transexpression [12]. In the present research, we found that the expression of EZH2 was upregulated parallel with the accumulation of ROS and nitrotyrosine in lungs in PAH mice (Figures 3 and 4(a) and 4(b)). In addition, we also found that H3K27Me3 accumulation on the SOD1 promoter, likely mediated by EZH2, might be responsible for SOD1 transrepression in the lungs following TAC-induced PAH. EPZ005687 has been previously reported acting as an anticancer drug [32, 33] and attenuating osteoarthritis progression [34]. The present research broadens the scope of pharmacological applications of EPZ005687.

This study has some limitations. First, in the present study, RVSBP was evaluated at day 28 after TAC, by which time plenty of leukocytes would have infiltrated the lungs was extremely serious [35]. The leukocyte infiltration cannot be ignored when we try to interpret the current dataset, especially given the fact that EPZ005687 treatment was a systemic EZH2 inhibition mouse model. In view of the fact that the targeted cell type which could cause adverse oxidative reaction was not confirmed in the present study. It invites the question as to whether EZH2 inhibition in leukocytes could suppress ROS generation and, if so, via what mechanism(s). These issues need further investigation preferably with lineage-specific SUV39H knockout mice. Second, to create a severe heart failure for the following PAH progression, some of mice in TAC group did not survive at the end of experiment. Third, because left heart failure-induced PAH caused other lung injuries like pulmonary edema, the results of the present study could not identify the other injuries caused by TAC. Fourth, although we provide a single transcription event, mediated by EZH2-SOD1-ROS axis, which may be linked to TAC-induced PAH, there lacks a clear delineation as to how EZH2 coordinates genome-wide transcription to manipulate this process. Fifth, 10 mg kg^{-1} (i.p.) for 4 times for four consecutive days might be sufficient to suppress the expression EZH2 in the present study; strict toxicity and dose experiments are necessary for further application of EPZ005687 in vivo.

EZH2 is important in cell cycle progression, cell proliferation, differentiation, apoptosis, DNA damage repair, and stem cell fate determination; loss of EZH2 leads to early embryonic lethality [36]. And the role of EZH2 in regulating oxidative stress is conflictive in different systems, for example, Yu et al. reported that inhibition of EZH2 against LPS-induced oxidative response in sepsis [37], whereas decreased EZH2 resulted in over-expression of a proapoptotic gene Bim and activation of oxidative reaction in erythroid cells [13]. The present study shows that inhibition of EZH2 by EPZ005687 reversed transcriptional repression of SOD1 in lung and delayed PAH progression in mouse TAC model. Given the diversity of EZH2 functions in regulation of oxidative reaction, a lineage or organ-specific EZH2 knockout or transgenic model might be more convincible. But, our results still provide some clues about pharmacologic targeting EZH2 in protection against PAH induced by TAC.

5. Conclusion

To sum up, increased EZH2 expression contributes to the progression of TAC-induced PAH by simulating ROS production and inhibiting SOD1 expression. The specific inhibitor of EZH2, EPZ005687, might reverse this deterioration of TAC-induced PAH. Ideally, using both RNA-seq and ChIP-seq techniques, in different types of cells in the context of TAC-induced PAH, then verified by a lineage or organ-specific EZH2 knockout or transgenic model, would hopefully render a more solid decision to target EZH2 for drug development.

Abbreviations

EZH2:	Enhancer of zeste homolog 2
TAC:	Transverse aortic constriction
PAH:	Pulmonary arterial hypertension
DMSO:	Dimethyl sulfoxide
RVSBP:	Right ventricular systolic blood pressure
PABP:	Pulmonary arterial systolic blood pressure
DHE:	Dihydroethidium
Real-time PCR:	Real-time polymerase chain reaction
ChIP:	Chromatin immunoprecipitation
ROS:	Reactive oxygen species
SOD1:	Superoxide dismutase 1
HF:	Heart failure
CVDs:	Cardiovascular diseases
H3K27me3:	Histone H3 lysine 27 trimethylation
HW:	Heart weight
LW:	Lung weight
BW:	Body weight
LV:	Left ventricle
RV:	Right ventricle
NT:	Nitrotyrosine.

Acknowledgments

This work was supported by the Natural Science Foundation of Zhejiang Province (no. LY13H290008) and the Medical Scientific Research Foundation of Zhejiang Province (no. 2011KYB075), China.

References

[1] H. I. Lu, T. H. Huang, P. H. Sung et al., "Administration of antioxidant peptide SS-31 attenuates transverse aortic constriction-induced pulmonary arterial hypertension in mice," *Acta Pharmacologica Sinica*, vol. 37, no. 5, pp. 589–603, 2016.

[2] J. L. Vachiéry, Y. Adir, J. A. Barberà et al., "Pulmonary hypertension due to left heart diseases," *Journal of the American College of Cardiology*, vol. 62, no. 25, pp. D100–D108, 2013.

[3] Y. Sotomi, N. Sato, K. Kajimoto et al., "Impact of pulmonary artery catheter on outcome in patients with acute heart failure syndromes with hypotension or receiving inotropes: from the ATTEND Registry," *International Journal of Cardiology*, vol. 172, no. 1, pp. 165–172, 2014.

[4] H. Wang, D. Kwak, J. Fassett et al., "Role of bone marrow-derived CD11c+ dendritic cells in systolic overload-induced left ventricular inflammation, fibrosis and hypertrophy," *Basic Research in Cardiology*, vol. 112, no. 3, p. 25, 2017.

[5] X. Weng, L. Yu, P. Liang et al., "A crosstalk between chromatin remodeling and histone H3K4 methyltransferase complexes in endothelial cells regulates angiotensin II-induced cardiac hypertrophy," *Journal of Molecular and Cellular Cardiology*, vol. 82, pp. 48–58, 2015.

[6] M. Gasparini, C. Leclercq, C. M. Yu et al., "Absolute survival after cardiac resynchronization therapy according to baseline QRS duration: a multinational 10-year experience: data from the Multicenter International CRT study," *American Heart Journal*, vol. 167, no. 2, pp. 203.e1–209.e1, 2014.

[7] D. Chen, Y. Yang, X. Cheng et al., "Megakaryocytic leukemia 1 directs a histone H3 lysine 4 methyltransferase complex to

regulate hypoxic pulmonary hypertension," *Hypertension*, vol. 65, no. 4, pp. 821–833, 2015.

[8] P. Dorfmuller, M. C. Chaumais, M. Giannakouli et al., "Increased oxidative stress and severe arterial remodeling induced by permanent high-flow challenge in experimental pulmonary hypertension," *Respiratory Research*, vol. 12, p. 119, 2011.

[9] G. Yang, X. Weng, Y. Zhao et al., "The histone H3K9 methyltransferase SUV39H links SIRT1 repression to myocardial infarction," *Nature Communications*, vol. 8, p. 14941, 2017.

[10] L. Yu, G. Yang, X. Weng et al., "Histone methyltransferase SET1 mediates angiotensin II-induced endothelin-1 transcription and cardiac hypertrophy in mice," *Arteriosclerosis, Thrombosis, and Vascular Biology*, vol. 35, no. 5, pp. 1207–1217, 2015.

[11] F. Lu, X. Cui, S. Zhang, T. Jenuwein, and X. Cao, "Arabidopsis REF6 is a histone H3 lysine 27 demethylase," *Nature Genetics*, vol. 43, no. 7, pp. 715–719, 2011.

[12] Z. Wang, X. J. Zhang, Y. X. Ji et al., "The long noncoding RNA Chaer defines an epigenetic checkpoint in cardiac hypertrophy," *Nature Medicine*, vol. 22, no. 10, pp. 1131–1139, 2016.

[13] M. Gao, Y. Liu, Y. Chen, C. Yin, J. J. Chen, and S. Liu, "miR-214 protects erythroid cells against oxidative stress by targeting ATF4 and EZH2," *Free Radical Biology and Medicine*, vol. 92, pp. 39–49, 2016.

[14] F. S. Siddiqi, S. Majumder, K. Thai et al., "The histone methyltransferase enzyme enhancer of zeste homolog 2 protects against podocyte oxidative stress and renal injury in diabetes," *Journal of the American Society of Nephrology*, vol. 27, no. 7, pp. 2021–2034, 2016.

[15] J. T. Poirier, E. E. Gardner, N. Connis et al., "DNA methylation in small cell lung cancer defines distinct disease subtypes and correlates with high expression of EZH2," *Oncogene*, vol. 34, no. 48, pp. 5869–5878, 2015.

[16] R. Zuo, X. Liu, W. Wang, W. Li, H. Ying, and K. Sun, "A repressive role of enhancer of zeste homolog 2 in 11beta-hydroxysteroid dehydrogenase type 2 expression in the human placenta," *Journal of Biological Chemistry*, vol. 292, no. 18, pp. 7578–7587, 2017.

[17] G. Laible, A. Wolf, R. Dorn et al., "Mammalian homologues of the Polycomb-group gene Enhancer of zeste mediate gene silencing in Drosophila heterochromatin and at *S. cerevisiae* telomeres," *EMBO Journal*, vol. 16, no. 11, pp. 3219–3232, 1997.

[18] P. Mathiyalagan, J. Okabe, L. Chang, Y. Su, X. J. Du, and A. El-Osta, "The primary microRNA-208b interacts with Polycomb-group protein, Ezh2, to regulate gene expression in the heart," *Nucleic Acids Research*, vol. 42, no. 2, pp. 790–803, 2014.

[19] M. Shao, G. Chen, F. Lv et al., "LncRNA TINCR attenuates cardiac hypertrophy by epigenetically silencing CaMKII," *Oncotarget*, vol. 8, no. 29, pp. 47565–47573, 2017.

[20] S. K. Knutson, T. J. Wigle, N. M. Warholic et al., "A selective inhibitor of EZH2 blocks H3K27 methylation and kills mutant lymphoma cells," *Nature Chemical Biology*, vol. 8, no. 11, pp. 890–896, 2012.

[21] S. Zhou, M. T. Li, Y. Y. Jia et al., "Regulation of cell cycle regulators by SIRT1 contributes to resveratrol-mediated prevention of pulmonary arterial hypertension," *BioMed Research International*, vol. 2015, p. 762349, 2015.

[22] X. Weng, L. Yu, P. Liang et al., "Endothelial MRTF-A mediates angiotensin II induced cardiac hypertrophy," *Journal of Molecular and Cellular Cardiology*, vol. 80, pp. 23–33, 2015.

[23] S. Zhang, J. Xue, J. Zheng et al., "The superoxide dismutase 1 3′UTR maintains high expression of the SOD1 gene in cancer cells: the involvement of the RNA-binding protein AUF-1," *Free Radical Biology and Medicine*, vol. 85, pp. 33–44, 2015.

[24] S. Woodhouse, D. Pugazhendhi, P. Brien, and J. M. Pell, "Ezh2 maintains a key phase of muscle satellite cell expansion but does not regulate terminal differentiation," *Journal of Cell Science*, vol. 126, no. 2, pp. 565–579, 2013.

[25] L. Yu, X. Weng, P. Liang et al., "MRTF-A mediates LPS-induced pro-inflammatory transcription by interacting with the COMPASS complex," *Journal of Cell Science*, vol. 127, no. 21, pp. 4645–4657, 2014.

[26] X. Lu, X. Guo, C. D. Wassall, M. D. Kemple, J. L. Unthank, and G. S. Kassab, "Reactive oxygen species cause endothelial dysfunction in chronic flow overload," *Journal of Applied Physiology*, vol. 110, no. 2, pp. 520–527, 2011.

[27] G. S. Reis, V. S. Augusto, A. P. Silveira et al., "Oxidative-stress biomarkers in patients with pulmonary hypertension," *Pulmonary Circulation*, vol. 3, no. 4, pp. 856–861, 2013.

[28] Y. Hoshikawa, S. Ono, S. Suzuki et al., "Generation of oxidative stress contributes to the development of pulmonary hypertension induced by hypoxia," *Journal of Applied Physiology*, vol. 90, no. 4, pp. 1299–1306, 2001.

[29] H. Wu, X. Chen, J. Xiong et al., "Histone methyltransferase G9a contributes to H3K27 methylation in vivo," *Cell Research*, vol. 21, no. 2, pp. 365–367, 2011.

[30] M. T. McCabe, H. M. Ott, G. Ganji et al., "EZH2 inhibition as a therapeutic strategy for lymphoma with EZH2-activating mutations," *Nature*, vol. 492, no. 7427, pp. 108–112, 2012.

[31] R. Cao, L. Wang, H. Wang et al., "Role of histone H3 lysine 27 methylation in Polycomb-group silencing," *Science*, vol. 298, no. 5595, pp. 1039–1043, 2002.

[32] E. Miele, S. Valente, V. Alfano et al., "The histone methyltransferase EZH2 as a druggable target in SHH medulloblastoma cancer stem cells," *Oncotarget*, vol. 8, no. 40, pp. 68557–68570, 2017.

[33] S. Idris, C. Lindsay, M. Kostiuk et al., "Investigation of EZH2 pathways for novel epigenetic treatment strategies in oropharyngeal cancer," *Journal of Otolaryngology Head and Neck Surgery*, vol. 45, no. 1, p. 54, 2016.

[34] L. Chen, Y. Wu, Y. Wu, Y. Wang, L. Sun, and F. Li, "The inhibition of EZH2 ameliorates osteoarthritis development through the Wnt/beta-catenin pathway," *Scientific Reports*, vol. 6, p. 29176, 2016.

[35] Y. Chen, H. Guo, D. Xu et al., "Left ventricular failure produces profound lung remodeling and pulmonary hypertension in mice: heart failure causes severe lung disease," *Hypertension*, vol. 59, no. 6, pp. 1170–1178, 2012.

[36] H. Kobayashi, K. Ogawa, N. Kawahara et al., "Sequential molecular changes and dynamic oxidative stress in high-grade serous ovarian carcinogenesis," *Free Radical Research*, vol. 51, no. 9-10, pp. 755–764, 2017.

[37] Z. Yu, A. Rayile, X. Zhang, Y. Li, and Q. Zhao, "Ulinastatin protects against lipopolysaccharide-induced cardiac microvascular endothelial cell dysfunction via downregulation of lncRNA MALAT1 and EZH2 in sepsis," *International Journal of Molecular Medicine*, vol. 39, no. 5, pp. 1269–1276, 2017.

Time to Exhale: Additional Value of Expiratory Chest CT in Chronic Obstructive Pulmonary Disease

Joshua Gawlitza,[1] Frederik Trinkmann,[2] Hans Scheffel,[1] Andreas Fischer,[1] John W. Nance,[3] Claudia Henzler,[1] Nils Vogler,[1] Joachim Saur,[2] Ibrahim Akin,[2,4] Martin Borggrefe,[2,4] Stefan O. Schoenberg,[1,4] and Thomas Henzler[1,4]

[1] *Institute of Clinical Radiology and Nuclear Medicine, University Medical Center Mannheim, Medical Faculty Mannheim, Heidelberg University, Heidelberg, Germany*
[2] *Department of Medicine (Cardiology, Angiology, Pulmonary, and Intensive Care), University Medical Center Mannheim, Medical Faculty Mannheim, Heidelberg University, Heidelberg, Germany*
[3] *Department of Radiology and Radiological Science, Medical University of South Carolina, Charleston, SC, USA*
[4] *DZHK (German Center for Cardiovascular Research), Partner Site Mannheim, Berlin, Germany*

Correspondence should be addressed to Frederik Trinkmann; frederik.trinkmann@umm.de

Academic Editor: Jörg D. Leuppi

Objectives. Diagnostic guidelines for chronic obstructive pulmonary disease (COPD) are based on spirometry and clinical criteria. However, this does not address the pathophysiological complexity of the disease sufficiently. Until now, inspiratory chest computed tomography (CT) has been considered as the preferred imaging method in these patients. We hypothesized that expiratory CT may be superior to demonstrate pathophysiological changes. The aim of this prospective study was to systematically compare lung function tests with quantified CT parameters in inspiration and expiration. *Materials and Methods.* Forty-six patients with diagnosed COPD underwent spirometry, body plethysmography, and dose-optimized CT in maximal inspiration and expiration. Four quantified CT parameters were acquired in inspiration, expiration, and their calculated delta values. These parameters were correlated with seven established lung function parameters. *Results.* For inspiratory scans, a weak-to-moderate correlation with the lung function parameters was found. These correlations significantly improved when adding the expiratory scan ($p < 0.05$). Moreover, some parameters showed a significant correlation only in expiratory datasets. Calculated delta values showed even stronger correlation with lung function testing. *Conclusions.* Expiratory quantified CT and calculated delta values significantly improve the correlation with lung function parameters. Thus, an additional expiratory CT may improve image-based phenotyping of patients with COPD.

1. Introduction

Chronic obstructive pulmonary disease (COPD) is a common and largely avoidable disease that is characterized by irreversible airway obstruction, predominantly due to inhaled noxae and particles. COPD was listed as the third leading cause of death by the World Health Organization in 2012 and has surpassed epidemiological estimations by the Global Burden of Disease Project, now causing over 3.1 million deaths per year [1, 2].

Traditionally, the diagnosis of COPD is based on spirometric measurements of forced expiratory volume in one second (FEV_1) and forced vital capacity (FVC), as specified by the Global Initiative for Chronic Obstructive Lung Disease (GOLD) [3]. However, recent studies have shown several shortcomings of this approach. While Hardie et al. showed a risk of overdiagnosis of COPD among the elderly using common spirometry criteria, Cerveri et al. were able to demonstrate an underestimation of airflow obstruction among young adults when using spirometric measurements

[4, 5]. Other pulmonary function tests, such as multiple-breath washout, provide a better differentiation of healthy controls and COPD patients, even with preserved lung function in spirometry [6–8].

Chest computed tomography (CT) is currently not listed as an obligate diagnostic tool in patients with suspected COPD by GOLD [3]. Nevertheless, imaging provides additional information as compared to spirometry by detection of pathological changes that directly contribute to the airflow limitations [9]. Emphysema, bronchial wall thickening, and air trapping are the key pathologic findings of COPD on chest CT that are associated with increased mortality [9–12]. Moreover, fibrotic changes of the lungs, which have significant symptom overlap with COPD, can only be differentiated from COPD using imaging [13].

Despite these benefits, CT has not become a recommended examination in newly diagnosed COPD yet since the clinical impact is not fully understood [9]. In this context, the American Thoracic Society and the European Respiratory Society proposed to evaluate the role of routine chest CT [14].

Several prior studies have correlated quantified chest CT measurements with functional lung parameters [15–17]. However, most studies to date have focused on the correlation of spirometry and quantified CT. In addition to the previously described limitations, spirometry does not provide residual volume, which is pathologically altered in COPD. Another limitation of recent studies is the quantified CT acquisition itself, which is most frequently performed only during maximal inspiration [16]. COPD mainly limits airflow during expiration, possibly limiting the diagnostic yield of inspiratory-only protocols; accordingly, the Fleischner Society has suggested the potential additive value of expiratory acquisitions [18].

Thus, the aim of this prospective study was to investigate the correlation of functional lung parameters beyond FEV_1 and FVC with quantified CT parameters acquired during maximum inspiration as well as maximum expiration.

2. Materials and Methods

2.1. Subjects. The HIPAA compliant study protocol, which is in accordance with the Declaration of Helsinki, was approved by our local ethics committee (*blinded for review*). The study was registered at http://www.clinicaltrials.gov (*blinded for review*).

We prospectively enrolled 49 patients with previously diagnosed COPD and a clinical indication for unenhanced chest CT in a single-center, all-comer approach. Written informed consent was obtained from all patients following a full explanation of the purpose of the study and of potential risks and discomforts associated with their participation.

2.2. Study Protocol

2.2.1. Lung Function Testing. All patients underwent spirometry and whole-body plethysmography (MasterScreen® Body, CareFusion, Höchberg, Germany) yielding the following parameters: vital capacity (VC), FEV_1, Tiffeneau index (FEV_1%VC), residual volume (RV), total lung capacity (TLC), ratio of residual volume to TLC (RV%TLC), and specific total airway resistance (sR_{tot}). Except for FEV_1%VC and RV%TLC, all values are given as percent of predicted, as calculated according to current ATS/ERS recommendations or GLI equations, respectively [19, 20].

2.2.2. CT Examinations. A noncontrast chest scan was performed in maximum inspiration and maximum expiration using a 3rd generation dual-source CT (Somatom FORCE, Siemens Healthineers, Forchheim, Germany) at 100 kVp with a dedicated tin filter for dose reduction [21]. The scan parameters were as follows: 100 kVp tube voltage, 96 mAs reference tube current using automated tube current modulation (effective mAs = 166.5 ± 105), 0.25 s rotation time, pitch 1.2, and 192 mm × 0.6 mm detector collimation. All images were reconstructed with a slice thickness of 1.5 mm, using a dedicated reconstruction kernel for quantitative lung analysis (Br32) and a novel iterative reconstruction technique (Adaptive Model-based Iterative Reconstruction (ADMIRE), Siemens Healthineers, Germany). The algorithm of ADMIRE was substantially explained in a recent work [22]. An iterative level of four was chosen for the present study as recommended by the CT vendor for quantitative lung analysis. The average CTDI (computed tomography dose index) was 0.48 ± 0.19 mGy and the mean DLP (dose length product) 17.2 ± 6.5 mGy·cm.

2.2.3. Image Analysis. Inspiratory and expiratory datasets were analyzed using dedicated semiautomatic software (SyngoViaVB10, Pulmo3D, Siemens Healthineers, Forchheim, Germany). Lung segmentation was automated and manually revised if necessary (Figure 1). Four quantitative parameters were acquired: total lung volume (volume), mean lung density (MLD), full width half max (FWHM), and low attenuation volume (LAV). The LAV threshold for emphysema was set to −950 HU. This cutoff had been extensively evaluated in previous studies and strongly correlates with microscopic and gross emphysema [23–25]. FWHM marks the width at the half maximum of the voxel count to specific HU value curve (voxel-density histogram) representing the density distribution of the lung parenchyma. An exemplary voxel-density histogram with its corresponding FWHM can be found in the Supplementary Materials (available here). The difference in the values between inspiratory and expiratory scans was defined as delta value.

2.3. Statistical Analysis. A total of 28 correlation pairs (four quantified CT parameters and seven lung function parameters) were analyzed for inspiratory, expiratory, and delta values. The Pearson product-moment correlation coefficient was calculated for each pair using JMP 11 (SAS, Cary, USA). The correlation coefficients of inspiratory and expiratory scans were compared by Pearson and Filon z test, using cocor Software [26]. Based on previously published data, we assumed a correlation of $r = -0.252$ between LAV and FEV_1

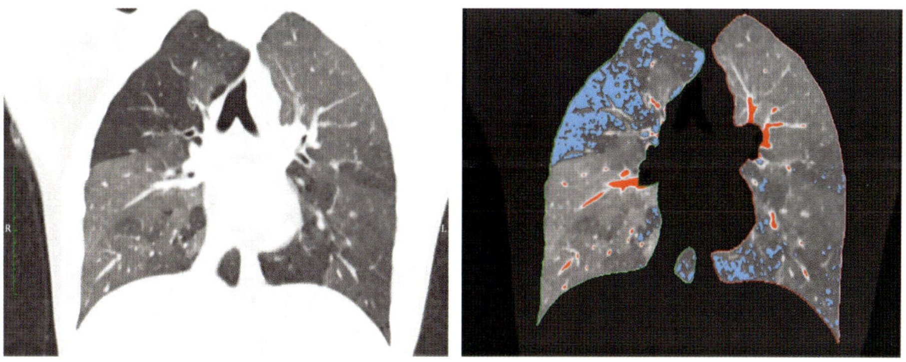

FIGURE 1: Automatic detection of lung borders and lung parenchyma. Blue areas: low attenuation volume (LAV) with HU values below −950; red areas: high attenuation volume (HAV) with HU values above −200.

TABLE 1: Patient characteristics.

n	♂/♀	Age, years (range)	Size, cm (range)	Weight, kg (range)	Smokers/ex-smokers
46	26/20	66 ± 10 (44–87)	166 ± 7 (153–190)	76 ± 18 (34–117)	20/26

[27]. Based on this correlation, we calculated that a planned sample size of 34 patients would give the study a power of 90% at a five percent significance level to detect a significant correlation. A p value of less than 0.05 was considered statistically significant.

3. Results

The study population consisted of 46 patients (26 male) with previously diagnosed COPD. Twenty patients were active smokers at the date of examination. The remaining 26 patients had smoked in the past (Tables 1–3).

Regarding inspiratory, expiratory, and delta values, we were able to show statistically significant correlations between every quantified CT parameter and each lung function parameter in either of one of the analyses (inspiration, expiration, and delta values; Tables E1–E3 in the Supplementary Materials). However, there was a strong difference in correlation distribution between quantitative parameters from the inspiratory and the expiratory CT scan as well as the delta values, as seen in the correlation heat maps (Figures 2–4). As substantiated in Figure E1 in the Supplementary Materials focusing on MLD, expiratory and delta parameters show improved correlation with spirometric data as compared to inspiratory parameters.

3.1. Inspiratory Quantified CT Values. The fewest significant correlations were found when using data from the inspiratory acquisition (14 out of 28 correlated pairs; Table E1 in the Supplementary Materials). The significant correlations of inspiratory values to lung function values had a range from −0.5098 to 0.5293 (p values 0.0415 to 0.0001). The strongest correlation was found between MLD and RV ($r = 0.5293$; CI: 0.2885 to 0.7071; $p = 0.0001$). No single significant correlation between FWHM and the functional lung parameters could be shown. No quantified CT parameter from the inspiratory scan correlated with VC.

TABLE 2: Lung function parameters.

Parameter	Mean	SD	Range
VC (%)	70	23.3	22.2–128.6
FEV_1 (%)	49.4	20.8	16.1–100.4
FEV_1%VC	53.4	13	32.7–90.9
RV (%)	210.9	81.9	35.3–405.7
TLC (%)	125	31.6	54.4–205
RV%TLC	65	14.8	16.4–87.6
sR_{tot} (%)	337.4	241	47.8–1054.8

VC: vital capacity; FEV_1: forced expiratory volume in one second; FEV_1%VC: Tiffeneau index; RV: residual volume; TLC: total lung capacity; sR_{tot}: specific total airway resistance.

3.2. Expiratory Quantified CT Values. The most significant correlations were found when using data from the expiratory acquisition (25 out of 28 correlated pairs; Table E2 in the Supplementary Materials). As visualized in Figures 2 and 3, the underlying correlation pattern is equal to the inspiratory values. Correlation coefficient analysis showed 17 significantly higher correlations in the expiratory scan compared to the inspiratory scan (Table 4). Every quantified CT parameter correlated with every functional lung parameter except for VC. Only LAV showed a significant negative correlation to VC ($r = -0.346$; CI: −0.5717 to −0.0718; p value = 0.0149). Overall, the significant correlations had a range from −0.6378 to 0.6466 (p values: 0.0188 to <0.0001). The strongest correlation was found between total volume and RV ($r = 0.6466$; CI: 0.444 to 0.7863; p value < 0.0001).

3.3. Delta-Quantified CT Values. As seen in Figure 4, the correlations for the delta values are contrary to the ones for the inspiratory and expiratory values. Twenty-one correlation pairs showed a significant correlation in the calculated quantified CT delta values (Table E3 in the Supplementary

Table 3: Quantified CT parameters.

Parameter	Mean		SD		Range	
	Inspiration	Expiration	Inspiration	Expiration	Inspiration	Expiration
Volume (ml)	5421	4417	1441	1279	2528 to 8541	1859 to 7792
MLD (HU)	−840	−803	48	66	−915 to −715	−910 to −663
FWHM (HU)	94	123	32	43	27 to 230	71 to 231
LAV (%)	12	9	15	14	0 to 50	0 to 50

MLD: mean lung density; FWHM: full width half max; LAV: low attenuation volume.

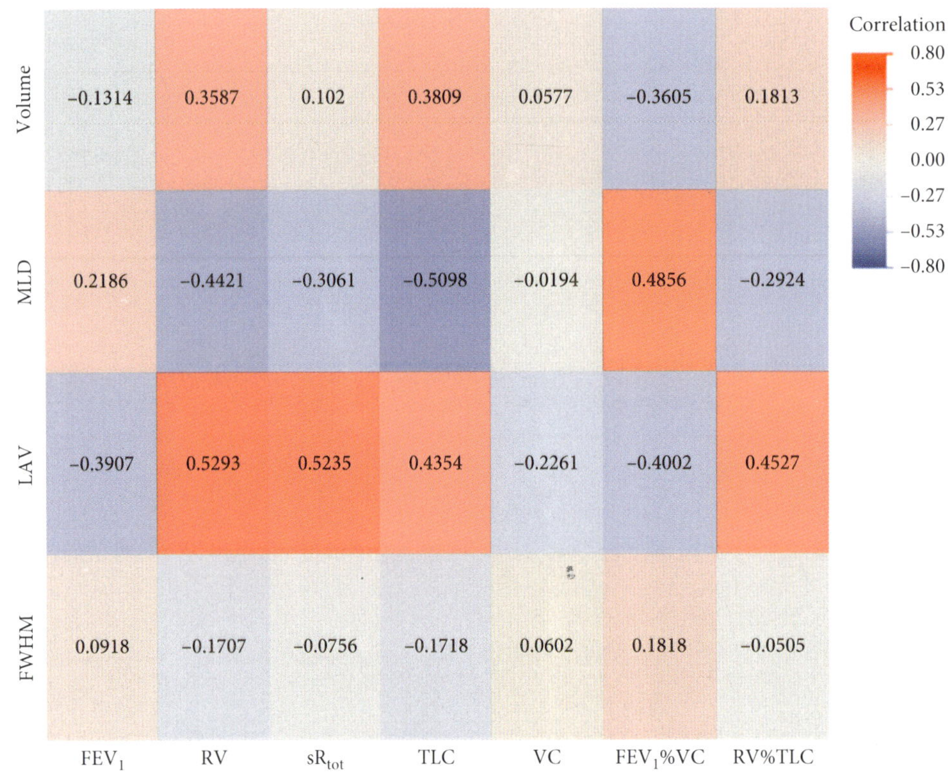

Figure 2: Heat map of correlations for inspiratory values. MLD: mean lung density; FWHM: full width half max; LAV: low attenuation volume; VC: vital capacity; FEV_1: forced expiratory volume in one second; $FEV_1\%VC$: Tiffeneau index; RV: residual volume; TLC: total lung capacity; sR_{tot}: specific total airway resistance.

Materials). The correlations had a range from −0.5098 to 0.6728 (p values: 0.8049 to <0.0001). In contrast to the inspiratory and the expiratory values, every quantified CT parameter showed a correlation to VC. The strongest correlation was found between MLD and RV%TLC ($r = 0.6728$; CI: 0.483 to 0.8022; p value < 0.0001). The LAV did not correlate with any lung parameters for the delta-quantified CT values.

4. Discussion

Our study found significant correlations for quantified CT parameters and functional lung parameters beyond the commonly used FEV_1 and VC. The additional scan performed in end-expiration showed overall stronger correlations compared to the inspiratory scan. These findings were consistent for both static and dynamic lung function parameters.

Every quantified CT parameter significantly correlated with the functional lung parameters in all of the three different analyses. Nevertheless, there was a strong difference in the extent and the number of significant correlations between the inspiratory, expiratory, and delta of the quantified CT parameters.

Stronger correlations were found between static parameters of lung volume, such as TLC and RV, as compared to the dynamic parameters FEV_1, $FEV_1\%VC$, and sR_{tot}. This finding could be reasonably expected, as the acquisitions were also static and provided predominantly anatomic information. Likewise, LAV correlated with these static parameters on all three analyses (i.e., there was no additive value of the expiratory scan or delta values), which can be expected, given the LAV was relatively fixed between inspiratory and expiratory acquisitions.

Our findings align with the 2015 Fleischner Society statement on CT-definable subtypes of COPD, in which they

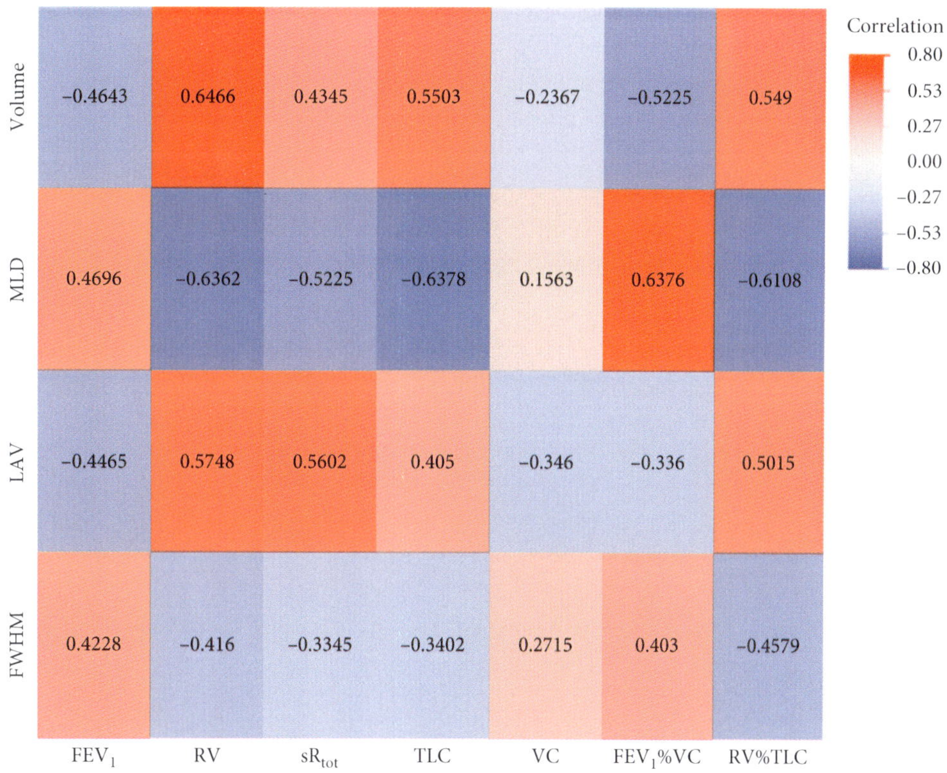

FIGURE 3: Heat map of correlations for expiratory values. MLD: mean lung density; FWHM: full width half max; LAV: low attenuation volume; VC: vital capacity; FEV_1: forced expiratory volume in one second; FEV_1%VC: Tiffeneau index; RV: residual volume; TLC: total lung capacity; sR_{tot}: specific total airway resistance.

noted the potential additive information of end-expiratory acquisitions in patients with COPD [18]. A combination of inspiratory and expiratory quantified CT values has already been shown to correlate well with air trapping and COPD grading [15, 28]. Nevertheless, neither inspiratory nor expiratory scans significantly correlate with VC. These findings are in accordance with the weak correlations of VC and LAV found by Timmins et al. [29]. Only the calculated delta values showed a correlation with VC, although they do have limitations. Delta LAV values did not show significant correlations with lung function parameters. This was expected due to the previously mentioned constancy of the LAV in inspiratory and expiratory scans (i.e., delta values were very small). Several studies have already correlated ratios of inspiratory and expiratory quantified CT scans with functional lung parameters. For example, Nambu et al. demonstrated a correlation between the MLD ratio, calculated from inspiratory and expiratory scans, and functional lung parameters such as FEV_1 [30]. Schroeder et al. compared emphysema and bronchial wall thickness to spirometry and found a strong correlation between the percentage of emphysema and FEV_1 as well as FEV_1/FVC [31]. The SPIROMICS investigators showed a correlation of small airway abnormalities and emphysema with FVC, FEV_1, and FEV_1/FVC among 580 individuals between the ages of 40 and 80 [32]. Decreased MLD is associated with hyperinflation and structural damage caused by COPD and correlates with parameters of functional emphysema such as RV or RV%TLC. Correlations of the latter steadily increase from inspiratory to expiratory to delta values. The strongest relation of the dynamic parameters FEV_1, FEV_1%VC, and sR_{tot} with delta values of MLD may relate to the dynamic information provided by delta values. Previously, FWHM of the Hounsfield distribution was suggested to be associated with parenchymal or emphysematous heterogeneity [17]. We found significant correlations between FWHM and functional parameters of emphysema (e.g., RV%TLC) and obstruction (e.g., FEV_1%VC) in expiratory but not inspiratory scans. From a pathophysiological standpoint, this may be explained by increasing differences between normal parenchyma and emphysematous areas in COPD patients compared to pulmonary healthy subjects. This effect may become more apparent during expiration due to increased geographic air trapping in patients with COPD.

TLC% and inspiratory volume showed only a weak correlation (0.38), despite the fact, that both parameters should measure the same volume. Beyond the weak correlation, the absolute values differed. One reason for this difference is the quantification process of the CT images. The software automatically ads a distance of 1 cm between the quantified lung volume and pleura to eliminate errors occurring through pleural irregularities. This led to a reduced total lung volume in the qCT when compared to lung function tests. Further, total lung volume was acquired in supine position in qCT rather than sitting TLC in body plethysmography. As shown previously, posture has an effect on measured lung volumes and thereby might have strengthened the named difference [33].

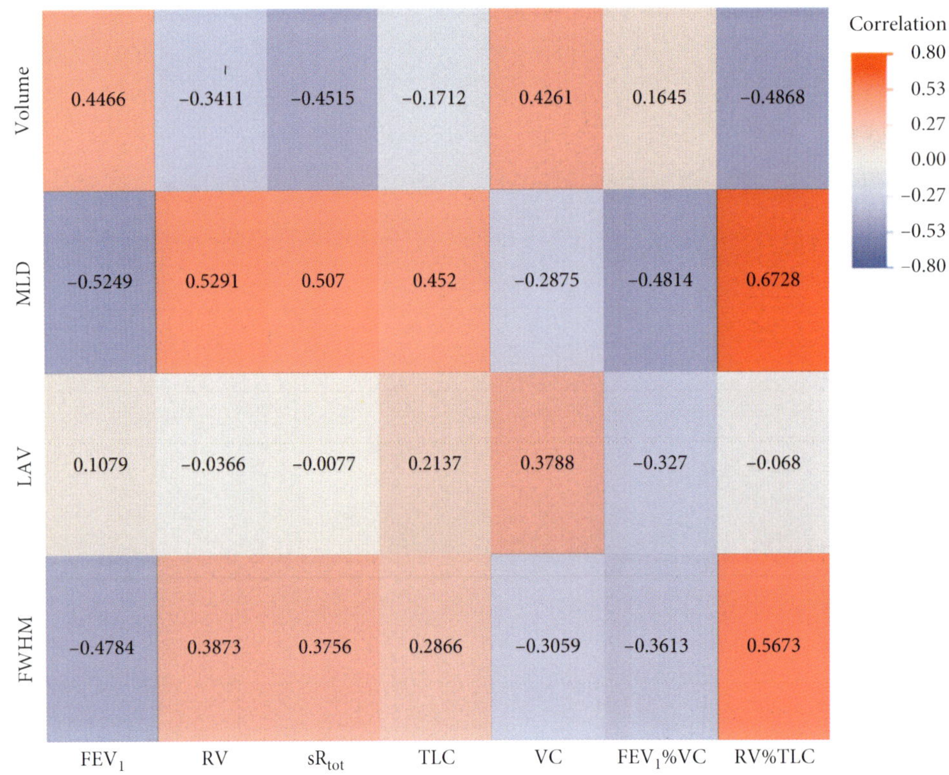

FIGURE 4: Heat map of correlations for delta values. MLD: mean lung density; FWHM: full width half max; LAV: low attenuation volume; VC: vital capacity; FEV_1: forced expiratory volume in one second; FEV_1%VC: Tiffeneau index; RV: residual volume; TLC: total lung capacity; sR_{tot}: specific total airway resistance.

Our study has several limitations that must be considered. First, we did not perform spirometric triggering during CT. Thereby, we cannot verify that all patients strictly followed the breathing commands. There was a mean volume difference of 1 liter between maximal inspiration and expiration, and we believe that our data are representative of functional inspiration and expiration. Second, since we only included patients with clinical indications for unenhanced chest CT, severe stages of COPD might be overrepresented in our cohort. Third, the number of subjects included in our study was rather small.

The strength of our study is the systematic evaluation of expiratory values, stand-alone delta values, and their respective correlations with lung function testing. As mentioned before, previous studies have correlated qCT parameters and lung function tests. But they did not take the expiratory and stand-alone delta values into account as we did in this work. Moreover, we focused on lung function parameters acquired by body plethysmography, which has advantages compared to traditional spirometry: While RV and TLC cannot be measured by spirometry, both are altered in COPD due to the loss of elastic recoil, airway closure, and hyperinflation of the lung [34]. Our study mainly addressed the relation of qCT and spirometric parameters. As stated initially, spirometry might not be ideal for COPD characterization. Nevertheless, we believe that the coherence of image data and lung function parameters is worth pointing out and need to be shown as a foundation for further research. Therefore, future studies should evaluate a qCT-based COPD characterization also considering expiratory and delta values. This would be particularly interesting in context of small airway disease. However, spirometry and body plethysmography used in our investigation are not ideal techniques and therefore further investigation including, for example, impulse oscillometry is warranted.

Overall, our study confirms three major presumptions. First, quantified CT parameters correlate with lung function parameters beyond the commonly used FEV_1 and VC. Second, a single acquisition in maximum inspiration alone is an incomplete approach for comparison of quantified CT parameters and functional lung parameters in COPD. Again, from a pathophysiological standpoint, these findings are related to the fact that COPD, as an *obstructive* lung disease, is most manifest at expiration. An additional scan in maximal expiration does not only provide a wider significant correlation profile but also allows the calculation of the delta value. These delta values have to be seen as an equivalent and discrete parameter. This becomes most evident for FWHM, with dynamic lung function parameters correlating significantly with delta and expiratory values, yet not with inspiratory values.

Consequently, the additional acquisition of an expiratory scan does not only provide a wider range of significant correlations with lung function parameters itself but also allows the calculation of the delta values. This does not only leads to more significant correlations to functional lung parameters but might also be important for future phenotyping of COPD with combined quantified CT and pulmonary function tests. Thereby, the expiratory and the delta values contain additional

Table 4: Comparison between inspiratory and expiratory correlation coefficients.

Quantified CT parameter	Lung function parameter	Correlation inspiration	Correlation expiration	z value	p value
Volume	VC	0.0577	−0.2367	3.1409	0.0017
Volume	FEV_1	−0.1314	−0.4643	3.631	0.0003
Volume	FEV_1%VC	−0.3605	−0.5225	1.8699	0.0615
Volume	RV	0.3587	0.6466	−3.3049	0.001
Volume	TLC	0.3809	0.5503	−1.9779	0.0479
Volume	RV%TLC	0.1813	0.549	−4.0252	0.0001
Volume	sR_{tot}	0.102	0.4345	−3.6152	0.0003
MLD	VC	−0.0194	0.1563	−1.9585	0.0502
MLD	FEV_1	0.2186	0.4696	−2.9337	0.0033
MLD	FEV_1%VC	0.4856	0.6376	−2.005	0.045
MLD	RV	−0.4421	−0.6362	2.4796	0.0132
MLD	TLC	−0.5098	−0.6378	1.7201	0.0854
MLD	RV%TLC	−0.2924	−0.6108	3.7492	0.0002
MLD	sR_{tot}	−0.3061	−0.5225	2.5933	0.0095
FWHM	VC	0.0602	0.2715	−1.8312	0.0671
FWHM	FEV_1	0.0918	0.4228	−2.9634	0.003
FWHM	FEV_1%VC	0.1818	0.403	−1.9774	0.048
FWHM	RV	−0.1707	−0.416	2.1972	0.028
FWHM	TLC	−0.1718	−0.3402	1.4834	0.138
FWHM	RV%TLC	−0.0505	−0.4579	3.6813	0.0002
FWHM	sR_{tot}	−0.0756	−0.3345	2.2735	0.023
LAV	VC	−0.2261	−0.346	3.1849	0.0014
LAV	FEV_1	−0.3907	−0.4465	1.5801	0.1141
LAV	FEV_1%VC	−0.4002	−0.336	−1.7761	0.0757
LAV	RV	0.5293	0.5748	−1.3982	0.1621
LAV	TLC	0.4354	0.405	0.8695	0.3846
LAV	RV%TLC	0.4527	0.5015	−1.4274	0.1535
LAV	sR_{tot}	0.5235	0.5602	−1.1266	0.2599

MLD: mean lung density; FWHM: full width half max; LAV: low attenuation volume; VC: vital capacity; FEV_1: forced expiratory volume in one second; FEV_1%VC: Tiffeneau index; RV: residual volume; TLC: total lung capacity; sR_{tot}: specific total airway resistance.

information and should be considered as mandatory correlation parameters in future studies.

Disclosure

An abstract containing preliminary analyses of the underlying data has been presented at the 2017 Annual European Congress of Radiology (C-2635, March 1 to 5) in Vienna, Austria.

Authors' Contributions

Joshua Gawlitza, Frederik Trinkmann, and Thomas Henzler conceived and designed the study. Andreas Fischer, Nils Vogler, Ibrahim Akin, Hans Scheffel, John W. Nance, Claudia Henzler, and Joachim Saur drafted the work. Martin Borggrefe and Stefan O. Schoenberg provided the final approval.

Supplementary Materials

Figure E1: correlations of mean lung density (MLD) and forced expiratory volume in one second (FEV_1) for inspiratory, expiratory, and calculated delta values. Figure E2: voxel-density histogram from a qCT. Table E1: correlation of quantified CT and lung function parameters for inspiration scan. Table E2: correlation of quantified CT and body plethysmography parameters for expiration scan. Table E3: correlation of quantified CT and body plethysmography parameters for delta values. (*Supplementary Materials*)

References

[1] *The Top 10 Causes of Death. Fact Sheet N°310*, 2014, http://www.who.int/mediacentre/factsheets/fs310/en/.

[2] A. S. Buist, W. M. Vollmer, and M. A. McBurnie, "Worldwide burden of COPD in high- and low-income countries. Part I. The burden of obstructive lung disease (BOLD) initiative," *International Journal of Tuberculosis and Lung Disease*, vol. 12, no. 7, pp. 703–708, 2008.

[3] J. Vestbo, S. S. Hurd, A. G. Agusti et al., "Global strategy for the diagnosis, management, and prevention of chronic obstructive pulmonary disease: GOLD executive summary," *American Journal of Respiratory and Critical Care Medicine*, vol. 187, no. 4, pp. 347–365, 2013.

[4] J. A. Hardie, A. S. Buist, W. M. Vollmer et al., "Risk of over-diagnosis of COPD in asymptomatic elderly never-smokers," *European Respiratory Journal*, vol. 20, no. 5, pp. 1117–1122, 2002.

[5] I. Cerveri, A. G. Corsico, S. Accordini et al., "Underestimation of airflow obstruction among young adults using FEV1/FVC <70% as a fixed cut-off: a longitudinal evaluation of clinical and functional outcomes," *Thorax*, vol. 63, no. 12, pp. 1040–1045, 2008.

[6] F. Trinkmann, T. Henzler, and J. Saur, "Symptoms in smokers with preserved pulmonary function," *New England Journal of Medicine*, vol. 375, no. 9, pp. 895-896, 2016.

[7] F. Trinkmann, D. Saur, K. Roth et al., "Multiple breath washout (MBW) using sulfur hexafluoride-proof of concept in COPD," *European Respiratory Journal*, vol. 48, no. 60, p. PA3440, 2016.

[8] P. G. Woodruff, R. G. Barr, E. Bleecker et al., "Clinical significance of symptoms in smokers with preserved pulmonary function," *New England Journal of Medicine*, vol. 374, no. 19, pp. 1811–1821, 2016.

[9] K. Ostridge and T. M. Wilkinson, "Present and future utility of computed tomography scanning in the assessment and management of COPD," *European Respiratory Journal*, vol. 48, no. 1, pp. 216–228, 2016.

[10] A. Haruna, S. Muro, Y. Nakano et al., "CT scan findings of emphysema predict mortality in COPD," *Chest*, vol. 138, no. 3, pp. 635–640, 2010.

[11] A. Johannessen, T. D. Skorge, M. Bottai et al., "Mortality by level of emphysema and airway wall thickness," *American Journal of Respiratory and Critical Care Medicine*, vol. 187, no. 6, pp. 602–608, 2013.

[12] P. M. Jairam, Y. van der Graaf, J. W. Lammers, W. P. Th. M. Mali, and P. A de Jong, "Incidental findings on chest CT imaging are associated with increased COPD exacerbations and mortality," *Thorax*, vol. 70, no. 8, pp. 725–731, 2015.

[13] M. D. Jankowich and S. I. Rounds, "Combined pulmonary fibrosis and emphysema syndrome: a review," *Chest*, vol. 141, no. 1, pp. 222–231, 2012.

[14] B. R. Celli, M. Decramer, J. A. Wedzicha et al., "An official American Thoracic Society/European Respiratory Society statement: research questions in COPD," *European Respiratory Review*, vol. 24, no. 136, pp. 159–172, 2015.

[15] K. Murphy, J. P. Pluim, E. M. van Rikxoort et al., "Toward automatic regional analysis of pulmonary function using inspiration and expiration thoracic CT," *Medical Physics*, vol. 39, no. 3, pp. 1650–1662, 2012.

[16] H. K. Koo, K. N. Jin, D. K. Kim et al., "Association of incidental emphysema with annual lung function decline and future development of airflow limitation," *International Journal of Chronic Obstructive Pulmonary Disease*, vol. 11, pp. 161–166, 2016.

[17] S. Baldi, M. Miniati, C. R. Bellina et al., "Relationship between extent of pulmonary emphysema by high-resolution computed tomography and lung elastic recoil in patients with chronic obstructive pulmonary disease," *American Journal of Respiratory and Critical Care Medicine*, vol. 164, no. 4, pp. 585–589, 2001.

[18] D. A. Lynch, J. H. Austin, J. C. Hogg et al., "CT-definable subtypes of chronic obstructive pulmonary disease: a statement of the Fleischner Society," *Radiology*, vol. 277, no. 1, pp. 192–205, 2015.

[19] P. H. Quanjer, S. Stanojevic, T. J. Cole et al., "Multi-ethnic reference values for spirometry for the 3-95-yr age range: the global lung function 2012 equations," *European Respiratory Journal*, vol. 40, no. 6, pp. 1324–1343, 2012.

[20] R. Pellegrino, G. Viegi, V. Brusasco et al., "Interpretative strategies for lung function tests," *European Respiratory Journal*, vol. 26, no. 5, pp. 948–968, 2005.

[21] M. Weis, T. Henzler, J. W. Nance Jr. et al., "Radiation dose comparison between 70 kvp and 100 kvp with spectral beam shaping for non-contrast-enhanced pediatric chest computed tomography: a prospective randomized controlled study," *Investigative Radiology*, vol. 52, no. 3, pp. 155–162, 2017.

[22] S. Gordic, F. Morsbach, B. Schmidt et al., "Ultralow-dose chest computed tomography for pulmonary nodule detection: first performance evaluation of single energy scanning with spectral shaping," *Investigative Radiology*, vol. 49, no. 7, pp. 465–473, 2014.

[23] P. A. Gevenois, V. de Maertelaer, P. De Vuyst, J. Zanen, and J. C. Yernault, "Comparison of computed density and macroscopic morphometry in pulmonary emphysema," *American Journal of Respiratory and Critical Care Medicine*, vol. 152, no. 2, pp. 653–657, 1995.

[24] P. A. Gevenois, P. De Vuyst, V. de Maertelaer et al., "Comparison of computed density and microscopic morphometry in pulmonary emphysema," *Journal of Respiratory and Critical Care Medicine*, vol. 154, no. 1, pp. 187–192, 1996.

[25] A. Madani, J. Zanen, V. de Maertelaer, and P. A. Gevenois, "Pulmonary emphysema: objective quantification at multi-detector row CT–comparison with macroscopic and microscopic morphometry," *Radiology*, vol. 238, no. 3, pp. 1036–1043, 2006.

[26] B. Diedenhofen and J. Musch, "cocor: a comprehensive solution for the statistical comparison of correlations," *PLoS One*, vol. 10, no. 4, article e0121945, 2015.

[27] F. A. Mohamed Hoesein, P. A. de Jong, J. W. Lammers et al., "Contribution of CT quantified emphysema, air trapping and airway wall thickness on pulmonary function in male smokers with and without COPD," *COPD*, vol. 11, no. 5, pp. 503–509, 2014.

[28] O. M. Mets, P. Zanen, J. W. Lammers et al., "Early identification of small airways disease on lung cancer screening CT: comparison of current air trapping measures," *Lung*, vol. 190, no. 6, pp. 629–633, 2012.

[29] S. C. Timmins, C. Diba, C. E. Farrow et al., "The relationship between airflow obstruction, emphysema extent, and small airways function in COPD," *Chest*, vol. 142, no. 2, pp. 312–319, 2012.

[30] A. Nambu, J. Zach, J. Schroeder et al., "Quantitative computed tomography measurements to evaluate airway disease in chronic obstructive pulmonary disease: relationship to physiological measurements, clinical index and visual assessment of airway disease," *European Journal of Radiology*, vol. 85, no. 11, pp. 2144–2151, 2016.

[31] J. D. Schroeder, A. S. McKenzie, J. A. Zach et al., "Relationships between airflow obstruction and quantitative CT measurements of emphysema, air trapping, and airways in subjects with and without chronic obstructive pulmonary disease," *American Journal of Roentgenology*, vol. 201, no. 3, pp. W460–W470, 2013.

ELISA Development for Serum Hemeoxygenase-1 and Its Application to Patients with Acute Respiratory Distress Syndrome

Yu Hara[1] **Masaharu Shinkai**[1] **Masataka Taguri,**[2] **Kenjiro Nagai,**[1] **Satoru Hashimoto,**[3] **and Takeshi Kaneko**[1]

[1]*Department of Pulmonology, Yokohama City University Graduate School of Medicine, Yokohama, Japan*
[2]*Department of Biostatistics, Yokohama City University School of Medicine, Yokohama, Japan*
[3]*Division of Intensive Care Unit, Kyoto Prefectural University of Medicine, Kyoto, Japan*

Correspondence should be addressed to Yu Hara; bronchiole0723@yahoo.co.jp

Academic Editor: Vito Fanelli

Background. Hemeoxygenase-1 (HO-1) is an essential enzyme in heme catabolism and has been proposed as a biomarker of lung disease prognosis. We modified a commercial HO-1 enzyme-linked immunosorbent assay (ELISA) kit to achieve higher sensitivity and evaluated if serum HO-1 could be a biomarker to predict the prognosis of acute respiratory distress syndrome (ARDS) patients. *Methods.* Serum samples were collected from 15 healthy volunteers to validate the modified ELISA. In the 22 patients with ARDS who were enrolled, serum HO-1 was measured upon diagnosis (D0) and at 7 days after diagnosis (D7). *Results.* The serum HO-1 concentration could be measured in all healthy volunteers. The intra- and interassay tests and the percentage recovery test were acceptable. Compared with normal control subjects, patients with ARDS had significantly higher D0 HO-1 concentrations (75.4 ng/mL versus 31.7 ng/mL, $P < 0.001$). The 28-day survival was significantly better in patients with low D0 HO-1 (<75.8 ng/mL) than in those with high D0 HO-1 (≥75.8 ng/mL) (mortality rate: 18% versus 73%, $P = 0.016$). Nonsurvivors had significantly higher D0 and D7 HO-1 concentrations than survivors ($P < 0.05$). *Conclusion.* Serum HO-1 may be a useful biomarker to predict the prognosis of patients with ARDS.

1. Introduction

Hemeoxygenase-1 (HO-1) is a 32 kDa heat shock protein that converts heme to carbon monoxide, iron, and bilirubin [1–3]. HO-1 is released from alveolar macrophages, bronchial epithelial cells, and inflammatory cells after stimulation by cytokines, hypoxia, exogenous nitric oxide, or diesel exhaust particles [4, 5]. Its expression in lung tissue was reported to increase in patients with diffuse alveolar damage (DAD), desquamative interstitial pneumonia, pulmonary sarcoidosis, and silicosis, whereas its expression decreased in patients with usual interstitial pneumonia (UIP) and chronic pulmonary obstructive disease (COPD) [5–9]. Peripheral blood HO-1 measured by enzyme-linked immunosorbent assay (ELISA) was reported to be useful in monitoring disease activity in patients with hemophagocytic syndrome and adult-onset Still's disease and is a predictor of lung function decline in patients with silicosis [10, 11]. However, there is no commercial detection kit to accurately measure serum HO-1 because the previously used kit was designed to measure HO-1 in cell lysates and tissue extracts and can be affected by factors contained in serum [11]. Therefore, we developed a new method of serum HO-1 measurement using an optimized assay buffer and validated the sensitivity of this ELISA technique of serum HO-1 measurement in predicting the clinical outcomes in patients with acute respiratory distress syndrome (ARDS).

2. Materials and Methods

2.1. Study Subjects for the Researches on Assay Validation and ARDS. For the research on assay validation, we recruited 15 healthy volunteers (mean age, 34.9 ± 8.6 years) from the medical staff of the Respiratory Disease Center, Yokohama

City University Medical Center. For the research on ARDS, 22 patients who met the Berlin definition for ARDS [12] during ICU stay were recruited from April 2011 to March 2014. Normal control subjects comprised healthy adults who were admitted to the National Defense Medical College Hospital for health exam.

2.2. Serum HO-1 ELISA. Serum HO-1 concentrations were measured using the HO-1 ELISA kit (Enzo, Farmingdale, NY, USA) and the ImmunoSet™ HO-1 ELISA development set (Enzo, Farmingdale, NY, USA), according to the manufacturers' instructions. The former kit used undiluted serum samples or samples diluted at 1 : 2 (commercial ELISA), whereas the latter kit used a modified assay buffer and serum samples diluted at 1 : 20 (modified ELISA).

2.3. Buffer Formulations and Reagent for the Modified ELISA. The buffer formulations used were coating buffer (phosphate-buffered saline (PBS)); blocking buffer (PBS containing 1% bovine serum albumin (BSA) and 0.05% Tween 20); assay buffer (PBS containing 1% BSA, 0.05% Tween 20, 0.1 M NaCl, 5 mM ethylenediaminetetraacetic acid (EDTA), and 50 μg/mL mouse IgG); wash buffer (PBS containing 0.1% *v/v* Tween 20); and 2% mouse serum added to the standard diluents. The reagents were ImmunoSet HO-1 ELISA development set (Cat#ADI-960-800, Enzo, Farmingdale, NY, USA); 3, 3′, 5, 5′ tetramethylbenzidine solution (Cat#T0440); stop solution (Cat#S5814); IgG from mouse serum (Cat#I5381); mouse serum (#CatM5905); BSA fraction V (Cat#A9647, Sigma, St. Louis, MO, USA); 10 × PBS buffer (pH 7.4, Wako Pure Chemical Industries, Ltd., Chuo-ku, Osaka, Japan); Ultra-Pure Tween 20 (Cat#EC-607, National Diagnostics, Atlanta, Georgia, USA); Nunc Immunoplate MaxiSorp 96-well ELISA plates (#Cat439454, Thermo Fisher Scientific Inc., Waltham, MA, USA); and ImmunoMini NJ-2300 Microplate reader (BIOTEC CO., Ltd., Tokyo, Japan).

2.4. Data Collection. The extracted data included age, gender, body mass index, and ARDS severity and etiology. The acute physiology and chronic health evaluation (APACHE) II was recorded during ICU visit [13]. The outcomes including the duration of mechanical ventilation and length of ICU stay were recorded.

We divided the patients into the survivors group (survived for >28 days) and the nonsurvivors group (survived for ≤28 days). Each patient was evaluated for peripheral blood HO-1, lactate dehydrogenase (normal < 225 U/L), C-reactive protein (normal < 0.3 mg/dL); PaO_2/F_IO_2; and lung injury score at the time of diagnosis, which was designated as D0, and at 7 days after diagnosis, which was designated as D7. The lung injury score (Murray score), which is a commonly utilized measure of lung injury severity, is calculated by adding the chest radiograph score (0–4), positive end-expiratory pressure score (0–4), hypoxemia score (0–4), and respiratory system compliance score (0–4) and dividing the sum by the number of components; a Murray score of 0 indicates no lung injury, and a score of >2.5 indicates severe lung injury [14]. ΔHO-1 was defined as D7 serum HO-1 concentration minus D0 serum HO-1 concentration.

2.5. Statistical Analysis. Data were expressed as median with 25th to 75th percentiles or mean ± standard deviation (SD). We compared the results between the commercial ELISA and the modified ELISA using Assay Blaster® software (Enzo, Farmingdale, NY, USA). Statistical analysis was performed using JMP10 and SAS version 9.3 (SAS Institute Inc., North Carolina, USA). Group comparisons were made using Wilcoxon's rank-sum test or chi-square test, as appropriate. Spearman correlation coefficients were calculated to assess the relationship between serum HO-1 and APACHE II score. The applicability of serum HO-1 in predicting survival was evaluated using the area under a receiver operating characteristic (ROC) curve; the sensitivity and specificity were calculated at several cutoff points. Survival curves were generated using the Kaplan–Meier method and were compared using the log-rank test. A P value of <0.05 was considered significant.

2.6. Study Approval. All aspects of this research were approved by the institutional review board of Yokohama City University Medical Center (approval number: D1303019) and the National Defense Medical College (approval number: 913). In the research on ARDS, the severely ill condition or deep sedation of the patients precluded us from obtaining informed consent from the patients themselves. Therefore, informed consent was obtained from the patients' relatives or their legal guardians instead. The other subjects of this research, including the normal control, provided informed consent prior to participation in this research.

3. Results

3.1. The Research on Assay Validation

3.1.1. Detecting Serum HO-1 Using the Commercial ELISA. The serum interference in detecting HO-1 was measured by the spike and recovery test. Using the commercial ELISA kit, we found a serum interference of 63% ± 17% (range, 39%–93%) in 11 samples (Figure 1). The ImmunoSet ELISA development set without modified buffers was also tested, and the interference with HO-1 detections was 48% ± 19% (range, 21%–80%) in 10 samples.

3.1.2. Assay Validation for the Modified ELISA. The modified ELISA was validated for its performance in detecting serum HO-1. A typical ELISA standard curve for HO-1 is shown in Figure 2(a). Seven calibration standards that were prepared using the modified assay buffer with 2% mouse serum were analyzed using a four-parameter logistic regression algorithm to fit the optical density as a function of the HO-1 concentration. The mean correlation coefficient from these 7 standard curves was 0.998 ± 0.002. The lower limit of detection was determined to be 0.038 ng/mL by interpolation at 2 SD above the mean background signal.

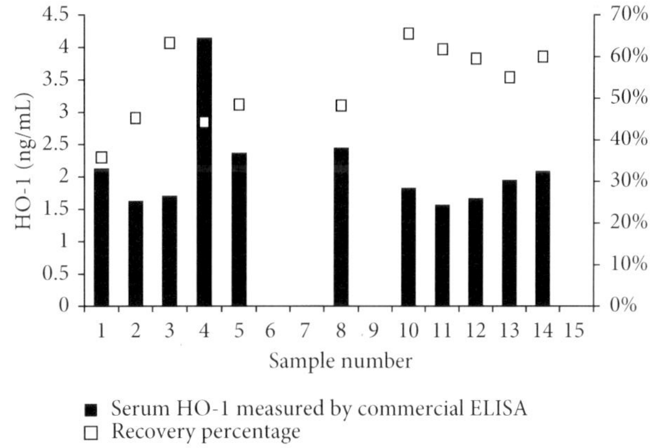

FIGURE 1: Measurement of serum HO-1 in healthy volunteers using a commercial ELISA kit (HO-1 ELISA kit; Enzo, Farmingdale, NY, USA). Serum HO-1 at 1 : 1 dilution (×1) is plotted against the % recovery, which was calculated by spiking the samples with 3.13 ng/mL of the recombinant human HO-1 protein at a dilution of 1 : 2. ELISA, enzyme-linked immunosorbent assay; HO-1, hemeoxygenase-1.

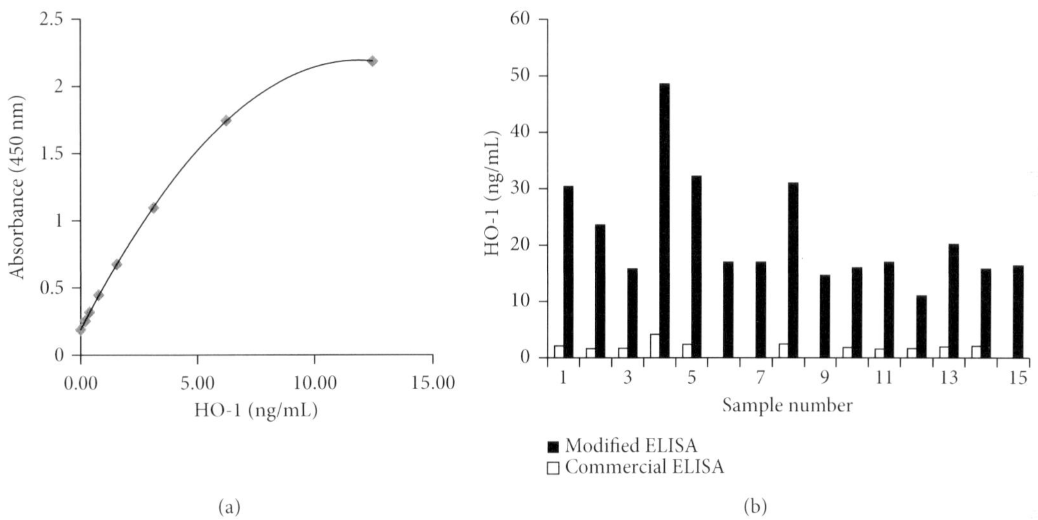

FIGURE 2: Validation of serum HO-1 ELISA. (a) In a typical standard curve using modified ELISA, the correlation coefficient from 7 standard curves was 0.998 ± 0.002. The lower limit of detection was 0.038 ng/mL. (b) Comparison shows that the average serum HO-1 of 15 healthy samples was 17.2 ± 9.5 ng/mL by modified ELISA (all with measurable concentrations) and 2.1 ± 0.7 ng/mL by commercial ELISA (undetectable concentrations in 4 of 15 samples). ELISA, enzyme-linked immunosorbent assay; HO-1, hemeoxygenase-1.

TABLE 1: Intra- and interassay test.

$N = 6$	Serum HO-1 (ng/mL)	% coefficient variations (%)
Intra-assay test	36.3 ± 1.6	7
Interassay test	32.5 ± 3.0	10

Values are reported as mean ± SD or number (%). The acceptable range of coefficient variation is less than 10%. HO-1, hemeoxygenase-1.

Intra-assay precision was tested in 1 run using 6 samples in 10 replicates, whereas interassay precision was tested in 6 separate runs, twice daily, using 6 samples in duplicates. The average coefficient intra-assay and interassay variations were 7% (serum HO-1 concentration, 36.3 ± 1.6 ng/mL) and 10% (serum HO-1 concentration, 32.5 ± 3.0 ng/mL), respectively (Table 1). The possible interference by other compounds in measuring serum HO-1 was investigated by spiking the serum with known concentrations of purified HO-1 (1, 5, and 10 ng/mL) and comparing the measured values with the expected values; we found an average recovery of 98%, 105%, and 104% respectively, with less than 10% coefficient of variation (Table 2).

3.1.3. Comparison of the Modified ELISA and the Commercial ELISA. Detection of serum HO-1 was compared between the commercial ELISA and the modified ELISA using serum from 15 healthy volunteers (Figure 2(b)). The modified ELISA yielded higher HO-1 concentrations than the

TABLE 2: Evaluation of influence of serum interferences using the spike and recovery test.

$N = 13$	Serum HO-1 (ng/mL)	% coefficient variations (%)[b]
Low, 1 ng/mL[a]	98	10
Middle, 5 ng/mL[a]	105	8
High, 10 ng/mL[a]	104	9

[a]Low, middle, and high mean known concentrations of purified HO-1; [b]the acceptable range of coefficient variation is less than 10%. HO-1, hemeoxygenase-1.

TABLE 3: Clinical characteristics of patients with ARDS.

Characteristics	Overall cases ($N = 22$)	Survivors ($N = 12$)	Nonsurvivors ($N = 10$)	P values, survivors versus nonsurvivors
Age, years	68.5 (62.0–75.0)	68.5 (56.5–75.0)	67.5 (63.0–76.0)	0.741
Male sex, N (%)	16 (73)	6 (50)	10 (100)	0.009
Body mass index	21.1 (18.6–23.1)	21.5 (20.3–23.4)	20.5 (18.3–23.1)	0.410
APACHE II score	25.5 (18.0–31.0)	23.0 (17.0–31.0)	26.5 (19.0–29.0)	0.644
Severity of ARDS, N (%)				0.548
Mild	7 (32)	5 (42)	2 (20)	
Moderate	11 (50)	5 (42)	6 (60)	
Severe	4 (18)	2 (17)	2 (20)	
Etiology of ARDS, N (%)				0.145
Infection	14 (64)	6 (42)	8 (80)	
Other causes	8 (36)	6 (58)	2 (20)	
Respiratory parameters				
D0 PaO_2/F_IO_2 ratio	165 (118–262)	176 (131–302)	141.5 (105.0–185.0)	0.291
D7 PaO_2/F_IO_2 ratio	198 (123–280)	260 (183–365)	140.5 (97.5–212.5)	0.019
D0 LIS	2.5 (2.0–2.8)	2.3 (1.6–2.5)	2.8 (2.5–3.5)	0.015
D7 LIS	2.3 (1.8–2.8)	2.0 (1.5–2.3)	3.0 (2.5–3.3)	0.008
Blood parameters				
D0 HO-1, ng/mL	75.4 (39.1–111.6)	61.7 (28.7–96.2)	100.5 (69.0–167.2)	0.027
D7 HO-1, ng/mL	74.5 (22.1–130.6)	32.5 (18.4–88.4)	123.8 (72.2–148.4)	0.008
D0 LDH, U/L	307 (242–437)	307 (253–448)	305 (237–437)	0.843
D7 LDH, U/L	326 (263–448)	326 (270–473)	329 (245–418)	0.847
D0 CRP, mg/dL	14.8 (9.7–24.1)	12.8 (9.2–26.6)	16.5 (11.4–20.3)	0.921
D7 CRP, mg/dL	6.9 (2.5–13.8)	7.7 (1.9–13.6)	5.7 (4.9–16.6)	0.642
Outcomes				
Mechanical ventilation, days	11.5 (7.0–21.0)	9.5 (7.5–17.0)	14.0 (5.0–24.0)	0.668
Length ICU stay, days	13.0 (9.0–26.0)	11.5 (10.0–27.0)	14.0 (5.0–26.0)	0.741

Values are reported as median with 25–75th percentiles or %, unless otherwise indicated. Two of the 10 nonsurvivors died within 7 days. APACHE, acute physiology and chronic health evaluation; ARDS, acute respiratory distress syndrome; LIS, lung injury score; HO-1, hemeoxygenase-1; LDH, lactate dehydrogenase; CRP, C-reactive protein.

commercial ELISA (17.2 ng/mL ± 9.5 ng/mL versus 2.1 ng/mL ± 0.7 ng/mL). The modified ELISA detected HO-1 in all samples, whereas the commercial ELISA did not detect HO-1 in 4 samples.

3.2. The Research on ARDS

3.2.1. Comparison of Serum HO-1 Concentrations between Patients with ARDS and Normal Control Subjects. The clinical characteristics of the 22 patients with ARDS, including 12 survivors and 10 nonsurvivors, are summarized in Table 3. The patients with ARDS had significantly higher D0 HO-1 concentrations than the normal control subjects (75.4 ng/mL versus 31.7 ng/mL, $P < 0.001$) (Figure 3).

3.2.2. Survival in Patients with ARDS. In the evaluation of the applicability of serum HO-1 in predicting survival, the area under the ROC curve was 0.76. The best cutoff concentration of serum HO-1 for estimating 28-day survival was 75.8 ng/mL, with sensitivity of 72% and specificity of 73%. Using this cutoff concentration of 75.8 ng/mL, the 22 patients with ARDS were divided into 2 groups, the low serum HO-1 group ($N = 11$) and the high serum HO-1 group ($N = 11$). The Kaplan–Meier survival curves of the 2 groups were significantly different on the log-rank test ($P = 0.016$) (Figure 4). The mortality rate was 18% for the former group and 73% for the latter group.

3.2.3. Correlations between ΔHO-1/D0 HO-1 and the Clinical Parameters. Two of the 10 nonsurvivors died within 7 days; therefore, we calculated the values of ΔHO-1/D0 HO-1 for 12 survivors and 8 nonsurvivors. As shown in Figure 5, ΔHO-1/D0 HO-1 was significantly correlated with the APACHE II score ($r = 0.58$, $P = 0.007$). The patient with the outlier on the top-right of Figure 5 was a survivor and this patient had 17.4 of ΔHO-1/D0 HO-1 and 45 of the APACHE II score. Also, the duration of mechanical ventilation was 49 days which was the longest duration of all enrolled patients.

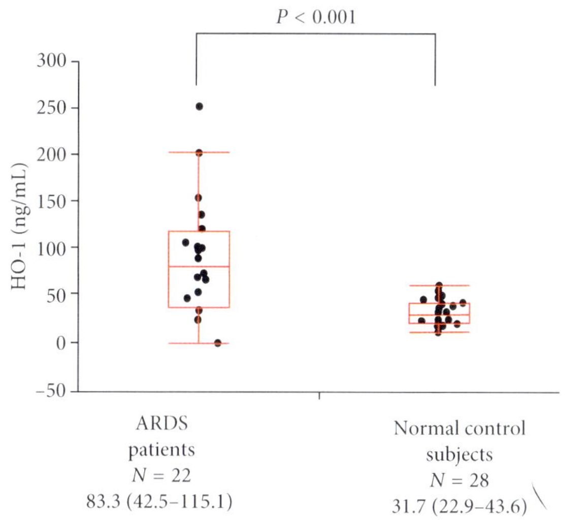

Figure 3: Comparison of serum HO-1 concentrations between patients with ARDS and normal control subjects. The patients with ARDS had significantly higher D0 HO-1 concentrations than the normal control subjects (75.4 ng/mL versus 31.7 ng/mL, $P < 0.001$). The center bold line is the median value; the bottom and top of the boxes represent the 25th to 75th percentiles, respectively; and the whiskers are 95% confident intervals. ARDS, acute respiratory distress syndrome; HO-1, hemeoxygenase-1.

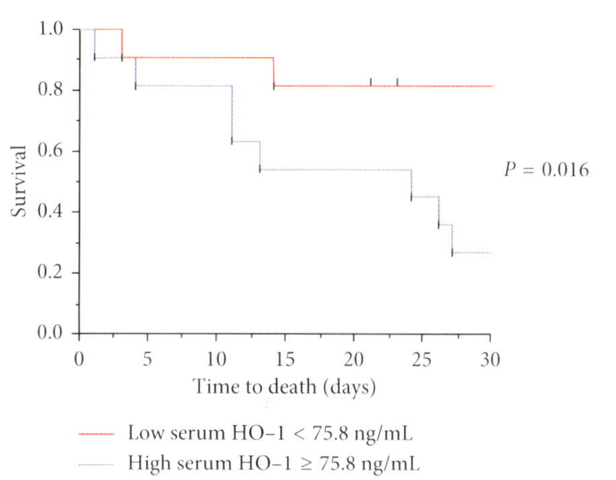

Figure 4: Comparison of patients according to serum HO-1 concentrations. The 28-day survival was significantly better in the low serum HO-1 group ($N = 11$) than in the high serum HO-1 group ($N = 11$) ($P = 0.016$). HO-1, hemeoxygenase-1.

3.2.4. Comparison of Serum HO-1 Concentrations at D0 and D7 between Nonsurvivors and Survivors. As shown in Figure 6, the serum HO-1 concentration was significantly higher in nonsurvivors than in survivors on D0 (100.5 ng/mL versus 61.7 ng/mL, $P = 0.027$) and on D7 (123.8 ng/mL versus 32.5 ng/mL, $P = 0.008$).

4. Discussion

The HO-1 ELISA kit (Enzo, Farmingdale, NY), which was designed to measure HO-1 in cell lysates and tissue extracts, had low sensitivity for detecting serum HO-1. Although serum HO-1 measured by the HO-1 ELISA kit has been previously reported to be a predictor of lung function decline in patients with silicosis [11], this method could not detect serum HO-1 in 4 of the 15 healthy volunteers in this study (Figure 2(b)). Moreover, we estimated a relatively difficult detection of serum HO-1 in patients with UIP and COPD, in which lung tissue HO-1 was reported to decrease [5, 9]. Therefore, we attempted to improve the sensitivity of serum HO-1 detection by including mouse γ-globulin in the assay buffer, changing the concentration of NaCl in the buffer, and adding EDTA to decrease the detection of nonspecific serum proteins and found that a buffer containing 50 μg/mL mouse IgG, 0.1 M NaCl, and 5 mM EDTA with 5% serum was the best buffer in decreasing serum interference in the assay [15–19]. In this research, we measured serum HO-1 concentrations in patients with ARDS using the modified ELISA and evaluated the correlations between serum HO-1 concentrations and clinical outcomes. Considering low sensitivity and instability of recovery percentage of the commercial ELISA to detect serum HO-1, we did not try to measure serum HO-1 of patients with ARDS using the commercial ELISA.

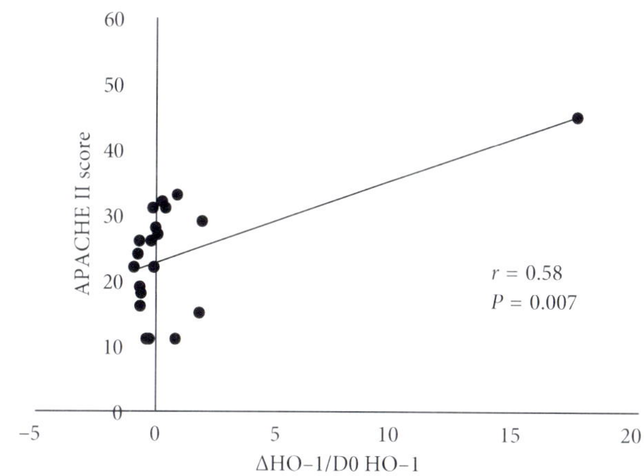

Figure 5: Correlations between ΔHO-1/D0 HO-1 and the clinical parameters. ΔHO-1/D0 HO-1 is significantly correlated with the APACHE II score. D0 HO-1 = HO-1 concentration measured upon diagnosis. D7 HO-1 = HO-1 concentration measured at 7 days after diagnosis. ΔHO-1 = D7 HO-1 minus D0 HO-1. APACHE, acute physiology and chronic health evaluation; D0, day 0; D7, day 7; HO-1, hemeoxygenase-1; ICU, intensive care unit.

In patients with DAD which is the typical pathological pattern of ARDS, HO-1 was reported to be overexpressed in lung tissues, including alveolar macrophages, epithelial cells, endothelial cells, and fibroblasts, reflecting a pulmonary cellular protective reaction [6]. In our preliminary data, we found that the arterial concentration of carboxyhemoglobin, which is the breakdown product of HO-1, was significantly higher in patients with acute exacerbation of idiopathic pulmonary fibrosis (IPF) (pathological DAD) than in patients with stable IPF [20, 21]. In the present study, the serum HO-1 concentration of patients with ARDS was significantly higher than that of normal control subjects. Therefore, we believe that serum HO-1 measurement is useful for detecting ARDS patients in the clinical setting.

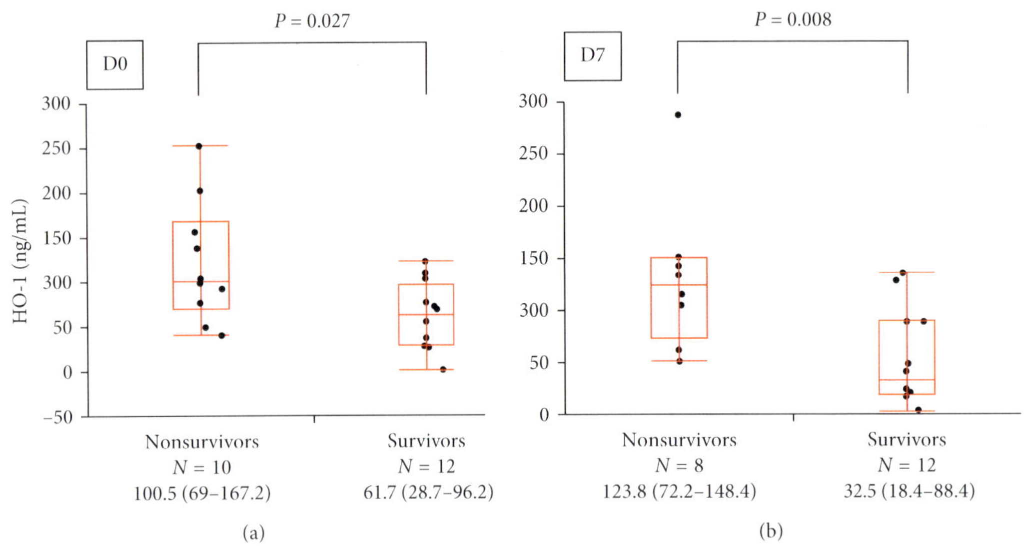

Figure 6: Comparison of serum HO-1 concentrations according to survival. The HO-1 concentrations were significantly higher in nonsurvivors than in survivors on day 0 (100.5 ng/mL versus 61.7 ng/mL, $P = 0.027$) and day 7 (123.8 ng/mL versus 32.5 ng/mL, $P = 0.008$). The center bold line is the median value; the bottom and top of the boxes represent the 25th to 75th percentiles, respectively; and the whiskers are 95% confident intervals. HO-1, hemeoxygenase-1.

The APACHE II score is frequently used to measure disease severity in the ICU, but has several limitations in predicting clinical outcome [13]. In the present study, we demonstrated significant correlations of ΔHO-1/D0 HO-1 with the APACHE II score. This result indicates that when the APACHE II score is high, serum HO-1 concentration increases from D0 to D7. Furthermore, we found that although the APACHE II score did not significantly differ between survivors and nonsurvivors, the serum HO-1 concentration of nonsurvivors was higher than that of survivors. Therefore, it may be important to follow up the D0 and D7 serum HO-1 concentration and this measurement may be more sensitive than the APACHE II score in predicting the outcome of patients with ARDS. However, further studies involving a large number of critically ill patients at risk for ARDS are needed to verify this hypothesis.

HO-1 induction is thought to represent a protective response to oxidative stress, which correlates with poor clinical outcome when persistent [1, 22]. In a previous report, we found that decreases in HO-1 concentrations in serum and bronchoalveolar lavage fluid reflected clinical improvement in patients with acute fibrinous and organizing pneumonia [23]. In another clinical research on patients with inflammatory pulmonary diseases, the concentrations of arterial carboxyhemoglobin decreased after treatment [24]. In this present study, we demonstrated that both D0 and D7 HO-1 concentration were significantly higher in nonsurvivors than in survivors. Therefore, we speculated that a high serum HO-1 concentration of both D0 and D7 reflects stronger oxidative stress and leads to poor clinical outcomes.

This study had several limitations. First, because we established a more sensitive ELISA method for serum HO-1 measurement than the commercial ELISA and validated the sensitivity of this new ELISA technique in patients with ARDS with high HO-1 production, we should examine the ability to detect serum HO-1 in patients with diseases with low HO-1 production, including COPD, UIP, and so on. In our preliminary data, we succeeded in detecting serum HO-1 in 40 of COPD patients (all patients with COPD were measurable and serum HO-1 concentration was 23.8 ± 11.9 ng/mL (a detailed data not shown)). Second, only univariate analysis could be performed because of the small number of patients with ARDS. It is important to do this study on a larger number of patients in the future. Third, the cause of ARDS in this population was heterogeneous; future studies should evaluate the clinical utility of serum HO-1 according to the cause of ARDS. Fourth, we could not analyze the correlation between serum HO-1 and the other previously established biomarkers of ARDS in this study.

5. Conclusions

The modified ELISA technique that we established for detecting serum HO-1 appeared to be more sensitive than the commercial ELISA used in previous publications. Serum HO-1 measurement can be useful for detecting ARDS patients. In addition, measurement of baseline and serial serum HO-1 concentrations is important in predicting the prognosis of patients with ARDS.

Abbreviations

APACHE: Acute physiology and chronic health evaluation
ARDS: Acute respiratory distress syndrome
BSA: Bovine serum albumin
COPD: Chronic pulmonary obstructive disease
DAD: Diffuse alveolar damage
EDTA: Ethylenediaminetetraacetic acid

ELISA: Enzyme-linked immunosorbent assay
HO-1: Hemeoxygenase-1
IPF: Idiopathic pulmonary fibrosis
PBS: Phosphate-buffered saline
ROC: Receiver operating characteristic
SD: Standard deviation.

Authors' Contributions

Yu Hara was responsible for study design, data analysis and interpretation, and manuscript drafting. Masaharu Shinkai and Takeshi Kaneko were responsible for study design and conception, data analysis and interpretation, and manuscript proofreading. Masataka Taguri, a professional statistician, double checked the statistical analysis. Kenjiro Nagai was responsible for data collection, analysis, and interpretation. All authors have read and approved the final manuscript.

References

[1] A. M. Choi and J. Alam, "Heme oxygenase-1: function, regulation, and implication of a novel stress-inducible protein in oxidant-induced lung injury," *American Journal of Respiratory Cell and Molecular Biology*, vol. 15, no. 1, pp. 9–19, 1996.

[2] S. W. Ryter, H. P. Kim, K. Nakahira, B. S. Zuckerbraun, D. Morse, and A. M. Choi, "Protective functions of heme oxygenase-1 and carbon monoxide in the respiratory system," *Antioxidants and Redox Signaling*, vol. 9, no. 12, pp. 2157–2173, 2007.

[3] Y. Hara, M. Shinkai, and B. K. Rubin, "Biomarkers for staging and evaluating therapy for idiopathic pulmonary fibrosis," *Clinical Pulmonary Medicine*, vol. 22, no. 4, pp. 165–171, 2015.

[4] N. Li, M. I. Venkatesan, A. Miguel et al., "Induction of heme oxygenase-1 expression in macrophages by diesel exhaust particle chemicals and quinones via the antioxidant-responsive element," *Journal of Immunology*, vol. 165, no. 6, pp. 3393–3401, 2000.

[5] M. Suzuki, T. Betsuyaku, Y. Ito et al., "Down-regulated NF-E2-related factor 2 in pulmonary macrophages of aged smokers and patients with chronic obstructive pulmonary disease," *American Journal of Respiratory Cell and Molecular Biology*, vol. 39, no. 6, pp. 673–682, 2008.

[6] S. Mumby, R. L. Upton, Y. Chen et al., "Lung heme oxygenase-1 is elevated in acute respiratory distress syndrome," *Critical Care Medicine*, vol. 32, no. 5, pp. 1130–1135, 2004.

[7] E. Lakari, P. Pylkas, P. Pietarinen-Runtti, P. Paakko, Y. Soini, and V. L. Kinnula, "Expression and regulation of hemeoxygenase 1 in healthy human lung and interstitial lung disorders," *Human Pathology*, vol. 32, no. 11, pp. 1257–1263, 2001.

[8] T. Sato, M. Takeno, K. Honma et al., "Heme oxygenase-1, a potential biomarker of chronic silicosis, attenuates silica-induced lung injury," *American Journal of Respiratory and Critical Care Medicine*, vol. 174, no. 8, pp. 906–914, 2006.

[9] Q. Ye, Y. Dalavanga, N. Poulakis, S. U. Sixt, J. Guzman, and U. Costabel, "Decreased expression of haem oxygenase-1 by alveolar macrophages in idiopathic pulmonary fibrosis," *European Respiratory Journal*, vol. 31, no. 5, pp. 1030–1036, 2008.

[10] Y. Kirino, M. Takeno, M. Iwasaki et al., "Increased serum HO-1 in hemophagocytic syndrome and adult-onset Still's disease: use in the differential diagnosis of hyperferritinemia," *Arthritis Research and Therapy*, vol. 7, no. 3, pp. R616–R624, 2005.

[11] T. Sato, Y. Saito, S. Inoue et al., "Serum hemeoxygenase-1 as a marker of lung function decline in patients with chronic silicosis," *Journal of Occupational and Environmental Medicine*, vol. 54, no. 12, pp. 1461–1466, 2012.

[12] ARDS Definition Task Force, V. M. Ranieri, G. D. Rubenfeld et al., "Acute respiratory distress syndrome: the Berlin definition," *JAMA*, vol. 307, no. 23, pp. 2526–2533, 2012.

[13] W. A. Knaus, E. A. Draper, D. P. Wagner, and J. E. Zimmerman, "APACHE II: a severity of disease classification system," *Critical Care Medicine*, vol. 13, no. 10, pp. 818–829, 1985.

[14] J. F. Murray, M. A. Matthay, J. M. Luce, and M. R. Flick, "An expanded definition of the adult respiratory distress syndrome," *American Review of Respiratory Disease*, vol. 138, no. 3, pp. 720–723, 1988.

[15] L. J. Kricka, "Human anti-animal antibody interferences in immunological assays," *Clinical Chemistry*, vol. 45, no. 7, pp. 942–956, 1999.

[16] L. Maple, R. Lathrop, S. Bozich et al., "Development and validation of ELISA for herceptin detection in human serum," *Journal of Immunological Methods*, vol. 295, no. 1-2, pp. 169–182, 2004.

[17] S. Hashida, K. Nakagawa, M. Imagawa et al., "Use of inorganic salts to minimize serum interference in a sandwich enzyme immunoassay for human growth hormone using Fab'-horseradish peroxidase conjugate," *Clinica Chimica Acta*, vol. 135, no. 3, pp. 263–273, 1983.

[18] L. E. DeForge, D. H. Shih, D. Kennedy et al., "Species-dependent serum interference in a sandwich ELISA for Apo2L/TRAIL," *Journal of Immunological Methods*, vol. 320, no. 1-2, pp. 58–69, 2007.

[19] K. Nielsen, L. Kelly, D. Gall et al., "The use of divalent cation chelating agents (EDTA/EGTA) to reduce non-specific serum protein interaction in enzyme immunoassay," *Veterinary Research Communications*, vol. 18, no. 6, pp. 433–437, 1994.

[20] R. Hyzy, S. Huang, J. Myers, K. Flaherty, and F. Martinez, "Acute exacerbation of idiopathic pulmonary fibrosis," *Chest*, vol. 132, no. 5, pp. 1652–1658, 2007.

[21] Y. Hara, M. Shinkai, S. Kanoh et al., "Arterial carboxyhemoglobin measurement is useful for evaluating pulmonary inflammation in subjects with interstitial lung disease," *Internal Medicine*, vol. 56, no. 6, pp. 621–626, 2017.

[22] S. Kanoh, H. Kobayashi, and K. Motoyoshi, "Exhaled ethane: an in vivo biomarker of lipid peroxidation in interstitial lung diseases," *Chest*, vol. 128, no. 4, pp. 2387–2392, 2005.

[23] Y. Hara, M. Shinkai, S. Kanoh et al., "Clinico-pathological analysis referring hemeoxygenase-1 in acute fibrinous and organizing pneumonia patients," *Respiratory Medicine Case Reports*, vol. 14, pp. 53–56, 2015.

[24] H. Yasuda, M. Yamaya, M. Yanai, T. Ohrui, and H. Sasaki, "Increased blood carboxyhaemoglobin concentrations in inflammatory pulmonary diseases," *Thorax*, vol. 57, no. 9, pp. 779–783, 2002.

30

Daily Chronic Intermittent Hypobaric Hypoxia Does Not Induce Chronic Increase in Pulmonary Arterial Pressure Assessed by Echocardiography

Jeremias Götschke,[1,2] Pontus Mertsch,[1,2] Nikolaus Kneidinger,[1,2] Diego Kauffmann-Guerrero,[1,2] Jürgen Behr,[1,2,3] Rudolf Maria Huber,[1,2] Frank Reichenberger,[2,3] and Katrin Milger[1,2]

[1]*Department of Internal Medicine V, Ludwig-Maximilians-University of Munich, Munich, Germany*
[2]*Comprehensive Pneumology Center (CPC-M), Member of the German Center for Lung Research (DZL), Munich, Germany*
[3]*Asklepios Fachkliniken München Gauting, Gauting, Germany*

Correspondence should be addressed to Katrin Milger; katrin.milger@med.uni-muenchen.de

Academic Editor: Sébastien Bonnet

Chronic hypoxia causes pulmonary vascular remodeling resulting in persistently increased pulmonary arterial pressures (PAP) even after return to normoxia. Recently, interest in chronic intermittent hypobaric hypoxia (CIHH) was raised because it occurs in subjects working at high altitude (HA) but living in lowland. However, effects of daily CIHH on PAP are unknown. In this pilot study, we included 8 healthy subjects working at (2650 m) each workday for 8-9 h while living and sleeping at LA and 8 matched control subjects living and working at LA. Cardiorespiratory measurements including echocardiography at rest and during exercise were performed at LA (Munich, 530 m) and HA (Zugspitze, 2650 m). Hemoglobin was higher in CIHH subjects. LA echocardiography showed normal right and left cardiac dimensions and function in all subjects. Systolic PAP (sPAP) and tricuspid annular plane systolic excursion (TAPSE) at rest were similar in both groups. Resting blood gas analysis (BGA) at HA revealed decreased pCO_2 in CIHH compared to controls (HA: 28.4 versus 31.7 mmHg, $p = 0.01$). During exercise, sPAP was lower in CIHH subjects compared to controls (LA: 28.7 versus 35.3 mmHg, $p = 0.02$; HA: 26.3 versus 33.6 mmHg, $p = 0.04$) and peripheral oxygen saturation (SpO_2) was higher. In sum, subjects exposed to CIHH showed no signs of pulmonary vascular remodeling.

1. Introduction

Acute and chronic physiologic reactions to altitude are observed starting at altitudes of 1400 m and have been studied in detail in the last decades [1]. Maladaptive diseases such as acute and chronic mountain sickness or high-altitude pulmonary edema and hypertension are observed at altitudes above 2500 m (high altitude) [2, 3]. The main causative factor for adaptive and maladaptive reactions is hypoxia. However, atmospheric pressure is also relevant, as differences between reactions to normobaric and hypobaric hypoxia have been demonstrated [4–7].

Acute hypoxia causes hypoxic pulmonary vasoconstriction (HPV) leading to an increase in pulmonary arterial pressure (PAP) with the level of altitude being inversely related to arterial oxygen saturation (SaO_2) and directly related to PAP [8]. Mean (m)PAP increases from 10 to 15 mmHg at lowland to values of 20–25 mmHg at altitudes of 2600–3600 m [9, 10]. Under chronic hypoxia, vascular remodeling occurs in the pulmonary arteries with thickening of the adventitia and media and muscularization of formerly nonmuscularized precapillary vessels, causing a sustained increase in PAP even weeks after return to normoxia [11].

PAP increases upon exertion because of rising cardiac output (CO). Yet, this increase is moderate in healthy subjects even under maximal exercise, because vasodilation and vascular recruitment are decreasing pulmonary vascular resistance (PVR) at the same time. A disproportionately high rise in PAP under exertion is considered a sign of early stages of pulmonary vascular remodeling and disease [12]. At altitude, PAP rises more sharply with the increase in CO upon exercise compared to sea level [13]. Thus, exercise at high altitude may unmask pulmonary vascular alterations that might not be noted at rest or at lowland.

A further important physiologic response to acute hypoxia is a rise in breathing rate and tidal volume, termed hypoxic ventilatory response (HVR). This hyperventilation increases alveolar and arterial oxygen pressure and decreases carbon dioxide pressure and is sustained during chronic exposure in healthy high-altitude dwellers, while a decrease in hyperventilation during chronic hypoxia is seen as an initial mechanism of maladaptation and development of chronic mountain sickness (CMS) [8].

In the course of the touristic exploitation of the Alps and other mountains as well as other activities such as research stations, an increasing number of people are working in higher altitudes while living in lowland and commuting between these altitudes every workday by gondola lift or cable car. Recently, interest in periodic exposure to high altitudes, also known as chronic intermittent hypobaric hypoxia (CIHH), as occurring in various working conditions, was raised. It has been shown that adjustments of ventilatory and cardiovascular responses, as well as hemoglobin (Hb) levels are similar to those observed under chronic hypoxia, but the acclimatization may take years instead of months [14, 15]. Interestingly, increased PAP at sea level with high prevalence of borderline pulmonary hypertension (PH) or, to a lower degree, even manifest PH was found in subjects exposed to CIHH for over 12 years [16].

So far, studies investigating CIHH focused on exposure–nonexposure durations of one to several weeks as occurring in mining or military workers [14, 16, 17]. Yet, the effect of daily CIHH is unknown. Therefore, we studied the effect of daily CIHH on cardiopulmonary physiology in subjects commuting every workday from 700 m to 2656 m asl for several years, focusing on the question whether this exposure induces pulmonary vascular remodeling and chronic increase in pulmonary arterial pressure. We further performed measurements during exercise to increase sensitivity of detecting pulmonary vascular alterations.

2. Methods

2.1. Study Population. In the CIHH group, we included 8 healthy Caucasian subjects (4 men and 4 women) working at high altitude (2650 m) on the Zugspitze (Wetterstein Mountains, Germany) with daily ascension by gondola lift or cable car from 700 m and an average high-altitude stay of 8-9 h per day, 5 days a week. Work activities of the staff were administrative work ($n = 2$), engineer and technician ($n = 3$), waitress and sale assistant ($n = 3$). Controls were matched according to age, gender, BMI, health, and physical activity status. All controls were living and working in lowland (Munich, Germany, 530 m asl) without any previous chronic or chronic intermittent exposure to high altitude and no acute hypoxia within the last 3 months. All subjects had previously traveled to similar heights and reported no history of acute mountain sickness. Work activities of controls were technician ($n = 3$), nurse ($n = 2$), physician ($n = 1$), housewife ($n = 1$), and secretary ($n = 1$). Prior written informed consent was obtained from all subjects. The study was approved by the institutional review board (IRB) of the University of Munich (number 328-16).

2.2. Study Design. The study overview is presented in Figure 1. Baseline low-altitude investigations of both groups were performed in Munich (low altitude 530 m asl; Department of Internal Medicine, University Hospital of the Ludwig-Maximilians-University, Munich, Germany). High-altitude measurements were performed two weeks later at the air-conditioned Environmental Research Station Schneefernerhaus (UFS, Zugspitze, Germany) at an altitude of 2650 m, located 300 m below the top of Germany's highest mountain, Zugspitze. The station was effortlessly reached by all participants by gondola lift and measurements started 2 h or later after arrival at high altitude. Blood withdrawal at low and high altitude was performed shortly before the exercise test.

2.3. Measurements. All measurements at low and high altitude were carried out at room temperature (19–22°C).

Baseline measurements at low altitude included venous blood analysis for hemoglobin, ferritin, pro-BNP, endothelin-1, pulmonary function testing using body-plethysmography, diffusion capacity for carbon monoxide, cycle ergometer exercise with capillary blood gas analysis, and echocardiography. Plethysmography was performed using Jaeger MasterScreen Body/Diff (Carefusion SN696373; Hoechberg, Germany). Peripheral oxygen saturation (SpO_2) was measured at fingertip (Criticare 504-US). Blood gas analysis (BGA) was performed from the arterialized earlobe sample using the Rapidpoint 405 (Siemens Healthineers, Erlangen, Germany). Ergometry was performed as bicycle ergometry in semi supine position tilted toward the left side for better visualization of the cardiac structures as described elsewhere [18]. We used a step-protocol using predefined steps of 50 W every two minutes at low altitude and 25 W every two minutes at high altitude. In addition to echocardiography, subjects were monitored during exercise by continuous measurement of heart rate and SpO_2 as well as blood pressure measurement every 2 min. All echocardiography measurements were performed by the same, experienced investigator (FR) using the Logic-e (GE healthcare). Exemplary echocardiographic tracing of sPAP measurements are shown in the Supplementary Figures S1(a)–(d). Human endothelin-1 was quantified with QuantiGlo Elisa (R&D systems Inc, Minneapolis, USA) following the manufacturer's instructions.

2.4. Statistics. Statistical analyses were performed using GraphPad 7 (LaJolla, California, USA). The Shapiro–Wilk test was used to test for normal distribution. Because data passed this test, parametric tests were used throughout the study (t-test, Pearson correlation). A $p < 0.05$ was considered

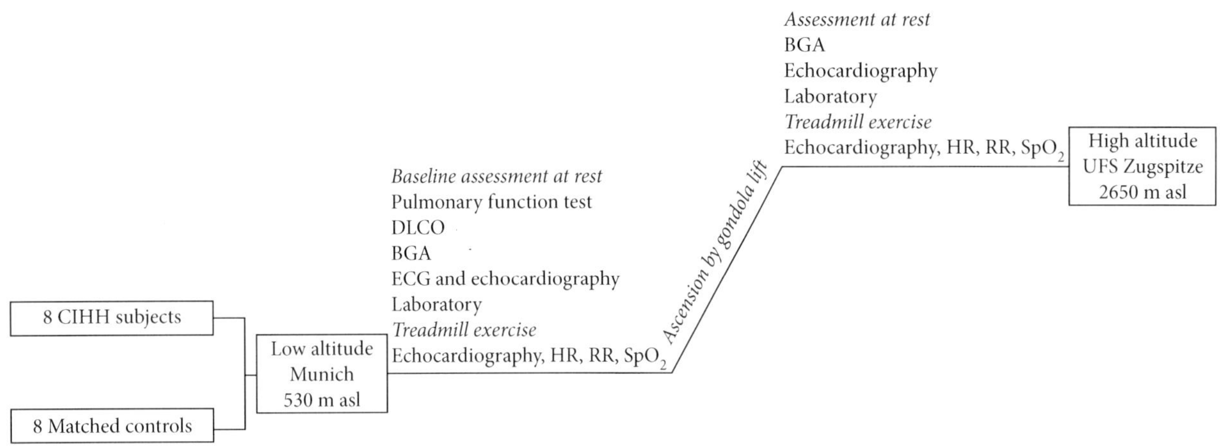

Figure 1: Study overview.

significant. As this was a pilot study, we did not perform correction for multiple testing and also reported tendencies ($p < 0.1$).

3. Results

The median age of subjects in the study was 34 years in both groups (Table 1). Further baseline characteristics including body mass index (BMI), physical activity, and preexisting medical conditions were not significantly different between the groups. The median duration of exposure to CIHH was 3.7 years (minimum 2.5 years and maximum 20 years; Table 1).

All subjects had a normal lung function and diffusion capacity with no significant differences between groups (Table 2). Baseline laboratory at low altitude showed a tendency toward higher Hb in CIHH subjects ($p = 0.05$). Pro-BNP levels were normal in all subjects and did not show significant difference between the groups.

At low altitude, resting echocardiography showed normal right and left cardiac dimensions and function and absence of cardiac disease in all subjects (Table 3). Of note, right heart function as measured by tricuspid annular plane systolic excursion (TAPSE) was similar in both groups. All subjects had either normal sPAP at rest or it was not possible to measure due to lack of tricuspid regurgitation (Table 3). sPAP at rest was not significantly different between CIHH subjects and controls. Low-altitude blood gas analysis at rest revealed a tendency toward increased hyperventilation with lower pCO_2 and decreased base excess (BE) in CIHH subjects (Table 3). During exercise at 150 W, CIHH subjects had a significantly lower sPAP and higher SpO_2 than controls, whereas TAPSE did not differ (Table 3).

At high altitude, there was a significantly lower pCO_2 at rest in CIHH subjects compared to controls, and BE tended to be lower (Table 4). Further, pO_2 at rest at high altitude tended to be higher with longer duration of exposure to CIHH (Supplementary Figure S2). Upon treadmill exercise at high altitude with 75 W, sPAP was significantly lower in CIHH subjects while SpO_2 was significantly higher than in controls (Figure 2 and Table 4). Again TAPSE was not significantly different between CIHH and control subjects. pCO_2 tended to be lower at exercise at high altitude (Supplementary Table 1); however, exercise BGA was not obtained at the same power level in all subjects.

As endothelin-1 has been shown to be of importance for hypoxic pulmonary vasoconstriction and chronic hypoxic PH [19], it was quantified in serum in low and high altitude. Here, endothelin-1 was increased at high altitude compared to low altitude in CIHH as well as in control subjects (Figure 3, $p < 0.01$). However, there were no significant differences between the groups. Similarly, pro-BNP was increased at high altitude compared to low altitude in the total study population ($p = 0.02$), but there were no significant differences between the groups (Tables 2 and 4).

Since sPAP was lower and SpO_2 higher in CIHH than in controls, we further investigated a possible correlation between sPAP and SpO_2 during exercise at high altitude and found a negative correlation that was not statistically significant (Figure 4).

4. Discussion

To our knowledge, this is the first study investigating the influence of daily CIHH on pulmonary arterial pressure. In contrast to chronic exposure to hypoxia, daily CIHH at an altitude of 2650 m did not lead to increases in sPAP compared to constant normobaric normoxia in lowlanders. Single breath diffusion capacity as well as Hb corrected Krogh factor were normal and similar to controls. Thus, there were no signs to suggest significant vascular remodeling in the CIHH subjects studied. Moreover, no signs of remodeling or altered function of the right heart were found.

While studies of chronic exposure have consistently shown chronic increases in PAP in high-altitude dwellers [2, 11, 20], results obtained for CIHH are less clear [14–16, 21, 22]. Antezana et al. prospectively investigated Chilean miners exposed to weekly CIHH at 4500 m asl for 3 years and found no signs of PH apart from increased PAP during hypoxia [21]. In this setting, PAP was lower in CIHH subjects than in permanent residents [14]. In a study of monthly CIHH at 3700 m in Kyrgyzstan over two years,

Table 1: Baseline characteristics.

Matched characteristics	CIHH	Controls	p value*
Total subject number, n	8	8	
Female, n	4	4	
Age, years median (min; max)	34 (29; 50)	34.5 (28; 51)	
BMI, kg/m^2 (±SD)	25.30 ± 3.78	23.90 ± 6.19	0.57
Smoking (current/ex/never)	2/2/4	0/1/7	0.21
Packyears			
Current	8; 16		
Ex-smoker	0.5; 2	12	
Endurance sport activity (regular/sometimes/rarely)	2/6/0	2/5/1	0.58
Treated hypertension, n	2	2	
Treated hypothyreosis, n	0	1	>0.99
Duration of CIHH, years		—	
(i) Median (min; max)	3.7 (2.5; 20)		
(ii) Individual values	2.5, 3, 3.2, 3.4, 4, 5, 10, 20		

CIHH: chronic intermittent hypobaric hypoxia; *by t-test or chi-square test as appropriate. Endurance physical activity was defined as cardiac workout of at least 30 min: regular >1/week; sometimes 1–3x/month; rarely <1/month.

Table 2: Lowland pulmonary function tests and laboratory parameters.

Pulmonary function test	CIHH#	Control#	p value*
FEV1 pp	104.29 ± 5.85	110.56 ± 16.83	0.34
FVC pp	110.70 ± 12.99	111.01 ± 8.71	0.96
FEV1/FVC	78.30 ± 5.37	81.99 ± 5.39	0.19
MEF 75% pp	90.23 ± 19.50	107.57 ± 34.6	0.23
MEF 50% pp	82.6 ± 11.32	105.3 ± 40.65	0.17
MEF 25% pp	75.25 ± 14.47	88.48 ± 38.07	0.37
R tot (kPa*s/L)	0.20 ± 0.10	0.20 ± 0.07	0.95
TLC pp	107.68 ± 12.00	92.87 ± 36.78	0.30
DLCO-SB pp	97.69 ± 14.59	90.18 ± 11.41	0.27
DLCO/VA pp	97.41 ± 16.94	88.77 ± 12.01	0.26
DLCOc/VA pp	93.16 ± 15.28	88.45 ± 9.50	0.47
Baseline laboratory			
Hb (mg/dl)	14.95 ± 0.95	13.81 ± 1.28	**0.05**
Ferritin (μg/l)	127.25 ± 131.23	132.63 ± 119.47	0.93
Pro-BNP (pg/ml)	17.80 ± 13.48	39.39 ± 38.60	0.18
Endothelin-1 (pg/ml)	1.26 ± 0.59	1.54 ± 1.06	0.73

CIHH: chronic intermittent hypobaric hypoxia; FEV1: forced expiratory volume in 1 sec; pp: percent predicted; FVC: forced vital capacitiy; R: resistance; TLC: total lung capacity; DLCO: lung diffusion capacity for carbon monoxide; SB: single breath; VA: alveolar volume; c: corrected for Hb; Hb: hemoglobin; BNP: brain natriuretic peptide; MEF 75, 50, 25: maximal expiratory flow at 25/50/75% of forced VC; *by t-test; #±SD.

similar results were obtained [21]. Yet, in an observational study investigating subjects exposed to weekly CIHH at 3550 m for more than a decade, Brito et al. found echocardiographic signs of elevated PAP in 6 out of 50 subjects [16]. From these studies, it can be concluded that pulmonary vascular remodeling may occur in CIHH as well but possibly only after very long exposure duration for more than a decade. In contrast, in the present study we did not find signs of chronic increases in PAP or remodeling in any of the subjects. This may be due to a shorter exposure interval of daily versus weekly exposure but also a lower height of 2650 m versus 3700 m. Chronic hyperventilation in adapted subjects at 2650 m might still be sufficient to maintain pO_2 at a level that prevents pronounced hypoxic PAP increase, whereas this compensation might not be sufficient at a very high altitude resulting in long-term remodeling. Moreover, we included only two subjects with very long exposure duration over 10 years, and therefore, it cannot be excluded that in a larger population subjects with signs of PH may be found. Interestingly, pO_2 at rest at high altitude tended to be higher after longer exposure to CIHH, whereas dampening of HVR is observed in native Andean populations [23].

Of note, in the present study sPAP under exertion at low and high altitude was even lower in CIHH subjects compared to controls. One possible explanation for this is adaptation. Firstly, we observed moderately higher hemoglobin, possibly reflecting the adaptation to the chronic intermittent high-altitude exposure and confirming a relevant but moderate exposure to hypoxia. The Hb values we found were lower than what would be expected from chronic exposure to a similar height, in line with previous studies of CIHH [14, 16]. Secondly, pCO_2 was lower both at low and at high altitude while BE was lower and pH was unchanged as a sign of chronic hyperventilation as means of ventilatory adaptation. More pronounced hyperventilation increases pO_2, possibly resulting in reduced hypoxic vasoconstriction and therefore explaining the slightly lower sPAP that was observed. Even though SpO_2 under exertion in both, high altitude and low

Table 3: Lowland echocardiography and blood gas analysis at rest and during exercise ($p = 150$ W).

	CIHH	Control	p value*
Echocardiography at rest			
LVEDD (mm)	45.50 ± 3.42	43.75 ± 2.82	0.28
LV-EF (%)	67.63 ± 2.39	65.57 ± 2.37	0.11
RVEDD (mm)	35.25 ± 3.20	32.88 ± 2.36	0.11
sPAP, not measurable at rest (n)#	3	4	
sPAP (mmHg)#	20.20 ± 3.27	18.50 ± 2.08	0.39
TAPSE (mm)	23.88 ± 3.48	22.67 ± 2.58	0.48
Vital signs rest lowland			
HR (bpm)	78.28 ± 13.64	77.5 ± 11.64	0.91
Mean RR (mmHg)	94.95 ± 10.37	92.83 ± 8.31	0.69
Blood gas analysis rest lowland			
pO_2 (mmHg)	86.41 ± 4.55	85.49 ± 5.91	0.73
pCO_2 (mmHg)	33.63 ± 4.63	37.65 ± 3.17	**0.06**
pH	7.43 ± 0.03	7.43 ± 0.02	1.00
BE (mmol/l)	−0.90 ± 2.21	0.64 ± 1.08	**0.09**
SaO_2 (%)	97.29 ± 0.43	97.00 ± 0.74	0.37
$AaDO_2$	21.2 ± 5.5	17.1 ± 6.1	0.18
Exertion 150 W			
HR (bpm)	134.42 ± 12.71	142.5 ± 21.35	0.41
Mean RR (mmHg)	120.58 ± 13.66	110.27 ± 19.14	0.26
sPAP (mmHg)	28.75 ± 3.99	35.33 ± 2.89	**0.02**
TAPSE (mm)	30.00 ± 2.83	31.17 ± 5.23	0.59
SpO_2 (%)	99.33 ± 1.21	94.75 ± 2.60	**0.001**

CIHH: chronic intermittent hypobaric hypoxia; LVEDD: left ventricular end diastolic diameter; LV-EF: left ventricular ejection fraction; RVEDD: right ventricular end diastolic diameter; sPAP: systolic pulmonary arterial pressure; TAPSE: tricuspid annular plane systolic excursion; pO_2: oxygen partial pressure; pCO_2: carbon dioxide partial pressure; BE: base excess; SaO_2: arterial oxygen saturation; SpO_2: peripheral oxygen saturation; *by t-test; #due to lack of TI, sPAP was not measurable in all subjects at rest at lowland; mean sPAP is therefore calculated from the remaining subjects only. During exercise and at altitude, sPAP was measurable in all subjects.

Table 4: High-altitude echocardiography and blood gas analysis at rest and during exercise ($p = 75$ W).

High altitude	CIHH	Control	p value*
Laboratory			
Pro-BNP (pg/ml)	39.5 ± 27.2	43.0 ± 41.2	0.85
Endothelin-1 (pg/ml)	1.84 ± 0.45	2.27 ± 1.38	0.37
Echocardiography at rest			
sPAP, not measurable at rest (n)	0	0	
sPAP (mmHg)	19.6 ± 3.3	20.1 ± 4.1	0.82
TAPSE (mm)	21 ± 3.9	22.1 ± 4.5	0.80
Vital signs at rest altitude			
HR (bpm)	79.4 ± 21	88.9 ± 22.2	0.41
Mean RR (mmHg)	104.0 ± 9.4	98.4 ± 10.8	0.31
Blood gas analysis at rest altitude			
pO_2 (mmHg)	70.1 ± 7.3	63.2 ± 7.6	0.10
pCO_2 (mmHg)	28.5 ± 2.3	31.8 ± 2.4	**0.01**
pH	7.44 ± 0.01	7.44 ± 0.01	0.46
BE (mmol)	−3.64 ± 1.12	−2.30 ± 1.32	**0.05**
SaO_2 (%)	93.1 ± 1.0	91.4 ± 2.5	0.10
$AaDO_2$	8.1 ± 7.6	11.2 ± 6.8	0.43
Echocardiography exertion 75 W			
sPAP (mmHg)	26.3 ± 4.1	33.6 ± 7.2	**0.04**
TAPSE (mm)	26.2 ± 2.8	25.6 ± 4.6	0.80
SpO_2 (%)	91.83 ± 1.47	87.38 ± 4.41	**0.03**

CIHH: chronic intermittent hypobaric hypoxia; sPAP: systolic pulmonary arterial pressure; TAPSE: tricuspid annular plane systolic excursion; pO_2: oxygen partial pressure; pCO_2: carbon dioxide partial pressure; BE: base excess; SaO_2: arterial oxygen saturation; SpO_2: peripheral oxygen saturation; *by t-test.

altitude, was significantly higher in CIHH subjects compared to controls, a direct correlation between sPAP and SpO_2 could not be demonstrated. The reason for this could be the small number of subjects studied, but other confounding factors such as individual differences based on genetic predisposition or differences in vasoactive mediators or differences in cardiac output are also possible. Moreover, results of BGA at exercise are not conclusive, possibly

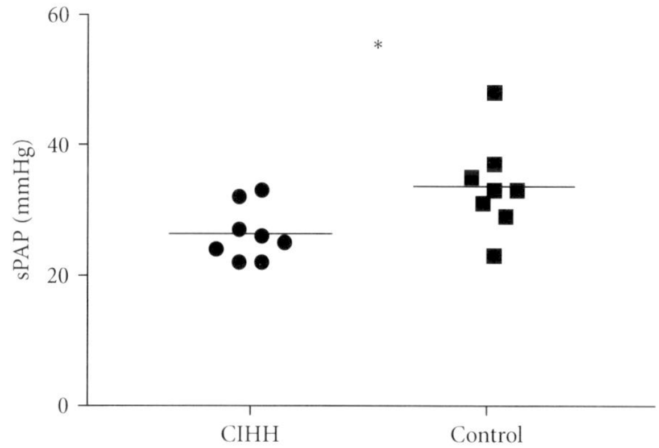

FIGURE 2: sPAP under exertion (75 W) at high altitude. sPAP was significantly higher in CIHH than in controls. CIHH: chronic intermittent hypobaric hypoxia. *By *t*-test.

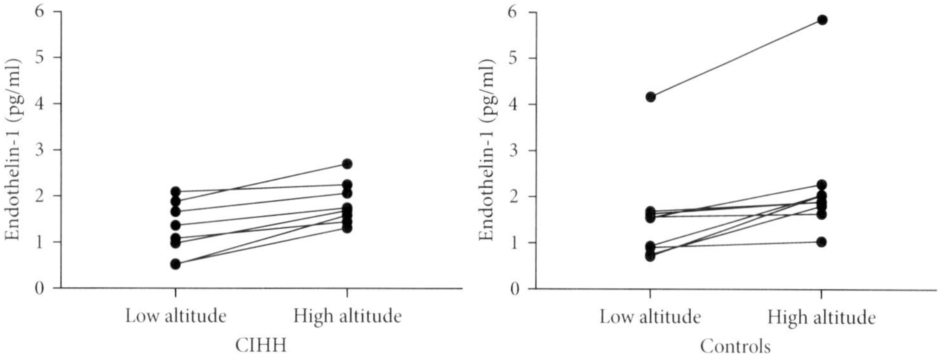

FIGURE 3: Endothelin-1 at lowland and high altitude. Endothelin-1 serum levels increased at high altitude compared to lowland in CIHH as well as in controls ($p < 0.01$ in both groups, by *t*-test, paired). There was no significant difference between CIHH and controls. Measurements at lowland and altitude from each individual are connected by a line.

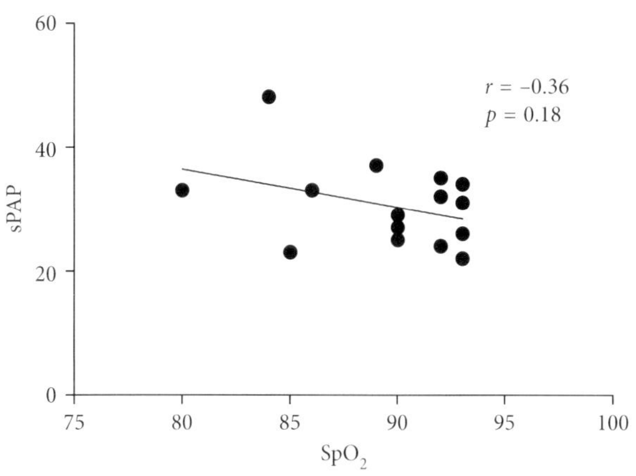

FIGURE 4: Correlation of sPAP and SpO_2 under exertion at high altitude. Each data point corresponds to one subject (CIHH or control). Correlation was not statistically significant.

because they were not measured at the same power level in all subjects (Supplementary Table S1).

Cardiac output was not measured in this study, but right heart function during exercise was assessed by TAPSE measurement. Here, we found that TAPSE in CIHH was increased as compared to resting measurement and not significantly different from controls at low as well as high altitude. We did not find any signs of decreased right heart function compared to controls. We further studied some of the vasoactive mediators that have been involved in the control of hypoxic pulmonary vasoconstriction and have also been linked long-term changes such as remodeling of the pulmonary vasculature and right heart. Brain natriuretic peptide (BNP) has diuretic, natriuretic, and hypotensive effects with cytoprotective and antiproliferative properties. It is clinically used as a marker of ventricular load, especially right ventricular load in pulmonary hypertension. Cardiac BNP release is increased under hypobaric hypoxia [24, 25], and disproportionately high increase of pro-BNP has been shown in HA pulmonary edema [26]. Endothelin-1 is a potent vasoconstrictor but also promotes vascular remodeling with migration and proliferation of vascular cells [24]. It increases in response to acute hypoxia [27] and hypoxia-induced PAP increase may be blunted by endothelin receptor blockade [28]. In our study, pro-BNP and endothelin-1 were increased at high altitude compared to low altitude but there were no significant differences between CIHH and control subjects. This supports our finding that there is no sign of chronic PH in CIHH. Further, there seems to be no adaptation to the HA exposure on this level.

Surprisingly, in our study hyperventilation was observed in CIHH subjects even at low altitude. Minute ventilation is increased in response to hypoxia by a rise in breathing frequency and tidal volume. This hypoxic ventilator response is triggered by the chemoreceptors in the bifurcation of the carotid arteries. In a study using 1 h of hypoxia per day for one week, it was found that HVR increased via augmented hypoxic sensitivity of chemoreceptors [29]. This enhanced HVR persisted after return to sea level for one week. In another study by Ricart et al., subjects were exposed to an altitude of 5000 m for 2 h per day for 2 weeks and subsequently exercised during hypoxia [30]. Here, it was found that ventilation and arterial oxygenation during exercise were higher than before the intermittent hypoxia and this is in line with our results. However, in that study resting ventilation was not altered, whereas we found hyperventilation also at rest even in lowland. Our low-altitude measurements were performed after all subjects had spent the night at normoxia as usual indicating hyperventilation is sustained for at least this time period without hypoxic stimulus.

This study should be interpreted in view of its limitations. It is an observational study of subjects exposed to daily CIHH for several years using matched controls for comparison. Therefore, subjects working at high altitude for years might be selected for those who adapt well and not correspond to the general population.

Further, in this pilot study we investigated a small number of subjects, and larger studies will be necessary to confirm the results obtained. Moreover, we used noninvasive assessment of PAP as well as heart structure and function. Invasive measurement of pulmonary hemodynamics is the gold standard providing a more exact and complete picture with measurement of CO and PVR in addition to PAP. However, reliability of echocardiographic sPAP measurement is high [31] and negative predictive value to exclude PH is high when parameters of RV structure and function and BNP are also considered [32]. Additionally, we used high-altitude exposure and exercise as challenges, and thus we are confident these results proof valid. Moreover, our techniques are comparable to other studies on this matter which also used echocardiographic assessment. In sum, the reliability of the finding of normal sPAP and right heart function in CIHH is high, whereas it is lower for the small differences in sPAP found between CIHH and controls warranting further investigations using more precise methods. Finally, we have not directly measured minute ventilation but can only conclude from pCO_2 levels and BE. Future studies should include more detailed and direct measurement of ventilation.

5. Conclusions and Outlook

Daily CIHH to an altitude of 2650 m leads to adaptation with moderately higher hemoglobin and chronic hyperventilation with higher O_2 saturation during exercise but no disproportionate increase in sPAP even during exercise. Meanwhile, there were no signs of chronic increase in PAP or altered RV structure and function. Larger studies are necessary to confirm results and obtain more insights into degree and mechanism of chronic hyperventilation that seems to persist even at lowland.

Authors' Contributions

Jeremias Götschke and Pontus Mertsch contributed equally to this work.

Acknowledgments

The authors thank Ulrike Schürmann, Christiane Donick, and Rosemarie Kiefl for excellent technical assistance. The study was funded by internal resources of Department of Internal Medicine V, Ludwig-Maximilians-University of Munich. There were no external funding resources.

Supplementary Materials

Supplementary Figure S1: exemplary echocardiographic tracings of sPAP measurements. (a) Lowland at rest. (b) Lowland exercise. (c) High altitude at rest. (d) High-altitude exercise. Supplementary Figure S2: correlation between pO_2 at high altitude at rest and years exposure to CIHH. Supplementary Table S1: BGA under exertion at lowland and high altitude.

References

[1] J. Grimminger, M. Richter, K. Tello et al., "Thin air resulting in high pressure: mountain sickness and hypoxia-induced pulmonary hypertension," *Canadian Respiratory Journal*, vol. 2017, Article ID 8381653, 17 pages, 2017.

[2] M. Maggiorini and F. Léon-Velarde, "High-altitude pulmonary hypertension: a pathophysiological entity to different diseases," *European Respiratory Journal*, vol. 22, no. 6, pp. 1019–1025, 2003.

[3] F. León-Velarde, M. Maggiorini, J. T. Reeves et al., "Consensus statement on chronic and subacute high altitude diseases," *High Altitude Medicine & Biology*, vol. 6, no. 2, pp. 147–157, 2005.

[4] J. A. Loeppky, R. C. Roach, D. Maes et al., "Role of hypobaria in fluid balance response to hypoxia," *High Altitude Medicine & Biology*, vol. 6, no. 1, pp. 60–71, 2005.

[5] R. Faiss, V. Pialoux, C. Sartori et al., "Ventilation, oxidative stress, and nitric oxide in hypobaric versus normobaric hypoxia," *Medicine & Science in Sports & Exercise*, vol. 45, no. 2, pp. 253–260, 2013.

[6] J. A. Loeppky, M. Icenogle, P. Scotto et al., "Ventilation during simulated altitude, normobaric hypoxia and normoxic hypobaria," *Respiration Physiology*, vol. 107, no. 3, pp. 231–239, 1997.

[7] N. A. Richard, I. S. Sahota, N. Widmer et al., "Acute mountain sickness, chemosensitivity, and cardiorespiratory responses in

humans exposed to hypobaric and normobaric hypoxia," *Journal of Applied Physiology*, vol. 116, no. 7, pp. 945–952, 2014.

[8] D. Penaloza and J. Arias-stella, "The heart and pulmonary circulation at high altitudes healthy highlanders and chronic mountain sickness," *Circulation*, vol. 115, no. 9, pp. 1132–1147, 2007.

[9] T. Yang, X. Li, J. Qin et al., "High altitude-induced borderline pulmonary hypertension impaired cardiorespiratory fitness in healthy young men," *International Journal of Cardiology*, vol. 181, pp. 382–387, 2015.

[10] P. Bärtsch and J. S. R. Gibbs, "Effect of altitude on the heart and the lungs," *Circulation*, vol. 116, no. 19, pp. 2191–2202, 2007.

[11] M. R. Wilkins, H.-A. Ghofrani, N. Weissmann et al., "Pathophysiology and treatment of high-altitude pulmonary vascular disease," *Circulation*, vol. 131, no. 6, pp. 582–590, 2015.

[12] B. I. Medarov, S. Jogani, J. Sun et al., "Readdressing the entity of exercise pulmonary arterial hypertension," *Respiratory Medicine*, vol. 124, pp. 65–71, 2017.

[13] B. N. Banchero and E. Marticorena, "Pulmonary pressure, cardiac output, and arterial oxygen saturation during exercise at high altitude and at sea level," *Circulation*, vol. 33, no. 2, pp. 249–262, 1966.

[14] J.-P. Richalet, M. V. Donoso, D. Jimenez et al., "Chilean miners commuting from sea level to 4500 m: a prospective study," *High Altitude Medicine & Biology*, vol. 3, no. 2, pp. 159–166, 2002.

[15] J. G. Farías, D. Jimenez, J. Osorio et al., "Acclimatization to chronic intermittent hypoxia in mine workers: a challenge to mountain medicine in Chile," *Biological Research*, vol. 46, no. 1, pp. 59–67, 2013.

[16] J. Brito, P. Siqués, F. León-Velarde et al., "Chronic intermittent hypoxia at high altitude exposure for over 12 years: assessment of hematological, cardiovascular, and renal effects," *High Altitude Medicine & Biology*, vol. 8, no. 3, pp. 236–244, 2007.

[17] D. Vinnikov, N. Brimkulov, and V. Krasotski, "Chronic intermittent hypoxia and blood pressure: is there risk for hypertension in healthy individuals?," *High Altitude Medicine & Biology*, vol. 17, no. 1, pp. 5–10, 2016.

[18] H. A. Ghofrani, F. Reichenberger, M. G. Kohstall et al., "Sildenafil increased exercise capacity during hypoxia at low altitudes and at Mount Everest base camp," *Annals of Internal Medicine*, vol. 141, no. 3, pp. 169–178, 2004.

[19] I. Pham, G. Wuerzner, J.-P. Richalet et al., "Endothelin receptors blockade blunts hypoxia-induced increase in PAP in humans," *European Journal of Clinical Investigation*, vol. 40, no. 3, pp. 195–202, 2010.

[20] M. A. Q. Pasha and J. H. Newman, "High-altitude disorders: pulmonary hypertension," *Chest*, vol. 137, no. 6, pp. 13S–19S, 2010.

[21] A.-M. Antezana, "Cardiovascular changes in chronic intermittent hypoxia," in *Health & Height*, G. Viscor and A. L. C. Ricart, Eds., pp. 151–155, Publicacions Universitat Barcelona, Barcelona, Spain, 2003.

[22] A. S. Sarybaev, G. Palasiewicz, D. A. Usupbaeva et al., "Effects of intermittent exposure to high altitude on pulmonary hemodynamics: a prospective study," *High Altitude Medicine & Biology*, vol. 4, no. 4, pp. 455–463, 2003.

[23] F. León-Velarde and J.-P. Richalet, "Respiratory control in residents at high altitude: physiology and pathophysiology," *High Altitude Medicine & Biology*, vol. 7, no. 2, pp. 125–137, 2006.

[24] K. Nakanishi, F. Tajima, H. Itoh et al., "Changes in atrial natriuretic peptide and brain natriuretic peptide associated with hypobaric hypoxia-induced pulmonary hypertension in rats," *Virchows Arch*, vol. 439, no. 6, pp. 808–817, 2001.

[25] A. Weidemann, B. Klanke, M. Wagner et al., "Hypoxia, via stabilization of the hypoxia-inducible factor HIF-1α, is a direct and sufficient stimulus for brain-type natriuretic peptide induction," *Biochemical Journal*, vol. 409, no. 1, pp. 233–242, 2008.

[26] M. Gao, R. Wang, and Z. Jiayong, "NT-ProBNP levels are moderately increased in acute high-altitude pulmonary edema," *Experimental and Therapeutic Medicine*, vol. 5, no. 5, pp. 1434–1438, 2013.

[27] S. Goerre, M. Wenk, P. Bärtsch et al., "Endothelin-1 in pulmonary hypertension associated with high-altitude exposure," *Circulation*, vol. 91, no. 2, pp. 359–364, 1995.

[28] I. Pham, G. Wuerzner, J. Richalet et al., "Randomized clinical trial Endothelin receptors blockade blunts hypoxia-induced increase in PAP in humans," *European Journal of Clinical Investigation*, vol. 40, no. 3, pp. 195–202, 2010.

[29] K. Katayama, Y. Sato, Y. Morotome et al., "Intermittent hypoxia increases ventilation and SaO_2 during hypoxic exercise and hypoxic chemosensitivity," *Journal of Applied Physiology*, vol. 90, no. 4, pp. 1431–1440, 2001.

[30] A. Ricart, H. Casas, M. Casas et al., "Acclimatization near home? Early respiratory changes after short-term intermittent exposure to simulated altitude," *Wilderness & Environmental Medicine*, vol. 11, no. 2, pp. 84–88, 2000.

[31] S. Greiner, A. Jud, M. Aurich et al., "Reliability of noninvasive assessment of systolic pulmonary artery pressure by doppler echocardiography compared to right heart catheterization: analysis in a large patient population," *Journal of the American Heart Association*, vol. 3, no. 4, pp. 1–8, 2014.

[32] N. Galiè, M. Humbert, J.-L. Vachiery et al., "2015 ESC/ERS guidelines for the diagnosis and treatment of pulmonary hypertension," *European Heart Journal*, vol. 37, no. 1, pp. 67–119, 2016.

Impact of Nasopharyngeal FilmArray Respiratory Panel Results on Antimicrobial Decisions in Hospitalized Patients

Kenneth K. Sakata,[1] Natalya Azadeh,[2] Anjuli Brighton,[1] M'hamed Temkit,[3] Christine L. Klassen,[4] Thomas E. Grys,[5] and Holenarasipur R. Vikram[6]

[1]*Division of Pulmonary Medicine, Mayo Clinic, Phoenix, AZ, USA*
[2]*Division of Pulmonary and Critical Care Medicine, Mayo Clinic, Rochester, MN, USA*
[3]*Division of Health Sciences and Research, Mayo Clinic Arizona, Scottsdale, AZ, USA*
[4]*Division of General Internal Medicine, Mayo Clinic, Rochester, MN, USA*
[5]*Department of Laboratory Medicine and Pathology, Mayo Clinic, Phoenix, AZ, USA*
[6]*Division of Infectious Diseases, Mayo Clinic, Phoenix, AZ, USA*

Correspondence should be addressed to Holenarasipur R. Vikram; vikram.hr@mayo.edu

Academic Editor: Alice M. Turner

Objective. To determine whether results of the nasopharyngeal FilmArray respiratory panel (NP-FARP) influenced antibiotic decisions. *Methods.* We reviewed the medical records of nonintensive care unit (ICU) inpatients that had an NP-FARP performed at our institution between June 2013 and June 2014. The inpatient records were reviewed 48 hours after the NP-FARP for the following data: demographic information; NP-FARP, serum procalcitonin, and methicillin-resistant *Staphylococcus aureus* nasal swab (MRSA NS) results; antibiotics prior and post-48 hours of the NP-FARP result; and the current immunosuppression status. Clinical outcome data were not obtained. Patients were categorized into those who had a positive (+) or a negative (−) NP-FARP. We further subdivided these two categories into groups A, B, and C based on the antibiotic modifications 48 hours after their NP-FARP result. Group A included patients who were never initiated on antimicrobial therapy. Patients whose antibiotics were discontinued or deescalated were placed in group B. Patients with antibiotic escalation or continuation without change constituted group C. We compared and analyzed groups A, B, and C in the (+) and (−) NP-FARP cohorts. *Results.* A total of 545 patients were included. There were 143 (26%) patients with positive and 402 (74%) patients with negative NP-FARPs. Comparison of groups A, B, and C between those with a (+) and (−) NP-FARP were as follows: (+) A and (−) A, 28/143 (20%) and 84/402 (21%); (+) B and (−) B, 59/143 (41%) and 147/402 (37%); and (+) C and (−) C, 56/143 (39%) and 171/402 (43%), respectively. We found no statistically significant differences between groups (+) A versus (−) A, (+) B versus (−) B, and (+) C versus (−) C with respect to age, gender, MRSA NS result, procalcitonin result, or concurrent immunosuppression. *Conclusion.* In non-ICU inpatients, NP-FARP alone or in combination with procalcitonin or MRSA NS did not influence antibiotic decisions during the study period.

1. Introduction

Respiratory tract infections remain the most common illness in humans for which urgent medical care is sought [1]. Early differentiation between bacterial infection and a self-limited viral infection is essential and continues to pose a major diagnostic challenge. Presenting symptoms of a viral respiratory illness may be indistinguishable from bacterial infections. Approximately three-quarters of all antibiotic doses are prescribed for acute viral respiratory tract infections [2]. Unnecessary antimicrobial therapy leads to increased healthcare costs, adverse events (such as *Clostridium difficile* infections), and the emergence of multidrug-resistant organisms [3]. A recent study describing the incidence of the antibiotic-associated adverse drug effect for adult inpatients receiving systemic antibiotic therapy showed that up to 20% of patients developed at least 1 antibiotic-associated adverse drug effect [4]. Twenty percent of nonclinically indicated antibiotic regimens were associated with an adverse drug effect, including 7 cases of *C. difficile* infection [4].

The nasopharyngeal FilmArray respiratory panel (NP-FARP) (BioFire Diagnostics, Salt Lake City, UT) was the first multiplex molecular panel approved in 2011 by the United States Food and Drug Administration for the detection of both bacterial and viral respiratory pathogens in nasopharyngeal swabs and was brought into our institution in February 2013. The NP-FARP targets 17 viruses and subtypes and 3 bacteria with high sensitivity and specificity. It has a fully automated sample-to-answer workflow with a turnaround-time of approximately 1 hour [5]. The performance characteristics, simplified workflow, and rapid turnaround-time have allowed its implementation in a wide range of laboratories and clinical settings.

We hypothesized that a positive NP-FARP for any of the 17 viral pathogens in the context of an absence of data supporting a bacterial infection would persuade clinicians to not initiate, discontinue, or deescalate antibiotic therapy. The primary aim of this retrospective observational study was to determine if the NP-FARP influenced antibiotic decisions. We also looked into whether the adjunctive use of serum procalcitonin, methicillin-resistant *Staphylococcus aureus* nasal swab (MRSA NS), or an immunosuppressed host impacted antibiotic decisions.

2. Materials and Methods

We reviewed the electronic medical records of all non-ICU inpatients that had an NP-FARP performed between June 1, 2013 and June 30, 2014. Inpatient progress notes and medication records were reviewed 48 hours after NP-FARP was performed to determine whether NP-FARP results led to a change in antibiotic regimens. When performed within 48 hours of the NP-FARP, procalcitonin was recorded as either not done or negative, and the MRSA NS was recorded as either not done, positive, or negative. For patients who were discharged < 48 hours after their NP-FARP, their discharge summary medication list was used. Outpatients, ICU patients, and patients with a positive procalcitonin (>0.25 μg/L) were excluded. Those who tested positive for any of the 3 atypical bacterial respiratory pathogens by NP-FARP (*Legionella* sp., *Chlamydia* sp., and *Mycoplasma* sp.) were excluded. Prophylactic antibiotic regimens in immunosuppressed patients were not considered in our analysis. Clinical outcomes were not assessed.

2.1. Definitions

2.1.1. Positive and Negative NP-FARP. A positive (+) NP-FARP identified a viral pathogen by multiplex PCR, and a negative (−) NP-FARP did not.

2.1.2. Antibiotic Decisions. All antibiotic decisions were documented based on what transpired within 48 hours of the NP-FARP result. Discontinuation of antibiotics was defined as the cessation of all empiric antimicrobial therapy. Narrowing of the antimicrobial spectrum (i.e., changing from a third-generation cephalosporin to a first-generation cephalosporin) or any decrease in the number of empiric antibiotics was termed deescalation. Patients who had their antimicrobial spectrum broadened (i.e., changing from a first-generation cephalosporin to a third-generation cephalosporin) or had any increase in the number of antibiotics after their NP-FARP results were referred to as escalation. Those who remained on the same antimicrobial regimen after the NP-FARP results were considered to continue therapy. Patients who were never initiated on antimicrobial therapy were labeled as no antibiotics and placed into group A. Discontinuation and deescalation were placed in group B. Escalation and continuation of therapy constituted group C.

2.1.3. Immunosuppression. Immunosuppression was defined as any hematologic malignancy, solid-organ or bone marrow transplantation, and/or receipt of any of the following immunosuppressive therapies at the time of the NP-FARP: cancer chemotherapy, systemic corticosteroids, therapeutic interferon preparations, tumor necrosis factor and interleukin inhibitors, azathioprine, methotrexate, calcineurin inhibitors, or mycophenolate mofetil.

2.1.4. Empiric Antimicrobial Therapy. Empiric antimicrobial therapy was defined as any antibiotic(s) apart from its prophylactic antibiotic regimen.

2.2. Statistical Methods. Our study patients were first divided into cohorts with a positive or negative NP-FARP. We further subdivided these cohorts into groups A, B, and C based on the patient's antibiotic modification 48 hours after their NP-FARP result. We compared and analyzed groups A, B, and C in the (+) and (−) NP-FARP cohorts.

The descriptives consist of frequencies and proportions for categorical variables, median, first and third quartiles, minimum, maximum, and range for continuous variables. The group comparisons were conducted using the Wilcoxon rank sum test to test for population mean shift between two groups for continuous variables. The Pearson chi-square and the Fisher's exact test were used in the presence of low frequencies to test for univariate associations between the categorical values. The significance level was at 0.05. Statistical analyses were performed using the statistical software packages SAS version 9.3 (SAS Institute, Cary, NC) and R version 3.1.2.

The study was approved by the Mayo Clinic Institutional Review Board.

3. Results

A total of 545 patients were included in the study analysis. There were 143 (26%) and 402 patients (74%) with positive and negative NP-FARPs, respectively. Comparison of groups A, B, and C between those with (+) and (−) NP-FARPs is detailed in Figure 1. In the total cohort, 64 (18%) and 226 (41%) patients underwent procalcitonin and MRSA NS testing, respectively. Within the group that had a positive NP-FARP, 17 (12%) and 53 (37%) patients had procalcitonin and MRSA NS performed, respectively. In the negative NP-FARP group,

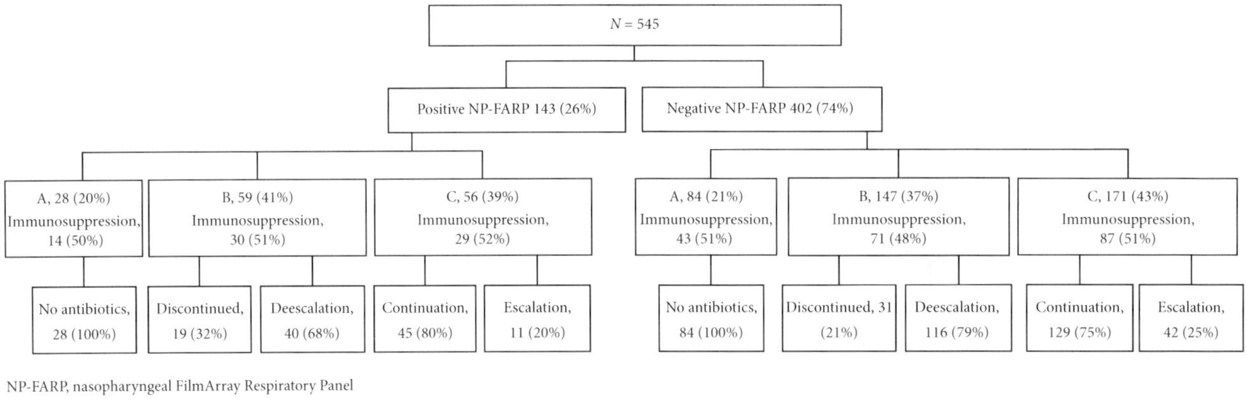

FIGURE 1: Flow diagram depicting positive and negative NP-FARP cohorts with subsequent antibiotic decisions. NP-FARP, nasopharyngeal FilmArray respiratory panel.

47 (12%) and 173 (43%) patients had procalcitonin and MRSA NS performed, respectively.

Basic demographic information, MRSA NS, and procalcitonin results, and underlying immunosuppression in groups A, B, and C are described in Table 1. We found no statistically significant differences between groups (+) A versus(−) A, (+) B versus (−) B, and (+) C versus (−) C with respect to age, gender, MRSA NS result, procalcitonin result, or concurrent immunosuppression.

Among groups B and C, the most common antibiotic regimens started prior to NP-FARP and then discontinued (group B) or added (group C) 48 hours after NP-FARP are listed in Table 2. In group B, the most common antibiotic regimen started prior to NP-FARP was the combination of anti-MRSA + β-lactam + atypical pathogen coverage. The most common antibiotic regimen discontinued after NP-FARP was the combination anti-MRSA + β-lactam. The most common antibiotic regimen started prior to NP-FARP in group C was atypical pathogen coverage, which was also the most common antibiotic added after the NP-FARP result.

Among group B, there were a total of 104 patients in whom antibiotics with anti-MRSA activity were discontinued. Of these, 67 (64%) patients had a concurrent negative MRSA NS, 6 (6%) patients had a concurrent positive MRSA NS, and 31 (30%) patients did not have an MRSA NS performed. Conversely, there were 12 patients in whom anti-MRSA antibiotic therapy was added: 8 (67%) patients did not have an MRSA NS performed, 3 (25%) patients had a negative MRSA NS, and 1 (8%) patient had a positive MRSA NS.

From group C, 150 of 227 (66%) patients had documented clinical reasons for their antibiotic continuation or escalation. The most frequently cited indications were clinical/radiographic deterioration or persistent signs and symptoms of infection. Seventy-one (31%) patients documented an identified pathogen by sputum culture or bronchoalveolar lavage, and 25 (11%) patients had an additional concurrent nonrespiratory tract infection.

4. Discussion

We hypothesized that, in non-ICU inpatients with a respiratory tract infection and the absence of evidence suggesting a bacterial etiology (i.e., positive procalcitonin or a positive bacterial culture), the identification of a viral pathogen by NP-FARP should prompt clinicians to consider withholding initiation, discontinuing, or deescalating antibiotics. ICU patients and those with a positive procalcitonin were excluded from our analysis because we felt that withholding, discontinuation, or deescalation of antibiotics would be unlikely regardless of the NP-FARP results. The similar proportions of patients between groups (+) A and (−) A, (+) B and (−) B, and (+) C and (−) C suggest that antibiotic decisions were made irrespective of NP-FARP results. Between each group, age and gender differences did not meet the statistical significance. Additional variables including MRSA NS, procalcitonin, or underlying immune suppression did not reach statistical significance, suggesting that these factors did not influence antibiotic decisions either. Therefore, NP-FARP used alone or in combination with adjunctive MRSA NS or procalcitonin does not appear to influence antibiotic decisions during the study time frame. Subgroup analysis revealed that the majority of patients who had their anti-MRSA antibiotic discontinued had a concurrent negative MRSA NS. A prior study from our institution showed that MRSA NS had a negative predictive value of 99% for excluding MRSA pneumonia [6]. The local awareness of the results of this study likely influenced a significant number of antimicrobial discontinuation decisions in group B when MRSA NS was negative.

Several studies have analyzed the clinical and economic impacts of multiplex respiratory testing [7]. In one study, comparison of outcomes of adult patients who tested positive for respiratory viruses across 2 influenza seasons was undertaken [8]. During the first season, conventional methods (viral culture, rapid antigen testing, and direct fluorescent antibody testing) were used and were compared to FARP obtained from the nasopharynx or bronchoalveolar lavage during the second season. FARP led to a significant decrease in the time to diagnosis of influenza (1.7 versus 7.7 hours) and noninfluenza viruses (1.5 versus 13.5 hours) compared to conventional methods. The study also found significantly lower odds for admission, duration of antimicrobial use, length of stay, and number of chest radiographs when influenza virus was detected by FARP [8]. Two additional studies in pediatric patients demonstrated better

Table 1: Demographics, MRSA NS, procalcitonin, and immunosuppression in groups A, B, and C.

	Group A				Group B				Group C			
	+A	−A	Total	p value	+B	−B	Total	p value	+C	−C	Total	p value
N	28	84	112		59	147	206		56	171	227	
Age				0.11[1]				0.36[1]				0.61[1]
Median	60.0	68.0	66.0		71.0	68.0	69.0		68.0	69.0	68.0	
Gender				0.44[2]				0.94[2]				0.18[2]
Female	17 (60.7%)	44 (52.4%)	61 (54.5%)		24 (40.7%)	59 (40.1%)	83 (40.3%)		33 (58.9%)	83 (48.5%)	116 (51.1%)	
Male	11 (39.3%)	40 (47.6%)	51 (45.5%)		35 (59.3%)	88 (59.9%)	123 (59.7%)		23 (41.1%)	88 (51.5%)	111 (48.9%)	
MRSA NS				0.43[3]				0.34[3]				0.67[3]
Not done	26 (92.9%)	67 (79.8%)	93 (83.0%)		31 (52.5%)	69 (46.9%)	100 (48.5%)		35 (62.5%)	94 (55.0%)	129 (56.8%)	
Negative	2 (7.1%)	16 (19.0%)	18 (16.1%)		26 (44.1%)	76 (51.7%)	102 (49.5%)		19 (33.9%)	68 (39.8%)	87 (38.3%)	
Positive	0 (0.0%)	1 (1.2%)	1 (0.9%)		2 (3.4%)	2 (1.4%)	4 (1.9%)		2 (3.6%)	9 (5.3%)	11 (4.8%)	
Procalcitonin				0.37[2]				0.52[2]				0.89[2]
Not done	25 (89.3%)	69 (82.1%)	94 (83.9%)		48 (81.4%)	125 (85.0%)	173 (84.0%)		53 (94.6%)	161 (94.2%)	214 (94.3%)	
Negative	3 (10.7%)	15 (17.9%)	18 (16.1%)		11 (18.6%)	22 (15.0%)	33 (16.0%)		3 (5.4%)	10 (5.8%)	13 (5.7%)	
Immunosuppression				0.91[2]				0.81[2]				0.91[2]
No	14 (50.0%)	41 (48.8%)	55 (49.1%)		29 (49.2%)	75 (51.0%)	104 (50.5%)		27 (48.2%)	84 (49.1%)	111 (48.9%)	
Yes	14 (50.0%)	43 (51.2%)	57 (50.9%)		30 (50.8%)	72 (49.0%)	102 (49.5%)		29 (51.8%)	87 (50.9%)	116 (51.1%)	

MRSA NS, methicillin-resistant *Staphylococcus aureus* nasal swab; [1]Wilcoxon; [2]chi-square; [3]Fisher's exact.

TABLE 2: Common antimicrobial regimens utilized to initiate (groups B and C), discontinue (group B), or escalate (group C) therapy in patients with positive (+) or negative (−) NP-FARP.

Group (+) B	
Antibiotics started	59
Anti-MRSA + β-lactam + atypical pathogen coverage	19
Atypical respiratory pathogen	14
β-lactam + atypical pathogen coverage	10
Antibiotics discontinued	59
Atypical respiratory pathogen	16
Anti-MRSA + β-lactam	14
β-lactam	9
Anti-MRSA	6
Group (−) B	
Antibiotics started	147
Anti-MRSA + β-lactam + atypical pathogen coverage	54
β-lactam + atypical pathogen coverage	29
β-lactam	27
Antibiotics discontinued	147
β-lactam	43
Anti-MRSA + β-lactam	43
Anti-MRSA	20
Group (+) C	
Antibiotics started	56
Atypical pathogen coverage	18
β-lactam	11
Anti-MRSA + β-lactam + atypical pathogen coverage	8
Antibiotics escalated	11
Anti-MRSA + β-lactam	2
β-lactam	2
Atypical pathogen coverage	2
Group (−) C	
Antibiotics started	171
Atypical pathogen coverage	49
β-lactam	27
β-lactam + atypical pathogen coverage	23
Anti-MRSA + β-lactam + atypical pathogen coverage	20
Anti-MRSA + β-lactam	18
Antibiotics escalated	42
Atypical pathogen coverage	12
β-lactam	11
Anti-MRSA	5

MRSA, methicillin-resistant *Staphylococcus aureus*.

sensitivity with NP-FARP, lower likelihood of antimicrobial therapy beyond 48 hours, decreased length of hospital stay, and isolation time [9, 10]. A single-center randomized controlled trial in adult patients presenting with acute respiratory illness found that point-of-care molecular testing with nasopharyngeal and oropharyngeal FARP led to shorter courses of antibiotics (<48 hours), shorter length of stay, and improved antiviral use for patients with influenza when compared to those in the control group who were tested by PCR assays at the discretion of the clinician [11]. Overall, there was no statistical difference in the mean duration of antibiotics and the proportion of patients who received antibiotics.

Another prospective randomized trial assessed the feasibility of using procalcitonin algorithms with nasopharyngeal and oropharyngeal FARP testing to guide antibiotic administration [12]. The investigators found no significant differences in overall antibiotic exposure or adverse events between the intervention and standard-of-care groups. Although the duration of antibiotic therapy was similar in the 2 groups, subgroup analyses of patients with the lowest risk for bacterial infection (patients with a positive FARP and a low procalcitonin level) revealed that significantly fewer patients were discharged on antibiotics and received a shorter duration of therapy compared to the nonintervention group. Importantly, investigators used a proactive communication strategy of text paging results while also simultaneously emailing the procalcitonin algorithm to providers. Such a strategy may not be feasible on a long-term basis outside the scope of a clinical trial, but some version of proactive communication will be critical to translate lab results to stewardship success.

Cost is an important consideration when utilizing novel testing strategies on a large scale. Multiplex PCR testing was the least expensive approach when compared to shell vial culture and direct fluorescent antibody testing when the prevalence of respiratory viral illness was >11% [13]. Multiplex PCR testing in the emergency room for children with influenza was cost-effective when compared with direct fluorescent antibody and traditional PCR [14]. The lab cost of each NP-FARP cartridge is approximately $125.00 USD at our institution.

Multiplex panels such as NP-FARP have several advantages and limitations. Advantages include excellent sensitivity, rapid result availability, detection of a multitude of respiratory viruses from a single sample, and ease of testing in the laboratory. They will allow better epidemiological descriptions of pathogens in a given hospital or community. They offer potential benefits such as antibiotic deescalation, shorter hospital stay, and decrease in the use of other invasive procedures for sample acquisition. Multiplex testing can identify other treatable atypical bacterial pathogens (*Chlamydia*, *Mycoplasma*, and *Bordetella pertussis*) which might otherwise be missed. Immunocompromised patients may shed respiratory viruses for a prolonged duration, and multiplex testing can identify such patients who will need to be placed in droplet isolation. However, the test result is only as good as the specimen submitted; a sample from the nose (instead of the nasopharynx) will provide a false-negative result. Viral detection will not distinguish between recent and active infection and may provide a false sense of security while masking an underlying nonviral infection as the cause of the patient's illness. Most panels do not allow for customizable ordering and testing for specific viruses and can be expensive.

There are several limitations of our study. This was a single-center retrospective observational study. Antibiotic decisions were entirely made by the clinical team, were not protocol driven, and were based on passive reporting of results to the chart since no proactive communication occurred. Patient outcomes were not recorded, and thus, we cannot comment on whether continuation, escalation, or discontinuation of antimicrobials resulted in either beneficial or adverse consequences. Impact on hospital length of stay was not determined. We did not differentiate the upper and lower respiratory tract infections in our cohort. This pilot study provided us with preliminary information pertaining to current practices and attitudes based on which future studies involving specific algorithm-driven interventions and patient outcomes can be designed. NP-FARP and procalcitonin became available at our institution in February and August 2013, respectively, and hence, providers may not have had adequate exposure and experience to fully understand and trust the utility of these tests in routine clinical practice during the study period (June 2013 to June 2014). Only 18% and 41% of patients in the total cohort, 12% and 37% of patients in the (+) NP-FARP, and 12% and 43% of patients in the (–) NP-FARP groups underwent PCT and/or MRSA NS testing, respectively. Hence, the exact contribution of each of these individual tests towards antimicrobial decisions cannot be ascertained. On the contrary, a study from our institution demonstrating an excellent negative predictive value of MRSA NS appears to have influenced provider's decision to discontinue anti-MRSA antibiotics if MRSA NS was negative with its widespread institutional publicity [6]. Repeating the current study at the present time utilizing a testing algorithm may provide us with different results.

How can the results of this study and others be utilized to improve patient outcomes and decrease unnecessary prescription of antibiotics in this era of rapidly escalating antimicrobial resistance? First, healthcare providers have to be educated about the indications for and appropriate utilization of noninvasive tests such as procalcitonin, NP-FARP, and MRSA NS to determine if a given patient has a self-limiting viral infection or another process that requires antimicrobial therapy. Algorithms involving these tests should be developed and validated in various populations (such as children, the elderly, and the immune suppressed) so that clinicians can feel confident about discontinuing or deescalating antibiotics in the absence of a bacterial infection. Such protocols will also prevent indiscriminate testing with multiplex PCR, as the cost per test is still expensive. Second, institutions should invest in a robust and all-encompassing antimicrobial stewardship program that carefully monitors antimicrobial usage, restricts indiscriminate use of broad spectrum antibiotics, and provides real-time feedback to providers. Stewardship programs can also provide guidance to clinicians regarding proper utilization of NP-FARP, procalcitonin, and other noninvasive tests and enforce early deescalation and discontinuation of antimicrobials in the appropriate clinical setting.

5. Conclusion

In our noninterventional retrospective observational study, NP-FARP alone, or in combination with procalcitonin, did not appear to influence antibiotic decisions. A negative MRSA NS appeared to have a stronger influence than positive NP-FARP as it pertains to deescalation and/or discontinuation of antibiotics. Incorporation of validated algorithms for appropriate test utilization, provider education, and antimicrobial stewardship program involvement to monitor and intervene when necessary can mitigate unnecessary NP-FARP testing and unwarranted antimicrobial therapy.

Abbreviations

HCAP: Healthcare-associated pneumonia
ICU: Intensive care unit
MRSA NS: Methicillin-resistant *Staphylococcus aureus* nasal swab
NP-FARP: Nasopharyngeal FilmArray respiratory panel.

References

[1] A. M. Fendrick, A. S. Monto, B. Nightengale, and M. Sarnes, "The economic burden of non-influenza-related viral respiratory tract infection in the United States," *Archives of Internal Medicine*, vol. 163, no. 4, pp. 487–494, 2003.

[2] J. Carlet, "Rapid diagnostic methods in the detection of sepsis," *Infectious Disease Clinics of North America*, vol. 13, no. 2, pp. 483–494, 1999.

[3] P. Schuetz, D. N. Amin, and J. L. Greenwald, "Role of procalcitonin in managing adult patients with respiratory tract infections," *Chest*, vol. 141, no. 4, pp. 1063–1073, 2012.

[4] P. D. Tamma, E. Avdic, D. X. Li, K. Dzintars, and S. E. Cosgrove, "Association of adverse events with antibiotic use in hospitalized patients," *JAMA Internal Medicined*, vol. 177, no. 9, pp. 1308–1315, 2017.

[5] N. Azadeh, K. K. Sakata, A. M. Brighton, H. R. Vikram, and T. E. Grys, "FilmArray respiratory panel assay: comparison of nasopharyngeal swabs and bronchoalveolar lavage samples," *Journal of Clinical Microbiology*, vol. 53, no. 12, pp. 3784–3787, 2015.

[6] B. Dangerfield, A. Chung, B. Webb, and M. T. Seville, "Predictive value of methicillin-resistant *Staphylococcus aureus* (MRSA) nasal swab PCR assay for MRSA pneumonia," *Antimicrobial Agents and Chemotherapy*, vol. 58, no. 2, pp. 859–864, 2014.

[7] P. Ramanan, A. L. Bryson, M. J. Binnicker, B. S. Pritt, and R. Patel, "Syndromic panel-based testing in clinical microbiology," *Clinical Microbiology Reviews*, vol. 31, no. 1, p. e00024-17, 2018.

[8] U. Rappo, A. N. Schuetz, S. G. Jenkins et al., "Impact of early detection of respiratory viruses by multiplex PCR assay on clinical outcomes in adult patients," *Journal of Clinical Microbiology*, vol. 54, no. 8, pp. 2096–2103, 2016.

[9] B. B. Rogers, P. Shankar, R. C. Jerris et al., "Impact of a rapid respiratory panel test on patient outcomes," *Archives of Pathology and Laboratory Medicine*, vol. 139, no. 5, pp. 636–641, 2015.

[10] A. Subramony, P. Zachariah, A. Krones, S. Whittier, and L. Saiman, "Impact of multiplex polymerase chain reaction testing for respiratory pathogens on healthcare resource utilization for pediatric inpatients," *Journal of Pediatrics*, vol. 173, pp. 196–201, 2016.

[11] N. J. Brendish, A. K. Malachira, and T. W. Clark, "Molecular point-of-care testing for respiratory viruses versus routine clinical care in adults with acute respiratory illness presenting to secondary care: a pragmatic randomised controlled trial protocol (ResPOC)," *BMC Infectious Diseases*, vol. 17, no. 1, p. 128, 2017.

[12] A. R. Branche, E. E. Walsh, R. Vargas et al., "Serum procalcitonin measurement and viral testing to guide antibiotic use for respiratory infections in hospitalized adults: a randomized controlled trial," *Journal of Infectious Diseases*, vol. 212, no. 11, pp. 1692–1700, 2015.

Impaired Hemorheology in Exacerbations of COPD

Erhan Ugurlu,[1] Emine Kilic-Toprak,[2] Ilknur Can,[1] Ozgen Kilic-Erkek,[2] Goksel Altinisik,[1] and Melek Bor-Kucukatay[2]

[1]*Faculty of Medicine, Department of Pulmonology, Pamukkale University, Denizli, Turkey*
[2]*Faculty of Medicine, Department of Physiology, Pamukkale University, Denizli, Turkey*

Correspondence should be addressed to Emine Kilic-Toprak; pt_emine@yahoo.com

Academic Editor: Franz Stanzel

Background. Chronic obstructive pulmonary disease (COPD) is characterized by progressive airflow limitation. Cardiovascular-related comorbidities are established to contribute to morbidity and mortality especially during exacerbations. The aim of the current study was to determine alterations in hemorheology (erythrocyte aggregation, deformability) in newly diagnosed COPD patients and their response to medical treatment and to compare with values of COPD patients with exacerbations. *Materials and Methods.* The study comprised 13 COPD patients, 12 controls, and 16 COPD patients with exacerbations. The severity of COPD was determined according to *Global Initiative for Chronic Obstructive Lung Disease* guidelines. Red blood cell (RBC) deformability and aggregation were measured by an ektacytometer. *Results.* RBC deformability of COPD patients with exacerbations was decreased compared to the other groups. Erythrocyte aggregation and plasma fibrinogen of COPD patients determined during exacerbations were higher than control. *Conclusion.* Decreased RBC deformability and increased aggregation associated with exacerbations of COPD may serve as unfavorable mechanisms to worsen oxygenation and thus clinical symptoms of the patient. Treatment modalities that modify rheological parameters might be beneficial.

1. Introduction

Chronic obstructive pulmonary disease (COPD) is a common, preventable, and manageable disease process that is characterized by progressive persistent airflow restrictions and related to increased chronic inflammatory reaction of the airways and lungs against harmful gases and particles [1]. Exacerbations of COPD are defined as the worsening of symptoms such as increment of dyspnea, phlegm volume, and phlegm purulence, usually accompanied by hypoxia and hypercapnia [2, 3]. The most common causes of COPD exacerbations are infections. Inflammation is an important component of the disease [4]. Macrophages and neutrophils play an important role in the inflammatory process [5]. On the other hand, RBC were proposed as biosensors for the stadium of COPD [6]. Nowadays, COPD treatment options include quitting smoking, pharmacological treatment (short-acting anticholinergic, short-acting beta$_2$-agonist, long-acting anticholinergic, long-acting beta$_2$-agonist, and inhaled corticosteroids), and nonpharmacological treatment (pulmonary rehabilitation) [7–9]. Aim of pharmacological treatment is to improve the quality of life and exercise tolerance beside achieving the reduction of symptoms and attacks [7, 8]. Inhaled corticosteroids specifically reduce the number of COPD exacerbations [10]. In COPD exacerbation first of all, it is important to identify the etiology. Viral and bacterial infections, air pollution, and environmental factors can initiate COPD exacerbation. Thus, antibiotics and oral steroids are choices of treatment [11].

Hemorheology is a branch of biorheology that focuses on blood and its interactions in both macro- and microcirculation under the influence of the applied constraints [12]. Erythrocyte deformability, red blood cell (RBC) aggregation, hematocrit (Hct), and blood viscosity are well-known components of hemorheology [12–14]. The flow properties of blood play significant roles in tissue perfusion. These properties are influenced by pathophysiological processes, including a variety of pulmonary diseases, thereby increasing the clinical relevance of blood rheology information [13, 15–17]. In COPD patients, RBC were shown to alter morphologically, like cytoskeleton changes, ultrastructural modifications, and reductions of glycophorin A, band 3, and RBC thiols [7, 18, 19]. Rheological blood properties were demonstrated to progressively deteriorate as pulmonary insufficiency increases in patients with chronic bronchitis [18]. There are limited number of studies exploring hemorheological alterations in COPD [16, 20–22]. The results of these studies were obtained either from COPD patients at different stages of the illness and age [18, 20, 22] or from patients receiving different types of therapy (medication, exercise) [16, 20, 23]. Additionally, different types of measurement techniques, some being rather old, were used in a variety of the studies mentioned above, which makes it difficult to compare the results [20, 21, 24]. Thus, we aimed to determine the possible alterations in RBC deformability and aggregation in newly diagnosed COPD patients and their response to medical treatment and to compare these parameters with values of COPD patients with exacerbations for the first time in the literature. The results of the current study are expected to contribute to the formation of alternative treatment options for COPD.

2. Materials and Methods

2.1. Subjects. Newly diagnosed patients with COPD as well as COPD patients with exacerbations according to the Global Initiative for Chronic Obstructive Lung Disease (GOLD) criteria at the Pulmonology Department of Pamukkale University were enrolled in the study. The severity of COPD was evaluated by the GOLD, the American Thoracic Society, and the European Respiratory Society. All subjects underwent respiratory function testing performed with the patient seated. Forced vital capacity (FVC), forced expiratory volume in the first second (FEV1), forced expiratory flow 25% to 75% (FEF 25/75), and peak expiratory flow (PEF) were measured with a clinical spirometer. We considered the predicted percentage value of air exhaled during the first second of forced expiration (pred FEV1%) and the Tiffeneau index (FEV1/FVC). In particular, pulmonary function test was evaluated in 13 newly diagnosed COPD patients before and after 1 month of medical treatment and in 16 COPD patients with exacerbations. The control group consisted of 12 subjects with comparable age and gender distribution. Among these subjects who had hypoxia (oxygen saturation $\leq 97\%$) on a pulse oximeter reading applied via the finger, smokers and patients with other systemic diseases were excluded from the study. Patients with no obvious medical problem were included in newly diagnosed group. COPD exacerbation group consisted of severe and hospitalized patients. FEV1/FVC $< 70\%$ with an expected FEV1 $> 80\%$ indicates stage 1 (mild) of the disease process; $50\% <$ FEV1 $< 80\%$ indicates stage 2 disease (moderate); $30\% <$ FEV1 $< 50\%$ indicates stage 3 disease (severe); and FEV1 $< 30\%$ indicates stage 4 disease (most severe) [1]. After obtaining pretreatment blood samples, patients were treated according to the stage of the illness. Posttreatment blood samples were taken after 1 month of treatment. Although 40 newly diagnosed patients were included in the beginning, 13 of them completed the study. Ethical approval was obtained from Pamukkale University Ethical Board on Human Experiments, with the approval number 60116787-020/35881. All participants gave their written informed consent to the study.

Treatment was in accordance with recently published guidelines. Combination of short-acting $beta_2$ agonists and/or short-acting anticholinergics was applied to stage I COPD patients, if necessary. Stage II patients were treated with long-acting anticholinergics for 1 month. COPD exacerbation group received antibiotics and oral or IV steroids.

2.2. Samples and Measurements. Venous blood samples of approximately 10 mL were drawn by venipuncture after 8 hours of fasting. Blood samples containing EDTA (1000/cs, 100/cp) were appropriately transported to the physiology laboratory and hemorheological tests were performed within 3 hours in accordance with "new guidelines for hemorheological laboratory techniques" [25]. Hematological parameters as complete blood count were determined by an electronic hematology analyzer (Siemens ADVIA® 2120i System, Siemens Healthcare Diagnostics, Japan). Sodium citrated blood samples were analyzed for plasma fibrinogen concentration using a fully automated coagulometer [Beckman COULTER Acl top 700, instrumentation laboratory (USA)].

2.3. Erythrocyte Deformability Measurements. RBC deformability was determined at various fluid shear stresses by laser diffraction analysis using an ektacytometer (laser assisted optical rotational cell analyzer (LORCA), RR Mechatronics, Hoorn, Netherlands). The system has been described elsewhere in detail [26]. Briefly, a low Hct suspension of RBC in an isotonic viscous medium (4% polyvinylpyrrolidone 360 solution; MW 360 kD; Sigma P 5288; St. Louis, MI) was sheared in a Couette system composed of a glass cup and a precisely fitting bob, with a gap of 0.3 mm between the cylinders. A laser beam was directed through the sheared sample, and the diffraction pattern produced by the deformed cells was analyzed by a microcomputer. On the basis of the geometry of the elliptical diffraction pattern, an elongation index (EI) was calculated as $EI = (L - W)/(L + W)$, where L and W are the length and width of the diffraction pattern, respectively. EI values were determined for 9 shear stresses between 0.3 and 30 Pa and similar patterns of RBC deformability alterations were obtained between groups at all stress levels. All measurements were carried out at 37°C. Subsequently, the shear stress for half-maximal deformation (SS1/2) was calculated using this nine-point data set for each measurement by employing a Lineweaver–Burk analysis as described elsewhere [27]. Briefly, the shear stress-EI curve was linearized by plotting the reciprocal of EI as a function of the reciprocal of shear stress: $1/EI = [(SS1/2/EImax)(I/SS)] + 1/EImax$, where SS is shear stress and EImax is the theoretical EI at infinite shear stress. The x-intercept of this line corresponds to the negative reciprocal value of shear stress causing half-maximal deformation (i.e., SS1/2); increased SS1/2 values indicate decreased RBC deformability.

2.4. Erythrocyte Aggregation Measurements. RBC aggregation was also determined by LORCA as described elsewhere [26]. The measurement is based on the detection of laser

Table 1: Laboratory data of the groups.

Parameter	Control group ($n = 12$)	Newly diagnosed patient group: Before treatment ($n = 13$)	Newly diagnosed patient group: After treatment ($n = 13$)	Exacerbation group ($n = 16$)	p_1	p_2
Hb (g/dl)	15.24 ± 1.75	15.54 ± 1.82	15.28 ± 1.51	**13.57 ± 2.27**$^{\beta}$	0.052	**0.033**
Hct (%)	44.95 ± 5.42	47.45 ± 6.17	45.78 ± 3.88	**40.93 ± 6.35**$^{\#,\beta}$	**0.013**	**0.045**
RBC (m/μL)	5.06 ± 0.61	5.21 ± 0.74	5.05 ± 0.55	4.57 ± 0.82	0.149	0.106
MCV (fL)	88.96 ± 3.73	91.41 ± 6.57	91.08 ± 5.81	90.13 ± 6.65	0.607	0.804
MCH (pg)	30.17 ± 0.97	29.98 ± 2.35	30.34 ± 2.07	29.83 ± 2.09	0.905	0.753
MCHC (g/dl)	33.95 ± 0.79	32.80 ± 1.07	33.32 ± 1.32	33.13 ± 1.41	0.060	0.246
WBC (K/uL)	7.41 ± 1.53	8.33 ± 1.85	8.66 ± 1.80	9.88 ± 5.40	0.228	0.231
Plt (K/uL)	214.64 ± 31.34	242.69 ± 49.77	242.38 ± 35.62	274.19 ± 154.62	0.263	0.175
Fibrinogen (mg/dL)	321.18 ± 115.24	312 ± 86.57	292.27 ± 74.51	**446.44 ± 193.65**$^{*,\#,\beta}$	**0.014**	**0.005**
RDW (%)	12.81 ± 0.77	13.99 ± 1.23	13.93 ± 1.34	**15.18 ± 1.62**$^{*,\#}$	**0.001**	**0.0001**

Values are expressed as means ± SD (Hb: hemoglobin, Hct: hematocrit, RBC: red blood cell, MCV: mean corpuscular volume, MCH: mean corpuscular hemoglobin, MCHC: mean corpuscular hemoglobin concentration, WBC: white blood cell, Plt: platelet count, and RDW: red blood cell distribution width). p_1: difference between the control group, before treatment of newly diagnosed COPD, and the exacerbation group; p_2: difference between the control group, after treatment of newly diagnosed COPD, and the exacerbation group; $^{*}p < 0.05$: difference from control, $^{\#}p < 0.05$: difference from before treatment of COPD, and $^{\beta}p < 0.05$: difference from after treatment of COPD.

backscattering from the sheared (disaggregated) and then unsheared (aggregating) blood, performed in a computer-assisted system at 37°C. Backscattering data were evaluated by the computer and the aggregation index (AI), aggregation half time ($t1/2$), and aggregation amplitude (AMP) were calculated on the basis that there is less light backscattered from aggregating red cells. Aggregation measurements were determined using RBC in autologous plasma adjusted to 40% Hct and blood was fully oxygenated before the measurements.

2.5. Statistical Analyses. Continuous variables were expressed as mean ± standard deviation (SD), median (minimum–maximum values), and categorical variables as number and percent. Shapiro-Wilk tests were used for testing normality. If parametric test conditions were satisfied, Analysis of Variance (ANOVA) was used for comparisons among groups. The post hoc Tukey test was used when the ANOVA determined a significant difference. If parametric test conditions were not satisfied, the Kruskal-Wallis Variance Analysis was used for comparisons among groups. The post hoc Mann–Whitney U Test with Bonferroni Correction was used when the Kruskal-Wallis Variance Analysis determined a significant difference. For pairwise comparisons, if parametric test conditions were satisfied, Paired Samples t-test was used and if parametric test conditions were not satisfied, Wilcoxon signed rank test was used. All statistical analyses were done by SPSS 21.0. Power of the study was found to be over 95% with 95% confidence ($\alpha = 0.05$).

3. Results

Table 1 shows the demographic characteristics and laboratory data of the groups. The study enrolled 13 newly diagnosed COPD patients (13 male) (mean age was 58.46 ± 9.72 years), 16 COPD patients with exacerbations (mean age was 67.75 ± 8.29 years), and 12 age and sex matched healthy controls (12 male) (mean age was 54.16 ± 11.4 years) ($p > 0.05$). The patients had a 48.8 ± 16.3 pack-years smoking history. RDW of COPD patients during exacerbations was higher compared to control and pretreatment of newly diagnosed patients groups ($p = 0.0001$ and $p = 0.039$, resp.), whereas fibrinogen level of this group was higher than all the other groups ($p < 0.05$). Additionally, Hb of COPD patients during exacerbations was less than posttreatment group ($p = 0.05$) and Hct of these patients were lower compared to both pre- and posttreatment groups ($p = 0.003$ and $p = 0.05$, resp.). There was no other statistically significant alteration between the parameters demonstrated in Table 1 ($p > 0.05$).

Table 2 shows pulmonary function test results of the subjects. Mean baseline predicted value of FEV1, FEV1/FVC, PEF, and FEF 25/75 of control group were significantly higher than COPD patients ($p < 0.05$). The treatment applied in newly diagnosed patients did not cause statistically significant alterations in pulmonary function test results. FVC ($p = 0.001$), FEV1, FEV1/FVC, and FEF 25/75 ($p = 0.0001$) of COPD patients with exacerbations were lower than control group while PEF of these patients were decreased compared to both control group and COPD patients receiving treatment ($p = 0.0001$ and $p = 0.031$, resp.).

Erythrocyte deformability (i.e., the elongation index, EI) for the RBC of the experimental groups was measured at nine shear stresses between 0.3 and 30.0 pascal (Pa) and shown in Table 3. RBC deformability of COPD patients with exacerbations measured at 0.53–30.00 Pa was decreased compared to control. On the other hand, EI of the same group measured at 0.30–9.49 Pa was lower than COPD patients receiving treatment ($p < 0.05$).

TABLE 2: Pulmonary function test results of the subjects.

Pulmonary function test	Control group ($n = 12$)	Newly diagnosed patient group: Before treatment ($n = 13$)	Newly diagnosed patient group: After treatment ($n = 13$)	Exacerbation group ($n = 16$)	p_1	p_2
FVC (%)	97.67 ± 14.07	82.23 ± 13.97	88.77 ± 16.10	**68.5 ± 30.63***	**0.005**	**0.006**
FEV_1 (%)	99.25 ± 12.83	**66.69 ± 13.83***	**75.54 ± 20.14***	**64.36 ± 16.10***	**0.0001**	**0.0001**
FEV_1/FVC ratio	82.58 ± 6.04	**63.85 ± 4.71***	**64.46 ± 8.66***	**60.93 ± 8.13***	**0.0001**	**0.0001**
PEF (%)	90.33 ± 12.06	**64.69 ± 16.12***	**70.54 ± 24.56***	**46.88 ± 29.38**$^{*,\beta}$	**0.0001**	**0.0001**
FEF 25–75 (%)	90.67 ± 20.83	**35.38 ± 9.40***	**42.08 ± 14.51***	**25.38 ± 16.20***	**0.0001**	**0.0001**

Values are expressed as means ± SD (FEV_1: forced expiratory volume in the first second, FVC: forced vital capacity, PEF: peak expiratory flow, and FEF 25/75: forced expiratory flow 25% to 75%). p_1: difference between the control group, before treatment of newly diagnosed COPD, and the exacerbation group; p_2: difference between the control group, after treatment of newly diagnosed COPD, and the exacerbation group; $^*p < 0.05$: difference from control, $^\#p < 0.05$: difference from before treatment of COPD, and $^\beta p < 0.05$: difference from after treatment of COPD. p_1 and p_2 are findings via ANOVA whereas other symbols are findings by comparison of two groups.

TABLE 3: The EI values of the groups at different shear stresses.

Shear stress (Pa)	Control group ($n = 12$)	Newly diagnosed patient group: Before treatment ($n = 13$)	Newly diagnosed patient group: After treatment ($n = 13$)	Exacerbation group ($n = 16$)	p_1	p_2
0.30	0.06 ± 0.03	0.06 ± 0.02	0.05 ± 0.02	**0.04 ± 0.01**$^\#$	**0.039**	0.333
0.53	0.12 ± 0.05	0.12 ± 0.05	0.08 ± 0.04	**0.05 ± 0.01**$^{*,\#}$	**0.010**	**0.001**
0.95	0.21 ± 0.08	0.21 ± 0.08	0.17 ± 0.057	**0.12 ± 0.02**$^{*,\#}$	**0.002**	**0.001**
1.69	0.33 ± 0.10	0.31 ± 0.09	0.26 ± 0.07	**0.22 ± 0.02**$^{*,\#}$	**0.002**	**0.001**
3.00	0.41 ± 0.07	0.40 ± 0.08	0.36 ± 0.06	**0.32 ± 0.02**$^{*,\#}$	**0.001**	**0.001**
5.33	0.49 ± 0.05	0.47 ± 0.06	0.45 ± 0.06	**0.42 ± 0.02**$^{*,\#}$	**0.001**	**0.001**
9.49	0.55 ± 0.04	0.54 ± 0.05	0.51 ± 0.05	**0.50 ± 0.02**$^{*,\#}$	**0.001**	**0.003**
16.87	0.60 ± 0.04	0.59 ± 0.04	0.57 ± 0.04	**0.55 ± 0.02***	**0.006**	**0.002**
30.00	0.63 ± 0.04	0.63 ± 0.04	0.61 ± 0.04	**0.59 ± 0.02***	**0.007**	**0.017**

Values are expressed as means ± SD; EI: elongation index and Pa: pascal. p_1: difference between the control group, before treatment of newly diagnosed COPD, and the exacerbation group; p_2: difference between the control group, after treatment of newly diagnosed COPD, and the exacerbation group; $^*p < 0.05$: difference from control, $^\#p < 0.05$: difference from before treatment of COPD, and $^\beta p < 0.05$: difference from after treatment of COPD. p_1 and p_2 are findings via ANOVA whereas other symbols are findings by comparison of two groups.

Table 4 demonstrates that EImax and SS1/2 of the exacerbation group were statistically significantly higher than the other groups ($p < 0.05$).

Erythrocyte aggregation parameters (AI and $t_{1/2}$) are demonstrated in Table 5. AI ($p = 0.0001$) of COPD patients determined during exacerbations was higher whereas $t_{1/2}$ ($p = 0.001$) was lower compared to control group. Increment of AI is in concordance with decrement of $t_{1/2}$ and indicates augmentation of RBC aggregation.

4. Discussion

COPD is a leading cause of mortality and morbidity with increasing prevalence worldwide [28, 29]. It is a progressive condition characterized by a poorly reversible airflow limitation associated with an abnormal inflammatory response of the lung. There is evidence that, in different lung diseases, including COPD, blood cells may undergo distinct alterations. Erythrocytes are affected at different levels in COPD, including structural alterations [23, 30]. Furthermore, emerging themes in RBC biology support the new concept that erythrocytes are also signalling cells [31, 32], with important roles in the regulation of biochemical interactions with other cells in (patho) physiology. Hypoxia is one of the prognostic factors in COPD [21]. Tissue oxygenation depends on three factors: (1) the functional integrity of the pulmonary, cardiac, and vascular system, (2) the quantity and quality of the hemoglobin molecule and binding of oxygen to hemoglobin, and (3) the flow characteristics of the blood (hemorheology) [33, 34]. Blood flow, RBC aggregation, and deformability are main components of hemorheology. In the microcirculation, RBC must collapse to pass through narrow capillaries; hence, RBC deformability and aggregation are major determinants of resistance to flow. The ability of the entire RBC to deform is critically important to perform its function of oxygen delivery and is also a determinant of cell

Table 4: The EImax and SS1/2 values of the groups.

	Control group ($n = 12$)	Patient group ($n = 13$) Before treatment	After treatment	Exacerbation group ($n = 16$)	p_1	p_2
EImax	0.64 ± 0.21	0.68 ± 0.24	0.66 ± 0.37	**0.83 ± 0.15**$^{*,\#,\beta}$	**0.001**	**0.0001**
SS1/2	2.06 ± 1.29	3.16 ± 3.65	4.64 ± 7,92	**6.17 ± 3.3**$^{*,\#,\beta}$	**0.0001**	**0.0001**

Values are expressed as means ± SD; EImax: theoretical EI at infinite shear stress and SS1/2: shear stress at half-maximal deformation. p_1: difference between the control group, before treatment of newly diagnosed COPD, and the exacerbation group; p_2: difference between the control group, after treatment of newly diagnosed COPD, and the exacerbation group; $^*p < 0.05$: difference from control, $^\#p < 0.05$: difference from before treatment of COPD, and $^\beta p < 0.05$: difference from after treatment of COPD. p_1 and p_2 are findings via ANOVA whereas other symbols are findings by comparison of two groups.

Table 5: The RBC aggregation measurements of the groups.

	Control group ($n = 12$)	Newly diagnosed patient group Before treatment ($n = 13$)	After treatment ($n = 13$)	Exacerbation group ($n = 16$)	p_1	p_2
AMP (au)	25.0 ± 2.91	25.1 ± 3.90	24.65 ± 3.18	**20.77 ± 3.59**$^{*,\#,\beta}$	**0.002**	**0.002**
AI (%)	68.15 ± 5.90	72.33 ± 6.16	73.16 ± 8.17	**79.96 ± 3.61***	**0.0001**	**0.007**
$t1/2$ (sn)	1.79 ± 0.55	1.45 ± 0.55	1.39 ± 0.68	**1.01 ± 0.37***	**0.001**	**0.003**

Values are expressed as means ± SD; AMP: amplitude of aggregation; AI: aggregation index; $t1/2$: aggregation half time. p_1: difference between the control group, before treatment of newly diagnosed COPD, and the exacerbation group; p_2: difference between the control group, after treatment of newly diagnosed COPD, and the exacerbation group; $^*p < 0.05$: difference from control, $^\#p < 0.05$: difference from before treatment of COPD, and $^\beta p < 0.05$: difference from after treatment of COPD.

survival time in the circulation [35, 36]. RBC aggregation is a reversible process meaning a temporary linear or branched aggregate formation of the erythrocytes under critically low shear stress conditions. The physiological importance of erythrocyte aggregation which is the reversible adhesion of adjacent erythrocytes in circulation is its tendency to increase the blood viscosity in low shear flow and to disturb the passage in capillary circulation [37, 38].

Current study demonstrates hemorheological parameters (i.e., RBC deformability and aggregation) in newly diagnosed stage 1-2 COPD patients and the alterations in these parameters in response to one-month medical treatment and compares these parameters with values of COPD patients during acute exacerbations. RDW of COPD patients during exacerbations was increased, and Hb and Hct decreased as expected [39, 40]. No statistically significant alteration was observed in deformability of the RBC of the newly diagnosed experimental groups measured at nine shear stresses between 0.3 and 30.0 Pa as well as Elmax and SS1/2 values. Similar to our results, Karul et al. found no difference in osmotic fragility of stable COPD patients compared to controls [21]. On the other hand, Coppola et al. measured erythrocyte filterability in 15 COPD patients of 67–79 years old and found it decreased [20]. Santini et al. demonstrated an increase in membrane rigidity in erythrocytes of COPD patients with respect to controls. According to the authors, this increase in red cell rigidity might be due to enhanced sphingomyelin values [30]. Index of RBC deformability was also found to be decreased in chronic cor pulmonale decompensation [18, 22]. The disparity in RBC deformability results seems to be due to the technique used, age of the patients, severity of the disease, and the presence of complications. LORCA (laser assisted optical rotational cell analyzer) which is an up-to-date device to measure RBC deformability and aggregation with a good repetition of consecutive measurements was used in our study. Results of the current study demonstrate for the first time in the literature that RBC deformability of COPD patients with exacerbations is lower than both healthy subjects (at 0.53–30.00 Pa) and newly diagnosed COPD patients receiving treatment (at 0.30–9.49 Pa). It was mentioned before that impaired RBC deformability leads to increased SS1/2 values. The shear stress level of normal pulmonary circulation was demonstrated to be around 2-3 Pa [41]. This information increases the importance of the reduced RBC deformability determined at 1.69 and 3 Pa in COPD exacerbations, herein. When EImax and SS1/2 values were evaluated, erythrocyte deformability of the COPD patients with exacerbations was also found to be lower compared to COPD patients before treatment. These reports support the suggestion that presentation and comparison of data via this approach may provide a more comprehensive view of RBC stress-deformation behavior compared to shear stress-EI curves since it utilizes the entire range of shear stress [27]. The relations between pressure and blood flow become more complex in the microcirculation as the vessel diameter approaches average RBC size [42]. In addition to the existing lung pathology, decreased RBC deformability in COPD patients during exacerbations may serve as an unfavorable factor to worsen the clinical condition of the patient by further disrupting tissue oxygenation.

Another hemorheological parameter measured in our study is the RBC aggregation. The aggregation index (AI) and aggregation half time ($t1/2$) of newly diagnosed COPD patients were not different from healthy subjects. One month of appropriate treatment did not cause any statistically significant alteration in the aggregation parameters of the patients nor the FVC, PEF, and FEV_1/FVC ratio. AI of COPD patients with exacerbations was higher whereas $t_{1/2}$ was lower than healthy subjects. Increment of AI is in concordance with decrement of $t_{1/2}$ and indicates augmentation of RBC aggregation. Similarly, Osipova et al. evaluated hemorheological properties by spontaneous aggregation of erythrocytes and observed a concurrently higher aggregation of erythrocytes in patients with COPD. The rheological blood properties worsened as hypertension of the small blood-circulation circle was increasing [43]. Index of RBC aggregation was found to increase in chronic cor pulmonale decompensation [18, 22]. Functional disturbances of erythrocytes in chronic bronchitis patients were shown to aggravate the course of the disease and need correction with membrane-stabilizing and membrane-repairing drugs [15, 18]. Plasma fibrinogen level is known as one of the most important determinants of RBC aggregation. The tendency to aggregate increases as fibrinogen concentration rises [34]. Thus, increased fibrinogen level observed in our COPD exacerbation group may provide an explanation for the augmentation of RBC aggregation in this group. Additionally, although not determined in our study, increases in plasma levels of inflammatory cytokines IL-6 and IL-8 were demonstrated in acute exacerbations of COPD [44] which may also alter RBC aggregation. It is also worth noting here that, in addition to decreased RBC deformability, increment of erythrocyte aggregation in COPD patients with exacerbation may also further play a role in diminishing circulation.

Oxidative stress represents one of the key mechanisms in the development of COPD [45]. Numerous studies have shown that oxidative stress is increased in lungs and systemic circulation of patients with COPD [46–50]. Markers of oxidative stress were found to increase even further during exacerbations of COPD [51] and in patients with very severe form of this disease [52]. Some studies have also demonstrated a marked decrease in plasma antioxidant capacity of COPD patients, while other studies have shown opposite findings [53]. RBC mechanical properties (i.e., erythrocyte deformability and aggregation) are known to be altered in response to oxidative stress [54, 55]. Although possible changes in oxidative stress parameters were not investigated in our study, due to the above information, it can be speculated here that impaired hemorheology herein may at least partly be due to increased oxidative stress in these patients.

5. Conclusion

In overview, the results of the current study indicate that exacerbations of COPD are characterized by significant hemorheological abnormalities known to adversely affect blood flow. The decrement observed in RBC deformability and the increment shown in erythrocyte aggregation during exacerbations might complement other pathophysiologic mechanisms, leading to worsening of oxygenation and thus clinical symptoms. The mechanisms of the hemorheological alterations could not be clarified. Oxidative stress and inflammation may be involved. Therapeutic approaches including antioxidants for normalizing hemorheological parameters during exacerbations of COPD may also be recommended. However, whether therapies to decrease RBC aggregation and enhance deformability directly and specifically can be developed and whether such therapies will relieve the patient's symptoms remain an area of active investigation. Further research with a larger number of patients to explain the mechanisms of hemorheological alterations may be necessary.

Disclosure

The funding organizations had no role in the design and conduct of the study; the collection, management, analysis, and interpretation of the data; the preparation, review, or approval of the manuscript; or the decision to submit the manuscript for publication. The abstract of this study was presented as an oral presentation in the 42nd National Physiology Congress (Düzce University, Konuralp Campus, Turkey, 5–8 September 2016) by Emine Kilic-Toprak and published in a supplement of the Acta Physiologica Journal (Sep 2016, vol 218 S709, p. 12).

Authors' Contributions

Erhan Ugurlu contributed to the study design and data collection, performed the statistical analysis, interpreted the data, drafted the manuscript, reviewed the radiology, assessed the severity of disease, and assisted with manuscript composition. Emine Kilic-Toprak contributed to the study design and data collection, performed the statistical analysis, interpreted the data, and drafted the manuscript. Ilknur Can contributed to the study design and data collection, performed the statistical analysis, interpreted the data, and drafted the manuscript. Ozgen Kilic-Erkek contributed to the study design, performed the data collection, and helped to draft the manuscript. Göksel Altinisik contributed to the study design, data acquisition, and reading and approving the final manuscript. Melek Bor-Kucukatay contributed to study design and writing the manuscript and revision of manuscript for important intellectual content and reading and approving the final manuscript.

References

[1] J. Vestbo, S. S. Hurd, A. G. Agustí et al., "Global strategy for the diagnosis, management, and prevention of chronic obstructive pulmonary disease," *American Journal of Respiratory and Critical Care Medicine*, vol. 187, no. 4, pp. 347–365, 2013.

[2] E. Merinopoulou, M. Raluy-Callado, S. Ramagopalan, S. Maclachlan, and J. M. Khalid, "COPD exacerbations by disease severity in England," *International Journal of COPD*, vol. 11, no. 1, pp. 697–709, 2016.

[3] Y. Duan, M. Zhou, J. Xiao et al., "Prediction of key genes and miRNAs responsible for loss of muscle force in patients during an acute exacerbation of chronic obstructive pulmonary disease," *International Journal of Molecular Medicine*, vol. 38, no. 5, pp. 1450–1462, 2016.

[4] S. Santos, A. Marin, J. Serra-Batlles et al., "Treatment of patients with COPD and recurrent exacerbations: the role of infection and inflammation," *International Journal of COPD*, vol. 11, no. 1, pp. 515–525, 2016.

[5] M. Decramer, W. Janssens, and M. Miravitlles, "Chronic obstructive pulmonary disease," *The Lancet*, vol. 379, no. 9823, pp. 1341–1351, 2012.

[6] G. Lucantoni, D. Pietraforte, P. Matarrese et al., "The red blood cell as a biosensor for monitoring oxidative imbalance in chronic obstructive pulmonary disease: An ex vivo and in vitro study," *Antioxidants and Redox Signaling*, vol. 8, no. 7-8, pp. 1171–1182, 2006.

[7] B. Han, W. J. Poppinga, H. Zuo et al., "The novel compound Sul-121 inhibits airway inflammation and hyperresponsiveness in experimental models of chronic obstructive pulmonary disease," *Scientific Reports*, vol. 6, Article ID 26928, 2016.

[8] M. Osthoffa, C. Jenkins, and J. D. Leuppi, "Chronic obstructive pulmonary disease-A treatable disease," *Swiss Medical Weekly*, vol. 143, Article ID w13777, 2013.

[9] K. J. Davis, S. H. Landis, Y.-M. Oh et al., "Continuing to confront COPD international physician survey: physician knowledge and application of COPD management guidelines in 12 countries," *International Journal of COPD*, vol. 9, pp. 597–611, 2014.

[10] J. Vestbo, R. Pauwels, J. A. Anderson, P. Jones, and P. Calverley, "Early onset of effect of salmeterol and fluticasone propionate in chronic obstructive pulmonary disease," *Thorax*, vol. 60, no. 4, pp. 301–304, 2005.

[11] Global Strategy for the Diagnosis, Management and Prevention of COPD: Global Initiative for Chronic Obstructive Lung Disease (GOLD) 2017, http://goldcopd.org/gold-2017-global-strategy-diagnosis-management-prevention-copd.

[12] A. V. Muravyov, S. V. Draygin, N. N. Eremin, and A. A. Muravyov, "The microrheological behavior of young and old red blood cells in athletes," *Clinical Hemorheology and Microcirculation*, vol. 26, pp. 183–188, 2002.

[13] M. J. Simmonds, H. J. Meiselman, and O. K. Baskurt, "Blood rheology and aging," *Journal of Geriatric Cardiology*, vol. 10, no. 3, pp. 291–301, 2013.

[14] I. A. Tikhomirova, A. O. Oslyakova, and S. G. Mikhailova, "Microcirculation and blood rheology in patients with cerebrovascular disorders," *Clinical Hemorheology and Microcirculation*, vol. 49, pp. 295–305, 2011.

[15] E. A. Stepovaya, V. V. Novitskiĭ, N. V. Ryazantseva, V. E. Gol'dberg, and etal., "Chronic bronchitis: participation of red cells in the pathologic process," *Klinicheskaia Meditsina*, vol. 82, pp. 53–56, 2004.

[16] B. Ahmad, N. Ferrari, G. Montiel et al., "Influence of a moderate physical activity intervention on red cell deformability in patients suffering from chronic obstructive pulmonary disease (COPD)," *Wiener Medizinische Wochenschrift*, vol. 163, no. 13-14, pp. 334–339, 2013.

[17] E. Ugurlu, E. Kilic-Toprak, G. Altinisik, and etal., "Increased erythrocyte aggregation and oxidative stress in patients with idiopathic interstitial pneumonia," *Sarcoidosis, Vasculitis and Diffuse Lung Diseases*, vol. 33, pp. 308–316, 2016.

[18] I. P. Danilov and A. E. Makarevich, "Mechanisms of blood rheological disorders and their role in the progression of chronic obstructive bronchitis," *Terapevticheskii Arkhiv*, vol. 57, no. 3, pp. 19–22, 1985.

[19] J. Zhou, D. Wu, Y. Zhu, D. Ding, and F. Peng, "Hemorrheological status in patients with silicosis and its clinical significance," *Zhonghua Yu Fang Yi Xue Za Zhi*, vol. 33, no. 6, pp. 348–350, 1999.

[20] L. Coppola, G. Verrazzo, G. Esposito et al., "Hemorheological and cardiovascular effects of exercise training in the rehabilitation of elderly patients with chronic obstructive pulmonary disease," *Archives of Gerontology and Geriatrics*, vol. 28, no. 1, pp. 1–8, 1999.

[21] A. B. Karul, F. Karadag, D. Kozaci, and C. Altun, "Erythrocyte fragility is not altered in stablechronic obstructive pulmonary diseasewith normal arterial pH," *Clinical Hemorheology and Microcirculation*, vol. 28, pp. 107–112, 2003.

[22] O. N. Verbitskii, I. V. Buturov, and T. Iu. Purkh, "hemodynamics, blood gas composition and viscosity in patients with chronic obstructive bronchitis complicated by chronic cor pulmonale," *Probl Tuberk Bolezn Legk*, vol. 7, pp. 42–45, 2004.

[23] E. Straface, P. Matarrese, L. Gambardella et al., "N-acetylcysteine counteracts erythrocyte alterations occurring in chronic obstructive pulmonary disease," *Biochemical and Biophysical Research Communications*, vol. 279, no. 2, pp. 552–556, 2000.

[24] M. Piagnerelli, K. Zouaoui Boudjeltia, D. Brohee et al., "Assessment of erythrocyte shape by flow cytometry techniques," *Journal of Clinical Pathology*, vol. 60, no. 5, pp. 549–554, 2007.

[25] O. K. Baskurt, M. Boynard, G. C. Cokelet, and etal., "International expert panel for standardization of hemorheological methods. New guidelines for hemorheological laboratory techniques," *Clinical Hemorheology and Microcirculation*, vol. 42, pp. 75–97, 2009.

[26] M. R. Hardeman, P. Goedhart, and S. Shin, "Methods in hemorheology," in *Handbook of Hemorheology and Hemodynamics*, O. K. Baskurt, M. R. Hardeman, M. R. Rampling, and H. J. Meiselman, Eds., pp. 242–266, IOS Press, Amsterdam, The Netherlands, 2007.

[27] O. K. Baskurt and H. J. Meiselman, "Analyzing shear stress-elongation index curves: comparison of two approaches to simplify data presentation," *Clinical Hemorheology and Microcirculation*, vol. 31, pp. 23–30, 2004.

[28] A. D. Lopez, K. Shibuya, C. Rao et al., "Chronic obstructive pulmonary disease: current burden and future projections," *European Respiratory Journal*, vol. 27, no. 2, pp. 397–412, 2006.

[29] Global strategy for the diagnosis, management, and prevention of COPD: Global Initiative for Chronic Obstructive Lung Disease (GOLD) 2014, http://www.goldcopd.org/.

[30] M. T. Santini, E. Straface, A. Cipri, M. Peverini, M. Santulli, and W. Malorni, "Structural alterations in erythrocytes from patients with chronic obstructive pulmonary disease," *Haemostasis*, vol. 27, no. 4, pp. 201–210, 1997.

[31] L. Yang, D. A. Andrews, and P. S. Low, "Lysophosphatidic acid opens a Ca^{++} channel in human erythrocytes," *Blood*, vol. 95, no. 7, pp. 2420–2425, 2000.

[32] J. R. Pawloski, D. T. Hes, and J. S. Stamler, "Export by red blood cells of nitric oxide bioactivity," *Nature*, vol. 409, no. 6820, pp. 622–626, 2001.

[33] O. K. Baskurt and H. J. Meiselman, "Blood rheology and hemodynamics," *Seminars in Thrombosis and Hemostasis*, vol. 29, no. 5, pp. 435–450, 2003.

[34] O. K. Baskurt, "Pathophysiological significance of blood rheology," *Turkish Journal of Medical Sciences*, vol. 33, pp. 347–355, 2003.

[35] Z. Y. Wen, L. C. Song, Z. Y. Yan et al., "An animal model to study erythrocyte, senescence with a narrow time window of

erythrocyte production: Alterations in osmotic fragility and deformability of erythrocytes during their life span," *Clinical Hemorheology and Microcirculation*, vol. 19, pp. 299–306, 1998.

[36] G. Cicco and A. Pirrelli, "Red blood cell (RBC) deformability, RBC aggregability and tissue oxygenation in hypertension," *Clinical Hemorheology and Microcirculation*, vol. 21, no. 3-4, pp. 169–177, 1999.

[37] B. Hiebl, C. Mrowietz, S. Lee et al., "Influence of rheological parameters on the velocity of erythrocytes passing nailfold capillaries in humans," *Microvascular Research*, vol. 48, pp. 129–139, 2011.

[38] O. K. Baskurt and H. J. Meiselman, "Erythrocyte aggregation: basic aspects and clinical importance," *Clinical Hemorheology and Microcirculation*, vol. 53, pp. 23–27, 2013.

[39] R. Farah, R. Ibrahim, M. Nassar, D. Najib, Y. Zivony, and E. Eshel, "Neutrophil lymphocyte ratio better addition to CRP than CD64 index as marker for infection in COPD," *Panminerva Med*, vol. 9, 2017.

[40] E. Günay, S. Sarinç Ulaşli, O. Akar et al., "Neutrophil-to-lymphocyte ratio in chronic obstructive pulmonary disease: a retrospective study," *Inflammation*, vol. 37, no. 2, pp. 374–380, 2014.

[41] M. Schäfer, V. O. Kheyfets, J. D. Schroeder et al., "Main pulmonary arterial wall shear stress correlates with invasive hemodynamics and stiffness in pulmonary hypertension," *Pulmonary Circulation*, vol. 6, no. 1, pp. 37–45, 2016.

[42] H. H. Lipowsky, "Microvascular rheology and hemodynamics," *Microcirculation*, vol. 12, no. 1, pp. 5–15, 2005.

[43] O. L. Osipova, V. E. Perleĭ, G. P. Orlova, A. I. U. Gichkin, and N. G. Iakovleva, "Blood rheological properties and their interrelation with pulmonary hypertension in patients with chronic dust bronchitis," in *Kliniceskaja Laboratornaja Diagnostika*, vol. 8, pp. 30-31, 2004.

[44] V. Austin, P. J. Crack, S. Bozinovski, A. A. Miller, and R. Vlahos, "COPD and stroke: are systemic inflammation and oxidative stress the missing links?" *Clinical Science*, vol. 130, no. 13, pp. 1039–1050, 2016.

[45] J. E. Repine, A. Bast, and I. Lankhorst, "Oxidative stress in chronic obstructive pulmonary disease," *American Journal of Respiratory and Critical Care Medicine*, vol. 156, no. 2 I, pp. 341–357, 1997.

[46] P. A. Kirkham and P. J. Barnes, "Oxidative stress in COPD," *Chest*, vol. 144, no. 1, pp. 266–273, 2013.

[47] U. Can, F. H. Yerlikaya, and S. Yosunkaya, "Role of oxidative stress and serum lipid levels in stable chronic obstructive pulmonary disease," *Journal of the Chinese Medical Association*, vol. 78, no. 12, pp. 702–708, 2015.

[48] R. C. J. Langen, S. H. Korn, and E. F. M. Wouters, "ROS in the local and systemic pathogenesis of COPD," *Free Radical Biology and Medicine*, vol. 35, no. 3, pp. 226–235, 2003.

[49] W. MacNee, "Pulmonary and systemic oxidant/antioxidant imbalance in chronic obstructive pulmonary disease," in *Proceedings of the American Thoracic Society*, vol. 2, pp. 50–60, Scotland, UK, 2005.

[50] W. Domej, K. Oettl, and W. Renner, "Oxidative stress and free radicals in COPD-implications and relevance for treatment," *International Journal of Chronic Obstructive Pulmonary Disease*, vol. 9, pp. 1207–1224, 2014.

[51] P. N. R. Dekhuijzen, K. K. H. Aben, I. Dekker et al., "Increased exhalation of hydrogen peroxide in patients with stable and unstable chronic obstructive pulmonary disease," *The American Journal of Respiratory and Critical Care Medicine*, vol. 154, no. 3, pp. 813–816, 1996.

[52] K. Kostikas, G. Papatheodorou, K. Psathakis, P. Panagou, and S. Loukides, "Oxidative stress in expired breath condensate of patients with COPD," *Chest*, vol. 124, no. 4, pp. 1373–1380, 2003.

[53] J. C. Mak, "Pathogenesis of COPD. Part II. Oxidative-antioxidative imbalance," *International Journal of Tuberculosis and Lung Disease*, vol. 12, pp. 368–374, 2008.

[54] O. K. Baskurt, A. Temiz, and H. J. Meiselman, "Effect of superoxide anions on red blood cell rheologic properties," *Free Radical Biology and Medicine*, vol. 24, no. 1, pp. 102–110, 1998.

[55] O. K. Baskurt and H. J. Meiselman, "Activated polymorphonuclear leukocytes affect red blood cell aggregability," *Journal of Leukocyte Biology*, vol. 63, no. 1, pp. 89–93, 1998.

Permissions

All chapters in this book were first published in CRJ, by Hindawi Publishing Corporation; hereby published with permission under the Creative Commons Attribution License or equivalent. Every chapter published in this book has been scrutinized by our experts. Their significance has been extensively debated. The topics covered herein carry significant findings which will fuel the growth of the discipline. They may even be implemented as practical applications or may be referred to as a beginning point for another development.

The contributors of this book come from diverse backgrounds, making this book a truly international effort. This book will bring forth new frontiers with its revolutionizing research information and detailed analysis of the nascent developments around the world.

We would like to thank all the contributing authors for lending their expertise to make the book truly unique. They have played a crucial role in the development of this book. Without their invaluable contributions this book wouldn't have been possible. They have made vital efforts to compile up to date information on the varied aspects of this subject to make this book a valuable addition to the collection of many professionals and students.

This book was conceptualized with the vision of imparting up-to-date information and advanced data in this field. To ensure the same, a matchless editorial board was set up. Every individual on the board went through rigorous rounds of assessment to prove their worth. After which they invested a large part of their time researching and compiling the most relevant data for our readers.

The editorial board has been involved in producing this book since its inception. They have spent rigorous hours researching and exploring the diverse topics which have resulted in the successful publishing of this book. They have passed on their knowledge of decades through this book. To expedite this challenging task, the publisher supported the team at every step. A small team of assistant editors was also appointed to further simplify the editing procedure and attain best results for the readers.

Apart from the editorial board, the designing team has also invested a significant amount of their time in understanding the subject and creating the most relevant covers. They scrutinized every image to scout for the most suitable representation of the subject and create an appropriate cover for the book.

The publishing team has been an ardent support to the editorial, designing and production team. Their endless efforts to recruit the best for this project, has resulted in the accomplishment of this book. They are a veteran in the field of academics and their pool of knowledge is as vast as their experience in printing. Their expertise and guidance has proved useful at every step. Their uncompromising quality standards have made this book an exceptional effort. Their encouragement from time to time has been an inspiration for everyone.

The publisher and the editorial board hope that this book will prove to be a valuable piece of knowledge for researchers, students, practitioners and scholars across the globe.

List of Contributors

Mazlum Sahin
Department of Cardiovascular Surgery, Haseki Teaching and Research Hospital, Istanbul, Turkey

Helin El
Department of Cardiovascular Surgery, Sisli Teaching and Research Hospital, Istanbul, Turkey

Ibrahim Akkoç
Department of Anesthesia and Reanimation, Haseki Teaching and Research Hospital, Istanbul, Turkey

Kathryn Fullmann, David F. Blackburn and Holly Mansell
College of Pharmacy and Nutrition, University of Saskatchewan, Saskatoon, SK, Canada

Mark E. Fenton
Division of Critical Care and Sleep Medicine, Department of Medicine, University of Saskatchewan, Saskatoon, SK, Canada

Xiang Zhang, Saihua Wang, Jun Luo, Zhihong Zhao and Changzhu Zheng
Shanghai Zhoupu Hospital, Shanghai, China

Xueming Zhang and Jieyan Shen
Renji Hospital, Shanghai Jiaotong University School of Medicine, Shanghai, China

Ali Cengiz
Pulmonology Department, Ağrı State Hospital, Ağrı, Turkey

Suat Konuk and Tuncer Tuğ
Pulmonology Department, Faculty of Medicine, Abant Izzet Baysal University, Bolu, Turkey
V. Madhu Chari and Robert Andrew McIvor McMaster University, Firestone Institute for Respiratory Health, Hamilton, ON, Canada

Sébastien Préville-Ratelle
Clinique de fibrose kystique, Centre hospitalier de l'Université de Montréal (CHUM), 1051 rue Sanguinet, Montréal, QC, Canada H2X 0C1

Adèle Coriati and Aurélie Ménard
Institut de recherches cliniques de Montréal (IRCM), 110 Avenue des Pins, Montréal, QC, Canada H2W 1R7

Isabelle Bourdeau
Centre de recherche Centre hospitalier de l'Université de Montréal (CRCHUM), 900 rue Saint-Denis, Montréal, QC, Canada H2X 0A9
Département de médecine, Faculté de médecine, Université de Montréal, 2900 boul. Édouard-Montpetit, Montréal, QC, Canada H3T 1J4

François Tremblay
Clinique de fibrose kystique, Centre hospitalier de l'Université de Montréal (CHUM), 1051 rue Sanguinet, Montréal, QC, Canada H2X 0C1
Département de médecine, Faculté de médecine, Université de Montréal, 2900 boul. Édouard-Montpetit, Montréal, QC, Canada H3T 1J4

Yves Berthiaume
Clinique de fibrose kystique, Centre hospitalier de l'Université de Montréal (CHUM), 1051 rue Sanguinet, Montréal, QC, Canada H2X 0C1
Institut de recherches cliniques de Montréal (IRCM), 110 Avenue des Pins, Montréal, QC, Canada H2W 1R7
Département de médecine, Faculté de médecine, Université de Montréal, 2900 boul. Édouard-Montpetit, Montréal, QC, Canada H3T 1J4

Kazushige Shiraishi , Torahiko Jinta, Naoki Nishimura , Hiroshi Nakaoka, Ryosuke Tsugitomi, Kohei Okafuji, Atsushi Kitamura, Yutaka Tomishima and Tomohide Tamura
Department of Pulmonary Medicine, St. Luke's International University, St. Luke's International Hospital, Tokyo, Japan

Gautam A. Deshpande
Center for Clinical Epidemiology, St. Luke's International University, St. Luke's International Hospital, Tokyo, Japan

Juliana Guarize, Monica Casiraghi, Stefano Donghi, Cristina Diotti, Nicolo Vanoni, Rosalia Romano and Daniela Brambilla
Division of Thoracic Surgery, European Institute of Oncology, Milan, Italy

Chiara Casadio
Division of Pathology, European Institute of Oncology, Milan, Italy

Patrick Maisonneuve
Division of Epidemiology and Biostatistics, European Institute of Oncology, Milan, Italy

Francesco Petrella and Lorenzo Spaggiari
Division of Thoracic Surgery, European Institute of Oncology, Milan, Italy
Department of Oncology and Hemato-Oncology, University of Milan, Milan, Italy

Ian Mitchell
Alberta Children's Hospital, 2888 Shaganappi Trail NW, Calgary, AB, Canada T6B 6A8

Isabelle Defoy
AbbVie Corporation, 8401 Trans-Canada Highway, Saint-Laurent, QC, Canada H4S 1Z1

ElizaBeth Grubb
AbbVie, Inc., 1 N. Waukegan Road, North Chicago, IL 60064, USA

Hampus Persson, Anne Lindberg and Nikolai Stenfors
Department of Public Health and Clinical Medicine, Division of Medicine, Umeå University, Östersund, Umeå, Sweden

R. Andrew McIvor
St. Joseph's Healthcare Hamilton, McMaster University, Hamilton, ON, Canada

Hollie M. Devlin
Hollie Devlin Consulting, Toronto, ON, Canada

Alan Kaplan
Family Physician Airways Group of Canada, Richmond Hill, ON, Canada
Department of Family and Community Medicine, University of Toronto, Toronto, ON, Canada
Health Quality Ontario COPD Community Standards Project, Toronto, ON, Canada

Xi Wang, Qian Li, Ruming Liu, Jin He, Di Wu, Yun Wang and Jun Zhang
The Department of Clinical Pharmacy, The First Affiliated Hospital of Kunming Medical University, Kunming, China

Wei-Liang Li and Yu-Bo Yang
Department of Respiratory and Critical Care Medicine, Mingzhou Hospital, Zhejiang University, No. 168 West Taian Road, Ningbo, Zhejiang 315199, China

Yong-Hua Li and Li-Hui Lv
Department of Respiratory and Critical Care Medicine, Donghai Hospital, Ningbo University, No. 377 Zhongshan East Road, Ningbo 315040, China

Katie Kinaschuk
Faculty of Medicine and Dentistry, University of Alberta, Edmonton, AB, Canada

Sabin J. Bozso
Department of Surgery, Division of Cardiac Surgery, Edmonton, AB, Canada

Kieran Halloran and Ali Kapasi
Department of Medicine, University of Alberta, Edmonton, AB, Canada

Kathy Jackson
Human Organ Procurement and Exchange Program, Edmonton, AB, Canada

Jayan Nagendran
Department of Surgery, Division of Cardiac Surgery, Edmonton, AB, Canada
Canadian National Transplant Research Program, Edmonton, AB, Canada
Alberta Transplant Institute, Edmonton, AB, Canada

Xingai Jiao, Jinxiang Wu, Jiping Zhao, Tian Liu, Jiawei Xu and Liang Dong
Department of Respiratory Medicine, Qilu Hospital of Shandong University, Jinan, Shandong, China

Yurong Xu and Lei Yang
Department of Respiratory Medicine, Shandong Chest Hospital, Jinan, Shandong, China

Xiaohui Ma
Department of Respiratory Medicine, Qilu Hospital of Shandong University, Jinan, Shandong, China
Department of Respiratory Medicine, Shandong Chest Hospital, Jinan, Shandong, China

Hong Lu, Meng-Wei Zhang and Xiang-Lei Li
Department of Oncology, Huaihe Hospital of Henan University, Kaifeng 475001, China

Yue-Hua Zhang
Department of Oncology, Huaihe Hospital of Henan University, Kaifeng 475001, China
Department of Oncology, "e First Affiliated Hospital of Henan University, Kaifeng 475001, China

Yuquan Lu
International Joint Research Laboratory for Cell Medical Engineering of Henan, Huaihe Hospital of Henan University, Kaifeng 475001, China

Yue-Min Zhou
International Joint Research Laboratory for Cell Medical Engineering of Henan, Huaihe Hospital of Henan University, Kaifeng 475001, China

Center of Translational Medicine Center, Huaihe Hospital of Henan University, Kaifeng 475001, China

Nikolić Emilija and Brandmajer Tijana
Faculty of Medicine, University of Montenegro, 81000 Podgorica, Montenegro

Nikolić Aleksandar
D.o.o. "NCG Inzinjering", 81000 Podgorica, Montenegro

Stević Ruža
Faculty of Medicine, University of Belgarde, 11000 Belgrade, Serbia

Mićanović Veselin and Mašnić Jelena
Faculty of Philosophy, University of Montenegro, 81000 Podgorica, Montenegro

Kwadwo Kyeremanteng
Department of Medicine, Division of Critical Care, University of Ottawa, Ottawa, ON, Canada

Louis-Philippe Gagnon
Department of Critical Care Medicine, Queen's University, Kingston, ON, Canada

Raphaëlle Robidoux and Dipayan Chaudhuri
University of Ottawa, Ottawa, ON, Canada

Kednapa Thavorn
Clinical Epidemiology Program, 'e Ottawa Hospital Research Institute, 'e Ottawa Hospital, Ottawa, ON, Canada
School of Epidemiology, Public Health and Preventive Medicine, University of Ottawa, Ottawa, ON, Canada
Institute of Clinical and Evaluative Sciences (ICES uOttawa), Ottawa, ON, Canada

Daniel Kobewka
Department of Medicine, Division of General Internal Medicine, University of Ottawa, Ottawa, ON, Canada

John P. Kress
University of Chicago Medicine, Chicago, IL, USA

Biing-Ru Wu
Division of Pulmonary and Critical Care Medicine, Department of Internal Medicine, China Medical University Hospital, Taichung, Taiwan

Chia-Hung Chen
Division of Pulmonary and Critical Care Medicine, Department of Internal Medicine, China Medical University Hospital, Taichung, Taiwan
Department of Respiratory "erapy, China Medical University, Taichung, Taiwan
Graduate Institute of Clinical Medical Science, China Medical University, Taichung, Taiwan

Wen-Chien Cheng, Chih-Yu Chen and Wei-Chun Chen
Division of Pulmonary and Critical Care Medicine, Department of Internal Medicine, China Medical University Hospital, Taichung, Taiwan
School of Medicine, China Medical University, Taichung, Taiwan
Department of Internal Medicine, Hyperbaric Oxygen "erapy Center, China Medical University, Taichung, Taiwan

Wei-Chih Liao
Division of Pulmonary and Critical Care Medicine, Department of Internal Medicine, China Medical University Hospital, Taichung, Taiwan
Graduate Institute of Clinical Medical Science, China Medical University, Taichung, Taiwan
Department of Internal Medicine, Hyperbaric Oxygen "erapy Center, China Medical University, Taichung, Taiwan

Chih-Yen Tu
Division of Pulmonary and Critical Care Medicine, Department of Internal Medicine, China Medical University Hospital, Taichung, Taiwan
School of Medicine, China Medical University, Taichung, Taiwan
Department of Life Science, National Chung Hsing University, Taichung, Taiwan

Andreas Hinz and Kristina Geue
Department of Medical Psychology and Medical Sociology, University of Leipzig, Leipzig, Germany

Markus Zenger
Faculty of Applied Human Studies, University of Applied Sciences Magdeburg and Stendal, Stendal, Germany
Integrated Research and Treatment Center (IFB) Adiposity Diseases-Behavioral Medicine,
Medical Psychology and Medical Sociology, University of Leipzig, Leipzig, Germany

Hubert Wirtz and Andrea Bosse-Henck
Department of Respiratory Medicine, University of Leipzig, Leipzig, Germany

Gord Blackhouse
Programs for Assessment of Technology in Health, The Research Institute of St. Joe's Hamilton,
St. Joseph's Healthcare Hamilton, Hamilton, ON, Canada
Department of Health Research Methods, Evidence, and Impact, Faculty of Health Sciences, McMaster University, Hamilton, ON, Canada

Jason R. Guertin
Programs for Assessment of Technology in Health, The Research Institute of St. Joe's Hamilton,
St. Joseph's Healthcare Hamilton, Hamilton, ON, Canada
Department of Health Research Methods, Evidence, and Impact, Faculty of Health Sciences, McMaster University, Hamilton, ON, Canada
Department of Social and Preventive Medicine, Université Laval, Quebec City, QC, Canada
Centre de Recherche du CHU de Québec, Université Laval, Axe Santé des Populations et Pratiques Optimales en Santé, Hôpital du St-Sacrement, Quebec City, QC, Canada

Carolyn Gosse, Emanuel Baltaga, Donna Johnson, Brandi Le Blanc, Jane Loncke, Ravi Sivakumaran and Laura Wheatley
St. Joseph's Healthcare Hamilton, Hamilton, ON, Canada

James M. Bowen and Daria J. O'Reilly
Programs for Assessment of Technology in Health, The Research Institute of St. Joe's Hamilton,
St. Joseph's Healthcare Hamilton, Hamilton, ON, Canada
Department of Health Research Methods, Evidence, and Impact, Faculty of Health Sciences, McMaster University, Hamilton, ON, Canada
St. Joseph's Healthcare Hamilton, Hamilton, ON, Canada

Gerard Cox, Stewart Pugsley and Kevin Smith
St. Joseph's Healthcare Hamilton, Hamilton, ON, Canada
Department of Medicine, DeGroote School of Medicine, McMaster University, Hamilton, ON, Canada

Jean-Eric Tarride
Programs for Assessment of Technology in Health, The Research Institute of St. Joe's Hamilton,
St. Joseph's Healthcare Hamilton, Hamilton, ON, Canada
Department of Health Research Methods, Evidence, and Impact, Faculty of Health Sciences, McMaster University, Hamilton, ON, Canada
St. Joseph's Healthcare Hamilton, Hamilton, ON, Canada
Center for Health Economics and Policy Analysis, McMaster University, Hamilton, ON, Canada

Xia Jing and Jianying Xu
Department of Respiratory Diseases, Shanxi Dayi Hospital Affiliated to Shanxi Medical University, Taiyuan, Shanxi, China

Yufeng Li
Department of Neurology, Shanxi Dayi Hospital Affiliated to Shanxi Medical University, Taiyuan, Shanxi, China

Seiko Miyamoto, Yoshiaki Minakata, Yuichiro Azuma, Kazumi Kawabe, Hideya Ono, Ryuta Yanagimoto and Tadatoshi Suruda
Department of Clinical Laboratory, National Hospital Organization Wakayama Hospital, 1138 Wada Mihama-cho, Hidaka-gun, Wakayama 644-0044, Japan

Buqi Na, Li Dai and Guoguang Xia
Department of Respiratory and Critical Care Medicine, Beijing Jishuitan Hospital, Beijing 100035, China

Hong Zhang and Guangfa Wang
Department of Respiratory and Critical Care Medicine, Peking University First Hospital, Beijing 100034, China

Francesco Feletti
Department of Diagnostic Imaging, AUSL Romagna, S. Maria delle Croci Hospital, Ravenna, Italy
Dipartmento di Elettronica, Informazione e Bioingegneria (DEIB), Politecnico di Milano, Milan, Italy

Andrea Aliverti
Dipartmento di Elettronica, Informazione e Bioingegneria (DEIB), Politecnico di Milano, Milan, Italy

Viviana Mucci
Antwerpen University Research Centre for Equilibrium and Aerospace (AUREA), Antwerp, Belgium

Ming-Xian Li
The First Affiliated Hospital of Jilin University, Changchun 130021, China

Jing Kang
The First Affiliated Hospital of Jilin University, Changchun 130021, China
Jilin Medical University, Jilin 132013, China

Zhan-Li Shi, Kun Fang , Zhi-Hui Li , Dan-Hong Ren , Jia-Ying Zhang and Jing Sun
Department of Intensive Care Unit, Hangzhou Red Cross Hospital/Zhejiang Chinese Medicine, Western Medicine Integrated Hospital, Hangzhou 310003, China

Joshua Gawlitza, Hans Scheffel, Andreas Fischer, Claudia Henzler and Nils Vogler
Institute of Clinical Radiology and Nuclear Medicine, University Medical Center Mannheim, Medical Faculty Mannheim, Heidelberg University, Heidelberg, Germany

Frederik Trinkmann and Joachim Saur
Department of Medicine (Cardiology, Angiology, Pulmonary, and Intensive Care), University Medical Center Mannheim, Medical Faculty Mannheim, Heidelberg University, Heidelberg, Germany

John W. Nance
Department of Radiology and Radiological Science, Medical University of South Carolina, Charleston, SC, USA

Ibrahim Akin and Martin Borggrefe
Department of Medicine (Cardiology, Angiology, Pulmonary, and Intensive Care), University Medical Center Mannheim, Medical Faculty Mannheim, Heidelberg University, Heidelberg, Germany
DZHK (German Center for Cardiovascular Research), Partner Site Mannheim, Berlin, Germany

Stefan O. Schoenberg and Thomas Henzler
Institute of Clinical Radiology and Nuclear Medicine, University Medical Center Mannheim, Medical Faculty Mannheim, Heidelberg University, Heidelberg, Germany
DZHK (German Center for Cardiovascular Research), Partner Site Mannheim, Berlin, Germany

Yu Hara, Masaharu Shinkai, Kenjiro Nagai and Takeshi Kaneko
Department of Pulmonology, Yokohama City University Graduate School of Medicine, Yokohama, Japan

Masataka Taguri
Department of Biostatistics, Yokohama City University School of Medicine, Yokohama, Japan

Satoru Hashimoto
Division of Intensive Care Unit, Kyoto Prefectural University of Medicine, Kyoto, Japan

Jeremias Götschke, Pontus Mertsch, Nikolaus Kneidinger, Diego Kauffmann-Guerrero, Rudolf Maria Huber and Katrin Milger
Department of Internal Medicine V, Ludwig-Maximilians-University of Munich, Munich, Germany
Comprehensive Pneumology Center (CPC-M), Member of the German Center for Lung Research (DZL), Munich, Germany

Jürgen Behr
Department of Internal Medicine V, Ludwig-Maximilians-University of Munich, Munich, Germany
Comprehensive Pneumology Center (CPC-M), Member of the German Center for Lung Research (DZL), Munich, Germany
Asklepios Fachkliniken München Gauting, Gauting, Germany

Frank Reichenberger
Comprehensive Pneumology Center (CPC-M), Member of the German Center for Lung Research (DZL), Munich, Germany
Asklepios Fachkliniken München Gauting, Gauting, Germany

Kenneth K. Sakata and Anjuli Brighton
Division of Pulmonary Medicine, Mayo Clinic, Phoenix, AZ, USA

Natalya Azadeh
Division of Pulmonary and Critical Care Medicine, Mayo Clinic, Rochester, MN, USA

M'hamed Temkit
Division of Health Sciences and Research, Mayo Clinic Arizona, Scottsdale, AZ, USA

Christine L. Klassen
Division of General Internal Medicine, Mayo Clinic, Rochester, MN, USA

Thomas E. Grys
Department of Laboratory Medicine and Pathology, Mayo Clinic, Phoenix, AZ, USA

Holenarasipur R. Vikram
Division of Infectious Diseases, Mayo Clinic, Phoenix, AZ, USA

Matthew J. Binnicker
Department of Laboratory Medicine and Pathology, Mayo Clinic, Rochester, MN, USA

Thomas E. Grys
Division of Clinical Microbiology, Mayo Clinic, Scottsdale, AZ, USA

Sy Duong-Quy
Bio-Medical Research Center, Lam Dong Medical College, Dalat, Vietnam
Division of Pulmonary, Allergy and Critical Care Medicine, Penn State College of Medicine, Hershey, PA, USA

Timothy J. Craig
Division of Pulmonary, Allergy and Critical Care Medicine, Penn State College of Medicine, Hershey, PA, USA

Huong Tran Van
Department of Health Science, Thang Long University, Hanoi, Vietnam

Anh Vo Thi Kim
Nam Anh General Hospital, Binh Duong Province, Vietnam

Quyen Pham Huy
Department of Clinical Immuno-Allergology, Hai Phong University, Haiphong, Vietnam

Che-Jui Chang
Institute of Occupational Medicine and Industrial Hygiene, National Taiwan University College of Public Health, Taipei, Taiwan
Department of Family Medicine, National Taiwan University Hospital, Taipei, Taiwan

Yu-Kang Tu
Department of Public Health, National Taiwan University College of Public Health, Taipei, Taiwan
Institute of Epidemiology and Preventive Medicine, College of Public Health, National Taiwan University, Taipei, Taiwan

Hsiao-Yu Yang
Institute of Occupational Medicine and Industrial Hygiene, National Taiwan University College of Public Health, Taipei, Taiwan
Department of Public Health, National Taiwan University College of Public Health, Taipei, Taiwan
Department of Environmental and Occupational Medicine, National Taiwan University Hospital, Taipei, Taiwan

Pau-Chung Chen
Institute of Occupational Medicine and Industrial Hygiene, National Taiwan University College of Public Health, Taipei, Taiwan
Department of Public Health, National Taiwan University College of Public Health, Taipei, Taiwan
Department of Environmental and Occupational Medicine, National Taiwan University Hospital, Taipei, Taiwan
Department of Environmental and Occupational Medicine, National Taiwan University College of Medicine, Taipei, Taiwan

Sabri Seyis
Department of Cardiology, Live Istinye University Hospital, Istanbul, Turkey

Adnan Kazım Usalan
Department of Chest Disease, Medical Park Hospital, Mersin, Turkey

Ibrahim Rencuzogullari
Department of Cardiology, Kafkas University Faculty of Medicine, Kars, Turkey

Özge Kurmuş
Department of Cardiology, Ufuk University, Ankara, Turkey

Adil Can Gungen
Department of Chest Disease, Live Istinye University Hospital, Istanbul, Turkey

Natalya Azadeh, Kenneth K. Sakata, Ali Saeed, John J. Mullon and Andrew H. Limper
Department of Pulmonary and Critical Care Medicine, Mayo Clinic, Rochester, MN, USA

Erhan Ugurlu, Ilknur Can and Goksel Altinisik
Faculty of Medicine, Department of Pulmonology, Pamukkale University, Denizli, Turkey

Emine Kilic-Toprak, Ozgen Kilic-Erkek and Melek Bor-Kucukatay
Faculty of Medicine, Department of Physiology, Pamukkale University, Denizli, Turkey